Textbook of Clinical Trials

Edited by

David Machin

*Division of Clinical Trials and Epidemiological Sciences,
National Cancer Centre, Singapore and UK Children's Cancer Study Group,
University of Leicester, UK and School of Health and Related Research, University of Sheffield, UK.*

Simon Day

*Medicines and Healthcare products Regulatory Agency,
London, UK*

Sylvan Green

Arizona Cancer Centre, Tucson, Arizona, USA

Section Editors

Brian Everitt

Institute of Psychiatry, London, UK

Stephen George

*Department of Biostatistics and Informatics,
Duke University Medical Centre, Durham, NC, USA*

John Wiley & Sons, Ltd

Other Wiley Editorial Offices

John Wiley & Sons Inc., 111 River Street, Hoboken, NJ 07030, USA

Jossey-Bass, 989 Market Street, San Francisco, CA 94103-1741, USA

Wiley-VCH Verlag GmbH, Boschstr. 12, D-69469 Weinheim, Germany

John Wiley & Sons Australia Ltd, 33 Park Road, Milton, Queensland 4064, Australia

John Wiley & Sons (Asia) Pte Ltd, 2 Clementi Loop #02-01, Jin Xing Distripark, Singapore 129809

John Wiley & Sons Canada Ltd, 22 Worcester Road, Etobicoke, Ontario, Canada M9W 1L1

Wiley also publishes its books in a variety of electronic formats. Some content that appears
in print may not be available in electronic books.

Library of Congress Cataloging-in-Publication Data

Textbook of clinical trials / edited by David Machin ... [et al.].
     p. cm.
  Includes bibliographical references and index.
  ISBN 0-471-98787-5 (alk. paper)
   1. Clinical trials. I. Machin, David.

  R853.C55T49 2004
  610′.72′4–dc22
                                    2003065147

British Library Cataloguing in Publication Data

A catalogue record for this book is available from the British Library

ISBN 0-471-98787-5

Typeset in 10/12pt Times by Laserwords Private Limited, Chennai, India
Printed and bound in Great Britain by Antony Rowe Ltd, Chippenham, Wiltshire
This book is printed on acid-free paper responsibly manufactured from sustainable forestry
in which at least two trees are planted for each one used for paper production.

Textbook of Clinical Trials

Contents

Contributors

TONY ARTHUR

School of Nursing, Faculty of Medicine and Health Sciences, University of Nottingham, Queens Medical Centre, Nottingham NG7 2UH, UK, Email: tony.arthur@nottingham.ac.uk

DONALD BERRY

Department of Biostatistics, UTMD Anderson Cancer Centre, 1400 Holcombe Blvd, Box 447, Houston, TX 77030, USA, Email: dberry@odin.mdacc.tmc.edu

S. BHATTACHARYA

Department of Obstetrics and Gynaecology, Aberdeen Maternity Hospital, Cronhill Road, Aberdeen AB25 2ZD, UK, Email: s.bhattacharya@abdn.ac.uk

ARMAN BUZDAR

Department of Breast Medical Oncology, The University of Texas, M.D. Anderson Cancer Centre, Texas, USA

SIMON DAY

Licensing Division, Medicines and Healthcare products Regulatory Agency, Room 13-205 Market Towers, 1 Nine Elms Lane, London SW8 5NQ, UK, Email: simon.day@mhra.gsi.gov.uk

GRAHAM DUNN

Biostatistics Group, School of Epidemiology and Health Sciences, Stopford Building, Oxford Road, Manchester M13 9PT, UK, Email: graham.dunn@man.ac.uk, chartell@man.ac.uk

FRED EDERER

The EMMES Corporation, 401 North Washington Street, Suite 700, Rockville, MD 20850, USA, Email: federer@emmes.com

BRIAN EVERITT — Box 20, Biostatistics Department, Institute of Psychiatry, Denmark Hill, London SE5 8AF, UK, Email: b.everitt@iop.kcl.ac.uk

LARRY FRIEDMAN — National Heart, Lung, and Blood Institute, Building 31, Room 5A03, Bethesda, MD 20892 2482, USA, Email: FriedmaL@hlbi.nih.gov

STEPHEN GEORGE — Department of Biostatistics and Bioinformatics, Duke University Medical Centre, Durham, NC 27710, USA, Email: george001@mc.duke.edu

RICH GOLDBERG — Medical Oncology, Mayo Clinic, 200 1st Street SW, Rochester, MN 55905, USA, Email: goldberg.richard@mayo.edu

SYLVAN GREEN — Arizona Cancer Centre, 1515 N Campbell Ave, PO Box 245024, Tucson, AZ 85724, USA, Email: sgreen@azcc.arizona.edu

CAROL JAGGER — Trent Institute for HSR, Department of Epidemiology and Public Health, University of Leicester, 22–28 Princess Road West, Leicester LE1 6TP, UK, Email: cxj@leicester.ac.uk

ANDERS KÄLLÉN — AstraZeneca R&D, Lund, Sweden, Email: Anders.Kallen@astrazeneca.com

JOHAN KARLBERG — Clinical Trials Centre, Faculty of Medicine, The University of Hong Kong, Hong Kong SAR, PR China, Email: jpekarl@hkucc.hku.hk

KYUNGMANN KIM — Department of Biostatistics & Medical Informatics, University of Wisconsin, 600 Highland Avenue, Box 4675, Madison, WI 53792, USA, Email: kmkim@biostat.wisc.edu

PHILIP LAVORI — VACSPCC (151K), 795 Willow Road, Menlo Park, CA 94025 2539, USA, Email: Philip.Lavori@med.va.gov

P.C. LEUNG — Department of Orthopaedics & Traumatology, The Chinese University of Hong Kong, Room 74026, 5th Floor, Clinical Sciences Building, Prince of Wales Hospital, Shatin, Hong Kong, Email: pingcleung@cuhk.edu.hk

PAUL LIMBURG — Gastroenterology and Hepatology, Mayo Clinic, 200 1st Street SW, Rochester, MN 55905, USA, Email: limburg.paul@mayo.edu

P.Y. LIU

SWOG Statistical Centre, MP 557, Fred Hutchinson Cancer Research Centre, 1100 Fairview Avenue North, PO Box 19024, Seattle, WA 98109 1024, USA, Email: pyl@swog.fhcrc.org

EDWARD LO

Dental Public Health, Faculty of Dentistry, The University of Hong Kong, 34 Hospital Road, Hong Kong, Email: edward-lo@hku.hk

DAVID MACHIN

Division of Clinical Trials and Epidemiological Sciences, National Cancer Centre Singapore, 11 Hospital Drive, Singapore 169610, Singapore, Email: ctedav@nccs.com.sg, david@machin-home.freeserve.co.uk

COLAMN MCGRATH

Dental Public Health, Faculty of Dentistry, The University of Hong Kong, 34 Hospital Road, Hong Kong, Email: mcgrath@hkucc.hku.hk

COSETTA MINELLI

Medical Statistics Group, Department of Epidemiology and Public Health, University of Leicester, 22–28 Princess Road West, Leicester LE1 6TP, UK, Email: cm109@le.ac.uk

JILL MOLLISON

Department of Public Health, University of Aberdeen, Polwarth Building, Foresterhill, Aberdeen AB25 2ZD, UK, Email: j.mollison@abdn.ac.uk

SHARON B. MURPHY

Children's Cancer Research Institute, The University of Texas Health Science Centre at San Antonio, 7703 Floyd Curl Drive, MC 7784, San Antonio, TX 78229-3900, USA, Email: murphysb@uthscsa.edu

LUIGI NALDI

Clinica Dermatologica, Ospedali Riuniti, L.go Barozzi 1, 24100 Bergamo, Italy, Email: luiginal@tin.it

GILDA PIAGGIO

Special Programme of Research, Development and Research Training in Human Reproduction, Department of Reproductive Health and Research, World Health Organisation, 1211 Geneva 27, Switzerland, Email: piaggiog@who.int

DANIEL SARGENT

Mayo Clinic, 200 First Street, SW, Kahler 1A, Rochester, MN 55905, USA, Email: sargent.daniel@mayo.edu

CHARLES SCHIFFER

Division of Oncology and Hematology/Oncology, Karmanos Cancer Institute, Wayne State University School of Medicine, Detroit, MI 48201, USA.

ELEANOR SCHRON

National Heart, Lung, and Blood Institute, Bethesda, MD 20892 2482, USA, Email: schrone@nhlbi.nih.edu

KATHERINE SHEAR

Panic Anxiety and Traumatic Grief Program, Western Psychiatric Institute and Clinic, 3811 O'Hara Street, Pittsburgh, PA 15213, USA, Email: shearmk@msx.upmc.edu, corcorannl@msx.upmc.edu

JON SHUSTER

PO Box 100212, College of Medicine, University of Florida, Gainesville, FL 32610 0212, USA, Email: jshuster@biostat.ufl.edu

TERRY SMITH

UTMD Anderson Cancer Centre, 1400 Holcombe Blvd, Box 447, Houston, TX 77030, USA, Email: tsmith@odin.mdacc.tmc.edu

VERNON K. SONDAK

University of Michigan Medical Centre, Division of Surgical Oncology, 1500 E Medical Centre Drive, 3306 Cancer/Geriatrics Ctr Box 0932, Ann Arbor, MI 48109 0932, USA, Email: vsondak@umich.edu

NICHOLAS TARRIER

University of Manchester, Academic Division of Clinical Psychology Education & Research Building, Wythenshawe Hospital, Southmoor Road, Manchester M23 9LT, UK, Email: ntarrier@man.ac.uk

LEON THAL

Department of Neurosciences, University of California, San Diego, 9500 Gilman Drive, San Diego, CA 92037, USA, Email: lthal@ucsd.edu

RONALD THOMAS

Department of Family and Preventative Medicine, and Neurosciences, UCSD 9500 Gilman Drive, La Jolla, CA 92039 0645, USA, Email: rgthomas@ucsd.edu

MAY C.M. WONG

Dental Public Health, Faculty of Dentistry, The University of Hong Kong, 34 Hospital Road, Hong Kong, Email: mcmwong@hkucc.hku.hk

TIL WYKES

Department of Psychiatry, De Crespigny Park, London SE5 8AF, UK, Email: t.wykes@iop.kcl.ac.uk

Preface

This *Textbook of Clinical Trials* is not a textbook of clinical trials in the traditional sense. Rather, it catalogues in part both the impact of clinical trials – particularly the randomised controlled trial –on the practice of medicine and allied fields and on the developments and practice of medical statistics. The latter has evolved in many ways through the direct needs of clinical trials and the consequent interaction of statistical and clinical disciplines. The impact of the results from clinical trials, particularly the randomised controlled trial, on the practice of clinical medicine and other areas of health care has been profound. In particular, they have provided the essential underpinning to evidence-based practice in many disciplines and are one of the key components for regulatory approval of new therapeutic approaches throughout the world.

Probably the single most important contribution to the science of comparative clinical trials was the recognition, more than 50 years ago, that patients should be allocated to the options under consideration at random. This was the foundation for the science of clinical trial research and placed the medical statistician at the centre of the process. Although the medical statistician may be at the centre, he or she is by no means alone. Indeed the very nature of clinical trial research is multidisciplinary so that a 'team' effort is always

needed from the concept stage, through design, conduct, monitoring and reporting.

Some of the developments impacting on clinical trials have been truly statistical in nature, for example Cox's proportional hazards model, while others such as the intention-to-treat (ITT) principle are – in some sense – based more on experience. Other important statistical developments have not depended on technical advancement, but rather on conceptual advancement, such as the now standard practice of reporting confidence intervals rather then relying solely on p-values at the interpretation stage. Of major importance over this same time period has been the expansion in data processing capabilities and the range of analytical possibilities only made possible by the tremendous development in computing power. However, despite many advances, the majority of randomised controlled trials remain simple in design – most often a comparison between two randomised groups.

On the medical side there have been many changes including new diseases that raise new issues. Thus, as we write, SARS has emerged: the final extent of the epidemic is unknown, diagnosis is problematical and no specific treatment is available. In more established diseases there have been major advances in the types of treatment available, be they in surgical technique, cancer chemotherapy or psychotropic drugs. Advances in medical and associated technologies are not confined to curative treatments but extend, for example, to diagnostic methods useful in screening for disease, vaccines for disease prevention, drugs and devices for female and male contraception, and pain relief and psychological support strategies in palliative care.

Clinical trials imply some intervention affecting the subjects who are ultimately recruited into them. These subjects will range from the very healthy, perhaps women of a relatively young age recruited to a contraceptive development trial, to those (perhaps elderly) patients in terminal decline from a long-standing illness. Each group studied in a clinical trial, from unborn child to aged adult, brings its own constraint on the ultimate design of the trial in mind. So too does the relative efficacy of the current standard. If the outcome is death and the prognosis poor, then bolder steps may be taken in the choice of treatments to test. If the disease is self-limiting or the outcome cosmetic then a more conservative approach to treatment options would be justified.

In all this activity the choice of clinical trial design and its ultimate conduct are governed by essential ethical constraints, the willingness of subjects to consent to the trial in question and their right to withdraw from the trial should they wish.

Thus the *Textbook of Clinical Trials* addresses some of these and many other issues as they impact on patients with cancer, cardiovascular disease, dermatological, dental, mental and ophthalmic health, gynaecology and respiratory diseases. In addition, chapters deal with issues relating to complementary medicine, contraception and special issues in children and special issues in older patients. A brief history of clinical trials and a summary of some pertinent statistical issues are included.

David Machin, Simon Day and Sylvan Green

INTRODUCTION

1

Brief History of Clinical Trials

S. DAY[1] AND F. EDERER[2]

[1]Licensing Division, Medicines and Healthcare products Regulatory Agency, London, UK
[2]The EMMES Corporation, Rockville, MD 20850, USA

The modern-day birth of clinical trials is usually considered to be the publication in 1948 by the UK Medical Research Council[1] of a trial for the treatment of pulmonary tuberculosis with streptomycin. However, earlier but less well documented examples do exist. The comparative concept of assessing therapeutic efficacy has been known from ancient times. Slotki[2] cites a description of a nutritional experiment involving a control group in the Book of Daniel from the Old Testament:

> Then Daniel said to the guard whom the master of the eunuchs had put in charge of Hananiah, Mishael, Azariah and himself, 'Submit to us this test for ten days. Give us only vegetables to eat and water to drink; then compare our looks with those of the young men who have lived on the food assigned by the king, and be guided in your treatment of us by what you see.' The guard listened to what they said and tested them for ten days. At the end of ten days they looked healthier and were better nourished than all the young men who had lived on the food assigned them by the king. So the guard took away the assignment of food and the wine they were to drink, and gave them only the vegetables.

Daniel lived around the period 800BC and although it may not be possible to confirm the accuracy of the account, what is clear is that when this passage was written–around 150BC–the ideas certainly existed.

The passage from Daniel describes not just a control group, but a *concurrent* control group. This fundamental element of clinical research did not begin to be widely practised until the latter half of the twentieth century.

Much later than the book of Daniel, but still very early, is an example from the fourteenth century: it is a letter from Petrarch to Boccaceto cited by Witkosky:[3]

> I solemnly affirm and believe, if a hundred or a thousand of men of the same age, same temperament and habits, together with the same surroundings, were attacked at the same time by the same disease, that if one followed the prescriptions of the doctors of the variety of those practicing at the present day, and that the other half took no medicine but relied on Nature's instincts, I have no doubt as to which half would escape.

The Renaissance period (fourteenth to sixteenth centuries) provides other examples including an

---

Textbook of Clinical Trials. Edited by D. Machin, S. Day and S. Green
© 2004 John Wiley & Sons, Ltd ISBN: 0-471-98787-5

unplanned experiment in the treatment of battle-field wounds. Packard[4] describes how the surgeon Ambroise Paré was using the standard treatment of pouring boiled oil over soldiers' wounds during a battle to capture the castle of Villaine in 1537. When he ran out of oil, he resorted to a mixture of egg yolks, oil of roses and turpentine. The superiority of the new 'treatment' became evident the next day:

> I raised myself very early to visit them, when beyond my hope I found those to whom I applied the digestive medicament feeling but little pain, their wounds neither swollen nor inflamed, and having slept through the night. The others to whom I had applied the boiling oil were feverish with much pain and swelling about their wounds. Then I determined never again to burn thus so cruelly by arquebusses.

Perhaps the most famous historical example of a planned controlled, comparative, clinical trial is from the eighteenth century: that where Lind[5] found oranges and lemons to be the most effective of six dietary treatments for scurvy on board ships. He wrote:

> On the 20th of May, 1747, I took twelve patients in the scurvy, on board the *Salisbury* at sea. Their cases were as similar as I could have them. They all in general had putrid gums, the spots and lassitude, with weakness of their knees. They lay together in one place, being a proper apartment for the sick in the fore-hold; and had one diet common to all, viz. water-gruel sweetened with sugar in the morning; fresh mutton-broth often times for dinner; at other times puddings, boiled biscuit with sugar etc. And for supper, barley and raisins, rice and currants, sago and wine, or the like. Two of these were ordered each a quart of cyder a day. Two others took twenty-five gutts of *elixir vitriol* three times a day, upon an empty stomach; using a gargle strongly acidulated with it for their mouths. Two others took two spoonfuls of vinegar three times a day, upon an empty stomach; having their gruels and their other food well acidulated with it, as also the gargle for their mouths. Two of the worst patients, with the tendons in the ham rigid (a symptom none of the rest had) were put under a course of sea-water. Of this they drank half a pint every day, and sometimes more or less as it

operated, by way of gentle physic. Two others had each two oranges and one lemon given them every day. These they eat with greediness, at different times, upon an empty stomach. They continued but six days under this course, having consumed the quantity that could be spared. The two remaining patients, took the bigness of a nutmeg three times a day of an electuary recommended by a hospital-surgeon, made of garlic, mustard-feed, *rad. raphan*, balsam of *Peru*, and gum myrrh; using for common drink barley-water well acidulated with tamarinds; by a decoction of which, with the addition of *cremor tartar*, they were greatly purged three or four times during the course.

> The consequence was, that the most sudden and visible good effects were perceived from the use of the oranges and lemons; one of those who had taken them, being at the end of six days fit for duty. The spots were not indeed at that time quite off his body, or his gums sound; without any other medicine, than a gargle of *elixir vitriol*, he became quite healthy before we came into Plymouth, which was on the 16th June. The other was the best recovered of any in his condition; and being now deemed pretty well, was appointed nurse, to the rest of the sick.

Pierre-Charles-Alexandre Louis, a nineteenth-century clinician and pathologist, introduced the numerical aspect to comparing treatments.[6] His idea was to compare the results of treatments on groups of patients with similar degrees of disease, i.e. to compare 'like with like':

> I come now to therapeutics, and suppose that you have some doubt as to the efficacy of a particular remedy: How are you to proceed?...You would take as many cases as possible, of as similar a description as you could find, and would count how many recovered under one mode of treatment, and how many under another; in how short a time they did so, and if the cases were in all respects alike, except in the treatment, you would have some confidence in your conclusions; and if you were fortunate enough to have a sufficient number of facts from which to deduce any general law, it would lead to your employment in practice of the method which you had seen oftenest successful.

'Like with like' was an important step forward from Lind's treatment of scurvy. Note, although early in Lind's passage he says that: 'Their cases were as similar as I could have them', later he acknowledges that the two worst cases both received the same treatment: 'Two of the worst patients, with the tendons in the ham rigid (a symptom none of the rest had) were put under a course of sea-water'. It remained for Bradford Hill, more than a century later, to use a formal method for creating groups of cases that were 'in all respects alike, except in the treatment'.

RANDOMISATION

The use of randomisation was a contribution by the statistician R.A. Fisher in agriculture (see, for example, Fisher,[7] Fisher and McKenzie[8]). Fisher randomised plots of crops to receive different treatments and in clinical trials there were early schemes to use 'group randomisation': patients were divided into two groups and then the treatment for each group was randomly selected. The Belgian medicinal chemist van Helmont[9] described an early example of this:

> Let us take out of the hospitals, out of the Camps, or from elsewhere, 200, or 500 poor People that have Fevers, Pleurisies, &c, Let us divide them into halfes, let us cast lots, that one half of them may fall to my share, and the others to yours,... we shall see how many funerals both of us shall have: *But* let the reward of the contention or wager, be 300 florens, deposited on both sides.

Amberson and McMahon[10] used group randomisation in a trial of sanocrysin for the treatment of pulmonary tuberculosis. Systematic assignment was used by Fibiger,[11] who alternately assigned diphtheria patients to serum treatment or an untreated control group. Alternate assignment is frowned upon today because knowledge of the future treatment allocations may selectively bias the admission of patients into the treatment group.[12] Diehl *et al.*[13] reported a common cold vaccine study with University of Minnesota students as subjects where blinding and random assignment of patients to treatments appears to have been used:

> At the beginning of each year... students were assigned at random... to a control group or an experimental group. The students in the control groups... received placebos... All students thought they were receiving vaccines... Even the physicians who saw the students... had no information as to which group they represented.

However Gail[14] points out that although this appears to be a randomised clinical trial, a further unpublished report by Diehl clarifies that this is another instance of systematic assignment:

> At the beginning of the study, students who volunteered to take these treatments were assigned alternately and without selection to control groups and experimental groups.

Bradford Hill, in the study of streptomycin in pulmonary tuberculosis,[1] used random sampling numbers in assigning treatments to subjects, so that the subject was the unit of randomisation. This study is now generally acknowledged to be the 'first properly randomised clinical trial'.

Later Bradford Hill and the British Medical Research Council continued with further randomised trials: chemotherapy of pulmonary tuberculosis in young adults,[15] antihistaminic drugs in the prevention and treatment of the common cold,[16] cortisone and aspirin in the treatment of early cases of rheumatoid arthritis[17,18] and long-term anticoagulant therapy in cerebrovascular disease.[19]

In America, the National Institutes of Health started its first randomised trial in 1951. It was a National Heart Institute study of adrenocorticotropic hormone (ACTH), cortisone and aspirin in the treatment of rheumatic heart disease.[20] This was followed in 1954 by a randomised trial of retrolental fibroplasia (now known as retinopathy of prematurity), sponsored by the National Institute of Neurological Diseases and Blindness.[21] During the four decades following the pioneering trials of the 1940s and 1950s, there was a large growth in the number of randomised trials not only in Britain and the US, but also in Canada and mainland Europe.

BLINDING

The common cold vaccine study published by Diehl *et al.*,[13] cited earlier, in which University of Minnesota students were alternately assigned to vaccine or placebo, was a masked (or blinded) clinical trial:

> All students thought they were receiving vaccines... Even the physicians who saw the students... had no information as to which group they represented.

Blinding was used in the early Medical Research Council trials in which Bradford Hill was involved. Thus, in the first of those trials, the study of streptomycin in tuberculosis,[1] the X-ray films were viewed by two radiologists and a clinician, each reading the films independently and not knowing if the films were of C (control, bed-rest alone) or S (streptomycin and bed-rest) cases.

Bradford Hill[22] (Reproduced with permission) noted in respect of using such blinding and randomisation:

> If [the clinical assessment of the patient's progress and of the severity of the illness] is to be used effectively, without fear and without reproach, the judgements must be made without any possibility of bias, without any overcompensation for any possible bias, and without any possible accusation of bias.

Not simply overcoming bias, but overcoming any possible *accusation of bias* is an important justification for blinding and randomisation.

In the second MRC trial, the antihistamine common cold study,[16] placebos, indistinguishable from the drug under test, were used. Here, Bradford Hill noted:

> ... in [this] trial... feelings may well run high... either of the recipient of the drug or the clinical observer, or indeed of both. If either were allowed to know the treatment that had been given, I believe that few of us would without qualms accept that the drug was of value–if such a result came out of the trial.

ETHICS

Experimentation in medicine is as old as medicine itself. Some experiments on humans have been conducted without concern for the welfare of the subjects, who have often been prisoners or disadvantaged people. Katz[23] provides examples of nineteenth-century studies in Russia and Ireland of the consequences of infecting people with syphilis and gonorrhoea. McNeill[24] describes how during the same period in the US, physicians put slaves into pit ovens to study heat stroke, and poured scalding water over them as an experimental cure for typhoid fever. He even describes how one slave had two fingers amputated in a 'controlled trial', one finger with anaesthesia and one without!

Unethical experiments on human beings have continued into the twentieth century and have been described by, for example, Beecher,[25] Freedman[26] and McNeil.[24] In 1932 the US Public Health Service began a study in Tuskegee, Alabama, of the natural progression of untreated syphilis in 400 black men. The study continued until 1972, when a newspaper reported that the subjects were uninformed or misinformed about the purpose of the study.[26] Shirer,[27] amongst others, describes how during the Nazi regime from 1933 to 1945, German doctors conducted experiments, mainly on Jews, but also on Gypsies, mentally disabled persons, Russian prisoners of war and Polish concentration camp inmates. The Nazi doctors were later tried for their atrocities in 1946–1947 at Nuremberg and this led to the writing, by three of the trial judges, of the Nuremberg Code, the first international effort to lay down ethical principles of clinical research.[28] Principle 1 of the Nuremberg Code states:

> The voluntary consent of the human subject is absolutely essential. This means that the person involved should have legal capacity to give consent; should be so situated as to be able to exercise free power of choice, without the intervention of any element of force, fraud, deceit, duress, overreaching, or other ulterior form of constraint or coercion; and should have sufficient knowledge and comprehension of the elements of the subject matter

involved as to enable him to make an understanding and enlightened decision.

Other principles of the Code are that experiments should yield results for the good of society, that unnecessary suffering and injury should be avoided, and that the subject should be free to withdraw from the experiment at any time and for any reason.

Other early advocates of informed consent were Charles Francis Withington and William Osler. Withington[29] realised, the 'possible conflict between the interests of medical science and those of the individual patient', and concluded in favour of 'the latter's indefensible rights'. Osler[30] insisted on informed consent in medical experiments. Despite this early advocacy, and the 1946–1947 Nuremberg Code, the application of informed consent to medical experiments did not take hold until the 1960s. Hill,[31] based on his experience in a number of early randomised clinical trials sponsored by the Medical Research Council, believed that it was not feasible to draw up a detailed code of ethics for clinical trials that would cover the variety of ethical issues that came up in these studies, and that the patient's consent was not warranted in all clinical trials. Gradually the medical community came to recognise the need to protect the reputation and integrity of medical research and in 1955 a human experimentation code was adopted by the Public Health Council in the Netherlands.[32] Later, in 1964, the World Medical Assembly issued the Declaration of Helsinki[33] essentially adopting the ethical principles of the Nuremberg Code, with consent being 'a central requirement of ethical research'.[34] The Declaration of Helsinki has been updated and amended several times: Tokyo, 1975; Venice, 1983; Hong Kong, 1989; Cape Town, 1996; and Edinburgh, 2000.

DATA MONITORING

In the modern randomised clinical trial, the accumulating data are usually monitored for safety and efficacy by an independent data monitoring committee. In 1968 the first such committee was established, serving the Coronary Drug Project, a large multicentre trial sponsored in the United States by the National Heart Institute of the National Institutes of Health.[35,36] In 1967, after a presentation of interim outcome data by the study co-ordinators to all participating investigators of the Coronary Drug Project, Thomas Chalmers addressed a letter to the policy board chairman expressing concern:

> that knowledge by the investigators of early nonstatistically significant trends in mortality, morbidity, or incidence of side effects might result in some investigators–desirous of treating their patients in the best possible manner, i.e., with the drug that is ahead–pulling out of the study or unblinding the treatment groups prematurely. (Canner[35], reproduced with permission from Elsevier)

Following this, a data and safety monitoring committee was established for the Coronary Drug Project. It consisted of scientists who were not contributing data to the study, and thereafter the practice of sharing accumulating outcome data with the study's investigators was discontinued. The data safety and monitoring committee assumed responsibility for deciding when the accumulating data warranted changing the study protocol or terminating the study.

The first formal recognition of the need for interim analyses, and the recognition that such analyses affect the probability of the type I error, came with the publication in the 1950s of papers on sequential clinical trials by Bross[37] and Armitage.[38] The principal advantage of a sequential trial over a fixed sample size trial, is that when the length of time needed to reach an endpoint is short, e.g. weeks or months, the sample size required to detect a substantial benefit from one of the treatments is less.

In the 1970s and 1980s solutions to interim analysis problems came about in the form of group sequential methods and stochastic curtailment.[39–41] In the group sequential trial, the frequency of interim analyses is usually limited to a small number, say between three and six. The Pocock boundaries[42] use constant nominal significance levels; the Haybittle–Peto boundary[43,44] uses stringent significance levels for all except the final test; in the O'Brien–Fleming method,[45] stringency gradually decreases; in the method by Lan and DeMets,[46] the total type I error probability is gradually spent in a manner that does not require the timing of analyses to be prespecified. More details of these newer methods in the development of clinical trials are given in the next chapter.

Recent years have seen a huge increase in the numbers of trials carried out and published, and in the advancement of methodological aspects relating to trials. Whilst many see the birth of clinical trials (certainly in their modern-day guise) as being the Medical Research Council streptomycin trial,[1] there remains some controversy (see, for example, D'Arcy Hart,[47,48] Gill,[49] and Clarke[50]). However, it is interesting to note that one of the most substantial reviews of historical aspects of trials is based on work for a 1951 M.D. thesis.[51] Bull cites 135 historical examples and other supporting references–but no mention of Bradford Hill and the Medical Research Council. The modern-day story of clinical trials perhaps begins where Bull ended.

ACKNOWLEDGEMENTS

This chapter is based heavily on work by F. Ederer in: Armitage P, Colton T, eds, *Encyclopedia of Biostatistics*. Chichester: John Wiley & Sons (1998).

REFERENCES

1. Medical Research Council. Streptomycin treatment of pulmonary tuberculosis. *Br Med J* (1948) **2**: 769–82.
2. Slotki JJ. *Daniel, Ezra, Nehemiah, Hebrew Text and English Translation with Introductions and Commentary* Soncino Press: London (1951) 1–6.
3. Witkosky SJ. *The Evil That Has Been Said of Doctors: Extracts From Early Writers* (translated with annotations by T.C. Minor). The Cincinnati Lancet-Clinic, Vol. 41, New Series Vol. 22 (1889) 447–8.
4. Packard FR. *The Life and Times of Ambroise Paré*, 2nd edn. New York: Paul B. Hoeber (1921) 27,163.
5. Lind J. *A Treatise of the Scurvy*. Edinburgh: Sands Murray Cochran (1753) 191–3.
6. Louis PCA. The applicability of statistics to the practice of medicine. *London Med Gazette* (1837) **20**: 488–91.
7. Fisher RA. The arrangement of field experiments. *J Min Agric* (1926) **33**: 503–13.
8. Fisher RA, McKenzie WA. Studies in crop variation: II. The manurial response of different potato varieties. *J Agric Sci* (1923) **13**: 315.
9. van Helmont JB. *Oriatrike or Physik Refined* (translated by J. Chandler). London: Lodowick Loyd (1662).
10. Amberson B, McMahon PM. A clinical trial of sanocrysin in pulmonary tuberculosis. *Am Rev Tuberc* (1931) **24**: 401.
11. Fibiger I. Om Serum Behandlung of Difteri. *Hospitalstidende* (1898) **6**: 309–25, 337–50.
12. Altman DG, Bland JM. Treatment allocation in controlled trials: why randomise? *Br Med J* (1999) **318**: 1209.
13. Diehl HS, Baker AB, Cowan DW. Cold vaccines: an evaluation based on a controlled study. *J Am Med Assoc* (1938) **111**: 1168–73.
14. Gail MH. Statistics in action. *J Am Stat Assoc* (1996) **91**: 1–13.
15. Medical Research Council. Chemotherapy of pulmonary tuberculosis in young adults. *Br Med J* (1952) **i**: 1162–8.
16. Medical Research Council. Clinical trials of antihistaminic drugs in the prevention and treatment of the common cold. *Br Med J* (1950) **ii**: 425–31.
17. Medical Research Council. A comparison of cortisone and aspirin in the treatment of early cases of rheumatoid arthritis – I. *Br Med J* (1954) **i**: 1223–7.
18. Medical Research Council. A comparison of cortisone and aspirin in the treatment of early cases of rheumatoid arthritis – II. *Br Med J* (1955) **ii**: 695–700.
19. Hill AB, Marshall J, Shaw DA. A controlled clinical trial of long-term anticoagulant therapy in cerebrovascular disease. *Q J Med* (1960) **29**(NS): 597–608.
20. Rheumatic Fever Working Party. The evolution of rheumatic heart disease in children: five-year report of a co-operative clinical trial of ACTH, cortisone, and aspirin. *Circulation* (1960) **22**: 505–15.
21. Kinsey VE. Retrolental fibroplasia. *AMA Arch Ophthalmol* (1956) **56**: 481–543.

22. Hill AB. *Statistical Methods in Clinical and Preventative Medicine*. Edinburgh: Livingstone (1962).

23. Katz J. The Nuremberg Code and the Nuremberg Trial. A reappraisal. *J Am Med Assoc* (1996) **276**: 1662–6.

24. McNeill PM. *The Ethics and Politics of Human Experimentation*. Cambridge: Press Syndicate of the University of Cambridge (1993).

25. Beecher HK. Ethics and clinical research. *New Engl J Med* (1966) **274**: 1354–60.

26. Freedman B. Research, unethical. In: Reich WT, ed., *Encyclopedia of Bioethics*. New York: Free Press (1995) 2258–61.

27. Shirer WL. *The Rise and Fall of the Third Reich*. New York: Simon and Schuster (1960).

28. US Government Printing Office. *Trials of War Criminals before the Nuremberg Military Tribunals under Control Council Law No. 10*, Vol. 2. Washington: US Government Printing Office (1949) 181–2.

29. Withington CF. *Time Relation of Hospitals to Medical Education*. Boston: Cupples Uphman (1886).

30. Osler W. The evolution of the idea of experiment. *Trans Congr Am Phys Surg* (1907) **7**: 1–8.

31. Hill AB. Medical ethics and controlled trials. *Br Med J* (1963) **1**: 1043–9.

32. Netherlands Minister of Social Affairs and Health. *4 World Med J* (1957) 299–300.

33. World Medical Assembly. *Declaration of Helsinki: recommendations guiding physicians in biomedical research involving human subjects*. World Medical Assembly, Helsinki (1964).

34. Faden RR, Beauchamp T, King NMP. *A History of Informed Consent*. New York: Oxford University Press (1986).

35. Canner P. Monitoring of the data for adverse or beneficial treatment effects. *Contr Clin Trials* (1983) **4**: 467–83.

36. Friedman L. The NHLBI model: a 25-year history. *Stat Med* (1993) **12**: 425–31.

37. Bross I. Sequential medical plans. *Biometrics* (1952) **8**: 188–295.

38. Armitage P. Sequential tests in prophylactic and therapeutic trials. *Q J Med* (1954) **23**: 255–74.

39. Armitage P. Interim analysis in clinical trials. *Stat Med* (1991) **10**: 925–37.

40. Friedman LM, Furberg CD, DeMets DL. *Fundamentals of Clinical Trials*, 2nd edn. Boston: Wright (1985).

41. Pocock SJ. *Clinical Trials: A Practical Approach*. Chichester: John Wiley & Sons (1983).

42. Pocock SJ. Group sequential methods in the design and analysis of clinical trials. *Biometrika* (1977) **64**: 191–9.

43. Haybittle JL. Repeated assessment of results of cancer treatment. *Br J Radiol* (1971) **44**: 793–7.

44. Peto R, Pike MC, Armitage P, Breslow NE, Cox DR, Howard SV, Mantel N, McPherson K, Peto J, Smith P. Design and analysis of randomized clinical trials requiring prolonged observation of each patient. 1. Introduction and design. *Br J Cancer* (1976) **34**: 585–612.

45. O'Brien PC, Fleming TR. A multiple testing procedure for clinical trials. *Biometrics* (1979) **35**: 549–56.

46. Lan KKG, DeMets DL. Discrete sequential boundaries for clinical trials. *Biometrika* (1983) **70**: 659–63.

47. D'Arcy Hart P. History of randomised controlled trials (letter to the Editor). *The Lancet* (1972) **i**: 965.

48. D'Arcy Hart P. Early controlled clinical trials (letter to the Editor). *Br Med J* (1996) **312**: 378–9.

49. Gill DBEC. Early controlled trials (letter to the Editor). *Br Med J* (1996) **312**: 1298.

50. Clarke M. Early controlled trials (letter to the Editor). *Br Med J* (1996) **312**: 1298.

51. Bull JP. The historical development of clinical therapeutic trials. *J Chron Dis* (1959) **10**: 218–48.

2

General Issues

DAVID MACHIN

National Cancer Centre, Singapore and United Kingdom Children's Cancer Study Group,
University of Leicester, UK and School of Health and Related Research, University of Sheffield, UK

INTRODUCTION

Just as in any other field of scientific and medical research, the choice of an appropriate design for a clinical trial is a vital element. In many circumstances, and for many of the trials described in this text, these designs may not be overly complicated. For example, a large majority will compare two therapeutic or other options in a parallel group trial. In which case the analytical methods used for description and analysis too may not be overly complicated. The vast majority of these are described in basic medical statistics textbooks and implemented in standard software packages. Nevertheless there are circumstances in which more complex designs, such as sequential trials, are utilised and for which specialist methods are required. There are also, often rather complex, statistical problems associated with monitoring the progress of clinical trials, their interim analysis, stopping rules for early closure and the possibility of extending recruitment beyond that initially envisaged.

Although the clinical trial itself may not be of complex design in the statistical sense, the associated trial protocol should carefully describe (and in some detail) the elements essential for its conduct. Thus the protocol will describe the rationale for the trial, the eligible group of patients or subjects, the therapeutic options and their modification should the need arise. It will also describe the method of patient allocation to these options, the specific clinical assessments to be made and their frequency, and the major endpoints to be used for evaluation. It will also include a justification of the sample size chosen, an indication of the analytical techniques to be used for summary and comparisons, and the proforma for data collection.

Of major concern in all aspects of clinical trial development and conduct is the ethical necessity which is written into the Declaration of Helsinki of 1964[1] to ensure the well-being of the patients or subjects under study. This in itself requires that clinical trials are well planned and conducted with due concern for the patient's welfare and safety. It also requires that the trial is addressing an important question, the answer to which will bring eventual benefit to the patients themselves or at least to future patients.

Textbook of Clinical Trials. Edited by D. Machin, S. Day and S. Green
© 2004 John Wiley & Sons, Ltd   ISBN: 0-471-98787-5

EVIDENCE-BASED MEDICINE

ʌ many circumstances trials have been conducted that are unrealistically small, some unnecessarily replicated while others have not been published as their results have not been considered of interest. It has now been recognised that to obtain the best current evidence with respect to a particular therapy, all pertinent clinical trial information needs to be obtained, and if circumstances permit, the overview is completed by a meta-analysis of the trial results. This recognition has led to the Cochrane Collaboration and a worldwide network of overview groups addressing numerous therapeutic questions.[2] In certain situations this has brought definitive statements with respect to a particular therapy. For others it has led to the launch of large-scale confirmatory trials.

Although it is not appropriate to review the methodology here, it is clear that the 'overview' process has led to many changes to the way in which clinical trial programmes have developed. They have provided the basic information required in planning new trials, impacted on an appropriate trial size, publication policy and very importantly raised reporting standards. They are impacting directly on decisions that affect patient care and questioning conventional wisdom in many areas.

TYPES OF CLINICAL TRIALS

In broad terms, the types of trials conducted in human subjects may be divided into four phases. These phases represent the stages in, for example, the development of a new drug which requires early dose finding and toxicity data in man, indications of potential activity, comparisons with a standard to determine efficacy and then (in certain circumstances) post-marketing trials. The nomenclature of Phase I, II, III and IV has been developed for drug development purposes and there may or may not be exact parallels in other applications. For example, a trial to assess the value of a health educational programme will

Table 2.1. Objectives of the trials of different phases in the development of drug (after Day[3])

Phase	Objective
I	The earliest types of studies that are carried out in humans. They are typically done using small numbers of healthy subjects and are to investigate pharmacodynamics, pharmacokinetics and toxicity.
II	Carried out in patients, usually to find the best dose of drug and to investigate safety.
III	Generally major trials aimed at conclusively demonstrating efficacy. They are sometimes called confirmatory trials and, in the context of pharmaceuticals, typically are the studies on which registration of a new product will be based.
IV	Studies carried out after registration of a product. They are often for marketing purposes as well as to gain broader experience with using the new product.

be a Phase III study, as will a trial comparing two surgical procedures for closing a cleft palate. In both these examples, any one of the Phase I, II or IV trials would not necessarily be conducted. The objectives of each phase in a typical development programme for a drug are summarised in Table 2.1.

Without detracting from the importance of Phase I, II and IV clinical trials, the main focus of this text is on Phase III comparative trials. In this context, reference will often be made to the 'gold standard' randomised controlled trial (RCT). This does not imply that this is the only type of trial worthy of conduct, but rather that it provides a benchmark against which other trial designs are measured.

PHASE I AND II TRIALS

The traditional outline of a series of clinical trials moving sequentially through Phases I to

IV is useful to consider in an idealistic setting, although in practice the sequential manner is not always followed (for reasons that will become clear).

Pocock[4] (pp. 2–3) also gives a convenient summary of the four phases while Temple[5] gives a discussion of them with emphasis from a regulatory perspective. Whether the sequential nature of the four phases is adhered to or not, the objectives of each phase are usually quite clearly defined.

As we have indicated in Table 2.1, Phase I studies aim to investigate the metabolism of a drug and its pharmacodynamics and pharmacokinetics. Typical pharmacokinetic data would allow, for example, investigation of peak drug concentrations in the blood, the half-life and the time to complete clearance. Such studies will assist in defining what doses should be used and the dosing frequency (once daily, twice daily, hourly) for future studies. These Phase I studies (certainly the very first ones) are almost always undertaken in healthy volunteers and would naturally be the very first studies undertaken in humans. However, later in a drug development programme it may be necessary to study its effects in patients with specific diseases, in those taking other medications or patients from special groups (infants, elderly, ethnic groups, pregnant women).

Most of the objectives of a Phase I study can often be met with relatively few subjects – many studies have fewer than 20 subjects. In essence, they are much more like closely controlled laboratory experiments than population-based clinical trials.

Broadly speaking, Phase II trials aim to set the scene for subsequent confirmatory Phase III trials. Typically, although exceptions may occur, these will be the first 'trials' in patients. They are also the first to investigate the existence of possible clinical benefits to those patients. However, although efficacy is important in Phase II it may often be in the form of surrogate, for example, tumour response rather than survival time in a patient with cancer. Along with efficacy, these studies will also be the first to give some detailed data on side effects.

Although conducted in patients, Phase II trials are typically still highly controlled and use highly defined (often narrow) patient groups so that extraneous variation is kept to a minimum. These are very much exploratory trials aimed at discovering *if* a compound *can* show useful clinical results. Although it is not common, some of these trials may have a randomised comparison group.

NON-RANDOMISED EFFICACY STUDIES

HISTORICAL CONTROLS

In certain circumstances, when a new treatment has been proposed, investigators have recruited patients in single-arm studies. The results from these patients are then compared with information on similar patients having (usually in the past) received a relevant standard therapy for the disease in question. However, such comparisons may well be biased in many possible ways, such that it may not be reasonable to ascribe the difference (if any) observed to the treatments themselves. Nevertheless it has been argued that using regression models to account for possible confounding variables may correct such biases,[6] but this is at best a very uncertain procedure and is not often advocated. Similar problems arise if all patients are recruited prospectively but allocation to treatment is not made at random. Of course, there will be situations in which randomisation is not feasible and there is no alternative to the use of historical controls or non-randomised prospective studies. One clear example of this is the early evaluation of the Stanford Heart Transplant Program in which patients could not be randomised to receive or not a donor heart. Many careful analyses and reviews of this unique data set have been undertaken and these have established the value of the programme, but progress would have been quicker (and less controversial) had randomisation been possible.

In the era of evidence-based medicine, information from non-randomised but comparative studies is categorised as providing weaker evidence than randomised trials (see Altman,[7] p. 3279).

PHASE III CONTROLLED TRIALS

EQUIPOISE AND UNCERTAINTY

As indicated, the randomised controlled trial is the standard against which other trial designs may be compared. One such trial, and there are many other examples described in subsequent chapters, compared conventional treatment, C, with a complementary medicine alternative in patients with severe burns.[8] The complementary medicine was termed Moist Exposed Burns Ointment (*MEBO*). One essential difference between the two treatments was that C covered the wounds (dressed) whilst *MEBO* left them exposed (not dressed). See Figure 2.1.

In this trial patients with severe burns were emergency admissions requiring immediate treatment, so that once eligibility was confirmed, consent obtained, randomisation immediately followed and treatment was then commenced. Such a trial is termed a two-treatment parallel group design. This is the most common design for comparative clinical trials. In these trials subjects are independently allocated to receive one of several treatment options. No subject receives more than one of these treatments.

In addition there is genuine uncertainty as to which of the options is best for the patient. It is this uncertainty which provides the necessary equipoise, as described by Freedman[9] and Weijer *et al.*[10] to justify random allocation to treatment after due consent is given. Enkin,[11] in a debate with Weijer *et al.*,[10] provides a counter view.

There are at least two aspects of the eligibility requirements that are important. The first is that the patient indeed has the condition (here severe burns) and satisfies all the other requirements. There must be no specific reasons why the patient should not be included. For example, in some circumstances pregnant or lactating women (otherwise eligible) may be excluded for fear of impacting adversely either on the foetus or the newborn child. The second is that all (here two) therapeutic options are equally appropriate for this particular patient. Only if both these aspects are satisfied should the patient be invited to consent to participate in the trial. There will be circumstances in which a patient may be eligible for the trial but the attending physician feels (for whatever reason) that one of the trial options is 'best' for the patient. In which case the patient should receive that option, no consent for the trial is then required and the randomisation would not take place. In such circumstances, the clinician should not randomise the patient in the hope that the patient will receive the 'best' option. Then, if he or she did not, withdraw the patient from the trial.

The consent procedure itself will vary from trial to trial and will, at least to some extent, depend on local ethical regulations in the country in which the trial is being conducted. The ideal is fully informed and written consent by the patient

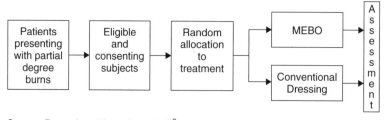

Source: Reproduced from Ang *et al.*,[8]

Figure 2.1. Randomised controlled trial to compare conventional treatment and Most Exposed Burns Ointment (MEBO) for the treatment of patients with partial degree burns

him or herself. However, departures from this may be appropriate. For example, such departures may concern patients with severe burns who may be unconscious at admission, very young children for whom a proxy must be used to obtain the consent for them, or patients with hand burns that are so severe that they affect their ability to write their signature.

Clearly, during the period in which patients are being assessed for eligibility and their consent obtained, both the attending physician and the patient will be fully aware of the potential options being compared in the RCT. However, neither must be aware, at this stage, of the eventual treatment allocation. It is important therefore that the randomisation list, for the current as well as for future patients, is held by a neutral third party. In most circumstances, this should be an appropriate trial office that is contacted by the responsible clinician once eligibility and consent are obtained. This contact may be made by telephone, fax, direct access by modem into a trial database, email or the web – whichever is convenient in the particular circumstance. It is then important that therapy is instituted as soon as practicable after the randomisation is obtained.

In specific cases, the randomisation can be concealed within opaque and sealed envelopes which are distributed to the centres in advance of patient recruitment. Once a patient is deemed eligible, the envelope is taken in the order specified in a prescribed list, opened and the treatment thereby revealed. Intrinsically, there is nothing wrong with this process but, because of the potential for abuse, it is not regarded as entirely satisfactory. However, in some circumstances it will be unavoidable; perhaps a trial is being conducted in a remote area with poor communications. In such cases, every precaution should be taken to ensure that the process is not compromised.

The therapeutic options should be well described within the trial protocol and details of what to do, if treatment requires modification or stopping for an individual patient should be given. Stopping may arise either when patients merely refuse to take further part in the trial or from safety concerns with a therapy under test.

STANDARD OR CONTROL THERAPY

In the early stages of the development of a new therapy it is important to compare this with the current standard for the disease in question. In certain circumstances, the 'new' therapy may be compared against a 'no treatment' control. For example, in patients receiving surgery for the primary treatment of head and neck cancer followed by best supportive care, the randomised controlled trial may be assessing the value of adding post-operative chemotherapy. In this case the 'control' group are those who receive no adjuvant treatment, whilst the 'test' group receive chemotherapy. In certain circumstances, patients may receive a placebo control. For example, in the randomised controlled trial conducted by Chow et al.[12] in those with advanced liver cancer, patients are randomised to receive either placebo or tamoxifen. In this trial both patients and the attending physicians are 'blinded' to the actual treatment given to individual patients. Such a 'double-blind' or 'double-masked' trial is a design that reduces any potential bias to a minimum. Such designs are not possible however in many circumstances and neither are those with a 'no treatment' control. In many situations, the 'control' will be the current best practice against which the new treatment will be compared. Should this turn out to be better than current practice then this, in its turn, may become standard practice against which future developments will be compared.

In general there will be both baseline and follow-up information collected on all patients. The baseline (pre-randomisation) information will be that required to determine eligibility together with other information required to describe the patients recruited to the trial together with those variables which are thought likely to influence prognosis. The key follow-up information will be that which is necessary to determine the major endpoint(s) of the randomised controlled trial. Thus in the example of the burns patients these may be when the unhealed body surface area finally closes or the size and severity of the resulting scars. To establish the first of these, the burns areas may have to be monitored on a daily basis to determine exactly when the endpoint is achieved, whereas the latter may be a single assessment at the anniversary of the initial burn accident. Pre-trial information on these end-points, possibly from clinical experience or other studies, will usually form the basis of the antic-ipated difference between treatments (the effect size), help determine the trial size and be the variables for the statistical comparisons.

LARGE SIMPLE TRIALS

It has become recognised over time, particularly in the fields of cardiovascular disease and cancer, that there are circumstances where small ther-apeutic advantages may be worthwhile demon-strating. In terms of trial size, the smaller the potential benefit, essentially the effect size, then the larger the trial must be in order to be rea-sonably certain that the small benefit envisaged really exists at all.

Trials of this size, often involving many thousands of patients, are a major undertaking. To be practical, they must be in common diseases in order to recruit the required numbers of patients in a reasonable time frame. They must be testing a treatment that has wide applicability and can be easily administered by the clinicians responsible or the patients themselves. The treatments must be relatively non-toxic else the small benefit will be outweighed by the side effects. The trials must be simple in structure and restricted as to the number of variables recorded, so that the recruiting clinicians are not overburdened by the workload attached to large numbers of trial patients going through the clinic. They also need to be simple in this respect, for the responsible trial centre to cope with the large amounts of patient data collected.

One example of such a trial tests the value of aspirin in patients with cardiovascular disease.[13] This trial concerned a very common disease using a very simple and low-cost treatment taken as tablets with very few side effects. The resulting estimates of absolute survival gain were (as expected) small but the benefits in public health

terms enormous. Similar types of trials have been conducted in patients with breast cancer, one in particular compared the three adjuvant treatment possibilities: tamoxifen, anastrozole or their combination.[14]

INTERVENTION AND PREVENTION TRIALS

The focus so far has been on randomised con-trolled trials in patients with medical conditions requiring treatment or a medical intervention of some sort. Such designs do apply to situa-tions such as trials in normal healthy women in which alternative forms of contraception are being tested.[15] However, there are quite different situations in which the object of a trial is to eval-uate alternative strategies for preventing disease or for detecting its presence earlier than is rou-tine. For example, intervention trials to encourage 'safe sex' to prevent the spread of AIDS or breast screening trials to assess the value of early detec-tion of the disease on subsequent treatment and prognosis. In such cases, it may be impossible to randomise on an individual subject basis. Thus an investigator may have to randomise communities to test out different types of health promotion or different types of vaccines, when problems of contamination or logistics, respectively, mean that it is better to randomise a group rather than an individual. This is the approach adopted by Donner et al.[16] in a trial to compare a reduced antenatal care model with a standard care model. For this trial, because of the clustered randomisa-tion of the alternatives on a clinic-to-clinic basis, the Zelen[17] single consent design was utilised.

PHASE IV TRIALS – POST-MARKETING SURVEILLANCE

Within a regulatory framework, Phase IV trials are generally considered as 'post-registration' trials: that is, trials of products that already have a marketing authorisation. However, within this post-registration period studies may be carried out for a variety of purposes, some within their existing licence and others out-with that licence. Studies may also be undertaken in countries where a marketing authorisation has not been approved, in which case they are regulatory or Phase III-type studies, at least for that country. Studies may be undertaken to expand the indications listed on a marketing authorisation either for a different disease or a different severity of the indicated condition. They may be undertaken to gain more safety data for newly registered products: this latter situation is more usually what is considered as a true Phase IV study.

Historically, pharmaceutical companies used to carry out studies that were solely for marketing purposes and answered very few (if any) research questions. These were termed 'seeding studies' although with tighter ethical constraints such studies are now very rare, if indeed they take place at all. Certainly the 'hidden' objective of many Phase IV studies carried out by pharmaceutical companies may be to increase sales, but if the means of doing so is via answering a useful scientific or medical question then this should be of benefit both to society and to the company.

Many trials organised by academic departments should also be considered as Phase IV studies. Classic examples such as the RISC Group trials[13] looking at the cardiovascular benefits of aspirin are studies of licensed products to expand their use.

ALTERNATIVE DESIGNS

For illustrative purposes we have used the two-arm parallel group RCT but these designs can be generalised to compare three or more groups as appropriate. In addition, there are other designs in common use which include 2×2 factorial and crossover designs.[18]

MORE THAN TWO GROUPS

Although not strictly a different design, a parallel group trial with more than two treatments to compare does pose some difficulties. For example,

how is the size of a trial comparing three treatments, A, B and C, determined, since there are now three possible anticipated effect sizes that one can use for planning purposes? These correspond to the treatment comparisons $A-B$, $A-C$ and $B-C$. The number of patients required for each of these comparisons may give three very different sample sizes. It is then necessary to decide which of these will form the basis for the final trial recruitment target, N. The trial will then randomise the patients equally into the three treatment groups. In many circumstances, a three-arm trial will tend to require some 50% more patients than a two-arm trial comparing two of the three treatments under consideration.

Once the trial has been completed, the resulting analysis (and reporting) is somewhat more complex than for a simple two-group comparison. However, it is the importance of the questions posed, rather than the ease of analysis, which should determine the design chosen. A good example of the use of such a design is the previously mentioned trial in post-menopausal patients with breast cancer in which three options are compared.[14]

Nevertheless practical considerations may rule out this choice of design. The design poses particular problems in data monitoring. For example, if an early advantage appears to favour one particular treatment and this suggests the trial might be stopped early as a consequence. Then it may not be clear whether the randomisation between the other treatment groups should or should not continue. Were the trial to stop early, then the questions relating to the other comparisons are unlikely to have been resolved at this stage. Should the (reduced) trial continue then there may be very complex issues associated with its analysis and reporting.

In addition, a potentially serious problem of bias can arise. At the onset of the trial, the clinician has to assess whether or not all the three options (A, B or C) available for treatment are suitable for the particular patient under examination. If any one of these were not thought to be appropriate (for whatever reason), then the patient's consent would not be sought to enter the trial and to be randomised. Suppose later in the trial, an interim analysis suggests recruitment to A is no longer necessary and that arm is closed. For future patients, the clinician now has to assess whether or not only the two options (B or C) are suitable for the particular patient under examination. As a consequence, the patients now going into the trial are no longer potentials for A and hence may be somewhat different than those entering at the earlier stages. Although this will not bias the final comparison between B and C, it does imply that there will be a bias if the patients entering at this stage are compared with those receiving A.

In the above, we have assumed that the three treatments A, B and C are, in a sense, unrelated albeit all suitable for the patients in mind. However, if they were related, for example, perhaps three doses of the same drug, then a note of this structure may change the approach to design from that outlined here.

FACTORIAL DESIGNS

In a trial conducted by Chan et al.[19] patients with dyslipidaemia in visceral obesity were randomised to either atorovastin alone, fish oil alone, both or neither (placebo) to investigate their influence on lipid levels. This trial may take the form of no treatment (**1**), atorovastin alone (**a**), fish oil alone (**f**) or both atorovastin and fish oil (**af**). These alternative options are summarised in Figure 2.2.

In contrast to the two-group parallel design of Figure 2.1, where *MEBO* is contrasted with conventional treatment C, the factorial design poses two questions simultaneously. Those patients assigned to groups I and II are compared with those receiving III and IV, to assess the value of fish oil. This estimates the effect of fish oil and is termed the 'main effect' of that treatment. Those assigned to I and III are compared to those receiving II and IV to assess the main effect of atorovastin. In most situations the final trial size will require fewer patients than would be necessary if the two questions were posed in two distinct parallel group trials of the format of Figure 2.2.

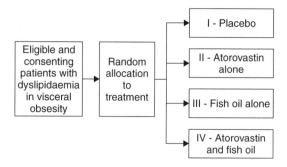

Figure 2.2. Randomised 2×2 factorial trial to determine the value of atorovastin, fish oil or both in patients with dyslipidaemia in visceral obesity. Reproduced from Chan et al.[19]

In addition, the factorial design allows the comparison of groups (I and IV) with (II and III) and this estimates the so-called fish oil by atorovastin interaction. For example, suppose both the main effect of fish oil alone and the main effect of atorovastin alone prove to be beneficial in this context, then an interaction would arise if the combination treatment fish oil–atorovastin gives a benefit greater (or lesser) than the sum of these constituent parts. As is the situation here, factorial designs can be of a double placebo type, where subjects of Group I of Figure 2.2 receive double placebo, one representing each treatment factor.

In principle, the 2×2 or 2^2 design can be extended to the 2^k ($k > 2$). Circumstances where this kind of design may be useful are if perhaps the first two factors are major therapeutic or curative options and the third is a factor for a secondary question not associated directly with efficacy but (say) to relieve pain in such subjects. However, the presence of a third factor of whatever type increases the complexity of the trial design (not itself a particularly difficult statistical problem) which may have implications on the patient consent procedures and the timing of randomisation(s). Nevertheless, a 2^3 design in a trial of falls prevention in the elderly has been successfully conducted by Day et al.[20] Piantadosi[21] describes several examples of the use of these designs.

However, Green[22] has issued a cautionary note that some of the assumptions behind the use of factorial designs may not be entirely justified and so any proposals for the use of such designs should be considered carefully.

CROSSOVER TRIALS

In contrast to the design of Figure 2.1, in the crossover trial each patient will receive both treatment options, one followed by the other in two periods of time. The two treatments will be given either in the order A followed by B (AB) or the reverse (BA). The essential features of a crossover design are summarised in Figure 2.3 for the trial conducted by Hong et al.[23] in patients with erectile dysfunction.

Typically, in the two-period, two-treatment crossover trial, for eligible patients there is a run-in stage in which the subject receives neither treatment. At the end of this randomisation to either AB or BA takes place. Following active treatment in Period I (in effect either A or B depending on the randomisation), there is a wash-out interval in which again no treatment is given, after which Period II commences and the (other) treatment of the sequence is given. The characteristics of this design, for example the possible run-in and the wash-out period, imply that only certain types of patients in which active treatment can be withheld in this way are suitable to be recruited. Further, there is an implication that the patient returns to essentially the same state at the beginning of Period II as he or she was in at the commencement of Period I. This ensures that the between-treatment comparison (A v B) within the patient remains unaffected by anything other than the change in treatment itself and random variation. These considerations tend to restrict the applicability of the design to patients with chronic conditions such as, for example, arthritis, asthma or migraine. Senn[24] describes in careful and comprehensive detail the role of crossover designs in clinical studies.

A clear advantage of the design is that the patient receives both options and so the analysis includes within-patient comparisons which are more sensitive than between-patient comparisons, implying that such trials would require fewer subjects than a parallel group design comparing the same treatment options.

EQUIVALENCE TRIALS

In certain situations, a new therapy may bring certain advantages over the current standard, possibly in a reduced side-effects profile, easier administration or cost. Nevertheless, it may not be anticipated to be better with respect to the primary efficacy variable. Under such conditions, the new approach may be expected to be at least 'equivalent' to the standard in relation to efficacy.

Trials to show that two (or more) treatments are 'equivalent' to each other pose special problems in design, management and analysis.[25] 'Proving the null hypothesis' in a significance testing scenario is never possible: the strict interpretation

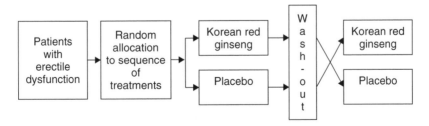

Source: Reproduced from Hong et al.,[23] with permission.

Figure 2.3. Randomised placebo controlled, two-period crossover trial of Korean red ginseng in patients with erectile dysfunction

when a statistically significant difference has *not* been found is that 'there is insufficient evidence to demonstrate a difference'. Small trials typically fail to detect differences between treatment groups but not necessarily because no difference exists. Indeed it is unlikely that two different treatments will ever exert truly identical effects.

A level of 'therapeutic equivalence' should be defined and this is a medical question, not a statistical one. For example in a study of weight gain in pre-term infants, if two treatments show mean increases in weight to within 25 g per week then they may be considered as therapeutically equivalent. Note that in this example 25 g is *not* the mean weight gain that is expected per week – we would hope that would be much more. But if infants receiving one feeding regimen had a mean increase of 150 g per week then we would consider an alternative treatment to be equivalent if the mean weight gain were between 125 and 175 g per week.

Conventionally, to show a treatment difference, we would state the null hypothesis as being that

there is no difference between the treatments and then look for evidence to refute that null hypothesis. In the case of equivalence we specify the range of equivalence, Δ (25 g per week in the above example) and then test *two* null hypotheses. We test that the observed difference is statistically significantly *greater* than $-\Delta$; and that the observed difference is statistically significantly *less* than $+\Delta$. In practice it is much easier to consider a confidence interval for the difference between the treatment means and draw this on a graph with the agreed limits of equivalence. Figure 2.4 shows various scenarios. Some cases show equivalence, some fail to show equivalence; some cases show a statistically significant difference, others fail to show a difference. Note that it is quite possible to show a statistically significant difference between two treatments yet also demonstrate therapeutic equivalence. These are not contradictory statements but simply a realisation that although there is evidence that one treatment works better than another, the size of the benefit is so small that it has little or no practical advantage.

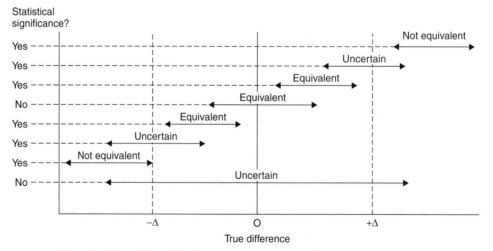

Examples of possible results of using the confidence interval approach: $-\Delta$ to $+\Delta$ is the prespecified range of equivalence; the horizontal lines correspond to possible trial outcomes expressed as confidence intervals, with the associated significance test result shown on the left; above each line is the decision concerning equivalence.

Source: Reproduced from Jones *et al.*,[86] with permission from the BMJ Publishing Group.

Figure 2.4. Schematic diagram to illustrate the concept of equivalence

The analysis and interpretation can be quite straightforward but the design and management of equivalence trials is often much more complex. In general, careless or inaccurate measurement, poor follow-up of patients, poor compliance with study procedures and medication all tend to bias results towards no difference. Since we are trying to offer evidence of equivalence, poor study design and procedures may therefore actually help to hide treatment differences. In general, therefore, the quality of equivalence trials should be demonstrably high.

One special subset of equivalence trials is termed 'non-inferiority' trials. Here we only wish to be sure that one treatment is 'not worse than' or is 'at least as good as' another treatment: if it is better, that is fine (even though superiority would not be required to bring it into common use). All we need is to get convincing evidence that the new treatment is not worse than the standard. We still have the same design and management considerations but here, looking at Figure 2.4, we would only be concerned with whether or not the *lower* limit of the confidence interval is *greater* than the non-inferiority margin $(-\Delta)$.

SEQUENTIAL TRIALS

There has been an implicit assumption in the trial designs discussed above, that the total (and final) sample size is determined at the design stage and before recruitment commences to the trial in question. This fixed sample size approach essentially implies that the data collected during the conduct of the trial will only be examined for efficacy once the trial has closed to patient accrual. However, the vast majority of Phase III trials will tend to recruit patients over perhaps an extended interval of time and so information on efficacy will be accumulated over this period. A sequential trial is one designed to utilise this accumulating knowledge to better effect. Perhaps to decrease the final trial size if the data are indicating an advantage to one of the treatments and this can be firmly established at an early stage or to extend the trial size in other circumstances.

In fact, Donaldson et al.[26] give examples where trials that had been conducted using a fixed sample size approach might have been curtailed earlier had a sequential design been utilised. Fayers et al.[27] describe the issues faced when designing a sequential trial using α-interferon in patients with renal carcinoma. The accumulating patient data from this trial crossed an early termination boundary which inferred an advantage to α-interferon.[28]

A fully sequential design will monitor the trial patient-by-patient as the information on the trial endpoint is observed from them. Alternatively, a 'group' sequential trial will utilise information from successive groups of patients. Computer programs to assist in the implementation of these designs are available[29] and a review of some of the issues is given by Whitehead.[30]

The solid lines of Figure 2.5 indicate stopping boundaries for declaring a statistically significant difference between treatments A and B. If the broken boundary is crossed, the trial stops, concluding that no significant difference was found between the treatments. Potentially, the number of preferences could continue indefinitely between the upper solid and broken lines or between the lower solid and broken lines; in such a case no conclusion would ever be reached.

In contrast to the open sequential design, the closed design of Figure 2.6 will continue to recruit to a pre-stated maximum or until a boundary is crossed. Thus this design has a finite size and a conclusion will always be drawn. Again the solid lines indicate stopping boundaries for declaring a statistically significant difference between treatments and if the broken line is crossed, concluding that no significant difference was found between the treatments.

For more complex designs implementing a sequential option remains possible. For example, a factorial structure of the treatments does permit a sequential approach to trial design as the two questions can be monitored separately. Nevertheless, if one of the factors, say the chemotherapy option in the example we discussed previously, is stopped by crossing a boundary during the sequential monitoring, then the recruiting clinician will only have to put two rather than four choices to the patients. Again, the subsequent

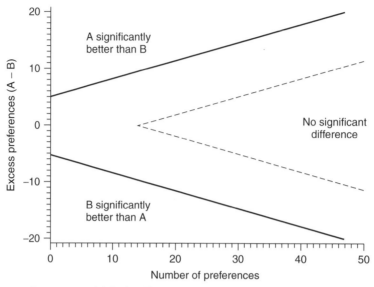

Open sequential design. The solid lines indicate stopping boundaries for declaring a statistically significant difference between treatments A and B. If the broken boundary is crossed, then the study stops, concluding that no significant difference was found between the treatments. Potentially the number of preferences could continue indefinitely between the upper solid and broken lines or between the lower solid and broken lines; in such a case no conclusion would ever be reached.

Source: Reproduced from Day[3] (Figure 24), with permission.

Figure 2.5. Open sequential design

patients recruited may then be somewhat different from those at the first stage of the trial. This will then impact on the form of the subsequent analysis.

In contrast, the three-arm trial cannot be so easily designed in a sequential manner although both Whitehead[31] and Jennison and Turnbull[32] address the problem. They do not however appear to give an actual clinical example of their use.

There are however several problems associated with the use of sequential designs. These range from difficulties of financing a trial of uncertain size, making sure the data is fully up-to-date as the trial progresses, to the more technical concerns associated with the calculation of the appropriate confidence intervals. However, Whitehead,[31] see also Jennison and Turnbull,[32] has argued very persuasively that all these objections can be resolved. Nevertheless, in relative terms the use of sequential designs is still somewhat limited.

ZELEN'S DESIGNS

Although not strictly an alternative 'design' in the sense of those of this section, Zelen's randomised consent design combines aspects of design with problems associated with obtaining consent from patients to participate in clinical trials. They were motivated by the difficulties expressed by clinicians in obtaining consent from women who they wished to recruit to trials with breast cancer.[17,33] Essentially subjects are randomised to one of two treatment groups. Those who were randomised to the standard treatment (conventional dressing in Figure 2.1) are all treated with it. For these patients no consent to take part in the trial is sought. On

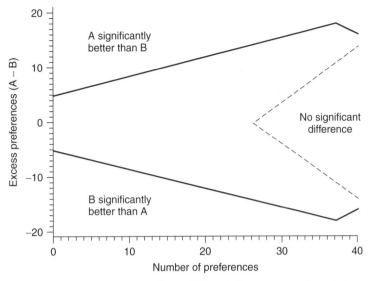

Closed sequential design. The solid lines indicate stopping boundaries for declaring a statistically significant difference between treatments A and B. For example, if out of ten patients expressing a preference for one or other treatment, nine preferred treatment B and only one preferred A, then the study would stop, concluding that B is significantly better than A. If the broken boundary is crossed, then the study stops and the conclusion is drawn that no significant difference was found between the treatments.

Source: Reproduced from Day[3] (Figure 4), with permission.

Figure 2.6. Closed sequential design

the other hand, those who are randomised to the experimental treatment (*MEBO* dressing in Figure 2.1) are asked for their consent; if they agree they are treated with the experimental treatment; if they disagree they are treated with the standard treatment. This is known as Zelen's single consent design. An alternative is that those randomised to the standard treatment may also be asked if they accept that treatment; again, they are actually given their treatment of choice. This latter double consent design is described in Figure 2.7; in either case, the analysis must be by intention-to-treat, that is based on the treatment to which patients were randomised, not the treatment they actually received.

The properties of these designs have been examined in some detail by Altman *et al.*[34] who concluded that: 'There are serious statistical arguments against the use of randomised consent designs, which should discourage their use'. In

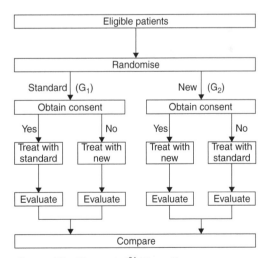

Source: After Altman *et al.*[34] (Figure 3).

Figure 2.7. The sequence of events to follow in Zelen's double randomised consent design, seeking consent in conjunction with randomisation

any event, they have rarely been used in practice although they continue to be advocated.[35] Nevertheless, in the large antenatal care trial described by Donner et al.[16] the Zelen single consent design is utilised. However, this is a cluster randomised trial and the issues are somewhat different.

BAYESIAN METHODS

The essence of Bayesian methodology in the context of the design of clinical trials is to incorporate relevant information into the design process. At a later stage, Bayesian methods may assist in data monitoring (as trial data accumulate) and with the final analysis and interpretation of the (now complete) trial data. In theory the information available and which is pertinent to the trial in question can be summarised into a prior distribution. This may include (hard) information from the published literature and/or elicited clinical opinion. The mean of such a distribution would correspond to the possible effect size which can then be assessed by the design team as clinically worthwhile in their context and hence used for sample size estimation purposes. The same prior, or that prior updated from new external evidence accumulated during the course of the trial, may be used by the trial Data Monitoring Committee (DMC) to help form the basis of recommendations with respect to future conduct of the trial. Perhaps to close the trial as efficacy has been clearly established or increase the planned size of the trial as appropriate. Finally once the trial data is complete, these can be combined with the prior (or updated prior) to obtain the posterior distribution, from which Bayesian estimates of treatment effect and corresponding credibility intervals can be calculated.

However, despite the feasibility of the above approach few trials to date have implemented a full Bayesian approach. A review of articles in the *British Medical Journal* from 1996 to November 1999 found no examples.[7] Nevertheless, Spiegelhalter et al.[36] show convincingly how the concept of optimistic and sceptical prior distributions obtained from the clinical teams may be of assistance in interpreting the results of a trial. Despite some technical difficulties, it is fairly certain that Bayesian methods will become more prominent in Phase II trial methodology. For example, Tan et al.[37] suggest how such ideas may be useful in a Phase II programme.

RANDOMISATION AND ALLOCATION TO TREATMENT

We have indicated above that randomisation of patients to the treatment they receive is an important part of the 'gold' standard. In fact it is the key element. The object of randomisation is to help ensure that the final comparison of treatment options is as unbiased as possible, that is, that any difference or lack of difference observed between treatments in efficacy is not due to the method by which patients are chosen for the options under study. For example, if the attending clinician chose which of *MEBO* or *C* should be given to each patient, then any differences observed may be due, at least in part, to the selection process itself rather than to a true difference in efficacy.

Apart from the possible effect of the allocated treatments themselves, observed differences may arise through the play of chance alone or possibly an imbalance of patients with differing prognoses in the treatment groups or both. The object of the statistical analysis will be to take account of any imbalance and assess the role of chance. Some of the imbalance in the major prognostic variables may be avoided by stratifying the randomisation by prognostic group and ensuring that an equal number of patients are allocated within each stratum to each of the options. This may be achieved by arranging the randomisation to be balanced within predetermined blocks of patients within each of the strata. Blocks are usually chosen as neither too small nor too large, four or six are often used. Sometimes the block size, perhaps between these options, is chosen at random for successive sequences of patients within a stratum of patient types.

Alternatively, the balance of treatments between therapeutic options can be made using a dynamic allocation procedure. In such schemes, during the randomisation procedure a patient is identified to belong to a predetermined category according to certain covariates. This category may, for example, be defined as those of a particular age, gender and tumour stage group. Once the category is determined, then randomisation to the treatment options may proceed as described above. One option, however, is to allocate the next patient to the treatment with the fewest patients already assigned within that category. In which case, the allocation at that stage is deterministic. A better option in such circumstances is to weight the randomisation, perhaps in the ratio of 3:2 in favour of the option with the fewest patients. Clearly, if numbers are equal, the randomisation would revert to 1:1.

We have implicitly assumed that, for two treatments, a 1:1 randomisation will take place. For all practical purposes, this will be statistically the most efficient. However, the particular context may suggest other ratios. For example, if the patient pool is limited for whatever reason, then the clinical team may argue that they should obtain more information within the trial from the test treatment rather than the well-known standard. Perhaps, there is a concern with the toxicity profile rather than just the efficacy *per se*. In such circumstances, a randomisation ratio of say 2:3 or 1:2 in favour of the test therapy may be decided. However, some loss of statistical power will ensue and this loss should be quantified before a decision on the allocation ratio is finally made.

ENDPOINTS

DEFINING THE ENDPOINT(S)

The protocol for every clinical trial will detail the assessments to be made on the patients recruited. Some of these assessments may focus on aspects of the day-to-day care of the patient whilst others may focus more on those measures which will be necessary in order to determine the trial endpoint(s) for each subject. It is important that these endpoints are unambiguously defined

so that they can be determined for each patient recruited to the trial. It is good practice to define which endpoint is the major endpoint of the trial as this will be used to determine trial size and be the main focus for the efficacy evaluation. In many situations, there may be several endpoints of interest, but in this case it is important to order them in order of priority or at least to identify those of primary or secondary importance. If there are too many endpoints defined, then the multiplicity of comparisons then made at the analysis stage may result in spurious statistical significance. This is a major concern if endpoints for health-related quality of life and health economic evaluations are added to the already established more clinical endpoints.

SINGLE MEASURES

In some trials a single measure may be sufficient to determine the endpoint in each patient. For example, the endpoint may be the diastolic blood pressure measured at a particular time, say 28 days post-randomisation in each patient. In this case the treatment groups will be summarised by the respective means. In some situations the endpoint may be patient response, for example, the patient becomes normo-tensive following a period of treatment. Those who respond are termed successes and those that do not failures. In this case, the treatment groups will be summarised by the proportion of responders. If, on the other hand, the patients are categorised as: normo-tensive, still hypotensive but diastolic blood pressure (DBP) nevertheless reduced, or still hypotensive and DBP not improved, then this would correspond to an ordered categorical variable. Alternatively, the endpoint may be defined as the time from randomisation and inception of treatment for the patient to become normo-tensive. In this situation repeated (say daily) measures of DBP will be made until the value recorded is normo-tensive (as defined in the protocol). The interval between the date of randomisation and the date of recording the first occurrence of a normo-tensive recording is the endpoint measure of interest. Such data are usually summarised using survival time methods.

A particular feature of time-to-event studies occurs when the endpoint cannot be determined. For example, in the trial monitoring the DBP it may be that a patient never becomes normo-tensive during the trial observation period. In which case the time from randomisation until the end of the trial observation period represents the time a patient has been under observation but has not yet become normo-tensive. Such a survival time is termed censored and is often denoted by, say, 28+, which here means the patient has been observed for 4 weeks but still remains hypotensive. In contrast, an observation of 28 means the patient has been observed for 4 weeks and became normo-tensive on the last observation day.

REPEATED MEASURES

In the trial taking repeated DBP assessments, these are recorded in order to determine a single outcome – 'time to becoming normo-tensive'. In other situations, the successive values of DBP themselves may be utilised in making the formal comparisons. If the number of observations made on each subject is the same, then the analysis may be relatively straightforward, perhaps using repeated measures analysis of variance. On the other hand, if the numbers of observations recorded varies or if the intervals between successive observations vary from patient to patient or if there is occasional missing data, then the summary and analysis of such data may be quite complex. One option is to calculate the area under the curve (AUC) and use this as a single measure for each patient, thus avoiding the use of more complex analytical methods.[38]

However, the AUC method is now being superseded somewhat in Phase III trials by the use of general estimating equations and multi-level modelling. The technical details are beyond the scope of this book but most good statistics packages[39] now include facilities for these types of analyses. Nevertheless, these methods have not yet had much impact on the reporting of clinical trials, although a good example of their use has been provided by Brown et al.[40]

QUALITY OF LIFE

In many trials, endpoints such as the percentage of patients responding to treatment, survival time or direct measures such as DBP have been used. In other situations, more psychosocial measures have been utilised such as pain scores, perhaps measured using a visual analogue scale, and emotional functioning scores, perhaps assessed by patients completing a questionnaire themselves. Such self-completed questionnaires have also been developed to measure aspects of quality of life (QoL) in patients undergoing treatment for their disease. One such instrument is the SF-36 of Ware and Sherbourne,[41] part of which is reproduced in Figure 2.8.

The QoL domains measured by these instruments may then be used as the definitive endpoints for clinical trials in certain circumstances. For example, in patients with terminal cancer the main thrust of therapy may be for palliation (rather than cure) so that aspects of QoL may be the primary concerns for any comparison of alternative approaches to management and care of such patients. If a single aspect of this QoL measured at one time point is to be used for comparison purposes, then no new principles are required either for trial design purposes or analysis. On the other hand, and more usually, there may be several aspects of the QoL instrument that may need to be compared between treatment groups and these features will usually be assessed over time. This is further complicated by often-unequal numbers of assessments available from each patient caused either by missing assessments in the series for a variety of reasons related or unrelated to their health status or perhaps in terminal patients by their death. Fayers and Machin[42] and Fairclough[43] discuss these features of QoL data in some detail.

As we have discussed previously, there is also a problem associated with the numerous statistical tests of significance of the multiple QoL outcomes. These pose problems of interpretation which have also been addressed by Fayers and Machin[42] (Chapter 14). In short, a cautious approach is needed to ensure apparently

---

The SF-36™ Health Survey

Instructions for Completing the Questionnaire

Please answer every question. Some questions may look like others, but each
one is different. Please take the time to read and answer each question
carefully by filling in the bubble that best represents your response.

EXAMPLE

This is for your review. Do not answer this question. The questionnaire
begins with the section *Your Health in General* below.

For each question you will be asked to fill in a bubble, in each line.

1.   How strongly do you agree or disagree with each of the following statements?

	Strongly agree	**Agree**	**Uncertain**	**Disagree**	**Strongly disagree**
a) I enjoy listening to music.	○	●	○	○	○
b) I enjoy reading magazines.	●	○	○	○	○

Please begin answering the questions now.

Your Health in General

---

1.   In general, would you say your health is:

Excellent	**Very good**	**Good**	**Fair**	**Poor**
○	○	○	○	○

2.   **Compared to one year ago**, how would you rate your health *now*?

Much better now than one year ago	**Somewhat better now than one year ago**	**About the same as one year ago**	**Somewhat worse now than one year ago**	**Much worse now than one year ago**
○	○	○	○	○

Please turn the page and continue

For permission to use contact: Dr John Ware, Medical Outcomes Trust, 20 Park Plaza
Suite 1014, Boston, MA 02116-4313, USA

Source: Reproduced from Ware and Sherbourne,[41] with permission.

Figure 2.8. 36-Item Short Form Health Survey (SF-36)

'statistically significant' differences are truly those. One way to overcome this problem is for the clinical protocol to rank the domains of QoL to be measured in terms of their relative importance and to confine the formal statistical tests and confidence intervals to these only.

ECONOMIC EVALUATION

Most trials are intended primarily to address questions of efficacy. Safety is frequently an important (though secondary) objective. Health economics is becoming increasingly important and is often now evaluated as part of a randomised controlled trial.

There are four main types of cost analyses that are usually considered:

- *cost minimisation*, simply to determine the best treatment to minimise the total cost of treating the disease;
- *cost effectiveness*, a trade-off between the cost of caring for a patient and the level of efficacy offered by a treatment;
- *cost benefit*, a trade-off between the cost of caring for a patient and the overall benefit (not restricted to efficacy);
- *cost utility*, the trade-off between costs and all measures of 'utility' which may include efficacy, quality of life, greater life expectancy or increased productivity.

One of the big difficulties with pharmacoeconomic evaluations is determining what *indirect costs* should be considered. *Direct costs* are usually easier: costs of medication, costs of those giving the care (doctors, nurses, health visitors) and the basic costs of occupation of a hospital bed. Indirect costs include loss of earnings and productivity, loss of earnings and productivity of spouses or other family members who may care for a sick relative and contribution to hospital/pharmacy overhead costs. Because of the ambiguity associated with these indirect costs, most pharmacoeconomic evaluations performed as part of a clinical trial tend to focus solely on direct costs.

If we were to design a trial primarily to compare costs associated with different treatments we would follow the basic ideas of blinding and randomisation and then record subsequent costs incurred by the patient and the health provider. A very careful protocol would be necessary to define which costs are being considered so that this is measured consistently for all patients. A treatment that is not very effective might, for example, result in the patient needing more frequent consultations. The increased physician, nurse and other paramedical personnel contact time would then be recorded as a cost but it needs to be clear whether patient travel costs, for example (still direct costs, but not to the health service) are included, or not. However, most trials are aimed primarily at assessing efficiency and a limitation of investigating costs in a clinical trial is that the schedule of, and frequency of, visits by the patient to the physician may be very different to what it would be in routine clinical practice. Typically patients are monitored more frequently and more intensely in a trial setting than in routine clinical practice. The costs recorded, therefore, in a clinical trial may well be different (probably greater but possibly less) than in clinical practice. This is sometimes put forward as a major objection to pharmacoeconomic analyses carried out in conjunction with clinical trials. The same limitation does, of course, apply to efficacy evaluations: the overall level of efficacy seen in clinical trials is often not realised in clinical practice. However, if we keep in perspective that, in a clinical trial, it is the *relative* efficacy of one treatment over another (even if one of them is a placebo) then this limitation, whilst still important, can be considered less of an overall objection. The same argument should be applied in pharmacoeconomic evaluations and the relative increase/decrease in costs of one treatment over another can be reported.

Recommendations on trials incorporating health economics assessment have been given by the BMJ Economic Evaluation Working Party.[44] Neymark et al.[45] discuss some of the methodological issues as they relate to cancer trials.

TRIAL SIZE

When designing a new trial, a realistic assessment of the potential benefit (the anticipated effect size) of the proposed test therapy must be made at the onset. The history of clinical trials research suggests that, in certain circumstances, rather ambitious or over-optimistic views of potential benefit have been claimed at the design stage. This has led to trials of inadequate size for the questions posed.

The retrospective review by Machin et al.[46] of the published trials of the UK Medical Research Council in solid tumour cancers is summarised in the funnel plot of Figure 2.9. The benefit observed, as expressed by the hazard ratio (HR) for the new treatment, is plotted against the number of deaths reported in the trial publication. Those trials within the left-hand section of the funnel have relatively few deaths observed and so will be of correspondingly low power. Of

these trials, some have an observed HR that is above the hatched horizontal line. This line has been drawn at a level that is thought to represent a clinically worthwhile advantage to the test treatment. These specific points would have been outside the funnel had they been estimated from more observed deaths. Thus we might conclude from Figure 2.9 that, had these trials been larger, the corresponding treatments may have been observed to bring worthwhile benefit, rather than being dismissed as 'not statistically' significant.

However, it is a common error to assume that the lack of statistical significance following a test of hypothesis implies no difference between groups. Conversely, a statistically significant result does not necessarily imply a clinically significant (important) result. Nevertheless, the message of Figure 2.9 is that potentially useful therapies may be overlooked if the trials are too small.

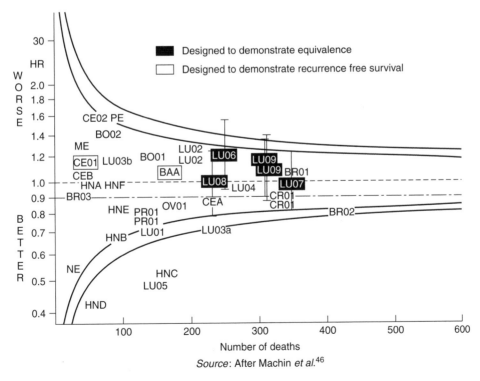

Source: After Machin et al.[46]

Figure 2.9. Retrospective review of UK Medical Research Council trials in solid tumours published prior to 1996

ANTICIPATED (PLANNING) EFFECT SIZE

A major factor in determining the size of a RCT is the anticipated effect size or clinically worthwhile difference. In broad terms if this is not large then it should be of sufficient clinical, scientific or public health importance to warrant the consequentially large trial that will be required to answer the question posed. If the anticipated effect is large, the RCT will be relatively small in which case the investigators may need to question their own 'optimistic' view of the potential benefit. In either case, a realistic view of the possible effect size is important. In practice, it is usually important to calculate sample size for a range of values of the effect size. In this way the sensitivity of the resulting sample sizes to this range of values will provide options for the investigating team.

Estimates of the anticipated effect size may be obtained from the available literature, formal meta-analyses of related trials or may be elicited from clinical opinion. In circumstances where there is little prior information available, Cohen[47] has proposed a standardised effect size, Δ. In the case when the difference between two treatments A and B is expressed by the difference between their means $(\mu_A - \mu_B)$ and σ is the standard deviation (SD) of the endpoint variable which is assumed to be a continuous measure, then $\Delta = (\mu_A - \mu_B)/\sigma$. A value of $\Delta \leq 0.1$ is considered a small standardised effect, $\Delta \approx 0.5$ as moderate and $\Delta \geq 1$ as large (see also Day[3]). Experience has suggested that in many clinical areas these can be taken as a good practical guide for design purposes. However, for large simple trials, the equivalent of effects sizes as small as $\Delta = 0.05$ or less may be clinically important.

SAMPLE SIZE

Once the trial has been concluded, then a formal test of the null hypothesis of no difference between treatments is often made. We emphasise later that it is always important to provide an associated confidence interval for the estimate of treatment difference observed. The test of the null hypothesis has an associated false positive rate

and the alternative hypothesis a false negative rate. The former is variously known also as the Type I error rate, test size or significance level, α. The latter is the Type II error rate β, and $1 - \beta$ is the power. When designing a clinical trial it is often convenient to think in hypothesis-testing terms and so set α and β and a specific effect size Δ for consideration. For determining the size of a trial, α and β are typically taken as small, for example $\alpha = 0.05$ (5%) and $\beta = 0.1$ (10%) or equivalently the power $1 - \beta = 0.9$ (90%) is large.

If the trial is ultimately to compare the means obtained from the two treatment groups, then with randomisation to each treatment in equal numbers, the total sample size, N, is given by

$$N = \frac{4(z_{1-\alpha/2} + z_{1-\beta})^2}{\Delta^2}, \qquad (2.1)$$

where $z_{1-\alpha/2}$ and $z_{1-\beta}$ are obtained from tables of the standardised normal distribution for given α and β.

If we set in equation (2.1) a two-sided $\alpha = 0.05$ and a power of $1 - \beta = 0.9$, then $z_{1-\alpha/2} = z_{0.975} = 1.96$ and $z_{1-\beta} = z_{0.9} = 1.2816$, so that $N = 42.028/\Delta^2 \approx 42/\Delta^2$. For large, moderate and small sizes of Δ of 1, 0.5 and 0.1 the corresponding sample sizes are 42, 168 and 4200, respectively. More realistically these may be rounded to 50, 200 and 4500. For a large simple trial with $\Delta = 0.05$, this implies 16 000 patients may be recruited.

This basic equation has to be modified to adapt to the specific trial design (parallel group, factorial, crossover or sequential), the type of randomisation, the allocation ratio, as well as the particular type of endpoint under consideration. Machin *et al.*[48] provide examples for many different situations.

A good clinical trial design is that which will answer the question posed with the minimum number of subjects possible. An excessively large trial not only incurs higher costs but is also unethical. Too small a trial size leads to inconclusive results, since there is a greater chance of missing the clinically important difference, resulting in a waste of resources. As Pocock[4] states, this too is unethical.

MONITORING TRIAL PROGRESS

DATA MONITORING COMMITTEES

It is clear that a randomised controlled trial is a major undertaking, which clearly involves human subjects in the process. Thus, as we have stated, it is important that some form of equipoise in respect to the treatments under test is required to justify the randomisation. However, once the trial is in progress, information accumulates and as it does so it may be that the initial equipoise becomes disturbed. Indeed the very point of a clinical trial is to upset the equipoise in favour of the best (if indeed one truly is) treatment.

Clearly there will be circumstances when such early information may be sufficient to convincingly answer the question posed by the trial. In which case the trial should close to further patient entry. One circumstance when this will arise is when the actual benefit far exceeds that which the design team envisaged. For example, Lau *et al.*[49] stopped a trial in patients with resectable hepatocellular carcinoma after early results on 43 patients suggested a substantial benefit to adjuvant intra-arterial iodine-131-labelled lipiodol. Their decision was subsequently criticised by Pocock and White,[50] who suggested the result was 'too good to be true' as early stopping may yield biased estimates of the treatment effect. A confirmatory trial is now in progress to substantiate or refute these findings.[51] Essentially, although very promising, in this case the trial results as published provided insufficient evidence for other clinical teams to adopt the test therapy for their patients.

Nevertheless in this, and for the majority of clinical trials, it is clearly important to monitor the accumulating data. It has also been recognised that such monitoring should be reviewed (not by the clinical teams involved in entering patients into the trial themselves) but by an independent DMC. The membership and remit of a DMC will usually depend on the particular trial(s) under review. For example, the European Organization for the Research on the Treatment of Cancer has a standing committee of three clinical and one statistical member, none of whom are involved in any way with the trials under review. This independent DMC reviews reports on trial progress prepared by the data centre teams and makes specific recommendations to the relevant trial coordinating group. Early thoughts on the structure of DMCs for the UK Medical Research Council Cancer Therapy Committee are provided by Parmar and Machin.[52] To emphasise the importance of 'independence', such committees sometimes choose the acronym IDMC.

SAFETY

Although an IDMC will be concerned with the relative efficacy of the treatments under test, issues of safety will also be paramount in many circumstances. In many cases, safety issues may dominate the early stages of a trial when relatively new and untested treatment modalities are first put into wider use, whereas in the later stages detailed review of safety may not be required as no untoward experiences have been observed in the early stages. In contrast, serious safety issues may force a recommendation for early closure of the trial even in situations where early indications of benefit in terms of efficacy are present. Clearly the role of the IDMC or (in view of the 'safety' aspects) the IDMSC is to provide a balanced judgement on these possibly conflicting aspects when making their report. This judgement will derive from the current evidence from the trial itself, external evidence perhaps on new information since the trial was inaugurated, and their own collective experience.

INTERIM ANALYSIS AND EARLY STOPPING RULES

At the planning stage of a clinical trial the design team will be aware of the need to monitor the progress of the trial by reports to an IDMSC. On these occasions the data centre responsible for the conduct of the trial will expect to prepare reports on many aspects of trial progress including especially safety and efficacy. This requirement is often detailed in the trial protocol. The detail may specify those aspects that are likely to be of major concern and also the timing (often expressed in terms of patient numbers or events observed) of such reports.

An interim report may include a formal (statistical) comparison of treatment efficacy. This comparison will then be repeated on the accumulating data for each IDMSC and finally following the close of the trial once the relevant data are to hand. These repeated statistical tests raise the possibility of an increased chance of falsely declaring a difference in efficacy between treatments. To compensate for this, methods of adjusting for the multiple looks at the accumulating data have been devised. Many of these are reviewed by Piantadosi[53] (Chapter 10).

Several of these methods of interim analysis also include 'stopping rules'; that is they incorporate procedures, or boundaries which once crossed by the data under review, imply that the trial should terminate. However, all these methods are predicated on obtaining timely and complete data, very rapid analysis and report writing and immediate review by the IDMSC.[54] They also focus on only one aspect (usually efficacy) and so do not provide a comprehensive view of the whole situation.

The nature of the essential balance required between a formal statistical approach to interim looks at the data and the less structured nature of IDMSC decision-making is provided by Ashby and Machin,[55] Machin[56] and Piantadosi[53] (Chapter 10.8). Parmar *et al.*[57] describe an approach for monitoring large trials using Bayesian methods.

REPORTING CLINICAL TRIALS

The first rule after completing a clinical trial is to report the results – whether they are positive, negative or equivocal. Selective reporting whereby results of positive studies tend to be published and negative studies tend not to be published presents a distorted view of the true situation. This approach to reporting is particularly important for clinical trial overviews and meta-analysis where it is clearly important to be able to include *all* relevant studies (not just the published ones) in the overall synthesis.

The second aspect of reporting is the standard of reporting, particularly the amount of necessary detail given in any trial report. The most basic feature that has repeatedly been emphasised is to give estimates (with confidence intervals) of treatment effects and not just *p*-values. Guidelines for referees (useful also for authors) have been published in several journals including the *British Medical Journal*.[58] The Consolidation of the Standards of Reporting Trials (CONSORT) statement is an international recommendation adopted by many leading medical journals.[59]

One particular feature of the CONSORT statement is that the outcomes of 'all' patients randomised to a clinical trial are to be reported. Thus a full note has to be provided on those, for example, who post-randomisation refuse the allocation and perhaps then insist on the competitor treatment. Two examples of how the patient flow through a trial is summarised are given in Figure 2.10.

It is of some interest to note that the writing team for Lau *et al.*[49] were encouraged by the journal to include information on late (post-interim analysis) randomisations in their report. It is clear that no such stipulation was required of the MRC Renal Cancer Collaborators.[28]

As indicated, the statistical guidelines referred to, and the associated checklists for statistical review of papers for international journals,[60] require confidence intervals (CIs) to be given for the main results. These are intended as an important prerequisite to be supplemented by the *p*-value from the associated hypothesis test. Methods for calculating CIs are provided in many standard statistical packages as well as the specialist software of Altman *et al.*[61]

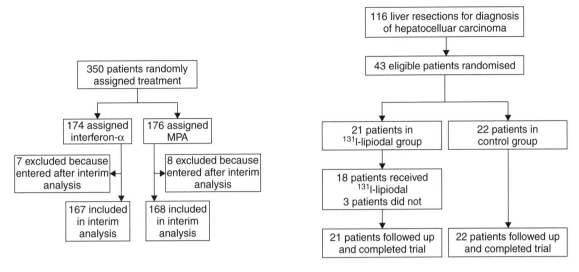

Source: After MRC Renal Cancer Collaborators;[28] Lau et al.[49]

Figure 2.10. Trial profiles following the CONSORT Guidelines

INTENTION-TO-TREAT (ITT)

As we have indicated, once patients have been randomised they should start treatment as specified in the protocol as soon as it is practicably possible. For the severely burnt patients either *MEBO* or *C* dressings can be immediately applied. On the other hand if patients, once randomised, have then to be scheduled for surgery, then there may be considerable delay before therapy is activated. This delay may provide a period in which the patients change their mind about consent or indeed in those with life-threatening illness some may die before the scheduled date of surgery. Thus, the number of patients actually starting the protocol treatment allocated may be less than the number randomised to receive it. The 'intention-to-treat' principle is that once randomised the patient is retained in that group for analysis whatever occurs, even in situations where a patient after consent is randomised to (say) *A* but then refuses and even insists on being treated by option *B*. The effect of such a patient is to dilute the estimate of the true difference between *A* and *B*. However, if such a patient was analysed as if allocated to treatment

B, then the trial is no longer properly randomised and the resulting comparison may be seriously biased.

However, in certain circumstances, the 'intention-to-treat' may be replaced or supplemented by a 'per protocol' summary.[62] For example, if the toxicity and/or side-effects profile of a new agent are to be summarised, any analysis including those patients who were randomised to the drug but then did not receive it (for whatever reason) could seriously underestimate the true levels. If this is indeed appropriate for such endpoints, then the trial protocol should state that such an analysis is intended from the onset.

One procedure that used to be in widespread use was, once the protocol treatment and follow-up were complete, and all the trial-specific information collected on a patient, to review these data in detail. This review would, for example, check that the patient eligibility criteria were satisfied and that there had been no important protocol deviations while on treatment. Any patients following this review, then found to be ineligible or protocol violators would then, in principle, be set aside and excluded from the trial results.

One particular problem is one in which patients are recruited to a trial on the basis of clinical examination during which a biopsy specimen is taken and sent for review. In the meantime the patient is randomised and treatment commenced but once the report is returned the patient is found not to comply with the eligibility criteria. The above review process would automatically exclude this patient, whereas Freedman and Machin[63] argue otherwise.

Usually, this review would not be blind to the treatment received – in fact even if the trial is double blind – there may be clues once the data are examined in this way as to which treatment is which. As a consequence, this process would tend to exclude more patients on the more aggressive treatment. For example, the review conducted by Machin et al.[46] of some early randomised trials in patients with cancer conducted by the UK Medical Research Council showed that the earlier publications systematically reported on fewer patients in the more aggressive treatment arm despite a 1:1 randomisation. The exclusion of a larger proportion of patients receiving the more aggressive therapy would tend to bias the results in its favour. Thus any patients who had 'difficulties' with the treatment, perhaps the more sick patients, were not included in the assessment of its efficacy. This type of exclusion was widespread practice, the consequences of which included the development of ITT policies and standards for reporting clinical trials. The latter policy insisting that the progress of all the randomised patients be reported.

In general, the application of ITT is conservative in the sense that it will tend to dilute between-treatment differences. Piaggio and Pinol[64] have pointed out that for equivalence trials ITT will not be conservative but will tend to favour the equivalence hypothesis.

SUMMARISING THE RESULTS

It is not relevant to review all the analytical techniques that may be utilised in summarising clinical trial data. Many of these are described in the texts we reference at the end of this chapter and many are covered in ICH E9 Expert Working Group.[65] However several aspects are fundamental and these include the statistical significance test, confidence intervals and analysis adjusted for confounding (usually prognostic) variables.

The form of these techniques will depend on the design and especially the type of endpoint variable under consideration. Thus if two means are to be compared then comparisons are made using the Student t-test, for two proportions it is the χ^2 test which might be extended for an ordinal endpoint to the χ^2 test for trend. In a survival time context, the difference between treatments may, under certain conditions, be summarised by use of the hazard ratio (HR) and tested using the logrank test.[66] Finally, whether the endpoint variable is binary, ordered categorical, continuous or a survival time, the corresponding between-treatment comparisons may be adjusted for baseline characteristics of the patients themselves using the appropriate regression techniques. These are made by logistic regression, ordered logistic regression, linear regression and Cox's proportional hazards regression respectively.

Should the design include cluster randomisation, then Bland and Kerry[67] state that the analysis is done by group rather than on an individual subject basis.

TESTS OF HYPOTHESES AND CONFIDENCE INTERVALS

If the data are continuous and can be summarised by the corresponding mean values in each of the two treatment groups A and B, then a simple comparison is made using the difference $d = \overline{x}_A - \overline{x}_B$ and the test of the null hypothesis is made using

$$z = \frac{d}{\text{SE}(d)} \qquad (2.2)$$

Formally, this tests the null hypothesis that the 'true' difference between treatments, δ, is zero. For large trials z will have, under the assumption that the null hypothesis of equal means is true, an approximately standard normal distribution from which the corresponding *p*-value can be obtained.

However, as has been pointed out it is very important to report the observed difference *d* together with an associated confidence interval for the true difference δ. In large samples, the $100(1 - \alpha)\%$ CI is given by

$$d - z_{1-\alpha/2}\mathrm{SE}(d) \quad \text{to} \quad d + z_{1-\alpha/2}\mathrm{SE}(d) \quad (2.3)$$

where $z_{1-\alpha/2}$ is obtained from tables of the normal distribution. For a 95% CI $z_{1-\alpha/2} = z_{0.975} = 1.96$.

Such a CI provides a sense of the precision with which the observed difference between the two treatments is provided by the data. In broad terms, the width of the interval is determined by the number of subjects recruited, the larger the number the narrower the corresponding CI. In general, the 95% CI will exclude the null value (zero in this instance) if the corresponding *p*-value <0.05.

Although *d* provides a simple summary of the between-treatment group differences it is important to verify if this remains unchanged when taking full account of baseline characteristics: sometimes termed confounding variables or covariates. This is often achieved by using regression techniques to adjust the observed difference, *d*, by the values of the baseline variables. In most circumstances, there will be some chance of imbalances in the values of the variables that may arise following randomisation. The adjustment may affect the value of *d* itself as well as the associated standard error, $\mathrm{SE}(d)$, and hence the CI. Such adjustments for important covariates affecting prognosis may result in the estimate *d* being reduced, essentially unchanged or increased – which of these occurs will depend on the trial data itself.

GRAPHS

Graphical presentation of data is invaluable to communicate results in published journal articles or in presentations or posters presented at scientific conferences. There are many types of graphics that can be used but careful thought should be given to the purpose of any graph. Graphs used for exploratory data analysis may include histograms, scatter plots, etc. but these may not be appropriate for the final presentation of data. When presenting the results of clinical trials, the comparative nature of trials should be kept in mind and graphics produced that help in the communication of differences between treatments. In trials using time as an endpoint measure the Kaplan–Meier survival curves provide an elegant summary (Figure 2.11).[66]

NUMBER NEEDED TO TREAT (NNT)

Although many summary measures, for example a difference in response rates or the hazard ratio, are utilised in clinical trials a measure unique to this context is the number needed to treat. This is one very convenient way of assessing the treatment benefit from trials with a binary outcome. From the result of a randomised trial comparing a new treatment with a standard treatment, the NNT is the number of patients who need to be treated with the new treatment rather than the standard (control) treatment in order for one additional patient to benefit. It can be obtained for any trial that has reported a binary outcome.

The NNT is calculated as the reciprocal of the difference between treatments where this is expressed as a difference of two proportions (say) p_T and p_C for test and control treatments under study. Thus $\mathrm{NNT} = 1/(p_T - p_C)$ and a large treatment effect thus leads to a small NNT. A therapy that will lead to one life saved for every 10 patients treated is clearly better than a competing treatment that saves one life for every 50 treated. When there is no treatment effects the risk difference is zero and the NNT is infinite.

A confidence interval for the NNT is obtained by taking reciprocals of the values defining the confidence interval for the treatment difference itself. However, as Altman[7] has pointed out there are some difficulties if the treatment effect that is not statistically significant and the confidence

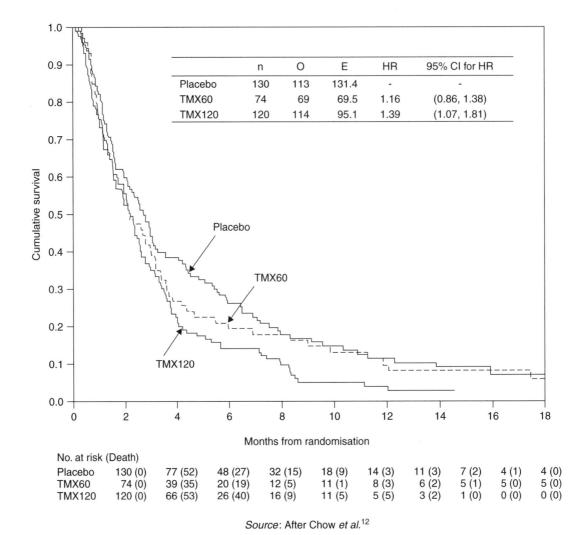

	n	O	E	HR	95% CI for HR
Placebo	130	113	131.4	-	-
TMX60	74	69	69.5	1.16	(0.86, 1.38)
TMX120	120	114	95.1	1.39	(1.07, 1.81)

No. at risk (Death)

Placebo	130 (0)	77 (52)	48 (27)	32 (15)	18 (9)	14 (3)	11 (3)	7 (2)	4 (1)	4 (0)
TMX60	74 (0)	39 (35)	20 (19)	12 (5)	11 (1)	8 (3)	6 (2)	5 (1)	5 (0)	5 (0)
TMX120	120 (0)	66 (53)	26 (40)	16 (9)	11 (5)	5 (5)	3 (2)	1 (0)	0 (0)	0 (0)

Source: After Chow *et al.*[12]

Figure 2.11. Kaplan–Meier estimates of survival in patients with inoperable hepatocellular carcinoma by double-blind treatment group

interval includes the null value of 0 (see also the comments by Hutton[68]). The NNT can also be obtained for survival analysis. For these studies the NNT is not a single number, but varies according to time since the start of treatment.

MULTIPLE COMPARISONS

In a clinical trial in which two groups are being compared, the formal statistical test of this comparison has an associated two-sided test size α. This is set as the boundary below which the p-value, calculated from the data for the primary endpoint of the trial, must fall to be declared statistically significant. In this case the null hypothesis of no difference between groups is then rejected.

When this approach is utilised in the analysis of a clinical trial comparing two groups and there is truly no difference between the two groups, despite this 'no difference' there is a $100\alpha\%$ probability of a statistically significant result and the false rejection of the null hypothesis.

If more than one endpoint is measured for the two-group study in question then the situation becomes more complex. For example, if a clinical trial is comparing two treatments (A and B) but there are three different independent outcomes being measured, then there are three comparisons to make between A and B and, in theory at least, three statistical tests. In this circumstance it can be shown that the false positive rate is no longer $100\alpha\%$ but approximately $300\alpha\%$. In fact for k (assumed independent) outcome measures the false positive rate is approximately $100k\alpha\%$. Clearly, the false positive rate increases as the number of comparisons made increases.

In order to retain the false positive rate as $100\alpha\%$ the Bonferroni correction is often suggested. This implies only declaring differences as statistically significant at the $100\alpha\%$ level if the observed p-value $< \alpha/k$. In the case of $\alpha = 0.05$ and $k = 3$, this implies p-value < 0.017. Equivalently, and preferably, multiply the observed p-value by k and declare this significant if less than α.[69]

Similar considerations apply equally to CIs. One approach that has been used to overcome this difficulty is to quote 99% CIs rather than 95% CIs whenever more than a single outcome is regarded as primary. Thus the UK Prospective Diabetes Study Group[70] report 21 distinct endpoints, ranging from fatal myocardial infarction to death from unknown cause, and provide the 99% confidence intervals for the corresponding 21 relative risks comparing tight with less tight control of blood pressure. This is a 'half-way house' proposal, since 0.01 ($= 1 - 0.99$) lies between taking no account of the multiplicity and retaining 0.05 to define significance and the Bonferroni corrected value of $0.05/21 = 0.0024$.

Similar considerations of multiplicity may also apply in situations other than trials with multiple endpoints. For example, Green[22] highlights this problem with respect to trials of a factorial design.

The problem of multiple comparisons is particularly acute in QoL assessments in clinical trials. Thus guidelines by Staquet *et al.*[71] on reporting such trials explicitly state: '. . . in the case of multiple comparisons, attention must be paid to the total number of comparisons, to the adjustment, if any, of the significance level, and to the interpretation of the results'. Perneger[72] concludes that: 'Simply describing what tests of significance have been performed, and why, is generally the best way of dealing with multiple comparisons'. In contrast the *American Journal of Public Health* recommend the use of a method of adjustment due to Holm.[73] From a clinical trials perspective these issues are reviewed by Proschan and Waclawiw.[74]

SUBGROUP ANALYSIS

In designing a RCT, sample size is usually determined by considering a clinically worthwhile effect which will be estimated from the trial data by a comparison of all patients randomised to one group as compared to the other. It is recognised that the precision with which this effect size is estimated may be improved by a stratified analysis adjusted for baseline prognostic variables which are known to influence outcome irrespective of the treatment received. However, if treatments are compared within these strata (thereby ignoring information on patients not in that stratum) it is clear that the patient numbers must be less than the RCT as a whole. Thus any such comparisons will usually lack sufficient statistical power and hence may be unreliable.

A common mistake is to observe a p-value in excess of 0.05 (and hence judged naively as not significant) but then to report subgroup analyses – perhaps repeating the treatment comparison within each disease stage group. In some circumstances, one of these subgroup comparisons may be 'significant' (p-value < 0.05) which will almost certainly imply that those within the other groups will not since the 'all-data-combined' analysis is not significant. In extreme cases, subgroup analysis can appear to favour one treatment in one subgroup and the other in the other subgroup(s). This may then lead to a false conclusion that the new treatment works for one group but not for the other. If a subgroup analysis is planned for at the design stage, adjustment for this should be built into the sample size considerations.

BASELINE COMPARISONS

Although the standard of reporting of randomised controlled trials has improved in many medical journals, there remain many who have not yet adopted the full rigours of the CONSORT Guidelines. There are also many situations in which inappropriate and substandard analyses are conducted. Particular examples include statistical significance tests of pre-randomisation (baseline) variables, often describing demographic and patient eligibility criteria in the different treatment groups, despite the allocation to groups having been made by randomisation so that any observed differences are by definition random.[75]

OTHER MISUSED APPROACHES TO ANALYSIS

Anderson[76] catalogues some commonly misused approaches used in the analysis of clinical trials. These include in, for example, cancer clinical trials with dual endpoints of tumour response and overall survival, the analysis of survival by tumour response itself. In these cases survival is compared between those patients who respond and those who do not. Such analysis may lead to a false conclusion that response 'caused' longer survival. Anderson states categorically that such comparisons are wrong unless an appropriate methodology such as one involving a landmark is used. Similar considerations apply if comparisons are made between groups established on the basis of the amount of (protocol defined) treatment received, dose intensity or toxicity. Anderson et al.[77] provide details of the landmark approach.

A common mistake is for investigators to provide treatment-specific CIs in their reports for the endpoint(s) of concern, rather than for a relevant measure of treatment comparison such as their difference or a hazard ratio.

COMPETING RISKS

In some situations, a patient may fail following apparently successful treatment from one of C (≥ 2) so-called competing risk types, for example, a local recurrence or a distant metastasis, which are competing causes of ultimate mortality in cancer patients. If relapse is the outcome of interest in the clinical trial, then usually it is the first event that is of primary importance to the clinician. Thus, in a randomised trial of adjuvant therapy in resected Dukes' C colorectal carcinoma, 17-1A monoclonal therapy was thought to be most effective against individually dispersed cells and less effective against local satellite tumour nodules or cell aggregates.[78] Since the 17-1A antibody should be most effective in preventing or delaying distant metastases after surgery, distant metastasis as a first event was thus a key endpoint in this trial.

In the analysis of competing patterns of failure, the Kaplan–Meier method and the associated logrank test are frequently used to estimate the comparative rates of, for example, local recurrence and distant metastasis in patients receiving alternative treatments for their cancer in two distinct calculations. In one, local recurrence as the first event is taken as the event of interest. In this situation, patients who do not have a local recurrence, or who have local recurrence as a second or subsequent event, irrespective of whether or not they have distant metastasis, are treated as censored observations in the calculations. In the other calculations, distant metastasis as the first event is taken as the event of interest.

A preferred method, described in detail by Tai et al.,[79] is to use the cause-specific cumulative incidence functions and comparisons between groups via the test developed by Gray.[80] Gelman et al.[81] have pointed out that the Kaplan–Meier method produces estimates that are appreciably higher than those of the competing risks method. Substantial differences have also been noted in data from patients with Ewing's sarcoma.[79] However a counter viewpoint on the use of the two approaches is given by Farley et al.,[82] using illustrations from clinical trials in contraceptive development.

SOFTWARE FOR STATISTICAL ANALYSIS

There are many statistical packages available for the summary and analysis of clinical trials and additional features are continually being added. Pertinent features that distinguish the packages are the flexibility and quality of graphical output and the presentation of statistical tables or results.

Over the last decades, there have been many statistical developments that have impacted on, for example, the endpoints that can be assessed, the design, size, analysis and summary. These include the Kaplan–Meier method for summarising survival time studies, the logrank test and most influential of all the associated Cox proportional hazards model which allows between-treatment comparisons adjusted for potentially confounding prognostic variables assessed at baseline. The Cox model can also accommodate time-dependent variables, that is variables that are assessed post-randomisation. These developments would have remained theoretical in nature but for parallel developments in statistical software.

CLINICAL DATA MANAGEMENT

GOOD QUALITY DATA

Although it is rather outside the scope of this text, a vital component to the eventual success of any clinical trial protocol is the quality of the associated clinical record forms (CRFs). Good CRFs will be pleasant to the eye, logical in layout, comprehensive yet focused on the key information required, easy to complete and easy to process.

A key feature of any scientific study is the implication that the data generated are of high quality. That is, that the observations made are carefully recorded at the point and time of observation, and then passed through to the analysis stage without change. All this is equally true for clinical trials of whatever design.

However, the problems associated with ensuring this process is indeed in place in, for example, a large multinational trial involving prolonged follow-up of subjects are considerable. Indeed a whole new industry of Clinical Research Organisations (CROs) has developed to guarantee this process. Further, the Regulatory Agencies rightly demand a guarantee of high quality data in any submission made to them for product registration.

Information from randomised controlled trials provides key information when the pharmaceutical and allied industries apply to register a new drug or device with the relevant regulatory authorities. The authorities themselves impose certain constraints on the way in which trials are conducted – these will include basics with respect to a justification of a sample size for the trial but will also specify standards.[65] These too have impacted on the ways that trials are designed, conducted, analysed and reported.

PRINCIPLES OF QUALITY DATA MANAGEMENT

In clinical trials, subjects are usually entered one at a time, and their responses to treatment monitored sequentially. Regular monitoring of trial progress, especially during the early stages, is advisable, and prompt attention to data errors, inconsistencies or missing items on the CRFs is required, so that corrections can be made immediately. If inadequate control is exercised in the management of clinical trials data, subsequent analysis may be delayed or at worst wrong.

The use of computers for data processing and statistical analysis requires careful planning and execution by experienced personnel. Errors are liable to happen in the recording of data in the CRFs, as well as in the transfer of data to the computer using a database management software.

In a typical trial the sequence of data collection might be registration and randomisation, a record of the patient's name or code, trial number, date of birth, date of randomisation and allocated treatment (if the trial is not blind) will be entered into the database. The on-study form, which contains other demographic and baseline clinical information would be completed and added to the database in due course. Patients are then anticipated to return for follow-up assessments often over an extended period of time. Since patients do not all enter the trial at the same time, the amount of data collected at any one time may vary considerably as the trial progresses, and the management of the data on a computer becomes increasingly complex and requires skilful intervention.

For repeated follow-up evaluations, a separate record is normally kept for each evaluation. For example, in a double-blind randomised placebo controlled trial on inoperable hepatocellular carcinoma,[12] information on ECOG performance status, Okuda staging, serum albumin and bilirubin is collected. In addition, QoL is evaluated not only on entry into the trial, but also at monthly intervals. Since patients may drop out of a trial at any time for a variety of reasons this further complicates the management of the database.

Quality data management via computers entails careful planning and execution by well-trained data managers. As the processes of data transcription and entry into computers are highly susceptible to producing errors, a series of checks for validity and completeness should be carried out immediately upon the return of CRFs. Items that are commonly verified include range checks for clinical parameters such as serum levels. These may be excessively high or extremely low (due to out-of-range or wrong units recorded), or in the case of qualitative variables, a non-permitted code.

Logical checks identify any inconsistency in information that may be captured in different parts of CRFs. For instance, dates of randomisation, follow-ups and death carry important information in clinical trials where survival is the endpoint. Thus it is important to check that these dates as well as other crucial ones have been recorded and entered correctly.

Routine checks on missing items or forms should also be undertaken, as any missing information could be due to oversight in data

transcription, electronic data entry or delay in returns of CRFs, rather than the information not having been collected. Queries should be raised for any discrepancies identified by these checks. The data should be edited accordingly after clarification with the investigator or comparison with source documents.

Although information in the CRF should be checked manually and discrepancies resolved by the data manager prior to data entry, on-line editing checks via computer provides an additional means of detecting errors or missing data. The validation rules would normally be specified and the associated data checks programmed in parallel with the building of the database.

SOFTWARE FOR CLINICAL DATA MANAGEMENT

Several specialised software tools for managing clinical trial data are commercially available. An early one written for the UK Medical Research Council was COMputer PAckage for Clinical Trails (COMPACT)[83] and this included many of the features necessary for handling ragged data sets which arise in clinical trails involving prolonged follow-up. However, current requirements of GCP demand, for example, more intensive audit trail facilities that were not part of the early systems. The newer systems, unlike standard spreadsheets, incorporate all the basic features of a good clinical data management system.

An ideal clinical data management process is one that delivers valid and accurate data which aid the maintaining of data integrity through facilities for verifying and validating data, as well as through the implementation of an audit trail to document database modifications. They also allow for automatic reporting of discrepancies, customised reports can be created and distributed to external sources such as the investigators for resolution and have the ability to efficiently handle repeated follow-up evaluations and track status of patients throughout the trial.

These systems also provide global libraries to store the definitions of standard code lists, and standard validation or derivation criteria, to optimise information input and access throughout the operation. Standard codes can easily be computed by defining appropriate derivation rules in the global libraries. These codes and rules can be tailored to meet the varying requirements of individual trials and can be re-used in subsequent databases.

In multi-centre trials involving diverse and distant locations, it is possible with these clinical data management systems to automatically propagate the study definitions, including amendments, to all study sites. At each site, the local data can then be independently managed using the same validation rules, derivation criteria and code lists. This is implemented by means of remote data entry.

With multiple sites and many users accessing the same network, possibly performing different tasks, for example database design, entry and resolution by data managers, data retrieval, query and analysis by statisticians, the security of the system is of primary concern. Thus a clinical trial system should allow network-wide security standards to be enforced by enabling system administrators to assign, monitor and control access to sensitive clinical data records.

For the purpose of statistical analyses, there should also be fast, flexible and easy extraction of data into a variety of user-defined file formats, such as those of the more commonly used statistical packages.

Ideally, a good clinical data management system should have facilities for randomising treatments, and registering all information captured at this stage directly into the database.

McFadden[84,85] provides further details on many aspects of clinical data management and associated areas.

SELECTED FURTHER READING ON CLINICAL TRIALS

GENERAL

Day S. *Dictionary for Clinical Trials*. Chichester: John Wiley & Sons (1999).

Redmond C, Colton T, eds. *Biostatistics in Clinical Trials*. Chichester: John Wiley & Sons (2000).

Senn SJ. *Statistical Issues in Drug Development*. Chichester: John Wiley & Sons (1997).

Williams CJ, ed. *Introducing New Treatments for Cancer: Practical, Ethical and Legal Problems*. Chichester: John Wiley & Sons (1992).

DESIGN AND CONDUCT OF CLINICAL TRIALS

Buyse ME, Staquet MJ, Sylvester RJ. *Cancer Clinical Trials: Methods and Practice*. Oxford: Oxford University Press (1984).

Crowley J, ed. *Handbook of Statistics in Clinical Oncology*. New York: Marcel Dekker (2000).

Jadad A. *Randomised Controlled Trials: A User's Guide*. London: British Medical Journal Books (1998).

Jennison C, Turnbull BW. *Group Sequential Methods with Applications to Clinical Trials*. Boca Raton: Chapman & Hall/CRC (2000).

Matthews JNS. *Introduction to Randomised Controlled Clinical Trials*. London: Arnold (2000).

McFadden ET. *Management of Data in Clinical Trials*. New York: John Wiley & Sons (1997).

Piantadosi S. *Clinical Trials: A Methodologic Perspective*. New York: John Wiley & Sons (1997).

Pocock SJ. *Clinical Trials: A Practical Approach*. Chichester: John Wiley & Sons (1983).

Senn SJ. *Cross-over Trials in Clinical Research*. 2nd edn. Chichester: John Wiley & Sons (2002).

Whitehead J. *Design and Analysis of Sequential Clinical Trials*, Revised 2nd edn. Chichester: John Wiley & Sons (1997).

Wooding WM. *Planning Pharmaceutical Clinical Trials*. New York: John Wiley & Sons (1994).

QUALITY OF LIFE

Fairclough DL. *Design and Analysis of Quality of Life Studies in Clinical Trials*. Andover: CRC Press (2002).

Fayers PM, Machin D. *Quality of Life: Assessment, Analysis and Interpretation*. Chichester: John Wiley & Sons (2000).

Staquet MJ, Hays R, Fayers PM. *Quality of Life Clinical Trials: Methods and Practice*. Oxford: Oxford Medical Publications (1998).

SAMPLE SIZE

Machin D, Campbell MJ, Fayers PM, Pinol APY. *Sample Size Tables for Clinical Studies*. Oxford: Blackwell Science (1997).

EVIDENCE-BASED MEDICINE

Altman DG, Chalmers I, eds. *Systematic Reviews*. London: British Medical Journal Books (1995).

Sutton AJ, Abrams KR, Jones DR, Sheldon TA, Song F. *Methods of Meta-Analysis in Medical Research*. Chichester: John Wiley & Sons (2000).

REFERENCES

1. World Medical Association. World Medical Association Declaration of Helsinki, 1996. Republished in *JAMA* (1997) **277**: 925–6.
2. Chalmers I, Sackett D, Silagy C. Cochrane collaboration. In: Redmond C, Colton T, eds, *Biostatistics in Clinical Trials*. Chichester: John Wiley & Sons (2000) 65–7.
3. Day S. *Dictionary for Clinical Trials*. Chichester: John Wiley & Sons (1999).
4. Pocock SJ. *Clinical Trials: A Practical Approach*. Chichester: John Wiley & Sons (1983).
5. Temple R. Current definitions of phases of investigation and the role of the FDA in the conduct of clinical trials. *Am Heart J* (2000) **139**: S133–5.
6. Gehan EA, Freireich EJ. Non-randomized controls in cancer clinical trials. *New Engl J Med* (1974) **290**: 198–203.
7. Altman DG. Statistics in medical journals: some recent trends. *Stat Med* (2000) **19**: 3275–89.
8. Ang ES-W, Lee S-T, Gan CS-G, See PG-J, Chan Y-H, Ng L-H, Machin D. Evaluating the role of alternative therapy in burn wound management: randomized trial comparing Moist Exposed Burn Ointment with conventional methods in the management of patients with second-degree burns. *Medscape Gen Med* (2001) **3**(2): 3.
9. Freedman B. Equipoise and the ethics of clinical research. *New Engl J Med* (1987) **317**: 141–5.
10. Weijer C, Shapiro SH, Glass KC. Clinical equipoise and not the uncertainty principle is the moral underpinning of the randomised controlled trial. *Br Med J* (2000) **321**: 756–8.
11. Enkin MW. Clinical equipoise and not the uncertainty principle is the moral underpinning of the randomised controlled trial. *Br Med J* (2000) **321**: 756–8.
12. Chow PK-H, Tai B-C, Tan C-K, Machin D, Johnson PJ, Khin M-W, Soo K-C. No role for high-dose tamoxifen in the treatment of inoperable hepatocellular carcinoma: an Asia–Pacific double-blind randomised controlled trial. *Hepatology* (2002) **36**: 1221–6.
13. RISC Group. Risk of myocardial infarction and death during treatment with low dose aspirin and intravenous heparin in men with unstable coronary artery disease. *Lancet* (1990) **336**: 827–30.
14. The ATAC (Arimidex, Tamoxifen Alone or in Combination) Trialists' Group. Anastrozole alone or in combination with tamoxifen versus tamoxifen alone for adjuvant treatment of postmenopausal women with early breast cancer: first results of the ATAC randomised trial. *Lancet* (2002) **359**: 2131–9.
15. Piya-Anant M, Koetsawang S, Patrasupapong N, Dinchuen P, d'Arcangues C, Piaggio G, Pinol A. Effectiveness of cyclofem® in the treatment of depo medroxyprogesterone acetate induced amenorrhea. *Contraception* (1998) **57**: 23–8.
16. Donner A, Piaggio G, Villar J, Pinol A, Al-Mazrou Y, Ba'aqeel H, Bakketeig L, Belizán JM, Berendes H, Carroli G, Farnot U, Lumbiganon P. Methodological considerations in the design of the WHO antenatal care randomised controlled trial. *Paediat Perinatal Epidemiol* (1998) **12**(Suppl. 2): 59–74.
17. Zelen M. A new design for randomized clinical trials. *New Engl J Med* (1979) **300**: 1242–5.
18. Wooding WM. *Planning Pharmaceutical Clinical Trials*. New York: John Wiley & Sons (1994).
19. Chan DC, Watts GF, Mori TA, Barrett PH, Beilin LJ, Redgrave TG. Factorial study of the effects of atorvastatin and fish oil on dyslipidaemia in visceral obesity. *Eur J Clin Invest* (2002) **32**: 429–36.
20. Day L, Fildes B, Gordon I, Fitzharris M, Flamer H, Lord S. Randomised factorial trial of falls prevention among older people living in their own homes. *Br Med J* (2002) **325**: 128–31.
21. Piantadosi S. Factorial designs. In: Redmond C, Colton T, eds, *Biostatistics in Clinical Trials*. Chichester: John Wiley & Sons (2000) 193–200.
22. Green S. Factorial designs with time-to-event end points. In: Crowley J, ed, *Handbook of Statistics in Clinical Oncology*. New York: Marcel Dekker (2000) Chapter 9, 161–71.
23. Hong B, Ji YH, Hong JH, Nam KY, Ahn Ty. A double-blind crossover study evaluating the efficacy of Korean red gingseng in patients with erectile dysfunction: a preliminary report. *J Urol* (2002) **168**: 2070–3.
24. Senn SJ. *Cross-over Trials in Clinical Research*. 2nd edn. Chichester: John Wiley & Sons (2002).
25. Simon R. Therapeutic equivalence trials. In: Crowley J, ed, *Handbook of Statistics in Clinical Oncology*. New York: Marcel Dekker (2000) Chapter 10, 173–87.
26. Donaldson AN, Whitehead J, Stephens R, Machin D. A simulated sequential analysis based on data from two MRC trials. *Br J Cancer* (1993) **68**: 1171–8.

27. Fayers PM, Cook PA, Machin D, Donaldson AN, Whitehead J, Ritchie A, Oliver RTD, Yuen P. On the development of the Medical Research Council trial of α-interferon in metastatic renal carcinoma. *Stat Med* (1994) **13**: 2249–60.

28. Medical Research Council Renal Cancer Collaborators. Interferon-α and survival in metastatic renal carcinoma: early results of a randomised controlled trial. *Lancet* (1999) **353**: 14–17.

29. MPS Research Unit. *PEST 4: Operating Manual*. Reading: University of Reading (1993).

30. Whitehead J. Use of the triangular test in sequential clinical trials. In: Crowley J, ed, *Handbook of Statistics in Clinical Oncology*. New York: Marcel Dekker (2000) Chapter 12, 211–28.

31. Whitehead J. *Design and Analysis of Sequential Clinical Trials*, revised 2nd edn. Chichester: John Wiley & Sons (1997).

32. Jennison C, Turnbull BW. *Group Sequential Methods with Applications to Clinical Trials*. Boca Raton: Chapman & Hall/CRC (2000).

33. Zelen M. Randomised consent trials. *Lancet* (1992) **340**: 375.

34. Altman DG, Whitehead J, Parmar MKB, Stenning SP, Fayers PM, Machin D. Randomised consent designs in cancer clinical trials. *Eur J Cancer* (1995) **31A**: 1934–44.

35. Machin D, Lee ST. The ethics of randomised trials in the context of cleft palate research. *Plastic Reconstruct Surg* (2000) **105**: 1566–8.

36. Spiegelhaleter DJ, Freedman LS, Parmar MKB. Bayesian approaches to randomized trials. *J R Statist Soc* (1994) **A 157**: 357–416.

37. Tan S-B, Machin D, Tai B-C, Foo K-F, Tan E-H. A Bayesian reassessment of two Phase II trials of gemcitabine in metastatic nasopharyngeal cancer. *Br J Cancer* (2002) **86**: 843–50.

38. Matthews JNS, Altman DG, Campbell MJ, Royston JP. Analysis of serial measurements in medical research. *Br Med J* (1990) **300**: 230–5.

39. StataCorp. *STATA Statistical Software: Release 7.0*. Stata Corporation, College Station, TX (2001).

40. Brown JE, King MT, Butow PN, Dunn SM, Coates AS. Patterns over time in quality of life, coping and psychological adjustment in late stage melanoma patients: an application of multilevel models. *Qual Life Res* (2000) **9**: 75–85.

41. Ware JE, Sherbourne CD. The MOS 36-Item Short Form Health Survey (SF-36) I: conceptual framework and item selection. *Med Care* (1991) **30**: 473–83.

42. Fayers PM, Machin D. *Quality of Life: Assessment, Analysis and Interpretation*. Chichester: John Wiley & Sons (2000).

43. Fairclough DL. *Design and Analysis of Quality of Life Studies in Clinical Trials*. Andover: CRC Press (2002).

44. BMJ Economic Evaluation Working Party. Guidelines for authors and peer reviewers of economic submissions to the BMJ. *Br Med J* (1996) **313**: 275–83.

45. Neymark N, Kiebert W, Torfs K, Davies L, Fayers P, Hillner B, Gelber R, Guyatt G, Kind P, Machin D, Nord E, Osoba D, Revicki D, Schulman K, Simpson K. Methodological and statistical issues of quality of life (QoL) and economic evaluation in cancer clinical trials: report of a workshop. *Eur J Cancer* (1998) **34**: 1317–33.

46. Machin D, Stenning SP, Parmar MKB, Fayers PM, Girling DJ, Stephens RJ, Stewart LA, Whaley JB. Thirty years of Medical Research Council randomized trials in solid tumours. *Clin Oncol* (1997) **9**: 20–8.

47. Cohen J. *Statistical Power Analysis for the Behavioral Sciences*, 2nd edn. New Jersey: Lawrence Earlbaum (1988).

48. Machin D, Campbell MJ, Fayers PM, Pinol APY. *Sample Size Tables for Clinical Studies*. Oxford: Blackwell Science (1997).

49. Lau WY, Leung TWT, Ho SKW, Chan M, Machin D, Lau J, Chan ATC, Yeo W, Mok TSK, Yu SCH, Leung NWY, Johnson PJ. Adjuvant intra-arterial iodine-131-labelled lipiodol for resectable hepatocellular carcinoma: a prospective randomised trial. *Lancet* (1999) **353**: 797–801.

50. Pocock SJ, White I. Trials stopped early: too good to be true? *Lancet* (1999) **353**: 797–801.

51. Tan SB, Machin D, Cheung YB, Chung YFA, Tai BC. Following a trial that stopped early: what next for adjuvant intra-arterial iodine-131-labelled lipiodol in resectable hepatocellular carcinoma? *J Clin Oncol* (2002) **20**: 1709.

52. Parmar MKB, Machin D. Monitoring clinical trials: experience of, and proposals under consideration by, the Cancer Therapy Committee of the British Medical Research Council. *Stat Med* (1993) **12**: 497–504.

53. Piantadosi S. *Clinical Trials: A Methodologic Perspective*. New York: John Wiley & Sons (1997).

54. Machin D. Discussion of 'The what, why and how of Bayesian clinical trials monitoring'. *Stat Med* (1994) **13**: 1385–9.

55. Ashby D, Machin D. Stopping rules, interim analysis and data monitoring committees. *Br J Cancer* (1993) **68**: 1047–50.

56. Machin D. Interim analysis and ethical issues in the conduct of trials. In: Williams CJ, ed, *Introducing New Treatments for Cancer: Practical, Ethical and Legal Problems*. Chichester: John Wiley & Sons (1992) Chapter 15.

57. Parmar MKB, Griffiths GO, Spiegelhalter DJ, Souhami RL, Altman DG, van der Scheuren E. Monitoring of large randomised clinical trials: a new approach with Bayesian methods. *Lancet* (2001) **358**: 375–81.

58. Altman DG, Gore SM, Gardner MJ, Pocock SJ. Statistical guidelines for contributors to medical journals. In: Altman DG, Machin D, Bryant TN, Gardner MJ, eds, *Statistics with Confidence*, 2nd edn. London: British Medical Journal Books (2000) 171–90.

59. Begg C, Cho M, Eastwood S, Horton R, Moher D, Olkin I, Pitkin R, Rennie D, Schultz KF, Simel D, Stroup DF. Improving the quality of reporting randomized controlled trials: the CONSORT statement. *J Am Med Assoc* (1996) **276**: 637–9.

60. Gardner MJ, Machin D, Campbell MJ, Altman DG. Statistical checklists. In: Altman DG, Machin D, Bryant TN, Gardner MJ, eds, *Statistics with Confidence*, 2nd ed. London: British Medical Journal Books (2000) 101–10.

61. Altman DG, Machin D, Bryant TN, Gardner MJ. *Statistics with Confidence*, 2nd edn. London: British Medical Journal Books (2000).

62. Lewis JA, Machin D. Intention to treat: who should use ITT. *Br J Cancer* (1993) **68**: 647–50.

63. Freedman LS, Machin D. Pathology review in cancer research. *Br J Cancer* (1993) **68**: 1047–50.

64. Piaggio G, Pinol APY. Use of the equivalence approach in reproductive health. *Stat Med* (2001) **20**: 3571–87.

65. ICH E9 Expert Working Group. Statistical principles for clinical trials: ICH harmonised Tripartite Guideline. *Stat Med* (1999) **18**: 1905–42.

66. Parmar MKB, Machin D. *Survival Analysis: A Practical Approach*. Chichester: John Wiley & Sons (1995).

67. Bland JM, Kerry SM. Statistics notes: trials randomised in clusters. *Br Med J* (1997) **315**: 600.

68. Hutton JL. Number needed to treat: properties and problems. *J Roy Stat Soc A* (2000) **163**: 381–402.

69. Altman DG. *Practical Statistics for Medical Research*. London: Chapman & Hall (1991).

70. UK Prospective Diabetes Study Group. Tight blood pressure control and risk of macrovascular and microvascular complications in type 2 diabetes: UKPDS 38. *Br Med J* (1998) **317**: 703–12.

71. Staquet MJ, Berzon RA, Osoba D, Machin D. Guidelines for reporting results of quality of life assessments in clinical trials. In: Staquet MJ, Hays RD, Fayers PM, eds, *Quality of Life Assessment in Clinical Trials: Methods and Practice*. Oxford: Oxford University Press (1998) 337–47.

72. Perneger TV. What's wrong with Bonferroni adjustments. *Br Med J* (1998) **316**: 1236–8.

73. Holm . A simple sequentially rejective multiple test procedure. *Scand J Public Health* (1979) **6**: 65–70.

74. Proschan MA, Waclawiw MA. Practical guidelines for multiplicity adjustment in clinical trials. *Contr Clin Trials*, (2000) **21**: 527–39.

75. Altman DG, Doré CJ. Randomisation and baseline comparisons in clinical trials. *Lancet* (1990) **335**: 149–53.

76. Anderson JR. Commonly misused approaches in the analysis of cancer clinical trials. In: Crowley J, ed, *Handbook of Statistics in Clinical Oncology*. New York: Marcel Dekker (2000) Chapter 24.

77. Anderson JR, Cain KC, Gelber RD. Analysis of survival by tumor response. *J Clin Oncol* (1983) **1**: 710–19.

78. Pugh RNH, Murray-Lyon IM, Dawson JL, Pietroni MC, William R. Transection of the oesophagus for bleeding oesophageal varices. *Br J Surg* (1973) **8**: 646–9.

79. Tai B-C, Machin D, White I, Gebski V. Competing risks analysis of patients with osteosarcoma: a comparison of four different approaches. *Stat Med* (2001) **20**: 661–84.

80. Gray R. A class of k-sample tests for comparing the cumulative incidence of competing risk. *Ann Stat* (1988) **16**: 1141–54.

81. Gelman R, Gelber R, Henderson IC, Coleman CN and Harris JR. Improved methodology for analyzing local and distant recurrence. *J Clin Oncol* (1990) **8**: 548–55.

82. Farley TMM, Ali MM, Slaymaker E. Competing approaches to analysis of failure times with competing risks. *Stat Med* (2001) **20**: 3601–10.

83. Chilvers CED, Fayers PM, Freedman LS, Greenwood RM, Machin D, Palmer N, Westlake AJ. Improving the quality of data in randomized clinical trials: the COMPACT computer package. *Stat Med* (1988) **7**: 1165–70.

84. McFadden ET. *Management of Data in Clinical Trials*. New York: John Wiley & Sons (1997).

85. McFadden ET. Data management and coordination. In: Redmond C, Colton CT, eds, *Biostatistics in Clinical Trials*, Chichester: John Wiley & Sons (2000) 158–67.

86. Jones B, Jarvis P, Lewis JA, Ebbutt AF. Trials to assess equivalence: the importance of rigorous methods. *Br Med J* (1996) **313**: 36–9.

3

Clinical Trials in Paediatrics

JOHAN P.E. KARLBERG

Clinical Trials Centre and Department of Paediatrics,
The University of Hong Kong, Hong Kong SAR

WHY SHOULD WE DO CLINICAL TRIALS IN CHILDREN?

Children are subject to many of the same diseases as adults, and are often treated with the same drugs and biological products. However, many drugs on the market used to treat children are inadequately labelled for use with paediatric patients; and many carry disclaimers stating that safety and effectiveness in paediatric patients have not been established. Information about the safety and effectiveness of treatments for some paediatric age groups is particularly difficult to find. Even today, no treatment is available for many of the thousands of rare and serious diseases that largely affect neonates, infants and children. Most drugs used to treat common diseases in both children and adults have not been investigated in children at all. Over 50% of all drugs prescribed in paediatric practice are either 'unlicensed' or 'off label'.

The paediatric medical community has for decades tried to persuade regulatory authorities and the pharmaceutical industry to test new drugs in the paediatric population in parallel with the adult studies. The motto of the campaign has been

'Children are not simply Small Adults' and its *Guidelines for the Ethical Conduct of Studies to Evaluate*, published in 1995, reported that:

- In 1973, 78% of medications included a disclaimer or lack of dose information for children.
- In 1991, 81% of listed drugs were restricted for certain age groups.
- In 1992, 79% of 19 new molecular entities approved were not labelled for use in children.

As a result of effectively being denied access to well-studied drugs, paediatricians either don't treat children with potentially beneficial medications, or treat them with medications based either on adult studies or anecdotal empirical experience in children. Such non-validated administration of medications may place more children at risk than if the drugs were administered as part of well-designed, controlled clinical trials. There is therefore a moral imperative to formally study drugs in children, so they can enjoy equal access to existing as well as new therapeutic agents.

The US National Institute of Health (NIH) published regulations in 1999 clearly defining what human studies could be funded by NIH

Textbook of Clinical Trials. Edited by D. Machin, S. Day and S. Green
© 2004 John Wiley & Sons, Ltd   ISBN: 0-471-98787-5

to the exclusion of paediatric subjects. The exclusionary circumstances were:

- Research topic irrelevant to children;
- Laws or regulations barring inclusion of children;
- The knowledge is available for children or will be obtained from another ongoing study;
- The relative rarity of the condition in children;
- The number of children is limited;
- Insufficient data are available in adults to judge potential risk in children.

Not until recently have children been more regularly included in clinical studies to investigate drugs. Considerable differences between the pharmacokinetics and pharmacodynamics of drugs in children and in adults frequently make it impossible to bridge conclusions from data obtained in adults. Children cannot even be considered a homogeneous group, since age groups differ in their absorption, distribution, metabolisation and excretion of drugs and their effect on developing organ systems. The anatomical structure of children's organs differ from adults, causing different pharmacodynamic characteristics observed during childhood.

The lack of paediatric safety information in product labelling exposes paediatric patients to the risk of age-specific adverse reactions unexpected from adult experience. The absence of paediatric testing and labelling may also expose paediatric patients to ineffective treatment through under-dosing, or may deny paediatric patients therapeutic advances. Failure to develop a paediatric formulation of a drug or biological product, where younger paediatric populations cannot take the adult formulation, may also deny paediatric patients access to important new therapies.

Three conclusions can therefore be drawn about paediatric drug studies: studies must be made in different age groups; describing the pharmacokinetics and pharmacodynamics is crucial; and the safety of drugs must be studied to identify potential severe side effects.

REGULATORY ISSUES OF CLINICAL TRIALS IN CHILDREN?

Regulatory authorities in the US and Europe have in recent years taken important steps to address the problem of inadequate paediatric testing and inadequate paediatric use information in drug and biological product labelling. But these efforts have, thus far, not substantially increased the number of products entering the marketplace with adequate paediatric labelling. The regulatory authorities have therefore concluded that additional steps are necessary to ensure the safety and effectiveness of drug and biological products for paediatric patients. Manufacturers of new and marketed drugs and biological products must now evaluate the safety and effectiveness of the products in paediatric patients if the product is likely to be used in a substantial number of children, or provide a more meaningful therapeutic benefit to paediatric patients than existing treatments.

Since 2000 in both the US and Europe, pharmaceutical companies have been obliged to include paediatric data in all new drug applications and licence extensions provided that substantial use of the drug in children and a meaningful therapeutic benefit is expected. The strength of this legislation is however different in the two regions–and so is the extension of market exclusivity.

In recent years an independent 'Orphan' drug regulation has been in force in the countries of the European Community as well as in the US. This creates incentives for the development of drugs for rare serious diseases, but is unlikely to achieve effective improvement in paediatric drug therapy. The Food and Drug Administration (FDA) Modernization Act established economic incentives for pharmaceutical manufacturers to conduct paediatric studies on drugs for which patent protection or exclusivity is available under the Drug Price Competition and Patent Term Restoration Act or the Orphan Drug Act. These provisions attach six additional months of marketing exclusivity to any existing exclusivity or patent protection of a drug for which FDA has requested paediatric studies.

However, there is likely to be a consensus during the coming years–at least in the ICH GCP regions–over requirements for conducting clinical trials on new drugs and other therapies in children. But before this consensus can be reached, a number of points have to be addressed and discussed, underlined by the following two examples.

EXAMPLE 1–ONGOING DISCUSSIONS OF THE CONSENT PROCESS IN PAEDIATRIC TRIALS

The significant increase in the number of children participating in clinical trials continues to raise ethical and procedural concerns. The FDA addressed this issue in April 2001, calling on institutional review boards to review study protocols that include children and ensure they adopt safeguards to protect young research participants. A group in the US is currently examining the 'best practices' related to research involving children. The study will address:

- Process for obtaining informed consent and assent from children and their parents or legal representatives.
- How well participants in paediatric studies and their guardians understand direct benefits and risks of study involvement?
- Definition of "minimal risk" related to healthy and ill child study participants.
- Whether regulations and policies should vary for children of different ages (for example, teenagers and infants)?
- Appropriateness of payments to children, parents, or legal representatives for participation in research.
- Role of IRBs in monitoring compliance with regulations related to paediatric studies.

EXAMPLE 2–ONGOING DISCUSSIONS OF THE LEGISLATION OF PAEDIATRIC TRIALS

Based on feedback from a consultation document, the European Commission was expecting to prepare draft legislation on paediatric medicinal development by Autumn 2002. This legislation is considered by many to be pressing, creating the conditions needed to improve medicines for children. Nearly all involved parties in Europe supported a legal and regulatory framework for improving child health, especially regarding the labelling of medicines. The consultation document concluded:

- A robust ethical framework for European paediatric research needs to be created, including guidance for informed consent, ethical review, recruitment of subjects, and safety and oversight.
- A robust paediatric clinical study infrastructure needs to be created in Europe, since as a result of reluctance to perform such studies up to now, there is a serious shortage of trained and experienced people and centres of excellence.
- Greater cooperation should be stimulated between public sector research and private sector research in paediatrics, in the interest of developing a European dimension to improving medicines for children.
- A clear framework should be developed for assembling international data and information regarding paediatric trials and medicines–to ensure that unnecessary trials are not carried out in Europe, and that European paediatricians have the benefit of up-to-date and comprehensive information regarding medicinal products for their patients, wherever in the world that information has been generated.
- A greater public dialogue is required in Europe regarding the benefits and risks of paediatric research for individual children participating in research, as well as for public health in general.

ICH GUIDELINE ON PAEDIATRIC STUDIES

The International Conference on Harmonisation (ICH) Guideline E11–Clinical Investigation of Medicinal Products in the Pediatric Population–became operational in January 2001 in the United States, Europe and Japan. The E11 guideline outlines critical issues in paediatric drug development. In summary, this new and important ICH document states that paediatric patients should be given medicines that have been appropriately evaluated for their use. It says safe and effective therapy in paediatric patients requires the timely development of information on the proper use of medicinal products in paediatric patients of various ages and, often, paediatric formulations of those products. The goal of this guideline is to encourage and facilitate timely paediatric medicinal product development internationally. This guideline addresses five issues, namely considerations when initiating a paediatric programme, the timing of its initiation, type of studies, age categories and ethics.

WHEN INITIATING A PAEDIATRIC PROGRAMME? (SUMMARY POINTS OF ICH GCP E11)

The decision to proceed with a paediatric development programme for a certain medicinal product requires consideration of factors such as:

- Prevalence of the condition in the paediatric population;
- Seriousness of the condition;
- Availability and suitability of alternative treatments;
- Unique paediatric indications;
- Unique paediatric-specific endpoints;
- Age ranges of paediatric patients likely to be treated;
- Unique paediatric safety concerns;
- Unique paediatric formulation development.

The most common considerations when discussing the need and timing of a paediatric programme are:

- Most important is the presence of a serious or life-threatening disease for which the medicinal product represents a potentially important advance in therapy. This situation suggests relatively urgent and early initiation of paediatric studies.

- For medicinal products for diseases predominantly or exclusively affecting paediatric patients, the entire development programme will be conducted in the paediatric population, except for initial safety and tolerability data, which will usually be obtained in adults.
- For medicinal products intended to treat serious or life-threatening diseases occurring in both adults and paediatric patients, for which there are currently no (or limited) therapeutic options, there is need for relatively urgent and early initiation of paediatric studies.
- For medicinal products intended to treat other diseases and conditions there is less urgency. Trials would usually begin at later phases of clinical development or, if a safety concern exists, even after a substantial post-marketing period in adults. Testing of these medicinal products in the paediatric population would usually not begin until Phase II or III–since very early initiation of testing in paediatric patients might needlessly expose them to a compound of no benefit.

TYPES OF STUDIES (SUMMARY POINTS OF ICH GCP E11)

Selection of the type of study should be on the same principles as studies planned for adults. However, several considerations are of specific importance for paediatric studies. Some of the most important are:

- When a medicinal product is to be used in the paediatric population for the same indication(s) as those studied and approved in adults, the disease process is similar in adults and paediatric patients, and the outcome is likely to be comparable, extrapolation from adult efficacy can be appropriate. In such cases, pharmacokinetic (PK) studies in all the age ranges of paediatric patients likely to receive the medicinal product, together with safety studies, may provide adequate information.
- When a medicinal product is to be used in younger paediatric patients for the same indication(s) as those studied in older paediatric

patients, the disease process is similar, and the outcome is likely to be comparable, extrapolation of efficacy from older to younger paediatric patients may be possible. In such cases, pharmacokinetic studies in the relevant age groups of paediatric patients together with safety studies may be sufficient.

- Many diseases in preterm and term newborn infants are unique or have unique manifestations precluding extrapolation of efficacy from older paediatric patients and call for novel methods of outcome assessment.
- Where the disease course/outcome of therapy in paediatric patients is expected to be similar to adults, but the appropriate blood levels are not clear, it may be possible to use measurements of a pharmacodynamic (PD) effect related to clinical effectiveness. Thus, a PK/PD approach combined with safety and other relevant studies could avoid the need for clinical efficacy studies.
- When unique indications are being sought for the medicinal product in paediatric patients, or when the disease course and outcome of therapy are likely to be different in adults and paediatric patients, clinical efficacy studies in the paediatric population are needed.

Pharmacokinetics

Pharmacokinetic studies generally should be performed to support formulation development and determine pharmacokinetic parameters in different age groups. Pharmacokinetic studies in the paediatric population are generally conducted in patients with the disease. Single-dose or steady-state studies are the choice of pharmacokinetic study:

- For medicinal products that exhibit linear pharmacokinetics in adults, single-dose pharmacokinetic studies in the paediatric population may be sufficient.
- When there is a nonlinearity in absorption, distribution and elimination in adults and difference in duration of effect between single and repeated dosing in adults suggests steady-state studies in the paediatric population.

Special considerations should be taken when blood is drawn more than once in paediatric subjects, such as in PK/PD studies. Several approaches can be used to minimise the amount of blood drawn and/or the number of venipunctures:

- Use of sensitive assays;
- Use of laboratories experienced in handling small volumes;
- Using routine clinical blood samples for pharmacokinetic analysis;
- Use of indwelling catheters;
- Use of population pharmacokinetics and sparse sampling.

Efficacy

The principles in study design, statistical considerations and choice of control groups are detailed in other ICH guidelines and apply to paediatric efficacy studies. But there are also certain features unique to paediatric studies.

- Extrapolation of efficacy from studies in adults to paediatric patients, or from older to younger paediatric patients, as mentioned above.
- For efficacy studies it may be important to employ different endpoints for specific age groups.
- Measurement of subjective symptoms requires different assessment instruments for patients of different ages.
- The response to a medicinal product may vary among patients because of the developmental stage of the patient.

Safety

ICH guidelines (E2 and E6) describe adverse event reporting and apply to paediatric studies. But there are certain safety aspects unique to paediatric studies.

- Medicinal products may affect physical and cognitive growth and development, and the adverse event profile may differ in paediatric patients, compared with adults.

- The dynamic processes of growth and development may not manifest an adverse event at once, but at a later stage of growth and maturation.
- Long-term studies or surveillance data may be needed to determine possible effects on skeletal, behavioural, cognitive, sexual and immune maturation and development.
- Post-marketing surveillance may provide important safety and/or efficacy information for the paediatric population.
- Age-appropriate, normal laboratory values and clinical measurements should be used in adverse event reporting.

AGE CLASSIFICATION OF PAEDIATRIC PATIENTS (SUMMARY POINTS OF ICH GCP E11)

Decisions on how to stratify studies and data by age need to take into consideration developmental biology and pharmacology. The identification of which ages to study should be medicinal product-specific and justified.

- *Preterm newborn infants:* Preterm newborn infants have a unique pathophysiology and responses to therapy. The complexity of and ethical considerations involved in studying preterm newborn infants requires a careful protocol development with expert input from neonatologists and neonatal pharmacologists. Only rarely can we extrapolate efficacy from studies in adults or in older paediatric patients to the preterm newborn infant.
- *Term newborn infants (0 to 27 days):* Newborn infants are more mature than preterm newborn infants, but many of the physiologic and pharmacologic principles for preterm infants also apply to them.
- *Infants and toddlers (28 days to 23 months):* This is a period of rapid CNS maturation, immune system development and total body growth. By 1–2 years of age, clearance of many drugs on a mg/kg basis may exceed adult values and then it may be dependent on specific pathways of clearance.

- *Children (2 to 11 years):* Most pathways of drug clearance are exceeding adult values. Changes in clearance of a drug may be dependent on maturation of specific metabolic pathways. The protocols should ascertain assessment of the effect of the medicinal product on growth and development. Recruitment of patients should ensure adequate representation across the age range in this category. Puberty can affect the activity of enzymes that metabolise drugs, and dose requirements for some medicinal products may decrease dramatically.
- *Adolescents (12 to 16–18 years (dependent on region)):* This is a period of sexual maturation and medicinal products may interfere with the actions of sex hormones. Medicinal products and illnesses that delay or accelerate the onset of puberty can have a profound effect and may affect final height. Many diseases are also influenced by the hormonal changes around puberty and hormonal changes may thus influence the results of clinical studies. Noncompliance is a special problem and compliance checks are important.

ETHICAL ISSUES IN PAEDIATRIC STUDIES (SUMMARY POINTS OF ICH GCP E11)

The paediatric population represents a vulnerable subgroup. Therefore, the following special measures are needed to protect the rights of paediatric study participants.

- Participants in clinical studies are expected to benefit from the clinical study, except under special circumstances.
- When protocols involving the paediatric population are reviewed, there should be IRB/IEC members or experts consulted by the IRB/IEC who are knowledgeable in paediatric ethical, clinical and psychosocial issues.
- Paediatric study participants are dependent on their parent(s)/legal guardian to assume responsibility for their participation in clinical studies. Participants of appropriate intellectual maturity should personally sign and date either

a separately designed, written assent form or the written informed consent.

- Information that can be obtained in a less vulnerable, consenting population should not be obtained in a more vulnerable population or one in which the patients are unable to provide individual consent.
- Studies in handicapped or institutionalised paediatric populations should be limited to diseases or conditions found principally in these populations, or when it is expected that the disease may alter the effects of a medicinal product.
- To minimise risk in paediatric clinical studies, those conducting the study should be trained and experienced in studying the paediatric population, including the evaluation and management of potential paediatric adverse events.
- In designing studies, every attempt should be made to minimise the number of participants and of procedures, consistent with good study design.
- To ensure that experiences of the study subjects are positive and to minimise discomfort and distress.

ETHICAL CONSIDERATIONS IN PAEDIATRIC STUDIES

Of all the problems surrounding research in children, the one that poses perhaps the most complex question is research ethics. Children are not legally able to provide consent and the extent to which children are able to understand the meaning, risks and potential benefits of participating in clinical trials varies enormously according to age and background. For this reason it may be appropriate to address some points related to the IRB review, including the informed consent process, in paediatric trials more specifically than outlined in the ICH GCP E11 guideline. One document that addresses this topic at more depth is the Review and Award Codes for the NIH Inclusion of Children Policy from 1999. The following partly originates from this document, but also incorporates sources listed at the end of this chapter.

First studies that promise no demonstrable benefits to the child participating in the study or to children in general should not be conducted, irrespective of the minimal nature of the attendant risks. The risks include discomfort, inconvenience, pain, fright, separation from parents or surroundings, effects on growth and development of organs, and size or volume of biological samples.

The proposed research must be of value to children in general and, in most instances, to the individual child subject:

- The research design must take into consideration the unique physiology, psychology and pharmacology of children and their special needs and requirements as research subjects.
- The design should minimise risk while maximising benefits.
- The study design must take into account the racial, ethnic, gender and socioeconomic characteristics of the children and their parents.
- A placebo/observational control group may be acceptable when there is no commonly accepted therapy, or the commonly used therapy is of questionable efficacy, or the commonly used therapy has high frequency of side effects, i.e. larger than the benefits.

PAEDIATRIC INFORMED CONSENT

Children are not legally able to provide consent and the extent to which children are able to understand the meaning, risks and potential benefits of participating in clinical trials varies enormously according to age and background. Children are counted as members of a vulnerable population at risk for exploitation and are given special protection in clinical research. In paediatric trials, just as in adult trials, materials in an understandable language, opportunities to discuss the trial, and freedom to withdraw without penalty must be provided to potential subjects.

Investigators are ultimately held responsible for ensuring adequate informed consent. More than two decades of inquiry into the process of consent have shown that adults are less than adequately informed about risks, benefits and participation in research. The process is even more problematic for research involving individuals with limited abilities in decision-making. The evolving psychological and emotional development of children and adolescents presents challenges to paediatric investigators not encountered when dealing with adult subjects. Unless opposing evidence is identified, capacity to understand and provide informed consent has long been assumed in adults. Results from studies in healthy and sick children suggest that also children have this capacity. Several investigators have evaluated the degree to which minors from school age through adolescence are capable of providing assent. Even very young children demonstrate inquisitiveness about the proposed research. By the age of nine, children can understand purpose, risk and the right to withdraw from the study. Even seven-year-old children can understand the purpose of a study. Such observations support the requirement by most ethics boards that assent be obtained in children aged seven and older. However, information regarding scientific versus therapeutic study objectives for both research and alternative treatment is not well understood in seven to 20-year-old subjects. Paediatric subjects can thus provide an informed agreement to participate, but the assent process should be conducted using discussions that encourage questions.

Obtaining Informed Permission–Assent–to Participate

Regulations permit studies involving minimal risk in children, with the provision that permission from parents and assent from subjects are obtained. Research involving greater than minimal risk, but providing potential direct benefit to the child, is also permitted with the same provision. There are some exceptions to the requirement for assent and consent. Assent is not necessary for research expected to directly benefit the child. Assent must be an active affirmation from any child with an intellectual age of seven years or older. Assent should be obtained from children who are competent to

understand; and the purpose, risks and benefits of a study should be explained to them. The following guideline has therefore been proposed:

No greater than minimal risk

- Assent of the child and permission of at least one parent.

Greater than minimal risk and prospect of direct benefit

- Assent of the child and permission of at least one parent.
- Anticipated benefit justifies the risk.
- Anticipated benefit is as least as favourable as alternative approaches.

Greater than minimal risk and no prospect of direct benefit

- Assent of the child and permission of both parents.
- Likely to yield generalisable knowledge about the child's disorder.

SPECIFIC PROBLEMS OF PAEDIATRIC STUDIES

SUBJECT RECRUITMENT

Insufficient enrollment of children is the most common reason for discontinuing paediatric studies. Creating and expanding networks for paediatric pharmacology studies, such as in the US and Europe, are steps in the right direction to recruit enough subjects. Many reasons for this poor recruitment rate for paediatric studies include:

- Strict inclusion and exclusion criteria;
- Limited size of the paediatric population;
- That each age group has to be considered separately;
- Inconvenience for the parents in having their children participate in a clinical study;
- Fear of making one's own child available as a 'guinea pig for research'.

- Doctors are wary of jeopardising the doctor–patient relationship, or losing the trust of parents.

EARLY TESTING

There are no healthy paediatric volunteers. The lack of volunteers for Phase I studies is a special problem and makes the planning of therapeutic studies in children difficult. The requirements for paediatric study designs are for this and other reasons different from studies in adults. Alternative study designs and alternative statistical methods are required.

STUDY MANAGEMENT

To obtain a sufficient number of subjects requires a large number of study centres. Moreover, the cost for each individual step of a paediatric study is usually higher than for studies in adults–both to pharmaceutical companies, as sponsors of the studies, and to the participating doctors. For instance, explaining the nature of a study–to obtain permission from parents and ensure their cooperation during the course of the study–is a very time-consuming process. Explanatory material and information has to be prepared not only for parents, but also adapted for the children. Caring for the children during their visits to the study centre also requires creativity, patience and time.

FINAL COMMENTS

Faced with heavy workloads, paediatricians may often be reluctant to assume what looks like the extra work of clinical trials. But a shortage of investigators is not the only problem that slows paediatric trials. It takes many subjects to satisfy the requirements for an adult drug to be adequately studied in children–and frequently the population of paediatrics with a certain disease does not exist. So not only do studies need to be designed to use small populations efficiently; they also need to be designed with children in mind.

Just taking adult protocols, then changing the age in the inclusion criteria and the dose, is not good enough. With a limited number of investigators and a limited number of potential subjects, study design is critical for successful development of new safe and life-saving therapeutic entities for paediatric usage.

FURTHER READING

PUBLICATIONS

- Shirkey H. Therapeutic orphans (editorial comment). *J Pediatr* (1968) **72**: 119–20.
- Rogers LC, Cocchetto DM. Labeling prescription drugs for pediatric use in the United States. *Appl Clin Trials* (1997) 50–6.
- Tarnowski KJ, Allen DM, Mayhall C, Kelly PA. Readability of pediatric biomedical research informed consent forms. *Pediatr* (1990) **85**: 58–62.
- Susman EJ, Dorn LD, Fletcher JF. Participation in biomedical research: the consent process as viewed by children, adolescents, young adults, and physicians. *J Pediatr* (1992) **121**: 547–52.
- Ethical Conduct of Studies to Evaluate Drugs in Pediatric Populations. Committee on Drug. *Pediatrics* (1995) **95**: 286–94.
- Wechsler J. Science, pediatric studies, and surrogates. *Appl Clin Trials* (1999) 28–33.
- Nahata MC. Lack of pediatric drug formulations. *Pediatrics* (1999) **104**: 607–9.
- Conroy S, McIntyre J, Choonara I. Unlicensed and off label drug use in neonates. *Arch Dis Childh: Fetal Neonatal Edit* (1999) **80**: F142–5.
- Conroy S, McIntyre J, Choonara I, Stephenson T. Drug trials in children: problems and the way forward. *Br J Clin Pharmacol* (2000) **49**: 93–7.
- Kauffman RE. Clinical trials in children: problems and pitfalls. *Paediatr Drugs* (2000) **2**: 411–18.
- Simar MR. Pediatric drug development; the International Conference of Harmonization Focus on Clinical Investigation in Children. *Drug Inform J* (2000) **34**: 809–19.

OFFICIAL DOCUMENTS/GUIDELINES

- Review and award codes for the NIH inclusion of children policy March 26, 1999.
- Regulation (EC) No. 141/2000 of the European Parliament and the Council of 16 December 1999 on orphan medicinal products.
- World Medical Association, Declaration of Helsinki (amended October 2000).

- Food and Drug Administration, Department of Health and Human Services, The Pediatric Exclusivity Provision January 2001 Status Report to Congress.
- Food and Drug Administration, Additional Safeguards of Children in Clinical Investigations of FDA-Regulated Products: Interim Rule, Federal Register 66 (79) 20589 (24 April 2001).
- Food and Drug Administration, Update of list of approved drugs for which additional paediatric information may produce health benefits in the paediatric population (May 20, 2001), Docket No. 98N0056ICH Topic Ell, 'Clinical Investigation of Medicinal Products in the Pediatric Population'. CPMP/ICH/2711/99, January 2001, adopted July 2000.
- European Commission, Better Medicines for Children: Proposed regulatory actions on paediatric medicinal products (European Commission, Brussels, Belgium, 2002).

4

Clinical Trials Involving Older People

CAROL JAGGER AND ANTONY J. ARTHUR

Department of Epidemiology and Public Health, University of Leicester, Leicester, UK

As few diseases or conditions present for the first time in later life, there are few treatments prescribed solely to older people. There is also little consensus on the definition of 'the elderly' since ageing can be considered a continuous process from birth to death. However the increasing likelihood of illness other than that under treatment and greater mental and physical frailty with ageing means that older people can be inherently different to younger adults and the numerous physiological changes that accompany the ageing process may alter the way in which older people respond to drugs.[1]

By 2010 in most of the developed countries, the 65+ age group will form over 15% of the total population and over 20% in Japan. In the UK, those aged 65 years and over make up 18% of the population but they receive nearly half of all prescriptions.[2] Despite this, few trials, unless specially designed and conducted in this age group, have sufficient numbers of older people, particularly the 'oldest-old', to provide evidence of efficacy, even for treatments of diseases and conditions that are seen predominantly in later life. A recent review of clinical trials in Parkinson's disease, where prevalence increases with age and incidence peaks between 70 and 80 years of age, found only 38% of studies included subjects over 75 years of age.[3]

Trials of the efficacy of interventions should cover the age groups who are affected.[4] Older people have been explicitly excluded through the use of a maximum age for eligibility and obviously such trials provide little information about the efficacy of treatments in older age groups. However implicit exclusion is also common, through criteria such as the presence of co-morbid conditions. In addition certain recruitment methods may result in study populations with older people an under-representation of the general population likely to be treated. In these cases it may be difficult for the clinician to be aware of the paucity of older people studied, resulting in the late recognition of serious side effects when drugs tested on predominantly younger adult populations are finally released and prescribed to larger numbers of older people. Perhaps the most famous, or infamous, case of this was benoxaprofen, a non-steroidal anti-inflammatory drug marketed as Opren, which was withdrawn after a report of the death of five elderly patients who had taken the drug.[5]

In this chapter we will explore, in more depth, the reasons why older people face a

Textbook of Clinical Trials. Edited by D. Machin, S. Day and S. Green
© 2004 John Wiley & Sons, Ltd ISBN: 0-471-98787-5

number of barriers at each stage of a trial: eligibility, recruitment, gaining informed consent and follow-up. In addition we will discuss strategies for increasing the number of older people in clinical trials, so that in future, those responsible for the treatment of older people will be able to base their practice on high-quality evidence.

ELIGIBILITY

Despite recommendations to the contrary, older people are still being excluded from clinical research on the basis of age alone, shown by an analysis of studies reported in four leading journals (*BMJ, Gut*, the *Lancet* and *Thorax*) which found 35% (170) excluded older people with no justifiable reason.[6] Reviews of trials in acute myocardial infarction[7] and Parkinson's disease,[3] conditions where prevalence and incidence are strongly related to advancing age, found that trials published later were more likely to exclude older subjects. Moreover, since more women than men survive to older age and in some cases, such as cardiovascular disease, women develop diseases later in life than men, exclusion on the basis of age disproportionately disadvantages women.[8]

Operating an upper age limit for trials has often been used to limit the problem of co-morbid conditions and drug interactions that may occur with increasing age, in the belief that most adverse drug reactions in older people are simply a consequence of advancing age. A review of pertinent studies suggests that this may be misguided since the physiological and functional characteristics of the patient, rather than chronological age *per se*, appear to be the most important in drug interactions.[9]

Even when age limits are not imposed, older patients are often implicitly excluded because of other exclusion criteria or because of investigator, cultural or other biases in enrollment.[8] In the review of acute myocardial infarction trials, comparison of the age distributions of patients in trials with and without age exclusions showed no differences, suggesting that factors other than explicit age restrictions were at play.[7]

The process of patient selection and recruitment mostly aims to produce an homogeneous study population with the purpose of increasing the statistical power to detect the effects of drugs.[10] The resulting clinical trial, conducted in 'sterile' conditions, bears little resemblance to practice and cannot be extrapolated to the general population. Indeed, although tight eligibility criteria may aim to produce very similar participants, inter-patient variability is such that a truly homogeneous group of patients is difficult, if not impossible, to identify. Important prognostic variables will be measured at baseline, but even if study participants are the same on these criteria, they will still vary in the course of their disease and on unmeasured prognostic factors.[11] Thus the gain in attempting to study a group of homogeneous patients is outweighed by the loss in generalisability and clinical applicability of the results. Even when treatment trials are specifically designed for older people, overly stringent exclusion criteria can produce highly skewed and non-representative patient populations. Many trials of treatments for Alzheimer's disease have excluded patients with behavioural problems despite such problems being common with increasing cognitive impairment. Since there is considerable scope for improving such symptoms with drugs that enhance cognition, these trials may well be missing opportunities.[12]

Studying a narrow group of patients also misses the potential to identify subgroups of patients who may respond particularly well to the drug under test. A trial comparing the efficacy of sertraline and nortriptyline in major depression included patients aged 60 years and over, but a subgroup analysis of the 76 patients aged 70 years and over suggested that treatment with sertraline may confer even greater benefit in this older age group than patients aged 60 years and over.[13] In trials of intervention packages or services rather than drugs, similar tensions exist between maximising the detection of a significant effect of the intervention in a population unencumbered with concurrent illness, and a need to assess effectiveness as close as possible to delivery in practice after the trial. The advantages of wide eligibility criteria for entering patients into clinical trials are summarised in Box 4.1.[11]

Box 4.1 Advantages of wide eligibility criteria for entering patients into clinical trials

1. Easier screening and recruitment. Large trials are more feasible and economical.
2. Large study sizes reduce random error, providing more reliable overall results.
3. Wider applicability of results. Therefore greater clinical and public health impact.
4. Greater opportunity to test subgroup hypotheses.

Source: Reproduced from Yusuf *et al.*[11]

RECRUITMENT

The recruitment, in sufficient numbers and within the desired time frame, of motivated and compliant subjects, representative of the wider group ultimately receiving treatment, is the goal of all who design and execute clinical trials. Recruiting motivated participants is a problem for all clinical trials but particular difficulties are evident when recruiting older patients. Clinical trials are likely to involve more regular monitoring and follow-up assessments than would routinely take place in practice and this in itself may be too burdensome for older people who may have other health problems, which they may perceive as more important, or lack access to transport. A longer enrollment phase, although deterring some older subjects, may allow a more complete collection of data and more accurate prediction of patient compliance, again highlighting the tension between pragmatic and explanatory trials.[14] If possible, assessments should be offered at home or, where this is impossible, transportation to clinics provided at times convenient to the subject.

Although the experience of earlier trials on strategies to maximise recruitment may not be immediately transferable across time and place, they may provide researchers with ideas. Experiences in recruiting older people to trials have been described in the treatment of hypertension with both pharmacological[15] and non-pharmacological interventions[16] and in trials of exercise.[17] Many of the reports simply describe the experience of one or two particular strategies, though mass mailing, media advertising, community-based screening, clinical practice screening, participant referrals and other recruitment methods have been compared in a trial of the efficacy of weight loss and sodium reduction for preventing hypertension in the elderly.[16] This study concluded that mass mailing of a brochure or letter describing the study resulted in the greatest yield in terms of percent randomised (76%; $N = 737$) though it is less clear whether this applied to all subgroups of the population. Trials recruiting volunteers, although producing a population who may be more likely to remain throughout the length of the study, provide little evidence of applicability to the general elderly population. Older volunteers tend to be more likely than younger ones to be healthy and living independently, of particular importance for trials of interventions involving exercise since volunteers may not be the subjects most likely to benefit.[17]

Rarely does one single strategy succeed in recruiting adequate numbers of representative patients. It is important therefore that the characteristics of participants are regularly monitored throughout the trial, and compared to the general population, so that, if necessary, specific demographic groups, such as the oldest-old or particular ethnic groups may be targeted. Such mixed-mode recruitment has produced representative samples of high-risk older people for a trial of geriatric evaluation and management.[18] The final sample should aim to be as representative as possible and a list of strategies that could be used if shortfalls occur during recruitment should be developed at the design stage of the trial.

GAINING INFORMED CONSENT

Obtaining informed consent from patients before randomisation is a universal requirement, although legal requirements across countries may differ. As with eligibility and recruitment, the means of gaining informed consent from subjects enrolling should be addressed at the design stage of the trial and the information that the patient requires to give informed consent is listed in Box 4.2. A synopsis of the practicalities in obtaining informed consent for clinical trials has been reported, stressing that gaining informed consent 'should not be seen as an exercise in bureaucratic form filling, but as an essential part of the trial requiring time, insight and communication skills'.[19]

Box 4.2 Patient information necessary for informed consent

1. Diagnosis.
2. Available treatments and treatment on trial.
3. Potential risks and benefits of treatment.
4. Concept of a clinical trial (including randomisation, use of placebos, double-blind procedures).
5. Discomforts or inconveniences associated with assessments.
6. Number of follow-up visits or extra travel for trial.

Clinicians may see relaying the concept of a randomised controlled trial as admittance of ignorance about the best treatment for the patient, or may make ageist assumptions concerning the ability of older people to consent to a trial. Furthermore, the clinical trial design is complex and even if explained carefully, patients may not understand fully enough to give true informed consent. A qualitative study, as part of a set of trials of the effectiveness of treatments for men with urinary retention and benign prostatic disease, found that, although information given was accurately

recalled, subjects found the concept of randomisation difficult to accept and were confused by terms such as 'trial' and 'random' which have different meanings to lay and professional groups.[20]

Studies examining significant predictors of enrollment into trials are equivocal in their findings. A systematic review of literature on informed consent found evidence of impaired understanding of the informed consent information in older subjects and those with less formal education,[21] whilst the Recruitment and Enrollment Assessment in Clinical Trials study, part of the Cardiac Arrythmia Suppression Trial (CAST), did not find education differences in enrollers and non-enrollers, although enrollers were more likely to have read the informed consent themselves and to have understood it.[22] The ability to understand information about clinical trials, particularly the randomisation process, may well be correlated with level of education.[23] An instrument to assess understanding of information given to ascertain informed consent for ambulatory trials has been developed, but its disadvantages are that it is study-specific and it was tested on relatively young and well-educated subjects.[24]

Family members have also been found to play an important role in the informed consent process, approval by family members, particularly spouses, being associated with successful enrollment in a cardiovascular trial.[25] This study also found that the majority (96%) of those approached by a physician agreed to enrol, compared to 66% of those approached by an experienced cardiovascular nurse. Reasons given by a subsample of those enrolled by the physician were predominantly the trust and respect subjects had for their doctor, though a small number admitted to agreeing through fear.

Much healthcare provision is imperialistic and this may re-enforce the belief, held by some older people, that all decisions relating to their treatment rest with their doctor. It should be remembered that not all older people however want active treatment in all cases and there may be reluctance to take medication for certain conditions. A recent trial of selective serotonin reuptake inhibitors in the treatment of depression and anxiety in community-dwelling older people found that, whilst 11 of 67 people with clinically diagnosed depression and/or a phobic anxiety disorder fulfilled one or more of the exclusion criteria, 89% of the remaining subjects eligible refused medication,[26] inferring that the process by which older people make decisions to participate in clinical trials is a complex one, meriting further research.

The nature of the trial may well be another important factor in the decision by older people to enrol. Trials including invasive procedures such as venepuncture, which may be necessary to determine compliance may not be seen as necessary to the subject and may therefore be more likely to lead to refusal.[27] Our experience of non-randomised studies of the health of older people suggests that, on the whole, older people will participate in lengthy interviews and are keen to assist with research that they perceive will help others,[28] confirming findings from cardiovascular trials.[25] When the study involves an assessment at an outpatients' clinic or an invasive procedure such as providing a blood sample, refusal rates can increase noticeably, making it necessary for trial personnel to explain clearly not only the need for randomisation but also the importance of subsequent assessments to monitor health. This should, of course, be balanced by any inconvenience the patient might incur by extra visits.

After World War II, the Nuremberg code required the 'voluntary consent of the human subject' in experimental research and that 'the person should have legal capacity to give consent'. Ethicists argue that to make a properly informed choice to enter a clinical trial, subjects should not only have been provided with the necessary information about the trial but should also have understood it. The two aspects of having sufficient understanding to give consent without coercion are key, but if taken literally, for example by being required to pass a test of competency, research on the efficacy of treatments and management strategies for dementia patients, particularly those with advanced dementia, would be impossible.[29] The increasing prevalence and incidence of dementia with advancing age may also pose problems for gaining informed consent generally for trials, not just those specifically for dementia treatments.

Currently, informed consent is usually gained from proxies on behalf of dementia patients, although technically only the subject may provide consent to be entered into a trial. Within clinical care there has been encouragement for patients to prepare advanced directives or living wills to cover the eventuality that they may not have the capacity to agree to treatment being given or withdrawn. At first sight this might appear a solution for dementia research also, but the strong motivational factors for individuals with clinical care are unlikely to be present for dementia research.[30] In addition, the number of people preparing living wills is still very small and tends to be the well-educated, higher social class groups. A more realistic future goal might be that people are encouraged to name proxies and state broad beliefs about research in advanced directives.

Rather than immediately approaching a proxy for consent with dementia patients, it may be best to promote the pragmatic view of decision-making capacity that if an individual appears competent then they are.[31] Dementia patients have been shown to be capable of understanding and differentiating the risk/benefit ratio between different treatments and of expressing their contentment with having a proxy make decisions on involvement in research although the proxies themselves tended to be more protective with their relatives than with themselves.[31] A more pressing problem is the lack of suitable proxies to provide informed consent on behalf of patients, one trial of palliative care of patients with advanced dementia who had been hospitalised finding that almost half (72/146) of eligible patients could not be enrolled.[32] In only four cases was this due to the proxy refusing consent, the proxies themselves lacking the capacity to understand the protocol in 18% of cases and in almost one-third no functional proxy being found. None of the patients for whom a proxy could not be found had made a living will.

It is when older people with dementia are resident in nursing homes–with their dependency and vulnerability–that the process of informed consent is most complex.[33] Certainly the high prevalence of dementia within long-term care settings exacerbates the problems already stated, although the more immediate barrier from a researcher's point of view may be the home-owner acting as gatekeeper. Experience of conducting censuses of older residents in all types of long-term care within Leicestershire over the last 20 years has shown, from the falling response rates of homes, the increasing difficulty over time in gaining access to residents or staff.[34,35] It is important that the inherent problems in conducting research within long-term care settings are recognised by researchers at the outset and that the shortage of staff time and often rigid regimes in homes are taken into consideration when designing trials, particularly those of interventions.[36] In these care settings, careful explanation to home-owners and staff of the purpose of the trial is likely to be vital to the success of the study.

FOLLOW-UP

Even when older people have been enrolled into trials, greater risk of the development of co-morbid conditions, cognitive impairment and polypharmacy will mean that they are more likely to withdraw before the final outcome assessment. To some extent this can be planned for in advance by allowing for a realistic withdrawal rate in the sample size calculation. Provision of information about the trial should not be considered a 'once and for all' activity at the commencement of the trial, and opportunities to re-enforce the importance of the participants' role in the success of the trial (for example at interim assessments) should be exploited. More flexible timing of follow-up visits may also help and these days should not pose any problems for analysis.

Missing data is still likely to be present and more complex data analysis techniques should be used to maximise the use of the data that are present. Some statistical packages for repeated measures data analysis—a common analysis for trials with regular follow-ups—ignore cases with data missing. Newer techniques such as multi-level modelling and random effects models can

accommodate incomplete data. Finally, outcomes such as mortality that may be easy to measure and important for younger populations may, in older people, be valued less than quality of life and the ability to function independently.[37]

CONCLUSIONS

If clinicians and other professionals caring for older people are to provide optimal treatment and the elderly are to benefit from new advances in treatments, decisions need to be based on firm evidence of efficacy in older people. At present this is noticeably lacking in many aspects of care. We have discussed the reasons why older people have been and are still being excluded both explicitly and implicitly from trials. We cannot give any definitive solutions to ensure that older people are recruited and enrolled in large numbers into trials, since the setting for the trial (community, nursing home, outpatient clinic) will influence the feasibility of different design options as well as the country in which the research is conducted. However we list below important features that should be considered when designing trials of future therapies that may ultimately be used by large numbers of older people:

- Aim for as wide eligibility criteria as possible to ensure smaller random error, a wider applicability of results and a greater opportunity to test pre-planned subgroup hypotheses.
- At the design stage, agree a list of strategies for recruiting specific subgroups (the very elderly, ethnic minorities) if these become under-represented during recruitment.
- Regularly monitor the characteristics of subjects enrolled to ensure good representation of the general population.
- Give careful thought to the information to be given to subjects and the method by which it will be given, to gain informed consent. Consider whether and when consent will need to be obtained from a proxy.
- If possible offer home assessments or, where this is impossible, provide transportation to

clinics at times convenient to the subject and their caregivers.

- Design a realistic withdrawal rate into the sample size calculation.

Finally, many clinical trials fail because of poor recruitment, lack of adherence to protocols and contamination between trial arms. The problems outlined in this chapter may mean that this is a particular issue for trials involving older people. There are useful lessons to be learnt from these experiences, yet by definition, these are rarely shared in the published literature. Methodological issues that arise from others' mistakes in carrying out clinical trials involving older people need to be aired and discussed in journals. If the quality of the evidence is improved then older people can expect to see an improvement in the quality of their health care.

REFERENCES

1. Stewart RB. Clinical research and the geriatric patient: an assessment of needs. *Clin Res Pract Drug Regulat Affairs* (1985) **3**: 477–500.
2. Statistical Bulletin. *Statistics of prescriptions dispensed in the Family Health Service Authorities: England 1984–1994* (1995).
3. Mitchell SL, Sullivan EA, Lipsitz LA. Exclusion of elderly subjects from clinical trials for Parkinson's Disease. *Arch Intern Med* (1997) **157**: 1393–8.
4. ICH Harmonised Tripartite Guidelines. *Studies in support of special populations: Geriatrics* (1993).
5. Taggart HMcA, Allardice JM. Fatal cholestatic jaundice in elderly patients taking benoxaprofen. *Br Med J* (1982) **284**: 1372.
6. Bugeja G, Kumar A, Banerjee AK. Exclusion of elderly people from clinical research: a descriptive study of published reports. *Br Med J* (1997) **315**: 1059.
7. Gurwitz JH, Col NF, Avorn J. The exclusion of the elderly and women from clinical trials in acute myocardial infarction. *JAMA* (1992) **268**: 1417–22.
8. Wenger NK. Exclusion of the elderly and women from coronary trials. Is their quality of care compromised? *JAMA* (1992) **268**: 1460–1.
9. Gurwitz JH, Avorn J. The ambiguous relation between aging and adverse drug reactions. *Ann Int Med* (1991) **114**: 956–66.

10. Yastrubetskaya O, Chiu E, O'Connell S. Is good clinical research practice for clinical trials good clinical practice? *Int J Geriat Psychiatry* (1997) **12**: 227–31.
11. Yusuf S, Held P, Teo K. Selection of patients for randomized controlled trials: implications of wide or narrow eligibility criteria. *Stat Med* (1990) **9**: 73–86.
12. Schneider LS, Olin JT, Lyness SA, Chui HC. Eligibility of Alzheimer's disease clinic patients for clinical trials. *J Am Geriatr Soc* (1997) **45**: 923–8.
13. Finkel SI, Richter EM, Clary CM. Comparative efficacy and safety of sertraline versus nortriptyline in major depression in patients 70 and older. *Int Psychogeriat* (1999) **11**: 85–99.
14. Applegate WB, Curb JB. Designing and executing randomized clinical trials involving elderly persons. *J Am Geriatr Soc* (1990) **38**: 943–50.
15. Petrovich H, Byington R, Bailey G, *et al.* Systolic Hypertension in the Elderly Program (SHEP) Part 2: Screening and recruitment. *Hypertension* (1991) **17**(Suppl II): 16–23.
16. Whelton PK, Bahnson J, Appel LJ, *et al.* Recruitment in the Trial of Nonpharmacologic Intervention in the Elderly (TONE). *J Am Geriatr Soc* (1997) **45**: 185–93.
17. Halbert JA, Silagy CA, Finucane P, Withers RT, Hamdorf PA. Recruitment of older adults for a randomized, controlled trial of exercise advice in a general practice setting. *J Am Geriatr Soc* (1999) **47**: 477–81.
18. Boult C, Boult L, Morishita L, Pirie P. Soliciting defined populations to recruit samples of high-risk older adults. *J Gerontol: Med Sci* (1998) **53**(5): M379–84.
19. Wager E, Tooley PJH, Emanuel MB, Wood SF. How to do it. Get patients' consent to enter clinical trials. *Br Med J* (1995) **311**: 734–7.
20. Featherstone K, Donovan JL. Random allocation or allocation at random? Patients' perceptions of participation in a randomised controlled trial. *Br Med J* (1998) **317**: 1177–80.
21. Sugarman J, McCrory DC, Hubal RC. Getting meaningful informed consent from older adults: a structured literature review of empirical research. *J Am Geriatr Soc* (1998) **46**: 517–24.
22. Gorkin L, Schron EB, Handshaw K *et al.* Clinical trial enrollers vs. nonenrollers: the Cardiac Arrhythmia Suppression Trial (CAST) Recruitment and Enrollment Assessment in Clinical Trials (REACT) project. *Contr Clin Trials* (1996) **17**: 46–59.
23. Pucci E, Belardinelli N, Signorino M, Angeleri F. Patients' understanding of randomised controlled

trials depends on their education. *Br Med J* (1999) **318**: 875.

24. Miller CK, O'Donnell DC, Searight HR, Barbarash RA. The Deaconess Informed Consent Comprehension Test: an assessment tool for clinical research. *Pharmacotherapy* (1996) **16**(5): 872–8.

25. DeLuca SA, Korcuska LA, Oberstar BH, Rosenthal ML, Welsh PA, Topol EJ. Are we promoting true informed consent in cardiovascular clinical trials? *J Cardiovasc Nurs* (1995) **9**(3): 54–61.

26. Stevens T, Katona C, Manela M, Watkin V, Livingston G. Drug treatment of older people with affective disorders in the community: lessons from an attempted clinical trial. *Int J Geriat Psychiatry* (1999) **14**: 467–72.

27. Ameer B, Burlingame MB. Difficulties enrolling elderly patients in pharmacokinetic studies. *J Geriatr Drug Ther* (1990) **4**: 61–7.

28. Clarke M, Jagger C, Anderson J, Battcock T, Kelly F, Campbell Stern M. The prevalence of dementia in a total population – the comparison of two screening instruments. *Age Ageing* (1991) **20**: 396–403.

29. Agarwal MR, Ferran J, Ost K, Wilson KCM. Ethics of 'informed consent' in dementia research – the debate continues. *Int J Geriat Psychiatry* (1996) **11**: 801–6.

30. Sachs GA. Advance consent for dementia research. *Alzh Dis Assoc Disord* (1994) **8**: 19–27.

31. Sachs GA, Stocking CB, Stern R, Cox DM, Hougham G, Sachs RS. Ethical aspects of dementia research: informed consent and proxy consent. *Clin Res* (1994) **42**: 403–12.

32. Baskin SA, Morriss J, Ahronheim JC, Meier D, Morrison RS. Barriers to obtaining consent in dementia research: implications for surrogate decision-making. *J Am Geriatr Soc* (1998) **46**: 287–90.

33. Becker D. Informed consent in demented patients: a question of hours. *Med Law* (1993) **12**: 271–6.

34. Campbell Stern M, Jagger C, Clarke M *et al*. Residential care for elderly people: a decade of change. *Br Med J* (1993) **306**: 827–30.

35. Lindesay J, Jagger C, Parker G *et al*. The Trent census of older people in residential care. Report to NHS Executive Trent (1999).

36. Eisch JS, Colling J, Ouslander J, Hadley BJ, Campbell E. Issues in implementing clinical research in nursing home settings. *J New York State Nurses Assoc* (1991) **22**: 18–21.

37. Grimley Evans J. Evidence-based and evidence-biased medicine. *Age Ageing* (1995) **24**: 461–3.

5

Complementary Medicine

PING-CHUNG LEUNG

Institute of Chinese Medicine, The Chinese University of Hong Kong, Hong Kong

INTRODUCTION

Medicine has been an art of healing. Although there is no absolute account on its history of development in the prehistorical and extreme primitive days, it must be closely related to the very ancient people's eating habits and animal behaviour. Ancient people fallen sick must prefer light meals with plenty of drinks. The latter might mean fruits and plant-related products, which are the forerunners of medicinal herbs.

Ancient people lived with animals: either keeping them as domestic friends or observing them closely in the fields. Animal instincts and behaviour lent the ancient people much wisdom of healing. When dogs and cats bit and ate up special grasses and leaves when they fell sick, followed by vomiting or diarrhoea, sometimes bringing out special unwanted ingested food or worms, the ancient people noted the special grasses and leaves. When they desired to clear up their guts under difficult circumstances, they recalled those grasses and leaves their animals ate and hence they imitated the animals, hoping to achieve the same healing. In this way, the primitive art of healing started.

What followed must have been more and more observations on more and more grasses and leaves which became considered as 'herbs'. Herb taking as a means to remove symptoms and ailments is, therefore, the standard early stage of the healing art in human history.[1,2] The valuable observations and experiences were kept until today.

All primitive tribal populations today are still using herb treatment, as the standard popular method of healing. The practice does not rule out trial uses of new herbs and their combinations, but the major practice depends on past experience and documentations. These early clinical trials were not the result of imagination but were initiated after observations on the anecdotal effects of different herbs.[3,4]

Traditionally there was no real need for large-scale clinical trials for complementary medicine. The need came only when scientific healers became interested in complementary medicine and started making use of herbs and other methods in their attempts to supplement modern medicine. They wanted to know whether, by utilising the same logic of analysis commonly practised in modern medicine, they could prove that

Textbook of Clinical Trials.   Edited by D. Machin, S. Day and S. Green
© 2004 John Wiley & Sons, Ltd   ISBN: 0-471-98787-5

herbal treatment constituted a logical substitution or supplement to scientific medicine.

This chapter explores the promises and fallacies of clinical trials in herbal medicine and some other complementary medicine; identifies the similarities and difficulties, the developments and limitations.

TYPES OF COMPLEMENTARY MEDICINE

The current main stream of medicine is the scientific variety. Other forms of health care outside the main stream fall into the category of complementary or alternative medicine.

If one uses history as the criterion of identification and considers ancient medicine was equivalent to complementary medicine, one sees four main systems of ancient healing. They are: Chinese, Indian, Greek and Egyptian. Geographically, the four systems are separated and yet, the nearby areas do carry similarities. China and India certainly did communicate. So did Greece and Egypt. China probably also obtained information from Greece, i.e. Europe, later in history through the 'silk route'.[5]

The four different systems have two main unique features. The Greek and Egyptian systems concentrate on the use of single herbs, while the Chinese and Indian systems use multiple combinations. Combined formulae are most commonly prescribed in Chinese herbal medicine.

After thousands of years, the four ancient systems of medicine still survive well. Greek medicine in Europe has established itself as a homeopathic healing art, while the other three systems enjoy persistent but varying popularities.

In the modern sense, alternative/complementary medicine includes not only the herbal streams, but any other form of medicine that is unrelated to the modern scientific stream. When the American Medical Association did a survey in the USA aimed at the revelation of the popularities and users of alternative medicine, 17 modalities were targeted.[6] These included the following:

1. Relaxation techniques
2. Herbal medicine
3. Massage
4. Chiropractice
5. Spiritual healing by others
6. Megavitamins
7. Self-help groups
8. Imagery
9. Commercial diets
10. Folk remedies
11. Lifestyle diets
12. Energy healing
13. Homeopathy
14. Hypnosis
15. Biofeedback
16. Acupuncture
17. Self-prayer

Of these varieties, the one that commanded the highest popularity was acupuncture as a form of pain control.

The author cannot possibly be knowledgeable about all the varieties of complementary medicine, and is not able to discuss all their clinical trials. Rather, he will concentrate on the two varieties that he is familiar with, herbal medicine and acupuncture. While discussions are being made, examples of clinical trials will be given, based on personal interests and experiences.

FUNDAMENTAL CONSIDERATIONS FOR CLINICAL TRIALS ON CHINESE MEDICINE

How should clinical trials of Chinese medicine be conducted? Are there differences between such trials and others designed for modern medicine?

We have explained earlier that originally, complementary medicine and its practitioners did not demand clinical trials. However, clinical trials are indicated for modern scientists because once the efficacy is proven, an alternative methodology of treatment can be endorsed.[7]

If modern medicine were not totally successful, there would be a real need for supplementing with alternative medicine. Generally speaking, the successes of modern medicine are well known in most areas. It is therefore necessary to look to complementary medicine only in those areas where the scientific main stream has deficiencies.

WHERE ARE THE DEFICIENCIES?

The deficient areas lie where modern medicine, in spite of recent advances, yet fails to get good solutions.

Modern medicine has developed from the logic of modern science which follows the deductive approach. The problem is first thoroughly understood by identifying the cause. The cause could then be removed by working out an effective means. In the situation of a disease when the cause is simple and straightforward, removing it would be easy. On the other hand, when the cause is either complicated, not well understood or multiple, removal becomes difficult or impossible. Simple disease-inducing causes include straightforward infections and simple hormonal deficiencies. The former is easily tackled with an efficient antibiotic while the latter could be treated with hormonal replacement.

When the causative agent is not yet thoroughly known, e.g. viral infections, treatment becomes difficult.

When the cause is complicated, e.g. in allergic conditions, treatment does not guarantee effective results.

When the cause is complicated, e.g. involving many factors such as physiological, social and psychological, modern scientific medicine becomes obviously deficient or incapable.[8-10]

Therefore the deficient areas in modern medicine that deserve contributions from complementary medicine include:

- Allergic conditions
- Autoimmune diseases
- Cancers
- Chronic pain
- Chronic derangements
- Degenerative diseases
- Nerve damages
- Viral infections
- Other areas that modern conventional therapy fails.

INDICATIONS AND PHILOSOPHY OF APPLYING COMPLEMENTARY MEDICINE

Current medical treatment emphasises the effectiveness and statistical chances of obtaining good results. Modern medicine has developed as direct corrective measures. Hence when it is effective, the probability of arriving at good results is very high. Unless not available, there is therefore no reason why modern medicine should not be endorsed as the primary mainline treatment.

Although there are still confident herbal practitioners who believe and declare that whatever the modern scientific practitioners can do, they could substitute with other herbal remedies, the number who remain that committed is getting less and less. Indeed today, most herbal practitioners accept the role of functioning as supplementary or alternative healers in a combined effort of cure and care.[11]

In this context, complementary herbal treatment is seldom used as the only healing modality. Instead, it is often given as an adjuvant treatment, either together with the mainline or after completion of the mainline. Users of herbal preparations, moreover, frequently look forward to a tonic supportive effect, rather than a curative effect.

HOW DOES HERBAL MEDICINE REALLY WORK?

Traditionally the system of herbal medicine was built on the rich experience of herb users or herbalists, accumulated over more than two thousand years in China since the early Chinese culture. For some reason, while basic medical sciences, e.g. anatomy and physiology, developed gradually in European territories around the Renaissance period, Chinese healers never felt the need to explore these basic medical sciences. Without sound knowledge of anatomy and physiology, i.e. biological structure and function of the human body, it would not be possible to explore abnormal structures and functions, i.e. pathology. Without understanding the pathology, it would not be possible to apply a direct means of removing the pathology. Herbal practitioners therefore try to heal, not by direct confrontation with the pathological problem, but by indirectly supporting the individual to overcome his own difficulties.[12,13]

HOW DOES THE INDIVIDUAL OVERCOME HIS OWN PATHOLOGICAL PROBLEMS?

Firstly by surviving the harmful disturbances imposed by the pathological processes. Secondly by supporting the unaffected organs and systems in their proper functions. Thirdly by preventing future pathological mishappenings while the current problem is being solved.

The herbal practitioner has means to suppress the symptoms which are manifestations of the pathology. Suppression of symptoms like cough, diarrhoea or dyspnoea helps the sick individual to survive.

While waiting for the pathological damages to heal naturally, the unaffected organs and systems need to be supported to maintain their efficient function, which in turn will support the overall function and metabolic harmony of the living individual.

Prevention in the modern biological sense frequently refers to an immunological mechanism through which the individual becomes more resistant to future attacks of similar pathological nature.

The main focus of disease management for Chinese medicine is often the control of adverse symptoms. The ultimate goal is maintaining the well-being of the biological system. The aetiological consideration is therefore not directed towards the actual cause of the disease (of which the herbal expert has no idea), but a general conceptual state of the biological balance of the human bodily functions. The ancient healers correlated this conceptual state with the Taoist philosophy and imagined that bodily function was kept at a balanced state between Yin and Yang (i.e. negative and positive). Any loss of balance led to ailment and disease.

The aim of treatment is therefore to maintain the balance. Yin and Yang includes other contrasting opposing forces like cold and heat,

superficial and deep, empty and solid. The causes of imbalance could be traced to a lack of balance of any pair of opposing forces. In the actual treatment, therefore, all efforts are spent on the maintenance of balance, by a supplement of the deficient force, or a decrement of the excessive.

Since the pathological causes of the symptomatology are unclear to the herbal expert, he would need to observe the changes of symptoms and adjust his day-to-day protocol accordingly. This approach differs very much from conventional modern medicine, which successfully identifies a pathological cause of disease, chooses a method of cure with good chance of success, then administers it with all effort and commitment, until the total removal of the pathology is achieved.

While the aetiology, epidemiology and natural course of a disease affect the design of clinical trials for modern medicine, it is now clear that in Chinese medicine, there is little analogy of aetiological and epidemiological considerations. The course of events in a disease, for a herbal expert, is the appearance of the symptoms: the loss of biological well-being due to the lack of balance between the vital forces. The aim of treatment is the re-establishment of balance; once balance is re-established, either naturally or through herbal intervention, well-being will be re-established. Treatment consists of a dynamic application of symptomatic relief with the goal of re-establishing the balance.[14]

Clinical trials for Chinese medicine or herbal medicine therefore could follow the line of thought for scientific planning on data collection and subsequent data meta-analysis. However, the pre-treatment data would be confined mainly to symptomatology. Other parameters would carry little weight for the herbal expert; but could still be included for more scientific knowledge in clinical trials.

GENERAL CONSIDERATIONS FOR CLINICAL TRIALS ON HERBS

In the modern scientific world, only up-to-date methodologies should be adopted. The set of common methodologies for conducting clinical trials on modern medicine has been logical, useful and has made wonderful contributions to the clinical testing of new drugs and new methods of clinical treatment. The proper analysis of data and the use of statistics have revealed the trustworthiness of certain accumulated experience, while at the same time the fallacies of some even well accepted and widely practised methods.[15]

The common methodology of random selection, blinding and placebo control, followed by statistical analysis, should be adopted. In the design of the trial, good clinical practice should be the aim. However, due to the nature of the herbs, which come from different origins and carry different species, it is not uncommon to encounter situations where basic principles that cannot be strictly kept.[16]

THE OLD APPROACHES

The herbal experts fervently respect case reports and anecdotal reports, particularly when results appear promising. Of course the reason behind it is that they don't make use of statistics. Moreover, they believe that treatment results are different with different patients. Once good results are known to be possible, the expert could try to achieve equally good results by wisely manipulating the varieties of treatment.

In this chapter, we do not endorse this traditional approach. We do want to apply modern assessment tools for a better understanding of herbal or Chinese medicine treatment while at the same time we need not argue against the value of anecdotal observations in Chinese medicine. After all, the development of this system of healing depends solely on anecdotal analysis.

Good clinical practice insists that the prescribed drug for the clinical trial should be thoroughly known and uniform. However, using herbal preparations for clinical trials faces difficulties of thorough technical knowledge and uniformity.

Pharmaceutical tests demand that details be known about the chemistry, the mode of action

and metabolic pathways before clinical tests be conducted. What is the chemistry of specific herbs? What are the pathways of action and metabolic degradation? Are there adverse effects in the process of metabolism? A lot of work has been done in the past 50 years on this basic understanding and not much has come out. Each and every herb contains so much complicated chemistry that many years of research might not yield much fruit. Actually at least four hundred herbs are popular and possess records of therapeutic action and impressive efficacy. To demand thorough knowledge on just this popular proportion of herbs is not practical, not to speak of the less commonly used extra one to two thousand varieties.[17]

Uniformity is another difficult area. Strictly speaking, since herbs are agricultural products, uniformity should start with the sites of agricultural production. The sites of production have different weather, different soil contents, and the methods of plantation are also different. At the moment, maybe over 50% of popular Chinese herbs are produced on special farms in China. However, these farms are scattered over different provinces, which have widely different climatic and soil environments. Good agricultural practice demands that environmental and nurturing procedures be uniformly ensured. Procedures include soil care, watering, fertilisers, pest prevention and harvests. When such procedures are not uniform and there are no means to ensure a common practice, good agricultural practice is not possible.

Not only is there a lack of uniformity in the mode of herb production, but different species of the same herb are found or planted in different regions and provinces. These different species may have different detailed chemical contents. Herbal experts have extensive experience and knowledge about some special correlations between the effectiveness of particular herbs and their sites of production. Some commonly used herbs are even labelled jointly with the best sites of production. With the development of molecular biology, coupled with modern means of assessment for active ingredients within a chemical product, species-specific criteria could be identified, using the 'finger-printing' technique. Uniformity today should include screening using 'finger-printing' techniques.

When we consider the other 50% of herbs that are only available from the wilderness, i.e. around mountains, highlands or swamps, and cannot be grown on agricultural farms, the insistence on product uniformity becomes even more difficult.

Putting together what we have discussed, to strictly insist on good clinical practice in clinical trials for herbal medicine is largely impossible. We have to accept a compromise. Indeed in the past 50 years, many attempts have been made at a proper analytical study of herbal preparations. The intention was: to put the herb to processes of extraction, analyse the important ingredients, then try to work out the chemical formulae which could be responsible for the clinical effects.

Extraction eliminates the useless components and concentrates the effective components, which not only cuts down the volume of herbs used but also intensifies the biological actions. Knowing the actual effective ingredients and working out the chemical formulae would be ideal for modernisation of herbal preparations with the aim of converting the preparations into proper pharmaceuticals.

In spite of the efforts and resources put into herbal extractions and chemical analyses in the past 50 years, successful examples have not been impressive. The results of such efforts certainly do not match the resources put in.[18]

The unsatisfactory outcome has initiated a new approach. Instead of following the scientific pathway already taken by pharmaceuticals, which has shown too many difficulties rather than promises, a more practical line has been endorsed. Since most, if not all, the herbs have been used for hundreds of years, there should be sufficient amount of reliability on the safety and efficacy of the herbs. The safety and efficacy of the herbs are already well documented, but their practical utilisation in specific clinical circumstances needs to be further established. The traditional use of the herbs had been focused on symptomatic control. Nowadays, the aim of clinical management is directed towards curing of a disease entity.

We need to acquire an updated understanding on the effectiveness of the herbal preparations on disease entities. That is why we could not be satisfied with records on efficacy alone, but should start a series of clinical trials to further prove the efficacy of the herbs.[19]

The National Institutes of Health of the United States have openly endorsed the approach of accepting traditional methods of healing as safe measures and then putting them to proper clinical trials.[20] The recognition of acupuncture as a practical effective means of pain control started in 1998.[21] The subsequent formation of a special section devoted to research on complementary/alternative treatment followed. The National Centre for Complementary, Alternative Treatment (NCCAM) was properly formed and given a substantially large budget.

Clinical trials to be discussed within this chapter follow the efficacy-driven principle. They are planned strictly according to the principles set out under the modern philosophy of clinical trials aimed at the production of objective evidence of the effectiveness of the methods used. It is however understood that product uniformity and quality could not be absolutely guaranteed and that although GMP (Good Manufacturing Process) could be assured, GCP (Good Clinical Practice) could not be absolutely ensured because of the lack of guarantee for any herbal preparations.

In our discussion full reference will be given to what is being recommended in China, which undoubtedly harbours most activity in Chinese medicine.

HERBAL DRUGS IN CHINA

In 1999 the National Bureau on Drug Control defined new drugs as 'a manufactured product for medical treatment that is produced for the first time or an old product reproduced with different formulation and different indications'.

New drugs are divided into five categories:

I. Group 1
   Artificial derivatives from Chinese herbs
   Newly discovered Chinese herbs and derivatives

Extracts from Chinese herbs and derivatives
Extracts from decortions of herbs
  II. Group 2
Herbal injections
Herbal preparations processed inside animals
Extracts from complex decortions
 III. Group 3
New preparations of decortions
Combined herbal and chemical preparations
Imported herbal preparations
 IV. Group 4
Converted formulary
Cultivated herbal and domestic animal preparations
  V. Group 5
Herbal preparations with extended uses

STAGES RECOMMENDED FOR HERBAL RESEARCH

The usual four stages are recommended.

Phase I: Study on the general acceptance of the human being after consumption of the herbal preparation. Normally Phase I refers to a toxicity study. The code of practice given under 'Code of Practice for the Scrutiny of New Drugs' in China, however, recommends that the general well-being of the individual after consumption be observed.[22] The logic of skipping toxicity tests is probably based on an assumption that Chinese herbal preparations have been used safely for centuries, therefore a special toxic screening is not necessary. The author has strong reservations on this attitude and would recommend that toxicity clearance should remain the first phase of clinical trials.

Phase II: Study on the safety and efficacy while working out the effective dosage.

Phase III: Expands on Phase II study, collecting more reliable confirmation on the safety and efficacy.

Phase IV: Further study on the safety and efficacy after the new drug is put to market. More observations on adverse effects are expected.

It has been pointed out that, as far as herbal medicine is concerned, it is not unusual to find that correlation does not exist between laboratory research and clinical trials. When studies on the pharmacology, pharmacodynamics and pharmacokinetics are carried out after the clinical trials, positive values, in support of the clinical observations, might not be impressive.

The possible explanation to this observation may lie in the fact that the clinical consumption of the herbal preparations involves multiple, complex *in vivo* biological interactions, whereas laboratory tests consist of only simple unidirectional biological interactions.

HOW DO CONCEPTS OF TRADITIONAL HEALING AFFECT CLINICAL TRIALS ON CHINESE MEDICINE?

Earlier in this chapter, the author has already touched on the unique concepts in Chinese medicine, which are different from modern scientific medicine. The application of modern concepts in the direction of clinical trials leads to the inevitable sacrifice of some of the fundamental principles. Experienced herbal experts, therefore, might not like to participate.

The following list includes the important concepts in Chinese medicine practice being sacrificed:

1. Symptom and syndrome Identification Principle
   Following this principle, the herbal expert adjusts details of his treatment according to observations on the day-by-day changes of symptomatology. He may then use different drugs for the same symptoms or use the same drug for different symptoms. Proper clinical trials could only use a uniform choice of treatment modality. This violates the symptom and syndrome identification principle.
2. Holistic Approach
   Chinese medicine emphasises holistic care and holistic response, whereas clinical trials prefer objective, specific data as endpoints. The inclusion of specific data into herbal research probably does not invite objection from the herbal expert, as long as general data like different aspects of well-being, i.e. quality of life, are included.

3. Response to Pathological Processes
   Chinese medicine emphasises the responses of healthy organs to diseases. The ability of the healthy organs to respond to pathological changes ensures that the individual would be able to better resist adversities. Modern clinical trials aim mostly at diseased organs.

4. Old System of Clinical Observation
   Herbal experts utilise a system of clinical observations which today might be considered obsolete and over-subjective. This system of clinical signs includes tongue observation, pulse detection and a collection of subjective feelings.[23] Modern clinical trials insist on objective data that could be monitored. We therefore have to either develop means to objectively assess the subjective signs in the tongue and the pulse or we sacrifice the whole system of observations. Herbal experts might not appreciate either choice.

5. Strong Tradition
   Herbal experts place genuine confidence on anecdotal observations and experience of single patients. Insisting on the need to investigate collective observations and condemning single-case experience would not be welcomed by herbal experts. This conceptual difference directly affects the participation and cooperation of the traditional and modern experts.

While thoroughly recognising the unique nature of Chinese medicine and having pointed out the lack of harmony between the old tradition and modern science, one realises that the current compromise adopted in China is to insist on a modern scientific approach as far as possible. Hence in standard textbooks, the following are advocated[24] as standard instructions for clinical trials:

1. Use the principles of randomisation, blinding and repetition.
2. Adopt good protocols for clinical trials.
3. Avoid bias at all cost.
4. Eliminate chance factors.
5. Establish new standards of clinical assessment.

6. Establish unique outcome studies.
7. Establish unique quality of life assessments.
8. Insist on using modern statistics.

ADVERSE EFFECTS

Historically, great herbal masters in China in the ancient days did produce records on adverse effects and toxic problems of some herbs. As early as the Han dynasty (second century) documents were produced on herbs that need to be utilised with care or extreme care.[25] This tradition was followed closely in the subsequent centuries.[26]

More reports were available on methods and means with which toxicities and adverse effects could be reduced.[27]

In spite of the good past experience, the prevalent belief is that Chinese medicinal herbs are safe. On the other hand, more and more reports appeared on adverse effects and toxicities, and non-users of herbs tend to exaggerate the reports.

When new preparations come into the market, the innovative processes of extraction and/or production might have produced or initiated new possibilities of adverse effects or toxicity. This experience is already well recorded in a number of modernised preparations, particularly those for injection.[28] Among the adverse effects, allergic reactions are commonest.

To date, standard instructions on clinical trials for Chinese medicine define adverse drug reaction in exactly the same way as modern scientific clinical trials, and explanations of the reactions have been identically identified.[29]

Categories of adverse reactions include the following:

1. Reactions to herbs
   Reactions are defined as harmful and unexpected effects while the standard dosages are used in certain drug trials. It is specially pointed out that for Chinese medicine, the harmful reactions could be due to the quality of the herb and poor choice of indication. These reactions do not include allergic responses.

2. Dosage-related adverse effects

   Using an unnecessarily high dose could induce excessive effects, side effects or even toxic effects. Secondary effects like electrolyte imbalance might also be observed.

3. Dosage-unrelated adverse effects

   These adverse effects could be the result of unfavourable preparation, contaminants in the herbs, sensitivity of the consumer, allergic reactions or specific inductive effects of the herb.

4. Drug interactions

   Classically, records are available in old Chinese medicinal literature on combined effects of herbs, their facilitatory and antagonistic effects. Nowadays, not only drug interactions between herbs are important, but possible interactions between herbs and commonly used pharmaceutical preparations are becoming issues of great concern since users of herbal preparations are greatly increasing. In the area of anaesthesia, drug interactions between herbs and modern medicine could induce life-threatening reactions. Table 5.1 illustrates some studies currently done on this issue.[30]

5. Delayed adverse effects

   Adverse effects of delayed nature include induction to cancer formation, foetal abnormalities and even blockage of bacterial sensitivities.

6. Drug dependence

   There might be suspicions that herbal preparations might lead to drug dependence. Apart from a few opium-related herbs, Chinese herbs in fact are well known to be non-addictive because of their gross lack of specificities.

From the above account it might appear obvious that adverse effects in clinical trials using Chinese medicine in fact follow closely the experience encountered in other drug trials.

As far as the grading of adverse effects is concerned, it would be appropriate to categorise the effects as mild, moderate and severe.

With regard to the overall assessment of adverse effects, a convenient recommendation for Chinese medicine trials is that of Naranjo.[31] Naranjo's system of grading adverse effects according to fact-finding results is shown in Table 5.2. Overall assessment:

ADR confirmed ≥ 9
ADR likely $5-8$
ADR possible $1-4$
ADR unlikely ≤ 0

Detection and recording of adverse effects should bear different emphases at different phases of the trial, e.g. Phase I trial aims at detection of adverse effects in relation to dosage, Phase II and III collect details, whereas Phase IV is concerned mainly with marketed drugs.

Whatever is the situation, detection of adverse effects should include both clinical observations and laboratory data, and detection should be followed with follow-up observations. The summation of observations should be thoroughly analysed so that explanations of the adverse effects may eventually be worked out.

REPORTING OF ADVERSE EFFECTS

It is currently required in China that adverse effects should be reported to the relevant monitoring body as soon as possible. Once a drug is marketed, adverse effects should be continuously reported to the National Control Bureau, within the first five years.

Adverse effects detected at the post-market Phase IV might be particularly important for Chinese medicine trials. Since herbal preparations do not have clear, definite information about the effective contents of the herbs, bias and chances might be more likely than other trials on simpler drugs at the early phases. The large trial population during Phase IV gives a better chance of elimination of bias and allows a better opportunity of objective detection of adverse effects. During the Phase IV trial, the following aspects would deserve particular attention:

1. Actual danger level of the adverse effects. Degree of danger of course depends on the

Table 5.1. Examples of Herb-Drug Interaction

Herb	Drug	Interaction	Mechanism
Radix Salviae Miltiorrhizae (Danshen)	Warfarin	Increased INR Prolonged PT/PTT	Danshen decreases elimination of Warfarin in rats
Radix Angelicae Sinensis (Danggui)	Warfarin	Increased INR and widespread bruising	Danggui contains coumarins
Ginseng (Radix Ginseng)	Alcohol	Increased alcohol clearance	Ginseng decreases the activity of alcohol dehydrogenase and aldehyde dehydrogenase in mice
Garlic	Warfarin	Increased INR	Post-operative bleeding and spontaneous spinal epidural haemorrhage
Herbal ephedrae (Ma Huang)	Pargyline, Isoniazid, Furazolidone	Headache, nausea, vomiting, bellyache, blood pressure increase	Pargyline, Isoniazid, and Furazolidone interfere with the inactivation of noradrenalin and dopamine; ephedrine in herbal ephedrine can promote the release of noradrenalin and dopamine
Ginkgo Biloba	Aspirin	Spontaneous hyphema	Ginkgolides are potent inhibitors of (PAF)
Cornu cervi pantotrichum Fructus crataegi	adrenomimetic	Strengthens the effect of increasing blood pressure	Natural MAOIs in Cornu cervi pantotrichum, Fructus crataegi and Radix polygoni multiflori inhibited the metabolism of adrenomimetic, levodopa and opium
Radix polygoni multiflori	Levodopa Opium	Increased blood pressure and heart rate Central excitation	
Bitter melon	Chlorpropamide	Decreased urea glucose	Bitter melon decreased the concentration of blood glucose
Liquorice	Oral contraceptives	Hypertension, oedema, hypokalaemia	Oral contraceptive may increase sensitivity to glycyrrhizin acid
St. John's wort	Warfarin Cyclosporin	Decreased INR Decreased concentration in serum	Decreased the activity of Warfarin

Table 5.1. (*continued*)

Herb	Drug	Interaction	Mechanism
Radix Isatidis (Banlangen)	Trimethoprin (TMP)	Significantly increase anti-inflammation effect	
Liu Shen pill	Digoxin	Frequent ventricular premature beat	
Tamarind	Aspirin	Increased the bioavailability of aspirin	
Yohimbine	Tricyclic antidepressants	Hypertension	

Note :

ACE	angiotension-converting enzyme	
INR	international normalised ratio	
PT	prothrombin time	
PTT	partial thromboplastin time	
PAF	platelet-activating factor	
AUC	area under the concentration/time curve	
MAOIs	monoamine oxidase inhibitors	

Source: Reproduced from De Smet and D'Arcy,[30] with permission from Springer-Verlag.

Table 5.2. Questions to be asked about adverse Drug Reactions

	Yes	No	Not clear
1. Are there decisive records about the ADR?	+1	0	0
2. Are the ADRs found after consumption of other drugs?	+2	−1	0
3. Are the ADRs improved after consumption of antidote?	+1	0	0
4. Are there repeated ADRs or repeated administration?	+2	−1	0
5. Are there other predisposing factors?	−1	+2	0
6. Are there ADRs after placebo?	−1	+1	0
7. Has the blood level of drug giving ADRs been investigated?	+1	0	0
8. Do the ADRs correlate to dosages?	+1	0	0
9. Is there past history?	+1	0	0
10. Is there objective proof	+1	0	0

incidence of occurrence. The requirement for treatment and the financial implications are also important.

2. More thorough studies at Phase IV should be considered according to epidemiological principles. Randomised controlled trials should be insisted on. Cohort studies might be convenient and useful, but there need to be markedly obvious differences between series of comparisons before results can be instructive. Case reports might still be useful, but might function as special warning signals to calls for more serious studies.[32]

QUALITY OF LIFE

While clinical trials aim at a thorough scientific understanding of the effectiveness of specific forms of treatment, endpoints of measurement are set to give objective standards of evaluation. Primary endpoints are unique, focused, specific criteria which indicate the situation of the target against which the trial is directed. Changes of primary endpoints illustrate the efficacy directly. Secondary endpoints are supplementary criteria created to support observations on changes and efficacy. Secondary endpoints become more important when, predictably, primary endpoints do not give clear-cut, impressive results. Secondary endpoints become more important when primary endpoints are expected to change slowly and would be particularly important when chronic problems are being faced.

Since Chinese medicine, under most circumstances, does not operate via a direct confrontation route but rather acts indirectly to support the healthy organs and helps to maintain vitality and prevent functional deterioration, critical and detailed assessment of the secondary endpoints is therefore of utmost importance.

Quality of life (QoL) is an important aspect on the assessment of care given to the chronically ill. QoL often measures the competency of the care and the ethical standard of the society in mental disorders and other disorders that demonstrate strong social orientations. Not infrequently, using technical endpoints as results of clinical trials a reasonable outcome is observed, and yet patients might not be satisfied with their QoL. QoL is therefore multifocal: it differs between developed and underdeveloped areas, it also differs under different cultural circles.[33] Different countries and regions therefore try to develop their own data to be included within their own studies on QoL.[34] Meanwhile global, generally acceptable QoL charts are also being planned, examined and validated.[35]

Before an acceptable general data chart is ready, one has to accept the achievements already revealed in different fields. Generally speaking, QoL data sheets take in information about physiological well-being, psychological well-being, social well-being and the individual's subjective feeling on the treatment received and the rehabilitation underway. Different specialties and special areas of concern have created charts of their own and all these provide valuable information when equivalent studies come up. Usually they are adopted right away or after validation. Hence there are charts already developed for children and the elderly, and different medical specialties and subspecialties likewise have created their own charts. Just to mention a few, special QoL charts are available for the mentally ill, cardiovascular diseases, rheumatological disease, respiratory problems, gynaecological problems and special infections.[36] QoL charts for Chinese medicinal studies need to be developed.

WHAT ARE THE RECOMMENDATIONS FOR CLINICAL TRIALS OF CHINESE MEDICINE?

The simplest thing to do is to make reference to the available charts in whichever clinical trial is being conducted and think about amendments to make them even more suitable.

ARE THERE UNIQUE FEATURES THAT NEED TO BE OBSERVED?

There are features related to health which are derived from the philosophy of Chinese medicine ever since its initial development. Chinese people in all walks of life are influenced by this philosophy without being aware of it at all stages of their life. The belief that health depends on a harmony between contrasting forces prompts the individual to feel either 'hot or cold', 'light' or 'heavy', 'sick inside' or 'sick outside'. After treatment, the feeling might remain, might reverse or might get balanced. The feeling is subjective, but in any clinical trial including the data of QoL, could one ignore the outcome of the philosophical guideline responsible for the whole system of healing art?

Henceforth, it is obvious the QoL studies are particularly important for clinical trials of Chinese medicine and research should be done on special inclusions of data which are unique for Chinese medicine.

EXAMPLES OF CLINICAL TRIALS ON CHINESE MEDICINE

To give more solid information about clinical trials on Chinese medicine being done in Hong Kong, the following paragraphs are devoted to summaries of such trials.

Synopsis I

Name of Study Medication: Phyllanthus SP. Compound

Title of Study: A Prospective Randomised, Double-Blind, Placebo-Controlled, Parallel Study to Evaluate the Effect of Phyllanthus SP. Compound in the Treatment of Chronic Hepatitus B Virus Infection.

Study Centre: Single-centre

Objective:

Primary

- To evaluate the efficacy of normalisation of liver enzyme, seroconversion of HbeAg and disappearance of HBV DNA in serum.
- To evaluate the safety of Phyllanthus SP. Compound in patients with hepatitis B.

Secondary

- Proportion of patients with end-of-treatment HbeAg seroconversion (HbeAg to anti-Hbe, normalisation of ALT and disappearance of HBV DNA at the end of treatment).
- Proportion of patients with HbeAg to anti-Hbe.
- Proportion of patients with sustained normalisation of ALT.
- Proportion of patients with undetectable HBV DNA.

Design: A single-centre, prospective randomised, double-blind, placebo-controlled, parallel study. Patients will be randomised to one of the four treatment groups and treated for a duration of 6 months.

Study Population: A minimum of 85 hepatitis B patients will be enrolled, 25 subjects per treatment group, 10 subjects in the control group, a total of four groups.

Definition of Endpoints:

- The primary safety endpoint is tolerability.
- Tolerability failure is defined as a permanent discontinuation of Phyllanthus PLUS as the result of an adverse event.
- The primary endpoint is a reduction in HBV DNA level from the baseline.
- The secondary endpoint is HbeAg negative, anti-Hbe positive and a decrease in ALT level from baseline.

Study Regimen: Subjects will be randomly and alternatively assigned to receive Phyllanthus PLUS or placebo for 6 months prospective parallel study.

Duration of Treatment: 6 months

Statistical Methods: Efficacy: Summary statistics for the change of HBV DNA, HbsAG, HbeAg and ALT from baseline will be generated and provided for each treatment group.

Safety

- The incidence of adverse events and laboratory toxicity will be summarised by treatment group and severity. Change from baseline in vital signs will be summarised by treatment group.
- Group differences with an error probability of less than 5% ($p < 0.05$) will be considered statistically significant.

- The statistical analyses will be made with SPSS for Windows 10.0.

Synopsis II

Name of Study TCM: Danggui Buxue Tang

Title of Study: A Randomised, Double-Blind, Comparison Study of the Effect of Danggui Buxue Tang with Oestradiol on Menopausal Symptoms and Quality of Life in Hong Kong Chinese Women.

Study Centre: Single-centre

Objective:

Primary

- To compare the effects of Danggui Buxue Tang with Oestradiol on menopausal symptoms of hot flushes and sweating.
- To evaluate the safety of Danggui Buxue Tang in patients with menopausal symptoms.

Secondary

- To evaluate the quality of life of the patients with menopausal symptoms.

Design: A single-centre, randomised, double-blind and comparison study. Subjects will be randomised to one of the two treatment groups and treated for a duration of 6 months with follow-up of 18 months.

Study Population: A minimum of 100 patients with menopausal symptoms will be enrolled, 50 subjects per treatment group.

Definition of Endpoints:

- The primary safety endpoint is tolerability. Tolerability failure is defined as

a permanent discontinuation of Danggui Buxue Tang as the result of an adverse event.
- The primary efficacy endpoint is the change in severity and frequency of hot flushes and night sweats.
- The secondary efficacy endpoint is the changes in score for the domains measured in the Menopause Specific Quality of Life Questionnaire.

Study Regimen: Subjects will be randomly and alternatively assigned to receive Danggui Buxue Tang or placebo for 6 months.

Duration of Treatment: 6 months treatment period and 18-month follow-up.

Statistical Methods:

- Data will be processed to give group mean values and standard deviations where appropriate.
- Mann–Whitney U-test will be used to compare the differences between the two groups of treatment. Group differences with an error probability of less than 5% ($p < 0.05$) will be considered statistically significant.
- The statistical analyses will be made with SPSS 10.0 for Windows.

Synopsis III

Name of Study TCM: Danggui Buxue Tang

Title of Study: A Randomised Comparison Study of the Effect of Danggui Buxue Tang with Tranexamic Acid on Dysfunctional Uterine Bleeding and Quality of Life in Hong Kong Chinese Women.

Study Centre: Single-centre

Objective:

Primary

- To compare the effects of Danggui Buxue Tang with Tranexamic acid on menstrual blood loss per month.
- To compare the patient's satisfaction between using Danggui Buxue Tang and Tranexamic acid.
- To evaluate the safety of Danggui Buxue Tang in patients with dysfunctional uterine bleeding.

Secondary

- To evaluate the improvement of anaemia.
- To evaluate the status of iron deficiency.
- To evaluate the unwanted side effects.

Design: A single-centre, randomised comparison study. Subjects will be randomised to one of the two treatment groups and treated for a duration of 6 months with follow-up of 24 months.

Study Population: A minimum of 125 patients with dysfunctional uterine bleeding will be enrolled, 63 subjects in the Danggui Buxue Tang group and 62 subjects in the Tranexamic acid group.

Definition of Endpoints:

- The primary safety endpoint is tolerability. Tolerability failure is defined as a permanent discontinuation of Danggui Buxue Tang as the result of an adverse event.
- The primary efficacy endpoint is change in frequency and severity of menstrual bleeding.
- The secondary efficacy endpoint is improving anaemia and iron deficiency.

Study Regimen: Subjects will be randomly and alternatively assigned to receive Danggui Buxue Tang or Tranexamic acid for 6 months treatment and 24 months follow-up.

Duration of Treatment: 6 months treatment and 24 months follow-up.

Statistical Methods:

- Data will be processed to give group mean values and standard deviations where appropriate.
- All the data in the outcome measure are continuous variables. Mann–Whitney U-test will be used to compare the differences between the two groups of treatment. The level of significance will be set at $p < 0.05$.
- The statistical analyses will be made with SPSS 10.0 for Windows.

Synopsis IV

Name of Study TCM: Formula A and Formula B

Title of Study: A Randomised, Double-Blind, Placebo-Controlled Study on the Clinical Effects of Integrated Western Medicine and Traditional Chinese Medicine for Diabetic Foot Ulcer.

Study Centre: Multi-centre

Objective:

Primary

- To evaluate the wound healing effect of Formula A and Formula B in patients with diabetic foot ulcer.
- To evaluate the safety of Formula A and Formula B in patients with diabetic foot ulcer.

Secondary

- To evaluate the effect of control of the local infection.

Design: A multi-centre, randomised, double-blind, placebo-controlled study. Subjects will be randomised to one of the two treatment groups and treated for a duration of 6 months.

Study Population: A minimum of 80 diabetic foot ulcer patients will be enrolled, 40 subjects per treatment group.

Definition of Endpoints:

- The primary safety endpoint is tolerability. Tolerability failure is defined as a permanent discontinuation of formula A and Formula B as the result of an adverse event.
- The primary efficacy endpoint is diabetic foot ulcer healing and to avoid leg amputation.
- The secondary efficacy endpoint is the control of local infection.

Study Regimen: Subjects will be randomly and alternatively assigned to receive Formula A and Formula B or placebo of a 6-month prospective parallel study.

Duration of Treatment: 6 months

Statistical Methods:

- Results will be presented as the mean ± SE per group.
- Group differences with an error probability of less than 5% ($p < 0.05$) will be considered statistically significant.
- The statistical analysis will be made with SPSS 10.0 for Windows.

Synopsis V

Name of Study TCM: Relieve Wheezing Tablet

Title of Study: A Randomised, Double-Blind, Placebo-Controlled Parallel Study of the Effect of Relieve Wheezing Tablet in the Treatment of Childhood Asthma.

Study Centre: Single-centre

Objective:

Primary

- To evaluate the medication score, including daily use of inhaled steroids.
- To evaluate the symptom score, including cough on daytime and nighttime, wheeze/chest tightness on daytime and nighttime, degree of shortness of breath on exertion.

Secondary

- To evaluate the spirometry lung function result.
- To evaluate the breakthrough attacks requiring medical attention from A/E doctors, family physicians on hospitalisation.
- To evaluate the degree of skin allergy.
- To evaluate the changes in peripheral blood and Eosinophilic Cationic Protein (ECP).

Design: A single-centre, randomised, double-blind, placebo-controlled, parallel study. Subjects will be randomised to one of the two treatment groups and treated for a duration of 6 months.

Study Population: A minimum of 80 patients with moderate to severe perennial asthma will be enrolled, 40 subjects per treatment group.

Definition of Endpoints:

- The primary safety endpoint is tolerability. Tolerability failure is defined as a permanent discontinuation of Relieve Wheezing Tablet as the result of an adverse event.
- The primary efficacy endpoint is a change in improving the symptoms of asthmatic children and use of inhaled steroids.
- The secondary efficacy endpoint is improvement of lung function.

Study Regimen: Subjects will be randomly and alternatively assigned to receive Relieve Wheezing Tablet or placebo for 6 months.

Synopsis VI

Name of Study Medication: Danshen and Radix Puerariae Compound

Title of Study: A Prospective Randomised, Double-Blind, Placebo-Controlled, Parallel Study to Evaluate the Effect of a Herbal Preparation with Compound Formula of Danshen and Radix Puerariae as Cardiovascular Tonic in Cardiac Patients.

Study Centre: Single-centre

Objective:

Primary

- To evaluate the safety of Danshen and Radix Puerariae Compound as adjunctive therapy in patients with coronary artery disease.
- To evaluate the efficacy of treatment and secondary prevention of cardiovascular diseases.

Secondary

- To evaluate the lipid and homocysteine-lowering effect of Danshen and Radix Puerariae Compound.

Design: A single-centre, prospective randomised, double-blind, placebo-controlled, parallel study. Patients will be randomised to one of the two treatment groups and receive Danshen and Radix Puerariae Compound or placebo for a duration of 24 weeks.

Study Population: A total of 100 patients with Coronary Artery Disease (CAD) will be enrolled, 50 subjects treated with Danshen and Radix Pruerariae Compound and 50 treated with placebo.

Definition of Endpoints:

- The primary safety endpoint is tolerability.
- Tolerability failure is defined as a permanent discontinuation of Danshen and Radix Puerariae Compound as the result of an adverse event.
- The primary endpoint is improving cardiovascular function (endothelial function and carotid intima-medial thickness) from the baseline.
- The secondary endpoint is decrease of plasma lipid and homocysteine levels.

Study Regimen: Subjects will be randomly assigned to receive Danshen and Radix Puerariae Compound (TCM) or placebo for 24 weeks in a prospective parallel study.

Duration of Treatment: 24 weeks

Duration of Project: 30 months

Statistical Analyses

- The statistical significance of changes between TCM and placebo groups will be assessed by one-way analysis of variance.
- Group differences with an error probability of less than 5% ($p < 0.05$) were considered statistically significant.
- The statistical analyses were made with SPSS for Windows 10.0.

ACUPUNCTURE

Acupuncture is a practical procedure using a special needle to enter special regions of the human body surface by which symptoms suffered by the patient are removed. Like other aspects of Chinese medicine, it aims at symptom control, not at the treatment of a specific disease entity. The most popular use must be in the field of pain control.

In 1998, the National Institutes of Health in the USA held a consensus conference on the use of acupuncture for pain control. The conclusion was that acupuncture should be accepted as an effective means of pain control for musculo-skeletal problems and under other specific situations.[21] Since then, interest in the use of acupuncture in the United States grew and many clinical studies were started.

Of course, acupuncture has been used for the control of other symptoms. Examples include nerve damages, allergic conditions like rhinitis, asthmatic attacks and general feelings of being 'unwell', often labelled as 'derangement'.

How are clinical trials on acupuncture being conducted? Could the clinical trials on acupuncture be put in line with modern epidemiological requirements? Or would it be even more difficult compared with herbal medicine? We have first of all, to look at the procedures involved and the explanations given to the effects produced.

Acupuncture involves the insertion of thin needles, through specific acupoints on the body surface, to varying depths of soft tissue, then allowing the needles to stay for some minutes. While the needles stay inside the soft tissue, the puncturist may give regular or occasional rotary movements on the nail. In recent years, acupuncturists have applied direct electrical current stimulation, so as to unify the stimulations, widen the effects and save manpower. Acupuncture is an invasive process directly aiming at the removal of symptoms. It is easy to imagine then, that patients would not agree to participate in a study where they would not be able to enjoy the puncture treatment and function as recipients of 'sham' puncture. Likewise, if there were other placebo punctures which fulfil the requirement of randomisation and placebo control, very few patents would be willing to participate.[37,38]

However, studies on placebo acupuncture have started and the varieties included the following:

1. Placebo points–entry points are sites outside the acupuncture meridians.
2. Sham puncture–puncture lightly then withdraw.
3. Hiding entry points–while entry points are hidden, it might be possible to achieve real placebo effect. Hiding of entry points may be achieved by puncturing through plastic tubes or soft plastic blocks.
4. Camouflage puncture by which a needle is just taped to the skin.

None of these methods could be endorsed because the requirements for placebo in the strict sense are far from being satisfied; most recipients could differentiate right away whether it is true or false puncture. The conventional application of acupuncture depends on a subjective feeling of 'numbness' felt within the punctured area. Puncturing without checking this feeling is not considered appropriate. This requirement makes 'placebo' puncture impossible. The use of electrical stimulation is a means to enhance the effects in modern situations where there is insufficient experience on acupoint identification and actual puncturing techniques. It is also considered as a method of modernising acupuncture. When electrical stimulation is used, placebo becomes absolutely impossible because the electrical stimulation is always felt.

The considerations are further complicated by the theories of acupuncture. There are two acceptable theories–the neurological and the humoral. The neurological theory observes that since some of the meridians and most of the acupuncture points are related to the peripheral nerves, stimulation of these points leading to physiological effects could be working via neurological pathways, possibly through proprioceptive receptors.[39] The humoral theory assumes that needle stimulation produces humoral (hormonal) reactions, manifested as serological appearance of functional factors which possess pain control effects and other regulatory functions.[40]

Whichever theory is at work, it specifies that the tiny area of puncture is producing chain reactions, either directly or indirectly. An apparently harmless, non-productive action on the skin and soft tissue, imitating acupuncture, might trigger off similar effects and would be far from being a placebo.

Therefore standard epidemiological planning for clinical trials in Chinese medicine including acupuncture would be very difficult, if at all possible. Randomisation would not be acceptable to patients, whereas in situations of acupuncture, if sham puncture is insisted on, it is both unacceptable to patients and falls short of the placebo requirements.

Carefully planned cohort studies aiming to compare the effects of different means of pain control and other treatment expectations are therefore the only reasonable means to objectively look at the clinical effects of acupuncture. Many cohort studies of this nature are being done for the study of back pain, neck pain, arthritis of the knee, etc. The effects of puncture were compared with conventional techniques using physiotherapy and other means.

Another common application for acupuncture is the restoration of nerve function. Damaged neurological tissues suffer from a real lack of regeneration. Peripheral damage feasible for repair carries reasonable promise. When cell bodies are involved, either intra-cranially or in the spinal cord, loss of neurological and secondary muscular functions becomes permanent. Acupuncture is widely used under such difficult situations. Although many reports of impressive results are available, it is difficult to realise the real value. Scientific data coming from well-planned cohort studies for the observation of functional restoration is still difficult to interpret, since the damage could not be uniform and the factors affecting the different aspects of rehabilitation and functional return are multiple and complicated.

We are therefore still relying on careful case studies. However, one does not need to get upset with the obvious limitations. After all, in the field of rehabilitation, experience in the last three decades has already shown that qualified, broad, trustworthy clinical trials are not possible.[41] Although meta-analysis has ruled out the absolute scientific justification for all the rehabilitation attempts like different forms of physiotherapy, massage, bracing and even invasive means like injections and surgery, we could still rely on them because we have to release our patients from suffering. We are all aware of the fact that we are not certain which patient is the best candidate to receive which treatment.[42]

CONCLUSION

Complementary medicine does not have any history of modern scientific development. It built up its knowledge relying on observations and experience. Now that we try to make use of this traditional stream of medicine in a scientific world, we need to explain why it works in the area of our concern. Very often, these areas are not well served by scientific medicine. This makes the scientific explanations even more important.

The way to go about giving scientific explanations to healing processes involves the application of methodologies that are well known and accepted by all clinical scientists. The standard way to start a scientific approach to clinical trials using traditional Chinese medicine would just be an application of the same methodologies. However this approach is not feasible and would probably remain unfeasible in spite of enthusiasms. We are barred from a smooth application of the scientific methodology, basically because of the different philosophy behind the traditional Chinese way of healing. Moreover, the lack of knowledge about the exact chemistry of the active component of the herbal remedy when herbal drug trials are being carried out further jeopardises the validity of the clinical trials.

In spite of the essential difficulties, efficacy-driven trials are still carried out, utilising principles of evidence-based medicine. As long as the scientific gap is successfully narrowed, the practical use of complementary medicine will become safer, more logical and would deserve wider applications. At the same time, workers on complementary medicine should workout a unique, relevant system of assessment for the clinical effects.

REFERENCES

1. Bensky D, Gamble A. *Chinese Herbal Medicine. Materia Medica.* Seattle: Eastland Press (1993).
2. Tang W, Eisenberg G. *Chinese Drugs of Plant Origin: Chemistry, Pharmacology and Use in Traditional and Modern Medicine.* New York: Springer-Verlag (1992).
3. Su WT. *History of Drugs.* Beijing: United Medical University Press (1992).
4. McGuire MB. *Ritual Healing in Suburban America.* Newbrunswick: Rutgers University Press (1988).
5. Kong YC. *Formulation's from South-West Asia.* Beijing: Chinese University Press (1998).
6. Eisenberg DM, Roger DB. Trends in alternative medicine use in the USA 1990–1997. *JAMA* (1998) **280**(18): 1569–75.
7. Lai SL. *Clinical Trials of Traditional Chinese Materia Medica,* Chapter 1. Guangdong: People's Publishing House (2000).
8. Leung PC. Editorial – Seminar series on evidence-based alternative medicine. *Hong Kong Med J* (2001) **7**(4): 332–4.
9. Kaptchuk TJ, Eisenberg DM. The persuasive appeal of alternative medicine *Ann Int Med* (1998) **129**(12): 1061–5.
10. Eisenberg DM, Kessler RC, Foster C. Unconventional medicine in the USA – prevalence, costs and patterns of use. *New Engl J Med* (1998) **328**(4): 246–52.
11. Fair WR. The role of complementary medicine in urology. *J Urol* (1999) **162**: 411–20.
12. Leung PC. Traditional Chinese Medicine in China. Seminar on Health Care in Modern China, Yale–China Association (2001).
13. Leung PC. Development of traditional Chinese medicine in Hong Kong and its implications for orthopaedic surgery. *Hong Kong J Orthopaed surg* (2002) **6**(1): 1–5.
14. Ho T. An anthropologist's view on traditional chinese medicine. In: *A Practical Guide to Chinese Medicine.* Singapore: World Scientific (2002).
15. Chalmers I. The Cochrane Collaboration: preparing, maintaining and disseminating systemic reviews of the effects of health care. *Ann NY Acad Sci* (1993) **203**: 166–72.
16. Tyler VE. *Herbs of Choice: The Therapeutic use of Phytomedicinals.* New York: Pharmaceutical Product Press (1994).
17. Ernst E. Harmless herbs? A review of the recent literature. *Am J Med* (1996) **104**: 170–8.
18. Bisset Ng. *Herbal Drugs and Phytopharmaceuticals.* Boca Raton: Medpharm Scientific Publisher (1982).
19. Leung PC. Clinical trials in Chinese medicine – the efficacy driven approach. Hospital Authority Convention, Hong Kong (2001).
20. NIH. National Centre for Complementary and Alternative Medicine Five Year Strategic Plan 2001–2005. NIH Document (2000).
21. NIH. Acupuncture. *NIH Consensus Statement* (1997) **15**(5): 1–34.
22. Wang PY. *New Chinese Medicine: Research, Production and Registration.* China: Chinese Medicine Press (1995).
23. Chen KC. *Research in Chinese Medicine.* Beijing: China Health Publisher (1996).
24. Lai SL, ed., *Clinical Trials of Traditional Chinese Materia Medica,* Chapter 2, 3, 4. Guangdong: People's Publishing House (2001).
25. Chang CK (Han Dynasty). *Discussions of Fever.* Classics.
26. Li ZC (Ming Dynasty). *Materia Medica.* Classics.
27. Suen TM (Tang Dynasty). *Important Prescriptions.* Classics.
28. National Bureau on Drug Supervision. *Regulations on Clinical Trials Using Drugs and Herbs.* Bureau Publication (1999).
29. Suen TY, Wang SF, Wang KL. *Adverse Effects of Drug Treatment.* Beijing: People's Health Press (1998).
30. De Smet P, D'Arcy PF, eds. Drug interactions with herbal and other non-toxic remedies. In: *Mechanisms of Drug Interactions.* Berlin: Springer-Verlag, (1996).

31. Sackett DL. *Clinical Epidemiology*, 2nd edn. Boston: Little, Brown & Co. (1991) 297–9.

32. Uppsala Monitoring Centre, WHO. *Safety monitoring of medicinal products: guidelines for setting up and running a pharmacovigilance centre* (2000).

33. Jaeschke R, Singer J. Measurement of health status. Ascertaining the minimally important difference. *Contr Clin Trials* (1989) **10**: 407–15.

34. Wyrwick KW, Nienaber NA. Linking clinical relevance and statistical significance in health related quality of life. *Med Care* (1999) **37**: 469–78.

35. Stewart AL, Greenfield GS, Hayo RD. Functional status and well-being of patients with chronic conditions. *JAMA* (1989) **262**: 907–13.

36. Keininger DL. Why develop IQOD? International Health Related Quality of Life Outcome Database. *QoL News* (1999) **Sept/Dec** (23): 2.

37. Park J, White AD, Lee H, Ernst ED. Development of a new sham needle. *Acupunct Med* (1999) **17**(2): 347–52.

38. Streiberger K, Kleinhenz J. Introducing a placebo needle into acupuncture research. *The Lancet* (1998) **352**: 364–5.

39. Godfrey CM, Morgan P. A controlled trial of the theory of acupuncture in musculoskeletal pain. *J Rheumatol* (1978) **5**: 121–4.

40. Lewith GT, Machin D. On the evaluation of the clinical effects of acupuncture. *Pain* (1983) **16**: 111–27.

41. Nachemson E. Causes and treatment of low back pain. *American Academy of Orthopaedic Surgery Lecture Series* (1989).

42. Spitzer WO, Leblanc FE. Scientific approach to the assessment and management of activity-related spinal disorders. *Spine* (1987) **12**(Suppl. 1): 51–9.

CANCER

6

Breast Cancer

DONALD A. BERRY, TERRY L. SMITH AND AMAN U. BUZDAR

Department of Biostatistics, The University of Texas M. D. Anderson Cancer Center, Houston, TX 77030, USA

INTRODUCTION

More than 200 000 women in the United States are diagnosed annually with breast cancer. About 40 000 women die from the disease each year. Among women, it is the most common malignancy, and is exceeded only by lung cancer as the leading cause of cancer death. Although the risk of breast cancer is substantially higher in older women, many cases occur in young women. Of cases diagnosed in the US in 1998, 5% occurred in women under the age of 35, 30% in women aged 35 to 49, 31% in women aged 50 to 64, and 33% in women aged 65 or older.[1] For US women, the lifetime risk of developing breast cancer is about 13%. About 0.1% of US women carry an inherited mutation of a breast/ovarian cancer susceptibility gene, BRCA1 or BRCA2, and so have a lifetime risk in excess of 50%.

From 1940 to the early 1980s, breast cancer incidence in the US increased by a fraction of a percent per year when adjusted for age. Chiefly because of the widespread dissemination of screening mammography beginning in the early 1980s, invasive breast cancer incidence has increased by 3–4% per year into the 1990s. Over the same period, the rate of ductal carcinoma in situ (DCIS) increased by about sixfold, from about 5 cases per 100 000 women in 1980 to more than 30 per 100 000 in 1998.

Despite the increasing incidence of breast cancer among US women since the early 1980s, and perhaps indirectly because of this increase, the annual age-adjusted rate of breast cancer mortality has decreased by almost 2% per year in the 1990s. Researchers generally attribute this improvement in breast cancer survival to increased use of screening mammography and to improvements in the treatment of breast cancer. Efforts are underway to better delineate the relative impacts of factors influencing breast cancer survival (see CISNET[2] for additional information).

An important development for breast cancer research in the 1980s and 1990s was not directly related to science. These years saw the formation of strong advocacy groups that worked to promote research in breast cancer. Federal funding has increased more than sixfold since 1990, and grass-roots action has resulted in an unprecedented programme of breast cancer research funding administered by the Department of Defense. In addition, patient advocates have become highly educated about research

Textbook of Clinical Trials. Edited by D. Machin, S. Day and S. Green
© 2004 John Wiley & Sons, Ltd ISBN: 0-471-98787-5

issues and many serve regularly alongside professional scientists on various governmental boards guiding the direction of research expenditures and treatment recommendations. Patient advocates also serve on cooperative group committees that plan clinical trials in breast cancer, institutional review boards, and data safety monitoring boards.

Advocacy groups have worked to increase the number of women who participate in clinical trials. The Clinical Trial Initiative of the National Breast Cancer Coalition Fund (NBCCF) maintains a registry of clinical trials and urges women with breast cancer to participate (see NBCCF[3]). Before a clinical trial can be included in their registry, experts from the NBCCF ascertain that it addresses an important, novel research question related to breast cancer, and that its design is scientifically rigorous and employs appropriate and meaningful outcomes.

STAGING

Breast cancer is staged using a system developed by the American Joint Committee on Cancer, and based on the size and other characteristics of primary tumour (T), the status of ipsilateral lymph nodes (N), and the presence or absence of distant metastases (M) (AJCC[4] and Singletary et al.[5]). The stage of disease, ranging from 0 to IV, is based on combinations of these TNM rankings.

Stage 0 consists of ductal and lobular carcinoma in situ (DCIS, LCIS), non-invasive and possibly non-malignant forms of the disease. Stages I to III are invasive stages in which the tumour is confined to the breast or its immediate vicinity. Higher stage indicates larger primary tumours or greater locoregional tumour involvement. Patients having evidence of distant metastasis are classified as Stage IV.

Distribution of disease stage at the time of breast cancer diagnosis varies by country, depending on the health care system's approach to diagnosis and reporting. In the US, the approximate proportions of women diagnosed with Stage

0 through Stage IV disease are 21%, 42%, 29%, 5% and 4%, respectively.[1] An additional tumour classification method based on histopathologic examination has limited discrimination ability because 70–80% of tumours are of a single type: infiltrating ductal carcinoma.

PROGNOSIS

Breast cancer is heterogeneous. Many breast cancers are slowly growing and their carriers survive for many years and die of other causes. Other tumours are very aggressive and may have spread to distant sites by the time the primary tumour is diagnosed. This heterogeneity has implications for research in all phases of the disease, beginning with screening and diagnostic methods through the evaluation of treatments for advanced disease.

Stage is the most widely recognised determinant of patient outcome. Stage IV disease is generally regarded to be incurable, with median survival in the range of 18 to 24 months, although a small fraction of patients with Stage IV disease achieve complete remission following systemic chemotherapy, and survive for many years.[6] On the other hand, patients with Stage I disease, consisting of a small primary tumour and no involved lymph nodes, have at least a 90% probability of being disease-free after five years. Lymph node involvement is associated with a worse prognosis, with five-year disease-free rates ranging from 50–75%. Tumour grade, proliferative activity and menopausal status play relatively minor roles.

Although stage is an important prognostic factor, it is of limited use as a determinant of treatment outcome. The relative benefits of treatment are reasonably consistent across stages – although the absolute benefit can be much greater for higher stage disease. Much current research focuses on factors that may predict clinical benefit from certain treatment approaches ('predictive factors') in contrast to the more conventional 'prognostic factors' which are regarded as indicators of general tumour aggressiveness, irrespective of type of therapy.

The best-studied predictive factor is oestrogen-receptor (ER) status, which is an important indicator of whether a tumour will respond to hormonal treatment. Tamoxifen and other selective oestrogen-receptor modulators (SERMs) are highly effective in patients with hormone-sensitive breast cancer, but they have no benefit in patients whose tumours are ER negative and progesterone-receptor negative (Early Breast Cancer Trialists' Collaborative Group [EBCTCG][7]). Patients who benefit from SERMs may also benefit from aromatase inhibitors.[8]

HER-2 (also referred to as HER-2/neu, ErbB2, c-erbB-2) is a member of the epidermal growth factor receptor family that is overexpressed in 20% to 40% of breast tumours, and has been cited in numerous reports as conveying poor prognosis.[9] Studies in early breast cancer have suggested that patients with HER-2 positive tumours are more likely to benefit from anthracycline therapy.[10–12] Trastuzumab, a monoclonal antibody against HER-2, is effective in delaying progression in Stage IV disease that overexpresses HER-2,[13] and is being evaluated for its efficacy in treating HER-2-overexpressing primary tumours.

HISTORICAL PERSPECTIVE ON CLINICAL TRIALS IN BREAST CANCER

SURGERY AND RADIOTHERAPY

Scientific understanding of the biology of breast cancer has changed radically in the past 50 years. Results of large randomised trials have played a major role in this transition. From the nineteenth century and up into the 1970s, breast cancer was understood to be a local/regional disease that spread by direct extension along lymphatic pathways to distant sites. This concept gave rise to the surgical methods promoted by W.S. Halsted[14–16] around the turn of the twentieth century, i.e., extensive resection of the breast, regional lymphatics, lymph nodes and muscle. This surgical technique, known as radical mastectomy, remained the principal approach to treatment of breast cancer throughout the first half of the century, sometimes combined with radiotherapy.

When the concept of large-scale randomised clinical trials to investigate alternative therapies was proposed in the 1960s, controversy arose among breast cancer researchers as well as in other medical fields. In a heated exchange, a prominent breast cancer surgeon denounced such studies as 'a great leap backward in the treatment of breast cancer'.[17] Despite such opposition, pioneers in the field persisted in designing trials to address important therapeutic questions of the time, and moreover, were able to persuade patients to participate in this novel idea of assigning treatment by randomisation. These early trials compared various surgical and radiotherapy approaches. In a trial of almost 1700 women implemented in 1971, there were no significant survival differences between conventional radical mastectomy, total mastectomy with radiation, and total mastectomy with removal of axillary nodes.[18,19] Results of this and other trials of the era challenged long-held views of the disease and gradually convinced researchers that their concept of breast cancer as a local disease which could best be treated by radical local treatment techniques was incorrect. Rather, breast cancer came to be understood as a systemic disease that could benefit from systemic therapy, and radical local therapies were no longer regarded as essential for prolonging survival.

CHEMOTHERAPY

Cytotoxic agents for treatment of solid tumours were first developed in the 1950s. Breast cancer proved to be highly sensitive to several of these, when used as single agents in small trials. Subsequently, combinations of these cytotoxic agents were evaluated, one of the earliest being the Cooper regimen (cyclophosphamide, methotrexate, 5-fluorouracil, vincristine and prednisone).[20] With the understanding of breast cancer as a systemic disease and the proven sensitivity of breast cancer cells to cytotoxic agents, the stage was set for the rapid development of adjuvant chemotherapy once this concept was introduced in the

1970s. A randomised trial comparing surgery followed by combination chemotherapy to surgery alone demonstrated that disease recurrence could be significantly reduced using this adjuvant therapy approach.[21]

The introduction of doxorubicin for treatment of breast cancer is illustrative of the series of clinical trials typically undertaken for the development of new agents. Small trials conducted in solid tumours in the early 1970s established safety and dosing, and these were quickly followed by Phase II trials of the agent in metastatic breast cancer. Subsequently, doxorubicin was evaluated in combination with other agents, and randomised trials established that higher response rates could be achieved in metastatic disease with combinations that included doxorubicin. These successes prompted the introduction of various doxorubicin and other anthracycline-containing combinations as adjuvant therapy for primary breast cancer. Known by such acronyms as 'FAC' = 'CAF', 'FEC', 'AC', these combinations continue to play a prominent role in the treatment of breast cancer.[22,23] Anthracycline-containing therapies further reduce the risk of recurrence and favourably impact survival in early breast cancer.[24]

HORMONAL THERAPY

Hormonal therapy is a key component of therapy when tumours are hormone-receptor positive. Early trials focused on ovarian ablation by surgery or chemical means. The anti-oestrogen agent tamoxifen was introduced in the 1970s, at a time when there was high regard for the potential of cytotoxic agents, but little interest in hormonal therapies. Early small trials in metastatic breast cancer were equivocal and could have led to abandoning the agent. However, the weight of evidence from laboratory studies and several small trials pointed to superior efficacy with prolonged administration in ER positive disease. After a series of large randomised trials, tamoxifen is now regarded as standard therapy for pre- and post-menopausal women with ER positive tumours.[25] Tamoxifen may be the single

most important advance in treating breast cancer. Questions remain about the optimum treatment duration even though a trial conducted by the National Surgical Adjuvant Breast and Bowel Project (NSABP) comparing 5 and 10 years of tamoxifen therapy concluded there was little or no advantage to longer therapy.[26]

HIGH-DOSE CHEMOTHERAPY WITH BONE MARROW TRANSPLANT OR STEM CELL SUPPORT

An unresolved question in therapy of breast cancer that has presented an unusual challenge for the conduct of clinical trials is that of high-dose chemotherapy supported by autologous bone marrow transplant or peripheral blood progenitor cells. Ten trials addressing the question of high-dose versus standard-dose chemotherapy have been reported. Two of these were subsequently discredited following an international investigation. Only two of the remaining eight trials entered more than 200 patients. Financial issues, patient and physician acceptance and competing treatment strategies have compromised accrual, and it is unclear if ongoing trials can be completed. The available evidence suggests that high-dose therapy provides little or no benefit for patients regardless of their disease stage.[27,28]

MAMMOGRAPHY

Eight large randomised trials conducted since 1963 assessed the value of screening mammography for reducing breast cancer mortality. These are of particular interest for the scrutiny they have undergone in recent years. The preponderance of evidence from the randomised trials indicates a benefit associated with screening mammography.[29–31] However, a meta-analysis concluded that six of the eight trials were seriously flawed and the remaining two trials showed insignificant breast-cancer mortality differences between the screened and non-screened groups.[32] The National Cancer Institute recommends screening mammography every 1 to 2 years for women aged 40 and older, while recognising that there are risks associated with false-positive results.

PREVENTION

Beginning in the 1990s, coinciding with the detection of methods for identifying women at high risk of breast cancer, the first large-scale trials were mounted to determine if the incidence of breast cancer could be reduced in targeted high-risk groups. These trials established that breast cancer incidence could be greatly reduced by daily doses of tamoxifen.[33,34] This reduction was due entirely to a lower incidence of ER positive tumours with no change in the incidence of ER negative tumours. This suggests that prophylactic tamoxifen will not have as great an impact on survival as it does on incidence, although none of the prevention trials address survival as an endpoint. An ongoing trial (STAR: the Study of Tamoxifen and Raloxifene) will recruit 22 000 women at high risk of breast cancer in order to compare the effects of tamoxifen and another SERM, raloxifene, on the incidence of primary breast cancer.[35]

MAJOR TRIAL GROUPS

One of the largest cooperative groups conducting trials in breast cancer in the US is the NSABP. Trials from this group are often referred to by their 'B' numbers, e.g., B-06, which established the equivalence of lumpectomy to total mastectomy.[36] Other major cooperative groups conducting clinical trials in breast cancer are the Eastern Cooperative Oncology Group (ECOG), Cancer and Leukemia Group B (CALGB), Southwest Oncology Group (SWOG), Breast Cancer International Research Group (BCIRG), European Organisation for Research and Treatment of Cancer (EORTC), North Central Cancer Treatment Group (NCCTG), and the National Cancer Institute of Canada (NCIC).

An important information resource regarding the benefits of treatment for early breast cancer is the Early Breast Cancer Trialists' Collaborative Group (EBCTCG). This group, based at Oxford University, serves as a centre for data synthesis rather than actual conduct of clinical trials. Beginning in 1983, this group has collected data from virtually all major randomised trials conducted in early breast cancer, published or not. Data from more that 200 000 women have been analysed, using statistical techniques for meta-analysis, with results published at the end of each five-year analysis cycle, beginning in 1985. These publications have addressed the role of radiation, ovarian ablation, polychemotherapy, tamoxifen and quality of life; these 'overview' articles are frequently cited in support of treatment approaches.[7,24,25,37–42] The weaknesses of meta-analysis have been widely discussed in the statistical literature, chief among these being the issue of heterogeneity among the trials being combined. For example, the overviewers combine various therapeutic regimens under the single rubric 'polychemotherapy'. However, these overview reports have allowed researchers to reliably assess moderate-size treatment effects which could not have been detected in individual trials. Treatments causing even moderate reductions in mortality, if implemented widely among women with breast cancer, could prevent or delay thousands of deaths due to the disease. The meta-analysis has also addressed questions of treatment efficacy within subsets, for example the confirmation of benefit of adjuvant tamoxifen in ER positive pre-menopausal women[7] as well as in post-menopausal women.

TIME-DEPENDENT HAZARDS

In this section we address a methodological issue that arises quite generally in survival analysis. Consider disease-free survival. This is the usual primary outcome measure in evaluating adjuvant therapies, with results presented in the form of Kaplan–Meier survival curves and compared using statistical tests that take into account the entire survival distributions. The simple hazard function, which is in effect the derivative of the survival curve, can serve as an effective graphical aid to understanding treatment and covariate effects. Moreover, it can reveal important effects that are not apparent in the survival curves, themselves.

We will use trial CALGB 8541 as an example.[43] This trial considered three different dose schedules of CAF (cyclophosphamide, doxorubicin and 5-fluorouracil) in node positive breast cancer. The schedules consisted of four cycles of CAF at 600, 60, 600 mg/m^2 (high dose), six cycles at 400, 40, 400 mg/m^2 (moderate dose) or four cycles at 300, 30, 300 mg/m^2 (low dose). The primary endpoint was disease-free survival, which is shown in Figure 6.1 for the three dose groups using Kaplan–Meier plots. Details of the comparison are provided in the original report, and will not be repeated here.

Time-to-event curves such as those in Figure 6.1 do not tell the whole story regarding any benefit of increasing dose and dose intensity. A clearer picture is contained in plots of hazard over time. The hazard in any particular time period is the proportion of events occurring during that time period in comparison with the number of patients who are at risk at the beginning of the period. For example, if there are 100 patients in a group and 10 of these recur in the first year, then the first-year hazard is 10%. Going into the second year, only 90 patients are at risk. If another 10 recur in the second year,

then the second-year hazard is $10/90 = 11\%$. When calculating hazards from survival plots such as those in Figure 6.1 (which incorporate censored observations), we subtract the current year's survival proportion from the previous year's survival proportion and divide by the previous year's survival proportion. The resulting yearly values are shown in Figure 6.2.

Some authors like to smooth hazard estimates over time. We prefer to show the raw estimates. The reason is that each time period provides a 'nearly independent' trial of therapeutic comparisons. Depending on what assumptions are made about the underlying survival distribution, these trials may not be truly independent, but events that have occurred previously are set aside and a 'new trial' is begun. Each time period has the potential for confirming observations made in other time periods.

A striking observation from Figure 6.2 is that all three hazards decrease over time (after year 2). This is a reflection of the heterogeneity of breast cancer. The most aggressive tumours recur early, yielding the high hazards evident in the first few years. Once their tumours have recurred, patients are removed from the at-risk population. The remaining tumours tend to be less aggressive and so they recur at a lower rate.

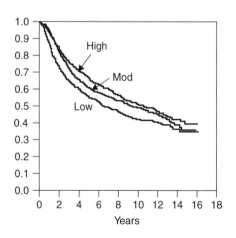

Figure 6.1. Disease-free survival proportion for the three CAF dose groups of CALGB 8541

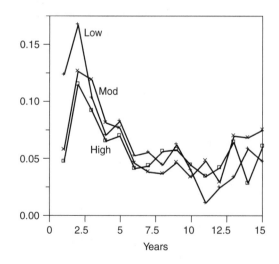

Figure 6.2. Hazards for the three CAF dose groups of CALGB 8541, derived from Figure 6.1

As regards treatment-arm effect, the apparent benefit of a regimen of high-dose chemotherapy is restricted to the first five years or so. Actually, the hazard for a high dose is lower than those of the other two arms in each of the first six years (although it is not much lower in years 4, 5 and 6, and it is not much lower than that for a moderate-dose regimen in any of the six years). In view of the 'near independence' of the six time periods, this observation is impressive. Another important observation from Figure 6.2 is that after five years the risks of all three groups come together, with the annual risk of recurrence being approximately 5% in all three groups.

The reduction in hazard of recurrence for high versus low doses is 14% over the 18 years of follow-up (95% confidence interval: 6–22%). This is an average over these years (weighted over time because of differences in at-risk sample sizes over time), but since there is no reduction at all in the later years, the overall reduction is being carried by the early years. Restricting to the first three years, the reduction is 24% (13–33%). A benefit of chemotherapy that is restricted to the first few years is typical in breast cancer trials. An implication is that a hazard reduction seen early in a trial, say one with a median of three years of follow-up, will deteriorate over time. This is because the comparison will eventually involve averaging over periods where there is no longer a treatment benefit.

In the later years, the hazards of about 5% are very similar to the annual hazard for node negative breast cancer patients. Interestingly, convergence to about 5% applies irrespective of the number of positive lymph nodes. Figure 6.3 shows this effect. It gives hazard plots for three categories of positive nodes: 1–3, 4–9 and 10 or more (for the three dose groups combined). Early in the trial, patients with 10+ positive nodes have a very high annual recurrence rate of 20–30%. However, after five years or so, the annual hazard is about 5% in all three groups. A patient with a large number of positive nodes who has not experienced recurrence in the first five years or so has the same updated prognosis as a patient with a small number of positive nodes, including

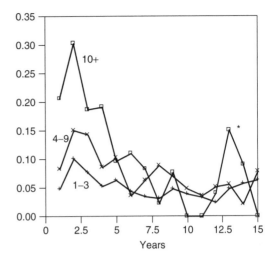

Figure 6.3. Hazards for the three categories of positive lymph nodes (1–3, 4–9 and 10 or more) for CALGB 8541. There are few patients at risk in the later years, especially in the 10+ group, and for two reasons. One is that this was the smallest group to start with (174 of the 1550 patients in the trial), and the other is that most recurred early. For example, the asterisk at 13 years indicates a time point at which there were only 24 patients at risk, and three of these recurred in the 13th year

no positive nodes. The effects of both the number of positive nodes and dose of CAF have elapsed after five years.

An important aspect of CALGB 8541 is the role of tumour HER-2/neu expression and in particular its interaction with dose of CAF.[10] HER-2/neu assessment was carried out for a subset of 992 patients from the original study. Its interaction with dose was shown to be significant in a multivariate proportional hazards model. But the manner of interaction is easiest to understand using hazards. Figure 6.4 shows the effect of dose of CAF separately for patients with HER-2/neu negative tumours ($n = 720$) and HER-2/neu positive tumours ($n = 272$). HER-2/neu negatives show no dose effect. The entire benefit of high dose over moderate dose and high dose over low dose that is observed in these patients is concentrated in patients whose tumours are HER-2/neu positive. Moreover, this

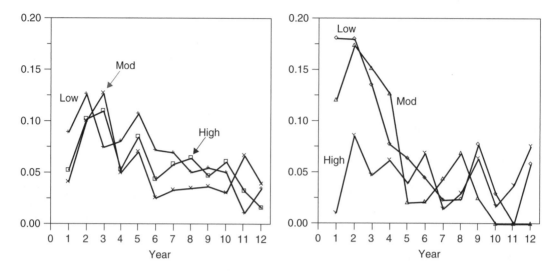

Figure 6.4. Annual disease-free survival hazards for a subset of patients ($n = 992$) in CALGB for whom expression of HER-2/neu in the patient's tumour was assessed. Patients in the left-hand panel had tumours that were HER-2/neu negative and the tumours of those in the right-hand panel were HER-2/neu positive

benefit occurs through a reduction in hazard in each of the first three to four years. Again, each year is a separate study and so each of these years provides a separate confirmation of the overall conclusion. The hazard reduction in the first three years for high dose as compared with the other two groups combined was 65% among patients whose tumours were HER-2/neu positive. HER-2/neu overexpression apparently conveys a poor prognosis for lower doses but not for a high dose – it might even provide a favourable prognosis for a high dose.

Many of the above conclusions would have been difficult or impossible without considering hazards over time. A final comment regarding hazards relates to the common problem of predicting survival results into the future for patients already accrued to a trial. Consider Figure 6.1. Some patients have as little as 10 years of follow-up information. As more follow-up information becomes available, there will be no change in these curves prior to the 10-year time point, but they may change subsequent to 10 years. Because the focus is on patients who have not yet recurred, the way the curves will change depends on the hazards beyond 10 years.

The information available about these hazards is shown in Figure 6.2. For predicting when and whether a patient recurs, hazards should be considered one year at a time, and based on the current year of follow-up.

ASSESSING LONG-TERM IMPACTS OF THERAPY

Showing that a cancer therapy is beneficial using logrank tests or proportional hazards regression models or whatever other analysis one uses, does not allow for concluding the nature of the benefit. It may be that some patients are cured of their disease; or the therapy may delay the disease's progress in some patients; or the effect may be a mixture of the two. Deciding among these possibilities may be possible when all or almost all events occur in a modest amount of follow-up time. In primary breast cancer, a goodly proportion of patients never recur. Therefore, such a decision is difficult or impossible to make.

Figure 6.5 illustrates the difficulty in discriminating between cure and prolonging survival in breast cancer trials. Consider a clinical trial that

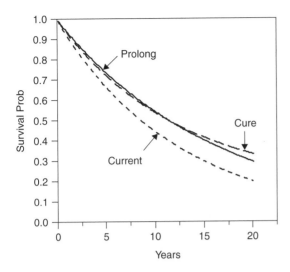

Figure 6.5. Hypothetical survival curves comparing cure and prolonging survival

long. Moreover, information beyond 20 years is relatively sparse because earlier events and competing risks (such as cardiovascular disease) will have removed patients from the at-risk population. To make inferential matters worse, there is an enormous array of possible curves that are similar to the two shown in the figure, with some having cure rates and others not. Finally, the 'current' survival distribution assumes that all breast cancer is fatal (although survival times vary). More realistically, some breast cancer (including some invasive as well as *in situ* breast cancer) will never kill the patient. Deciding whether a new therapy cures some patients is even more difficult if a proportion of patients is assumed to have non-fatal disease.

This inability to distinguish between curing patients and prolonging survival has further implications in the evaluation of screening and diagnostic methods. It is possible that breast cancers become lethal or not in their very early development, as suggested by studies of tumour markers purported to identify especially aggressive tumours. If this is so, then early detection may not help, and the observed benefits of therapy, however substantial, may be the result of slowing the progress of the disease rather than curing it. Such slowing may be beneficial whether it comes early or late in the disease.

is designed to evaluate a new therapy, one that may improve survival. Suppose further that in the population of interest, the current annual rate of breast cancer mortality is 8%. The corresponding survival distribution is shown by the dashed survival curve labelled 'current' in Figure 6.5. It assumes exponential survival (although the same effect holds for any parametric form) and so the current median survival is 8.66 years. The goal of the new therapy is to improve this by 1/3 to 11.55 years. If this happens then it may be through prolonging every patient's survival by reducing the annual mortality rate to 6% – the curve labelled 'prolong' – or by leaving the annual rate unchanged (at 8%) for most of the patients but curing a fraction of them – the curve labelled 'cure'. To have the same median (11.55 years) as 'prolong' implies a cure rate of 17.1%.

In view of the sampling variability present in empirical survival information, it is impossible to discriminate between the 'prolong' and 'cure' curves shown in Figure 6.5 on the basis of results of even impossibly large clinical trials. Indeed, the critical part of the follow-up period for this discrimination is 20 years and beyond, and few trials have followed patients for this

ADAPTIVE DESIGNS OF CLINICAL TRIALS

Adaptive designs have the dual goals of efficient learning from all relevant results and effective treatment of patients. They are more flexible than conventional designs, and have application in all phases of drug development. Such designs can be implemented using Bayesian methodology as a means to incorporate new information into the trial design.

Designs of clinical trials for breast cancer are usually static in the sense that the sample size and any prescription for assigning treatment, including the randomisation of patients, are fixed in advance. While designs may include stopping rules, such as the two-stage Phase II trial design of Simon,[44] or the interim comparisons in Phase III designs,[45,46] the criteria for early stopping are very conservative and therefore few trials actually stop early. The simplicity of trials with static design makes them solid inferential tools. The sample sizes tend to be large, with a straightforward treatment comparison as the objective. Despite their virtues, static trials result in slow and unnecessarily costly development of new therapeutic agents.

The tradition of drug development is to evaluate a single drug at a time. Given the fast pace of current new drug discovery (there are hundreds of known experimental drugs with potential benefits in breast cancer), these inefficient evaluation methods are no longer adequate. In addition to the traditional focus on false-positive and false-negative errors in standard drug testing, another kind of error applies to drugs not under investigation. Every such drug is a false neutral. Given the limited resources available to the medical establishment to develop new therapies, resource allocation must be approached in a more rational way. This is as true in breast cancer, for which a relatively large number of women are willing to participate in clinical trials, as it is for other forms of cancer. Pharmaceutical companies and medical researchers generally must be able to consider hundreds of drugs for development at the same time. Static trials inhibit the simultaneous processing of many drugs. They cannot efficiently address dose–response questions or prioritisation of similar agents when many drugs are under consideration. Dynamic designs that are integrated with the drug development process are necessary for reasonable progress in medical research.

Using an adaptive design means examining the accumulating data periodically – or even continually – with the goal of modifying the trial's design. These modifications depend on what the data show about the unknown hypotheses. Among the modifications possible are stopping early, restricting eligibility criteria, expanding accrual to additional sites, extending accrual beyond the trial's original sample size if its conclusion is still not clear, dropping arms or doses, and adding arms or doses. All of these

possibilities are considered in light of the accumulating information.

Adaptive designs also include unbalanced randomisation, in which the degree of imbalance depends on the accumulating data. For example, arms that give more information about the hypothesis in question or that are performing better than other arms can be weighted more heavily.[47] Current (Bayesian) probabilities that each of several doses or agents surpass standard or placebo therapy are calculated. These calculations use all information from patients treated to date. A new patient is then assigned to treatment randomly, with weights proportional to these probabilities. The assignments involve some degree of randomisation, but all patients are more likely to receive treatments that are performing better. Those that are doing sufficiently poorly become inadmissible in the sense that their assignment weight becomes 0. When and if we learn that a new agent is effective (or ineffective), we stop the trial. Patients in the trial benefit from data collected *in the trial*. The explicit goal is to treat patients more effectively, but in addition we learn about the new agents more efficiently. Initially we evaluate each design's frequentist operating characteristics using Monte Carlo simulation, possibly modifying the parameters of the assignment algorithm to achieve the desired characteristics.

Adaptive designs are being used increasingly in cancer trials. This is true for trials sponsored by pharmaceutical companies, and more generally. A variety of trials at The University of Texas M.D. Anderson Cancer Centre (MDACC) are prospectively adaptive. For example, we are building the foundation for a Phase II trial for evaluating drugs for breast cancer that is more a process than a trial. The idea is an extension of more general adaptive assignment strategies. We start with a number of treatment arms plus a control – possibly a standard therapy. We randomise to the arms and learn about their relative efficacy as the trial proceeds. Arms that perform better get used more often. An arm that performs sufficiently poorly gets dropped. An arm that does well enough graduates to Phase III, and if it does sufficiently well it might even replace the control. As more treatments become available, they are added to the mix and the process can continue indefinitely.

A trial of a new agent for treatment of metastatic breast cancer is being compared to the current standard therapy in a dynamic manner that allows the incorporation of newly available treatments in the randomisation process, as well as the elimination of treatments when a lack of improved efficacy can be established. Patients are randomised to treatments with weights proportional to the probability that a treatment is better than the standard therapy. The result is that superior therapies move through quickly and poorer therapies get dropped. Patients in the trial are provided with better treatment (when the arms are not equally good). Patients outside the trial get access to better treatments more rapidly.

Dose-finding trials of new agents are also conducted adaptively at MDACC, with dose assignment based on Bayesian updating of a model which relates dose and toxicity, using results from preceding patients. The model is the continual reassessment method or CRM.[48,49] Each patient is assigned to the dose having a probability of toxicity closest to some predetermined target value. This is the Bayesian posterior probability calculated from the data available up to that point (and so it is based on sufficient statistics).

The CRM more effectively finds the maximum tolerated dose (MTD) than does the conventional 3 + 3 design.[50] A way in which both the 3 + 3 and CRM designs are crude is the need to pause accrual while waiting for toxicity information.[51] Such pauses are inefficient and they cause logistical problems. Trials should be paused or stopped if there are safety concerns, not because the design cannot get out of its own way. In getting information about toxicity (or efficacy), there is seldom a magical dose that the next patient must get. All doses are potentially informative. Rather than stopping, one should use a design that models dose–response (toxicity and efficacy) and is able to assign a next dose even though patients previously treated are not

yet fully evaluable. Other improvements to dose-finding methods are underway. These include the simultaneous incorporation of efficacy results into the design, and the use of toxicity severity rather than the usual assumption that toxicity is dichotomous.

CONCLUSION

Breast cancer clinical trials are not fundamentally different from those of other cancers. However, breast cancer stands out for several reasons. First, it is common, and it is becoming even more common with the improvements in and greater use of detection methods. That implies a greater ability to investigate the potential for therapeutic agents and combinations. As a consequence, there have been hundreds of randomised clinical trials conducted in breast cancer, more by far than in any other cancer. Second, it is a disease that is fatal in only a minority of cases. Third, patient advocates in the breast cancer community have been very influential, both as a research force and a political force, in lobbying for research funding. Fourth, breast cancer has been shown to be sensitive to a number of chemotherapies and hormonal therapies. The advances that have been made in breast cancer therapy are more impressive than for any other type of cancer, except for testicular cancer and some forms of leukaemia that commonly affect children. These advances have been built on a foundation of clinical trials.

REFERENCES

1. Surveillance, Epidemiology, and End Results Program (SEER) Public-Use Data (1973–1998), National Cancer Institute, DCCPS, Surveillance Research Program, Cancer Statistics Branch, Bethesda, MD, August 2000 submission; released April 2001 [online database, available at http://seer.cancer.gov].
2. Cancer Intervention and Surveillance Modeling Network (CISNET) [online information site]. Available through the National Cancer Institute, US government, at http://cisnet.cancer.gov/about.
3. National Breast Cancer Coalition Fund (NBCCF). A patient guide to quality breast cancer care

[online information site]. Available at http://www.natlbcc.org/nbccf.

4. American Joint Committee on Cancer (AJCC) [online information site]. Available at http://www.cancerstaging.org.

5. Singletary SE, Allred C, Ashley P, Bassett LW, Berry D, Bland KI, Borgen PI, Clark G, Edge SB, Hayes DF, Hughes LL, Hutter RBP, Morrow M, Page DL, Recht A, Theriault RL, Thor A, Weaver DL, Wieand HS, Greene FL. Revision of the American Joint Committee on Cancer Staging System for Breast Cancer. *J Clin Oncol* (2002) **20**: 3628–36.

6. Greenberg PA, Hortobágyi GN, Smith TL, Ziegler LD, Frye DK, Buzdar AU. Long-term follow-up of patients with complete remission following combination chemotherapy for metastatic breast cancer. *J Clin Oncol* (1996) **14**: 2197–205.

7. Early Breast Cancer Trialists' Collaborative Group (EBCTCG). Tamoxifen for early breast cancer: an overview of the randomised trials. *Lancet* (1998) **351**: 1451–67.

8. Buzdar A, Howell A. Advances in aromatase inhibition: clinical efficacy and tolerability in the treatment of breast cancer. *Clin Cancer Res* (2001) **7**: 2620–35.

9. Yamauchi H, Stearns V, Hayes DF. When is a tumor marker ready for prime time? A case study of c-erbB-2 as a predictive factor in breast cancer. *J Clin Oncol* (2001) **19**: 2334–56.

10. Thor AD, Berry DA, Budman DR, Muss HB, Kute T, Henderson IC, Barcos M, Cirrincione C, Edgerton S, Allred C, Norton L, Liu ET. erbB-2, p53, and efficacy of adjuvant therapy in lymph node-positive breast cancer. *J Natl Cancer Inst* (1998) **90**: 1346–60.

11. Paik S, Bryant J, Tan-Chiu E, Yothers G, Park C, Wickerham DL, Wolmark N. HER2 and choice of adjuvant chemotherapy for invasive breast cancer: National Surgical Adjuvant Breast and Bowel Project Protocol B-15. *J Natl Cancer Inst* (2000) **92**: 1991–8.

12. Ravdin PM, Green S, Albain KS, Boucher V, Ingle J, Pritchard K, Shepard L, Davidson N, Hayes DF, Clark GM, Martino S, Osborne CK, Allred DC. Initial report of the SWOG biological correlative study of c-erbB-2 expression as a predictor of outcome in a trial comparing adjuvant CAF T with tamoxifen (T) alone. *Proc Am Soc Clin Oncol* (1998) **17**: 97a.

13. Slamon DJ, Leyland-Jones B, Shak S, Fuchs H, Paton V, Bajamonde A, Fleming T, Eiermann W, Wolter J, Pegram M, Baselga J, Norton L. Use of chemotherapy plus a monoclonal antibody against HER2 for metastatic breast cancer that overexpresses HER2. *N Engl J Med* (2001) **344**: 783–92.

14. Halsted WS. The results of operations for the cure of cancer of the breast performed at the Johns Hopkins Hospital from June 1889 to January 1894. *Ann Surg* (1894) **20**: 497–555.

15. Halsted WS. The results of radical operations for the cure of carcinoma of the breast. *Ann Surg* (1907) **SLVI**: 1–19.

16. Buchanan EB. A century of breast cancer surgery. *Cancer Invest* (1996) **14**: 371–7.

17. Haagensen CD. A great leap backward in the treatment of carcinoma of the breast. *JAMA* (1973) **224**: 1181–3.

18. Fisher B, Montague E, Redmond C, Barton B, Borland D, Fisher ER, Deutsch M, Schwarz G, Margolese R, Donegan W, Volk H, Konvolinka C, Gardner B, Cohn I, Lesnick G, Cruz AB, Lawrence W, Nealon T, Butcher H, Lawton R. Comparison of radical mastectomy with alternative treatments for primary breast cancer: a first report of results from a prospective randomized clinical trial. *Cancer* (1977) **39**: 2827–39.

19. Fisher B, Jeong J-H, Anderson S, Bryant J, Fisher ER, Wolmark N. Twenty-five-year follow-up of a randomized trial comparing radical mastectomy, total mastectomy, and total mastectomy followed by irradiation. *N Engl J Med* (2002) **347**: 567–75.

20. Cooper RG. Combination chemotherapy in hormone-resistant breast cancer. *Proc Am Assoc Cancer Res* (1969) **10**: abstr 57.

21. Bonadonna G, Brusamolino E, Valagussa P, Rossi A, Brugnatelli L, Brambilla C, DeLena M, Tancini G, Bajetta E, Musumeci R, Veronesi U. Combination chemotherapy as an adjuvant treatment in operable breast cancer. *N Engl J Med* (1976) **294**: 405–10.

22. Hortobágyi GN. Anthracyclines in the treatment of cancer. *Drugs* (1997) **54**(Suppl): 1–7.

23. Weiss RB. The anthracyclines: will we ever find a better doxorubicin? *Semin Oncol* (1992) **19**: 670–86.

24. Early Breast Cancer Trialists' Collaborative Group (EBCTCG). Polychemotherapy for breast cancer: an overview of the randomised trials. *Lancet* (1998) **352**: 930–42.

25. Early Breast Cancer Trialists' Collaborative Group (EBCTCG). Tamoxifen for early breast cancer (Cochrane Review) [online database, available at http://cochrane.de/cochrane]. *Cochrane Database Syst Rev* (2001) **1**: CD000486.

26. Fisher B, Dignam J, Bryant J, Wolmark N. Five versus more than five years of tamoxifen for lymph node-negative breast cancer: updated findings from the National Surgical Adjuvant Breast and Bowel Project B-14 randomized trial. *J Natl Cancer Inst* (2001) **93**: 684–90.

27. Farquhar C, Basser R, Hetrick S, Lethaby A, Marjoribanks J. High dose chemotherapy and

autologous bone marrow or stem cell transplantation versus conventional chemotherapy for women with metastatic breast cancer (Cochrane Review) [online database, available at http://cochrane.de/cochrane]. *Cochrane Database Syst Rev* (2003) **1**: CD003142.

28. Farquhar C, Basser R, Marjoribanks J, Lethaby A. High dose chemotherapy and autologous bone marrow or stem cell transplantation versus conventional chemotherapy for women with early poor prognosis breast cancer (Cochrane Review) [online database, available at http://cochrane.de/cochrane]. *Cochrane Database Syst Rev* (2003) **1**: CD003139.

29. Miller AB, Baines CJ, To T, Wall C. Canadian National Breast Screening Study: 1 – Breast cancer detection and death rates among women aged 40 to 49 years. *Can Med Assoc J* (1992) **147**: 1459–76.

30. Miller AB, Baines CJ, To T, Wall C. Canadian National Breast Screening Study: 2 – Breast cancer detection and death rates among women aged 50 to 59 years. *Can Med Assoc J* (1992) **147**: 1477–88.

31. Nystrom L, Andersson I, Bjurstam N, Frisell J, Nordenskjold B, Rutqvist LE. Long-term effects of mammography screening: updated overview of the Swedish randomised trials. [erratum in *Lancet* (2002) **360**: 724]. *Lancet* (2002) **359**: 909–19.

32. Gøtzsche PC, Olsen O. Is screening for breast cancer with mammography justifiable? *Lancet* (2000) **355**: 129–34.

33. Fisher B, Costantino JP, Wickerham DL, Redmond CK, Kavanah M, Cronin WM, Vogel V, Robidoux A, Dimitrov N, Atkins J, Daly M, Wieand S, Tan-Chiu E, Ford L, Wolmark N. Tamoxifen for prevention of breast cancer: report of the National Surgical Adjuvant Breast and Bowel Project P-1 Study. *J Natl Cancer Inst* (1998) **90**: 1371–88.

34. IBIS investigators. First results from the International Breast Cancer Intervention Study (IBIS-I): a randomised prevention trial. *Lancet* (2002) **360**: 817–24.

35. Vogel VG. Follow-up of the breast cancer prevention trial and the future of breast cancer prevention efforts. *Clin Cancer Res* (2001) **7**: 4413s–18s.

36. Fisher B, Anderson S, Bryant J, Margolese RG, Deutsch M, Fisher ER, Jeong J-H, Wolmark N. Twenty-year follow-up of a randomized trial comparing total mastectomy, lumpectomy, and lumpectomy plus irradiation for the treatment of invasive breast cancer. *N Engl J Med* (2002) **347**: 1233–41.

37. Early Breast Cancer Trialists' Collaborative Group (EBCTCG). Effects of adjuvant tamoxifen and of cytotoxic therapy on mortality in early breast cancer: an overview of 61 randomized trials among 28,896 women. *N Engl J Med* (1988) **319**: 1681–91.

38. Early Breast Cancer Trialists' Collaborative Group (EBCTCG). *Treatment of Early Breast Cancer*, Vol. I, *Worldwide Evidence 1985–1990*. Oxford: Oxford University Press (1990).

39. Early Breast Cancer Trialists' Collaborative Group (EBCTCG). Systemic treatment of early breast cancer by hormonal, cytotoxic, or immune therapy: 133 randomised trials involving 31,000 recurrences and 24,000 deaths among 75,000 women. *Lancet* (1992) **339**: 1–15; 71–85.

40. Early Breast Cancer Trialists' Collaborative Group (EBCTCG). Effects of radiotherapy and surgery in early breast cancer: an overview of the randomized trials. *N Engl J Med* (1995) **333**: 1444–55.

41. Early Breast Cancer Trialists' Collaborative Group (EBCTCG). Ovarian ablation in early breast cancer: overview of the randomised trials. *Lancet* (1996) **348**: 1189–96.

42. Early Breast Cancer Trialists' Collaborative Group (EBCTCG). Favourable and unfavourable effects on long-term survival of radiotherapy for early breast cancer: an overview of the randomised trials. *Lancet* (2000) **355**: 1757–70.

43. Budman DR, Berry DA, Cirrincione CT, Henderson IC, Wood WC, Weiss RB, Ferree CR, Muss HB, Green MR, Norton L, Frei III E. Dose and dose intensity as determinants of outcome in the adjuvant treatment of breast cancer. *J Natl Cancer Inst* (1998) **90**: 1205–11.

44. Simon R. Optimal two-stage designs for phase II clinical trials. *Control Clin Trials* (1989) **10**: 1–10.

45. O'Brien PC, Fleming TR. A multiple testing procedure for clinical trials. *Biometrics* (1979) **35**: 549–56.

46. Lan KKG, DeMets DL. Discrete sequential boundaries for clinical trials. *Biometrika* (1983) **70**: 659–63.

47. Berry DA, Fristedt B. *Bandit Problems: Sequential Allocation of Experiments*. London: Chapman-Hall (1985).

48. O'Quigley J, Pepe M, Fisher L. Continual reassessment method: a practical design for phase I clinical trials in cancer. *Biometrics* (1990) **52**: 673–84.

49. Goodman S, Zahurak M, Piantadosi S. Some practical improvements in the continual reassessment method for phase I studies. *Stat Med* (1995) **14**: 1149–61.

50. Ahn C. An evaluation of phase I cancer clinical trial designs. *Stat Med* (1998) **17**: 1537–49.

51. Thall PF, Lee JJ, Tseng C-H, Estey E. Accrual strategies for phase I trials with delayed patient outcome. *Stat Med* (1999) **18**: 1155–69.

7

Childhood Cancer

SHARON B. MURPHY[1] AND JONATHAN J. SHUSTER[2]

[1]Children's Cancer Research Institute, University of Texas Health Science Centre, San Antonio, TX 78229-3900, USA

[2]College of Medicine, University of Florida, Gainesville, FL 32610-0212, USA

INTRODUCTION

There are substantial differences in the conduct of clinical cancer research in children compared to adults. First, childhood cancer is comparatively rare. According to statistics released by the National Cancer Institute SEER programme in 1999,[1] it is estimated that approximately 12 400 children and adolescents, younger than 20 years of age, are diagnosed annually with cancer. Stated another way, the average annual age-adjusted incidence rate for all childhood cancers is 150 per million persons, aged <20. This is under 2% of the total cancers diagnosed in the USA. Despite the rarity and notwithstanding the spectacular success in treatment of paediatric cancer, compared to incidence and mortality rates of cancer occurring among adults, cancer is the leading cause of death from disease among children and adolescents. Only accidents and firearms kill more children than cancer. Further, the distribution of cancer diagnoses in children is very different from that in adults. There are a number of major

tumours, such as Wilm's tumour, retinoblastoma, rhabdomyosarcoma, neuroblastoma, Ewing's sarcoma and osteogenic sarcoma, for example, that are either exclusively or predominantly paediatric in nature. In contrast, carcinomas of differentiated epithelial tissues, like the aerodigestive tract or breast or prostate, do not occur in children. Thanks to the usual lack of co-morbid conditions and concomitant illnesses, children usually have a greater tolerance to cancer therapy than adults. Taken together with the differing spectrum of cancer seen, the host differences related to age necessitate that paediatric studies of anti-cancer drug dosage, efficacy and safety are needed. Recognising that children are not just small adults and that special considerations apply, the FDA has issued regulations mandating the testing of new drugs in paediatric patients.

Given the fact that modern treatments result in cure of 75–80% of all children and adolescents with cancer who are managed appropriately, the long-term consequences of therapy for children are also potentially much greater than in adults, as the therapy can interfere with normal growth and development, leaving them exposed for

---

Textbook of Clinical Trials. Edited by D. Machin, S. Day and S. Green
© 2004 John Wiley & Sons, Ltd ISBN: 0-471-98787-5

decades at risk for serious sequelae, major organ disturbance, such as cardiac damage and cognitive dysfunction, or second malignancies. Children diagnosed with cancer generally also have less of a problem with competing mortality risks, when compared to adult cancer.

Given these factors, to adequately size childhood cancer research studies, a substantial proportion of the incident cases must be enrolled. In fact, in some situations, such as randomised Phase III trials of new regimens compared to already effective front-line treatments, nationwide multi-institutional trials are a necessity. These trials will need to enroll nearly every child in the target population with the disease being studied for three to five years, with many years of follow-up needed to assess long-term outcomes. Accrual duration in childhood trials may be considerably longer than a corresponding adult trial. However, since clinical practice closely approximates that of the ongoing study, it is rare that progress from an external source ever renders the study question obsolete. Finally, given the rarity of childhood cancer, and the desirability of study designs of maximal efficiency, it is often desirable to conduct '2 × 2 factorial studies', where two interventions are used in the same trial (Standard vs. Standard + A vs. Standard + B vs. Standard + A + B). Such designs carry some risk where there is a qualitative interaction between the two interventions. For example, this would occur if the impact of A is highly dependent upon whether B is given or not. Hence the choice of randomised interventions needs to take this pitfall into account when such factorial designs are considered.

Based on previous trials and internal registry data of the major national paediatric cooperative oncology groups, Table 7.1 provides estimates of the potential accrual to the Children's Oncology Group (COG), a consortium of about 230 American, Canadian, European and Australasian medical centres. COG was formed in 2000 by the merger of the Pediatric Oncology Group (POG), the Children's Cancer Group (CCG), the Intergroup Rhabdomyosarcoma Study Group (IRSG) and the National Wilm's Tumor

Table 7.1. Major categories of paediatric cancer and projected annual accrual of the Children's Oncology Group

Leukaemia

Infant ALL[a]: 50
'Standard Risk' B-Precursor ALL[a]: 1100
'High Risk' B-Precursor ALL[a]: 600
T-Cell ALL[a]: 240
Philadelphia Chromosome Positive (Ph+) ALL[a]: 20
B-Cell (SIg+)ALL[a]: 45
ANLL[a]: 300

Lymphoma

Hodgkin's Disease: 250
'Early Stage' NHL[a]: 90
'Advanced Stage' Lymphoblastic NHL[a]: 90
'Advanced Stage' Large Cell NHL[a]: 80
'Advanced Stage' Small Non-Cleaved Cell NHL[a]: 125

Brain Tumours

Astrocytoma: 140
Medulloblastoma: 140
Glioma: 70
Ependymoma: 35

Sarcomas

Ewing's Sarcoma: 80
Osteosarcoma: 170
'Low Risk' Rhabdomyosarcoma: 64
'Intermediate Risk' Rhabdomyosarcoma: 99
'High Risk' Rhabdomyosarcoma: 21

Kidney

Wilm's Tumour: 480

Embryonal

'Low Risk' Neuroblastoma: 200
'Intermediate Risk' Neuroblastoma: 110
'High Risk' Neuroblastoma: 150
Hepatoblastoma: 65
Germ Cell Tumours: 25

[a]ALL = Acute Lymphoblastic Leukaemia
AML = Acute Non-Lymphoblastic Leukaemia
NHL = Non-Hodgkin's Lymphoma.

Study Group (NWTSG). Virtually every US or Canadian hospital with a childhood paediatric haematology/oncology division belongs to COG. Note that the anticipated annual accrual to COG trials does not mirror incidence figures, as there is a substantial gap between incident rates and rates of referral of newly diagnosed paediatric cancer patients to member institutions of COG and participation in clinical trials. Ross *et al.*[2] analysed 21 026 incident paediatric cancer cases, diagnosed from 1989–91, and compared observed to expected numbers of cases seen at member institutions of POG and CCG and found vastly different ratios (observed/expected) depending on age and site, and to a much less extent, geographic region. According to this survey, 92% of children aged less than 15 years in the US received their care at a CCG or POG institution, thereby providing at least a mechanism approximating population-based studies. However, the ratio (O/E) for 15–19 year olds was only 0.21, pointing to an adolescent gap in access to national cancer clinical trials at qualified institutions.

As seen in Table 7.1, the Children's Oncology Group runs Phase III clinical trials in a wide variety of tumours, with accrual ranging from as few as 20 patients per year to over 1000 per year. The Children's Oncology Group is also heavily involved in correlative science, pilot studies of potential Phase III interventions, as well as standard Phase I (dose escalation) studies and Phase II (early efficacy) studies. The group places special emphasis on translational research (biologic correlation studies) and cancer control (supportive care studies to limit long-term side effects and epidemiologic studies to learn about the aetiology of childhood cancer). Due to the presumably genetic origin of most forms of childhood cancer and the short lag time between symptoms and diagnosis, prevention trials and screening trials are difficult to do in paediatric cancer, with neuroblastoma,[3] which is based on urinary screening for elevated levels of catecholamines, a notable exception.

This chapter is organised into several sections. In the first section, major accomplishments in the area of childhood cancer treatment are discussed. In the following section, examples are cited where translational research has affected the design of paediatric cancer trials. In the succeeding section, the typical methods of designing trials for the Children's Oncology Group

are presented. A special section dealing with the ethical aspects and unique considerations affecting the conduct of clinical trials in children is also included. The final section is devoted to a look into the future.

HISTORY AND PERSPECTIVES ON IMPORTANT PAEDIATRIC CANCER CLINICAL TRIALS

Statistically and clinically significant improvements have been achieved in all major forms of childhood cancers through conduct of well-organised single institution and cooperative group clinical trials which have resulted in sequential and steady improvement in survival rates since the 1960s when curative treatments were first devised. SEER data document that the overall childhood cancer mortality rates have consistently declined throughout the 1975–95 time period.[1] Documentation of the overall progress achieved by POG investigators has been reported, demonstrating significant improvements in overall survival (OS) and event-free survival (EFS) for 8 of 10 disease areas, in a sample of over 7000 children and adolescents treated between 1976 and 1989.[4] Similar results have been achieved by CCG and by European national paediatric cooperative clinical trials organisations. There is also evidence that children and adolescents with acute lymphocytic leukaemia (ALL), non-Hodgkin's lymphoma (NHL), Wilm's tumour, medulloblastoma and rhabdomyosarcoma enjoy a significant survival advantage when treated according to well-defined protocols, compared to paediatric patients not enrolled on protocols and treated outside of paediatric cancer centres.[5] Most probably the inclusion benefit related to participation in clinical trials is a result of a number of factors, including the rigorous process of protocol development, incorporation of rapid pathology review and reference laboratories, defined staging practices and procedures, on-study review of radiotherapy port films, and close monitoring for toxicity and efficacy. Some of the important advances achieved in treatment of paediatric cancers are listed in Table 7.2.

Table 7.2. Examples of important advances resulting from paediatric cancer clinical trials

---

- Adjuvant chemotherapy improves survival from 20% to 70% in non-metastatic osteosarcoma of the extremity.[50]
- Doxorubicin improves outcome when added to other chemotherapy for Ewing's sarcoma[51] and the addition of ifosfamide and etoposide to vincristine, adriamycin, cyclophosphamide and actinomycin results in greater benefit.[52]
- Radiation therapy does not improve survival for patients receiving chemotherapy with Stage I and II, Wilm's tumour,[53,54] Stage I rhabdomyosarcoma[55] or localised non-Hodgkin's lymphoma.[56]
- Demonstration of improved event-free survival in high-risk neuroblastoma receiving myeloablative therapy in conjunction with autologous bone marrow transplantation and subsequent treatment with 13-cis-retinoic acid compared to chemotherapy alone.[57]
- Attainment of 80% 4-year event-free survival rates for standard risk B-precursor ALL.[58]
- Achievement of 78% EFS for patients with loco-regional embryonal rhabdomyosarcoma through intensification of chemotherapy in Intergroup Rhabdomyosarcoma Study (IRS)-IV.[59]

Success in treatment of the most common form of paediatric malignancy, acute lymphoblastic leukaemia (ALL), has been most gratifying. Indeed, a major reason for improvements in overall survival for childhood cancer in general is due to improvement in survival rates for ALL, which accounts for roughly a third of paediatric cancer.[1] With modern chemotherapy, 97–99% of children can be expected to attain complete remission, and it is not inconceivable to predict that modifications of the currently most successful protocols will boost long-term leukaemia-free survival rates to as high as 85–90%. Treatment success has been achieved through post-induction intensification/consolidation and re-induction treatments, effective treatments ('prophylaxis') for subclinical central nervous system leukaemia, and prolonged anti-metabolite-based continuation treatments of 24–36 months duration. Advances have been achieved by many single institutions and cooperative groups treating childhood leukaemias, including investigators at St. Jude Children's Research

Hospital in Memphis who pioneered a 'Total Therapy' curative approach beginning in the 1960s. It is beyond the scope of this chapter to review the treatment advances achieved through clinical trials for ALL by the BFM (Berlin–Frankfurt–Münster) Group, POG, CCG, the Dana Farber Consortium, the Medical Research Council/UKALL, the Dutch Childhood Leukaemia Study Group, the French Acute Lymphoblastic Leukaemia Cooperative Group (FRALLE) and the Italian Association of Paediatric Haematology–Oncology (AIEOP), but the interested reader may consult reviews summarising the spectacular progress achieved in treatment of ALL.[6]

The lymphomas, Hodgkin's disease (HD) and non-Hodgkin's lymphomas (NHL), are the third most common form of paediatric malignancy, next in frequency behind leukaemias and tumours of the central nervous system. Currently 80–90% of all children and adolescents with malignant lymphomas are curable with optimal multidisciplinary management, based on immunopathologic classification, staging for determination of disease extent, and design and selection of risk-adapted therapies. Paediatric investigators at Stanford, beginning in 1970, first pioneered combined modality treatment for children with HD and demonstrated that low-dose involved field radiotherapy combined with multiple cycles of chemotherapy (MOPP or MOPP/ABVD) resulted in cure of 90% of paediatric patients.[7] Similarly outstanding rates of disease control with combined modality management of paediatric HD have since been reported by others, establishing the curability of HD in nearly all cases, such that the thrust of current trials in paediatric HD is towards reduction of serious late effects of HD treatments, such as secondary malignancies, particularly leukaemia, infertility, pulmonary fibrosis and restrictive lung disease, serious cardiac problems and premature death.

The non-Hodgkin's lymphomas occurring among children and adolescents are virtually all high-grade, diffuse malignancies, differing markedly from the distribution of histologic types typically seen among older adults. Staging systems in use for childhood and adult NHL also differ.[8]

Ninety percent of localised NHLs, regardless of histology, are readily cured by nine weeks of chemotherapy without radiation.[9]

Progress in the treatment of paediatric solid tumours has been equally striking in the last 30 years as the progress in treating childhood leukaemias and lymphomas, and may be attributable to development of accurate diagnostic methods and systems of disease staging and effective multimodal treatments combining surgery, chemotherapy and radiation. Cure rates for rhabdomyosarcoma have increased from approximately 25% in 1970 to greater than 75% currently, to 60–70% for non-metastatic bone sarcomas, to over 80% for Wilm's tumour, over 90% for retinoblastoma, over 90% for infants and children with localised neuroblastoma, and to over half of all children with brain tumours.

Aims of current trials are to increase or preserve high cure rates, decrease acute toxicity and long-term adverse sequelae of treatment, decrease costs and improve the quality of life for children with readily curable cancers. Patients with high risk or metastatic disease at diagnosis or those who recur after front-line therapies continue to pose challenges and should properly benefit from pilot trials and Phase I or II studies of new treatments.

PROGNOSTIC FACTORS, TRANSLATIONAL RESEARCH AND THERAPEUTICALLY RELEVANT RISK GROUPS

Successful childhood cancer research is in large part dependent upon its translational research programme. Over the past three decades, initial diagnosis and classification of childhood cancer has become far more sophisticated, as laboratory scientists have collaborated closely with clinical investigators. In addition, special biological and pharmacological studies, conducted during and after treatment, offer tools to clinical investigators that were never previously available. As a result, paediatric oncologists, surgeons, pathologists and collaborating statisticians have the opportunity and the obligation to design and stratify trials specifically for biologically defined, risk-adapted subsets of patients. For example, the National Wilms' Tumor Study-5, a therapeutic trial and biology study, was designed to reduce treatment intensity for the subgroup(s) of patients with the most favourable prognosis and intensify treatment for the patients with the least favourable prognosis, based on stage, histology (favourable or unfavourable, anaplastic, rhabdoid and clear cell types), tumour size and bilaterality, and to investigate the impact of loss of heterozygosity (LOH) of chromosome 16q and 1p on two-year relapse-free survival through collection of tumour and normal kidney tissue for DNA analysis and banking.

Perhaps the best example of important translational research that has led directly to therapeutic implications is in the collection of bone marrow specimens for cytogenetic studies in childhood acute lymphocytic leukaemia (ALL).[10] While classical karyotype analysis is typically informative in 60–70% of the patients, important genetic markers can now be identified by probes, using FISH (fluorescence *in situ* hybridisation) or PCR (polymerase chain reaction) in virtually all patients. Translocations, such as the t(4;11),[11–13] t(9;22)[14–16] and t(1;19),[17,18] confer an adverse prognosis and lead to targeting the patients for more aggressive therapy. On the other hand, patients with the cryptic t(12;21) genetic lesion encoding the TEL-AML1 transcript,[19–21] with hyperdiploid leukaemia identified by flow cytometric measurement of DNA index (typically 53+ chromosomes in their primary clone),[22,23] or with specific trisomies detected by FISH, such as 4, 10 and 17,[23,24] have a more favourable outcome and can be targeted for less intensive treatment. As an example of the latter, POG investigators designed a trial (#9201) with less intense chemotherapy for ALL patients with lesser risk of relapse, defined by initial white blood cell counts <50 000, age between 1 and 10 years, absence of CNS disease, and presence of one or both of the following: DNA index >1.16, and/or trisomies of chromosomes 4 and 10 by FISH.

In addition to the well-recognised prognostic importance of initial white blood cell count, age at diagnosis, extramedullary disease and blast cell genetic features in B-precursor ALL and their significance for stratification and trial design, the early response to therapy, presence of minimal residual disease (MRD), and pharmacologic and pharmacokinetic variables are also predictive of outcome. Slow early response to induction treatment is predictive of an adverse outcome and can be defined in several ways: slow clearance of circulating blast cells to one week of prednisone or multiagent induction, or greater than 25% marrow blasts on day 7 (or day 14) of treatment. Quantitation of MRD by immunologic methods or PCR assay of rearranged T-cell-receptor or immunoglobulin heavy-chain genes of leukaemic blasts as clonal markers of leukaemia in patients in clinical remission has been shown to identify patients at elevated risk for relapse, a factor which (arguably) should be taken into account in assigning alternative treatment.[25,26] Wide variability in absorption of orally administered chemotherapy, such as 6-mercaptopurine, and inter-patient variability in systemic exposure to both methotrexate and 6-mercaptopurine are important determinants of outcome in ALL.[27,28] Graham et al.[29] uncovered a pharmacologic interaction between methotrexate and cytosine arabinoside when given simultaneously, and demonstrated a correlation between host drug levels and adverse outcome. Individual variability in response to cancer treatment is surely related to genetic polymorphisms in drug-metabolising enzymes, transporters, receptors and other drug targets, and suggests that these genetic differences may form a solid scientific basis for optimising therapies within the context of clinical trials.[30]

Given the plethora of prognostic factors now known for most paediatric malignancies, a pragmatic and rational approach to clinical trials design and stratification consists of risk assignment by a combination of clinical and biological factors identified through multivariate analysis to be of prognostic significance. Treatment is then tailored to risk status, commonly considering variables such as patient age, extent of disease and tumour biology. For example, the risk

assignments for the Intergroup Rhabdomyosarcoma Study V (shown in Table 7.3) are based on favourable prognostic factors identified in Studies I–IV, conducted from 1972 through 1991, and include (1) undetectable distant metastases at diagnosis; (2) primary sites in the orbit and non-parameningeal head/neck and genitourinary non-bladder/prostate regions; (3) grossly complete surgical removal of localised tumour at diagnosis; (4) embryonal/botryoid histology; (5) tumour size ≤ 5 cm; and (6) age younger than 10 years at diagnosis. Patients defined as shown into low, intermediate and high risk are predicted to have an estimated three-year EFS rate of 88%, 55–76% and <30%, respectively.[31]

Similarly, significant advances in translational research is neuroblastoma, which accounts for 8 to 10% of all childhood cancers, have resulted in a refined risk-related approach to therapy based on the age of the patient, the stage of the tumour according to the International Neuroblastoma Staging System (INSS), histopathologic features, the number of N-myc copy numbers and the ploidy of tumour cells (Table 7.4).

Because childhood cancer is rare, national reference laboratories have been established to analyse and store samples from the membership of the Children's Oncology Group as well as other large institutions and other international paediatric clinical trials organisations. Such laboratories help the research programme in terms of scientific expertise, quality control and correlative science. Few institutions can afford to maintain such laboratories solely for their own paediatric cancer patients, and web-based informatics applications afford access to the most sophisticated on-line resources and information even in smaller remote centres.

STUDY DESIGN FOR CHILDHOOD CANCER TRIALS

PHASE I STUDY DESIGN

Because childhood cancer is rare and the response to conventional treatment good, most children never experience recurrent disease and are thus

Table 7.3. Risk group assignments for intergroup Rhabdomyosarcoma Study Group study V

Risk (protocol)	Stage	Group	Site	Size	Age	Histology	Metastasis	Nodes	Treatment
Low, subgroup A (D9602)	1	I	Favourable	a or b	<21	EMB	M0	N0	VA
	1	II	Favourable	a or b	<21	EMB	M0	N0	VA + XRT
	1	III	Orbit only	a or b	<21	EMB	M0	N0	VA + XRT
	2	I	Unfavourable	a	<21	EMB	M0	N0 or NX	VA
Low, subgroup B (D9602)	1	II	Favourable	a or b	<21	EMB	M0	N1	VAC + XRT
	1	III	Orbit only	a or b	<21	EMB	M0	N1	VAC + XRT
	1	III	Favourable (excluding orbit)	a or b	<21	EMB	M0	N0 or N1 or NX	VAC + XRT
Intermediate (D9803)	2	II	Unfavourable	a	<21	EMB	M0	N0 or NX	VAC + XRT
	3	I or II	Unfavourable	a	<21	EMB	M0	N1	VAC (+XRT, Gp II)
	3	I or II	Unfavourable	b	<21	EMB	M0	N0 or N1 or NX	VAC (+XRT, Gp II)
	2	III	Unfavourable	a	<21	EMB	M0	N0 or NX	VAC ± Topo + XRT
	3	III	Unfavourable	a	<21	EMB	M0	N1	VAC ± Topo + XRT
	3	III	Unfavourable	b	<21	EMB	M0	N0 or N1 or NX	VAC ± Topo + XRT
	1 or 2 or 3	I or II or III	Favourable or unfavourable	a or b	<21	ALV/UDS	M0	N0 or N1 or NX	VAC ± Topo + XRT
	4	I or II or III or IV	Favourable or unfavourable	a or b	<10	EMB	M1	N0 or N1 or NX	VAC ± Topo + XRT
High (D9802)	4	IV	Favourable or unfavourable	a or b	≥10	EMB	M1	N0 or N1 or NX	CPT-11, VAC + XRT
	4	IV	Favourable or unfavourable	a or b	<21	ALV/UDS	M1	N0 or N1 or NX	CPT-11, VAC + XRT

Favourable = orbit/eyelid, head and neck (excluding parameningeal), genitourinary (not bladder or prostate) and biliary tract.
Unfavourable = bladder, prostate, extremity, parameningeal, trunk, retroperitoneal, pelvis, other.
a = tumour size ≤5 cm in diameter; b = tumour size >5 cm in diameter.
EMB = embryonal, botryoid, or spindle-cell rhabdomyosarcomas or ectomesenchymomas with embryonal RMS.
ALV = alveolar rhabdomyosarcomas or ectomesenchymomas with alveolar RMS, UDS = undifferentiated sarcomas.
N0 = regional nodes clinically not involved; N1 = regional nodes clinically involved; NX = node status unknown.
VAC = vincristine, actinomycin D, cyclophosphamide; XRT = radiotherapy; Topo = topotecan; Gp = Group; CPT-11 = irinotecan.

Source: Reproduced from Raney et al.[31] (p. 218), with permission.

Table 7.4. International Neuroblastoma Staging System (INSS)

Stage 1:   Localized tumour continued to the area of origin; complete gross resection, with or without microscopic residual disease; identifiable ipsilateral and contralateral lymph node negative for tumour.

Stage 2A: Unilateral with incomplete gross resection; identifiable ipsilateral and contralateral lymph node negative for tumour.

Stage 2B: Unilateral with complete or incomplete gross resection; with ipsilateral lymph node positive for tumour; identifiable contralateral lymph node negative for tumour.

Stage 3:   Tumour infiltrating across midline with or without regional lymph node involvement; or unilateral tumour with contralateral lymph node involvement; or midline tumour with bilateral lymph node involvement.

Stage 4:   Dissemination of tumour to distant lymph nodes, bone marrow, liver or other organs except as defined in stage 4S.

Stage 4S: Localized primary tumour as defined in stage 1 or 2, with dissemination limited to liver, skin or bone marrow

Risk group and protocol assignment schema: POG and CCG

INSS stage	Age (y)	N-*myc* status	Shimada histology	DNA ploidy	Risk group/study
1	0–21	Any	Any	Any	Low
2A and 2B	<1	Any	Any	Any	Low
	≥1–21	Nonamplified[a]	Any	NA	Low
	≥1–21	Amplified[b]	Favourable	NA	Low
	≥1–21	Amplified	Unfavourable	NA	High
3	<1	Nonamplified	Any	Any	Intermediate
	<1	Amplified	Any	Any	High
	≥1–21	Nonamplified	Favourable	NA	Intermediate
	≥1–21	Nonamplified	Unfavourable	NA	High
	≥1–21	Amplified	Any	NA	High
4	<1	Nonamplified	Any	Any	Intermediate
	<1	Amplified	Any	Any	High
	≥1–21	Any	Any	NA	High
4S	<1	Nonamplified	Favourable	>1	Low
	<1	Nonamplified	Any	1	Intermediate
	<1	Nonamplified	Unfavourable	Any	Intermediate
	<1	Amplified	Any	Any	High

[a] N-*myc* copy number ≤10.
[b] N-*myc* copy number >10.

POG, Pediatric Oncology Group; CCG, Children's Cancer Group; INSS, International Neuroblastoma Staging System; NA, not applicable.

Source: Reproduced from Castleberry,[60] (pp. 926, 930), with permission from Elsevier.

not eligible for trials of new agents. Phase I trials are designed to estimate the maximal tolerated dose of a drug, to determine the nature and frequency of toxicities, and to define the drug pharmacokinetics. While eligibility varies, patients have typically failed front-line therapy and usually they will also have failed second-line therapy. Because of the small number of paediatric patients eligible for Phase I trials, most

are accomplished as multi-institutional collaborations. Paediatric drug development requires separate Phase I studies (i.e., separate and distinct from studies done in adults) because paediatric patients may tolerate either higher or lower levels of drugs and may exhibit toxicities unique to children. Separate trials warranting emphasis may also reflect unique agents active in paediatric tumours, differing from agents that are of the highest priority for cancers common among adults.

The basic design is to begin at about 80% of the adult maximal tolerated dose. Patients are entered in cohorts and treated at increasing doses. At each level, three patients are typically accrued. If there is no dose-limiting toxicity amongst the three patients, the dose is raised to the next level (usually a 20–30% escalation), in successive cohorts of patients with no intrapatient dose escalation. If two or all three of these initially accrued patients experience dose-limiting toxicity (DLT), the maximum tolerated dose (MTD) will have been deemed exceeded. Finally, if one patient amongst the initial three patients experiences dose-limiting toxicity, an additional three patients are accrued. If six patients are needed, a dose escalation will occur if a total of one in six (i.e. zero of the next three) has dose-limiting toxicity. If two or more (i.e. one or more of the next three) experience dose-limiting toxicity, the maximal tolerated dose will be deemed to have been exceeded. The MTD is defined as the dose level immediately below the level at which two patients in three to six experience DLT. The definition of dose-limiting toxicity can vary from study to study, but it generally falls into two categories: (a) Grade 3, 4 or 5 non-haematologic toxicity other than (1) Grade 3 nausea/vomiting; (2) Grade 3 transaminase elevation; and (3) Grade 3 fever/infection and (b) Grade 4 myelosupression, that lasts more than 7 days, which requires transfusions twice in 7 days, or causes a delay in therapy exceeding 14 days. While the study is temporarily closed after accrual of each set of three patients in order to assess patient-specific responses and toxicities, a patient reservation system is used to obtain places when and if the study reopens. Phase I trials often require the evaluation of many dose levels. At a given dose level, the probabilities of declaring that the MTD has been exceeded are 9.3%, (50%) and [83%], when the true probabilities of dose-limiting toxicities are respectively 0.1, (0.3) and [0.5].

Consensus guidelines established by American and European investigators for the conduct of paediatric Phase I trials have been established.[32] A problem recently identified is the determination of MTDs in paediatric trials that are lower than those defined in adult patients, which may relate to differences in the intensity of prior therapy between adult and paediatric patients entered onto Phase I trials. There is a well-established association between prior therapy and reduced tolerance to myelotoxic drugs. If current paediatric Phase I trials in heavily pretreated patients define MTDs that tend to be lower than those determined in adult patients with minimal prior therapy, then application of the paediatric MTD to less heavily pretreated paediatric patients, e.g., in Phase II trials, may be problematic.

PHASE II STUDY DESIGN

The specific purpose of a Phase II trial is to determine activity, i.e., to develop estimates of the response rate of patients with specific tumour types to a particular drug or novel combination. Eligible patients typically will have relapsed on a front-line therapy, and the prospect of a cure is unlikely. Typically, the dependent variable is an objective all or none response variable such as achievement of a complete or partial (>50%) response. Interim results are masked from the participants until the study closes to accrual and response information for all patients has been established. There are three types of Phase II trial designs that depend upon the study objectives.

Testing Activity

The most common is 'proving activity'. For these studies, a fixed objective response rate is specified for activity (null hypothesis), and the goal is to reject the hypothesis in favour of the alternate hypothesis that the response rate is greater than this fixed figure. Generally, since the number of Phase II agents that can be tested is large in comparison to patient availability, sequential designs are preferred. However, as Simon[33] pointed out, it is rarely advantageous to go beyond two stages. Two excellent references with regard to Phase II design are Simon[33] and Shuster[34] The designs of Simon[33] stop at the first stage only if lack of activity is demonstrated. His argument is that patients should benefit from active drugs. However, in paediatrics, due to the relative scarcity of patients with recurrent disease, designs that stop early for either lack of activity or proven activity are preferred.

Historical Comparison

Another strategy for defining efficacy would be to prove a response rate is superior to that seen in an historical control study. The response rate of the new study is statistically compared to that of the control therapy. Makuch and Simon[35] have provided methods to determine the sample size requirements for these studies. Chang et al.[36] have extended this to two-stage designs (i.e., a sequential approach that could save patient resources).

Randomised Phase II Comparison

Due to a limited availability of patients, it is exceedingly rare that a randomised comparison of a new agent to a control is feasible in a paediatric Phase II study. However, such studies have been done. See McWilliams et al.[37] for an example from childhood neuroblastoma. As above, two-stage or group sequential designs are the preferred method. The programme EAST[38] can be used for designs that allow for both early acceptance and early rejection of the null hypothesis that the new treatment is equivalent to the control treatment.

In paediatric oncology, with limited patient numbers, only one or two cooperative Phase II trials are conducted with each new agent, and all malignancies refractory to standard therapy are typically combined into a single paediatric Phase II trial, usually stratified by histology. Not surprisingly, Phase II trials of novel multiagent regimens provide greater evidence of activity than single agent Phase II trials and offer considerable possibility of therapeutic benefit.[39]

PHASE III DESIGN

These studies typically ask a randomised question about either survival or event-free survival (the time from study entry to the earliest of induction failure, relapse, second cancer, or death of any cause). Intent-to-treat[40] is the analysis of choice for efficacy, with other analysis done as secondary supportive inference. For treatment questions where the randomised divergence is considerably after study entry or where a significant number of failures are expected to occur before divergence, a delayed randomisation is typically done as close to the divergence point as possible. For these randomisations, the dependent variable would be event-free survival from the randomisation date.

Phase III studies are typically designed assuming either proportional hazards or the cure model of Sposto and Sather.[41] In either case, the designs are group sequential in nature with planned interim analyses. In the case of proportional hazards, the O'Brien–Fleming method[42] is used. The reader is referred to Shuster[43] for specific details. Nearly all Phase III childhood cancer trials are run either as two-armed studies or as 2×2 factorial studies. It is rare that sufficient numbers of paediatric cancer patients are available to conduct three-armed studies, except perhaps in ALL, the most commonly occurring malignancy. The type of questions utilised in 2×2 factorial studies must be such that the expectation is for no 'qualitative interaction' between the two interventions. A qualitative interaction between treatments A and B would occur if a standard regimen plus A is superior to the standard regimen alone, but the standard plus A plus B is inferior to the standard plus B. For example, if a study is to randomise leukaemia patients to receive or not receive regimen A, designed to have an impact on the CNS, while at the same time to receive or not receive regimen B, designed to have an impact on marrow remission, a factorial design would seem appropriate. Essentially, we can run two studies for the price of one. If the two interventions have much in common, this would be a contraindication for a factorial design. In contrast, if we wished to ask if the same drug had an impact in induction therapy (first intervention) and in maintenance therapy (second intervention), there is, at least intuitively, the plausibility that the advantage of both interventions over just one may be zero or even harmful.

Phase III studies done in cooperative groups are required by the NCI to have a Data Safety and Monitoring Board which reviews the study at a minimum of every six months for toxicity and at planned intervals for efficacy, until it releases the study to the study committee. The release can occur no sooner than the earlier of (1) all subjects have completed the planned intervention or (2) the study was closed early and a new intervention is needed for patients on one or both arms. Any release prior to the planned date of final analysis requires approval of the board. Double-blind Phase III studies are rarely feasible due to the toxic nature of cancer treatment. However, they are encouraged for studies of supportive care, as long as the intervention is given in a pill form, and has no major known side effects requiring special medical monitoring.

Negative questions are often posed for paediatric cancer. For such studies, a very high cure rate of at least 85% has been shown possible on a conventional regimen. The question posed is can we do 'almost as well' with reduced therapy? To answer such questions with confidence requires large numbers, and it is rare that even the entire patient resources of COG are sufficient to address this in a randomised manner. For example, if a disease has a historical 4-year remission rate of 90%, and an accrual rate of 200 patients per year, a randomised study would take 6 years of accrual (10-year duration) to have 95% power to detect a degradation to 85% under reduced therapy at $p = 0.20$, one-sided. (Note that the typical values of type I error and power are reversed.) A single-arm study would require 315 patients to ask the same question of a fixed standard of 90% vs. a reduction to 85% (nearly a 75% reduction in sample size). While the benefits of reduced therapy may be obvious, such studies carry considerable risk and must be carefully monitored for early evidence that the reduction in therapy is unsafe and is associated with an inferior outcome.

ANCILLARY STUDIES

In paediatric cancer, there is considerable activity in translational research (see above). This can take the form of biologic studies, late effects, or in controlling acute side effects. These studies are designed on a case-by-case basis. Examples include the conduct of case–control 'tissue bank' studies to establish a promising prognostic marker. Cases are defined as patients failing a protocol (typically a relapse) and controls are long-term successes. These studies can be done using sequential designs, typically two-stage designs. Other typical studies might look at cognitive impairment (multivariate analysis of variance of neuropsychological variables), acute toxicity of a specified type (typical Chi-square test), the prognostic significance of serial pharmacologically measured drug levels (time-dependent covariate in survival analysis), or exploratory analysis (e.g. microarrays).

ETHICAL AND OTHER SPECIAL CONSIDERATIONS AFFECTING CONDUCT OF TRIALS IN CHILDREN WITH CANCER

Children and adolescents constitute a special vulnerable population of research subjects, often grouped with other special classes, like the mentally retarded, mentally ill and prisoners. There are special federal protections which apply to all research involving children as subjects which are covered by Subpart D of Part 46 of Title 45 of the Code of Federal Regulations (45 CFR 46), requiring that institutional review boards (IRBS) give consideration to the degree of risk, the benefit to child subjects, the nature of the knowledge to be gained, permission of the parent or guardian, and the concurrence of the child subjects, known as assent. A child's capacity to give assent is conditioned by his or her developmental level.[44,45]

Subsequent to the promulgation of the original rules, adopted in 1983 and modified in 1991, there has been nearly continuous debate and controversy surrounding safeguards for all human subjects of research and for children especially.

The tragic death of an 18-year-old research subject in 1999 in a gene-transfer trial at a major research university in which human subjects were not protected, adverse events had not been reported and financial conflicts of interest were involved, served to trigger several new federal initiatives to further strengthen protections of human research subjects in clinical trials,[46] including the imposition of sanctions on investigators who fail to adhere to regulations. As this chapter goes to press, the federal Office for Protection from Research Risks (OPRR) has been reorganised, expanded and renamed the Office for Human Research Protections (OHRP) and transferred to the Office of the Secretary, Health and Human Services (HHS) and the National Biothetics Advisory Commission, at the request of the President, has undertaken a sweeping examination of the ethical and policy issues in the oversight of human research in the United States (see www.bioethics.gov). As a result, the ethical and regulatory framework within which paediatric cancer clinical trials are conducted, now and in the future, will continue to evolve, and investigators must remain abreast.

Specific ethical issues impacting statisticians involved in collaborative research include ensuring confidentiality, data and safety monitoring, and problems and pitfalls in interpretation of interim analyses and planning studies to answer negative questions.[47] A negative question, e.g., what is the minimum therapy needed to produce cure?, has particular relevance for paediatric cancer trials which are (often) aimed at reduction of the acute or delayed effects of cancer treatment on the growing child.

Notwithstanding the strict ethical guidelines and regulations surrounding research in children, there is substantial and even increasing pressure to enroll children in clinical trials as a result of other federal policies and recent legislation, including the Food and Drug Administration's (FDA's) 1998 paediatric rule, the paediatric provisions of the FDA Modernization Act (FDAMA) of 1997, and the sweeping Children's Health Act of 2000 (PL 106–310), the sum of which is certain to increase paediatric clinical trials, particularly drug trials. Federal NIH policies promulgated in 1998 were aimed at increasing the participation of children in research so that adequate data would be developed to support the treatment for disorders affecting adults which also affect children, and rules mandated that children (i.e., individuals under age 21) must be included in all human subjects research unless there are scientific and ethical reasons not to include them. The FDA rules and regulations[48] require pharmaceutical manufacturers to assess the safety and effectiveness of new drugs and biologics in paediatric patients and established powerful economic incentives for manufacturers (six-months' extension of market exclusivity) on any drug for which FDA requested paediatric studies (see www.fda.gov/cder/cancer for further information on regulatory aspects of paediatric oncology drug development).

In addition to ethical and regulatory issues which impact the conduct of paediatric trials, there are also practical problems associated with clinical cancer research in children. Due to an understandably greater concern for long-term adverse consequences of treatment in a population of patients, the majority of whom are likely to be cured and alive for decades at risk for late effects, it is absolutely essential that long-term follow-up and serial surveillance of survivors is built into the studies. While follow-up is essential, it is also exceedingly difficult and expensive to maintain, as children and adolescents grow up, go away to school, leave home, marry, change name, etc. The frequency and severity of late effects also tend to progress with time off treatment, making follow-up beyond 15 or 20 or 30 years critical and identification of risk factors for the development of these late consequences of treatment essential. For example, Lipshultz et al.[49] studied 120 survivors of childhood ALL or osteogenic sarcoma who had been treated with doxorubicin a mean of 8.1 years earlier (range 2–14 years) and compared their cardiac function to a control population, and evaluated the impact of gender, age at diagnosis, length of time since completion of therapy, and dosage and cumulative dose of doxorubicin on cardiac status. Calculating sex-specific standardised scores or z scores (expressed as the number of standard deviations above or below the value for the normal controls) for cardiac contractility, wall thickness and afterload, the results of univariate and multivariate analysis showed that female sex and higher cumulative dose of doxorubicin were associated with depressed contractility, that there was an association between younger age at diagnosis and reduced left ventricular wall thickness and increased afterload, and that the prevalence and severity of abnormalities increased with longer follow-up.[49] Such studies typify the challenge of methodologic and statistical issues in the study of late effects of childhood cancer, the greatest challenge being data collection.

A LOOK INTO THE FUTURE OF CHILDHOOD CANCER RESEARCH

Despite the progress of the last half century there remain a number of challenges in childhood cancer. The focus of research in certain patient subsets with very high cure rates will be on quality of life endpoints. For example, retinoblastoma is curable in nearly 100% of cases, so preservation of sight and reduction of second malignances (not survival) are now considered to be the primary goals and endpoints, and trials avoiding enucleation and eliminating external beam therapy are now the norm.

One would hope that future therapies for childhood cancer will be developed which would be more rational, less empirical and less toxic, relying more on strategies for growth control (e.g., anti-angiogenesis) and regulation of gene expression and cell proliferation, and/or induction of apoptotic pathways or blocking of anti-apoptotic signals, than on cytotoxic or ablative treatments. Assuming that deregulated and/or mutated cellular proto-oncogenes or loss of tumour suppressor genes are the proximate cause(s) of most forms of childhood cancer, then the genes and/or their protein products will very likely be the targets for the next generation of paediatric anti-cancer agents, many of which will likely be orphan drugs for orphan diseases.

With advances in translational research, the pie (universe of childhood cancer patients) will be divided into smaller but more homogeneous slices than ever before. International collaboration will probably be required in a substantial segment of cancer types in order to obtain sufficient patient numbers to conduct randomised trials. Enlightened partnerships between industry and academia, with the assistance of the FDA and NCI, will be needed for efficient development of new agents.

Finally, the skill sets necessary to conduct paediatric cancer research are expanding. Traditionally the field involved paediatric haematologist/oncologists, surgeons, radiation oncologists, pathologists, nurses, clinical research associates, pharmacologists, epidemiologists and biostatisticians. Today, diagnostic imagers, bench scientists, geneticists, pharmacists, clinical psychologists, health economists and others also play significant roles in the research. In the future, other fields of expertise will surely need to be added to the team. The cooperation of a multidisciplinary team and prompt referral of patients to paediatric cancer centres participating in clinical trials will be critical to achieving future goals of refining and improving therapy.

REFERENCES

1. National Cancer Institute, SEER Program. *Cancer Incidence and Survival among Children and Adolescents: United States SEER Program 1975–1995.* NIH Publ. No. 99–4649. Bethesda, MD: National Cancer Institute (1999).
2. Ross JA, Severson RK, Pollock BH, Robison LL. Childhood cancer in the United States. A geographic analysis of cases from the Pediatric Cooperative Clinical Trials Groups. *Cancer* (1996) **77**: 201–7.
3. Woods WG, Tuchman M, Robison LL *et al*. A population-based study of the usefulness of screening for neuroblastoma. *Lancet* (1996) **348**: 1682–7.
4. Pediatric Oncology Group. Progress against childhood cancer: the Pediatric Oncology Group experience. *Pediatrics* (1992) **89**(4): 597–600.

5. Murphy SB. The national impact of clinical cooperative group trials for pediatric cancer. *Med Pediat Oncol* (1995) **24**: 279–80.

6. Pui CH. *Childhood Leukemias*. Cambridge: Cambridge University Press (1999).

7. Donaldson SS, Link MP. Combined modality treatment with low-dose radiation and MOPP chemotherapy for children with Hodgkin's disease. *J Clin Oncol* (1987) **5**(5): 742–9.

8. Murphy SB. Classification, staging, and end results of treatment of childhood non-Hodgkin's lymphomas: dissimilarities from adults. *Sem Oncol* (1980) **7**: 332–9.

9. Link M, Shuster J, Donaldson S, Berard CW, Murphy SB. Treatment of children and young adults with early-stage non-Hodgkin's lymphoma. *New Engl J Med* (1997) **337**(18): 1259–66.

10. Shuster JJ, Carroll AJ, Look TA *et al.* Management of cytogenetic data in multi-center leukemia trials. *Comput Methods Programs Biomed.* (1993) **40**: 269–77.

11. Pui CH, Frankel LS, Carroll AJ *et al.* Clinical characteristics and treatment outcome of childhood acute lymphoblastic leukemia with the t(4;11)(q21;q23): a collaborative study of 40 cases. *Blood* (1991) **77**: 440–7.

12. Pui CH, Carroll AJ, Raimondi SC *et al.* Childhood acute lymphoblastic leukemia with the t(4;11)(q21;q23): an update. *Blood* (1994) **83**: 2384–5.

13. Heerema NA, Sather HN, Ge J *et al.* Cytogenetic studies of infant acute lymphoblastic leukemia: poor prognosis of infants with t(4;11) – a report of the Children's Cancer Group. *Leukemia* (1999) **13**: 679–86.

14. Ribeiro RC, Broniscer A, Rivera GK *et al.* Philadelphia chromosome-positive acute lymphoblastic leukemia in children: durable responses to chemotherapy associated with low initial white blood cell counts. *Leukemia* (1997) **11**: 1493–6.

15. Uckun FM, Nachman JB, Sather HN *et al.* Poor treatment outcome of Philadelphia chromosome-positive pediatric acute lymphoblastic leukemia despite intensive chemotherapy. *Leukemia Lymphoma* (1999) **33**: 101–6.

16. Arico M, Valsecchi MG, Camitta B *et al.* Outcome of treatment in children with Philadelphia chromosome-positive acute lymphoblastic leukemia. *N Engl J Med* (2000) **342**: 998–1006.

17. Crist WM, Carroll AJ, Shuster JJ *et al.* Poor prognosis of children with pre-B acute lymphoblastic leukemia is associated with the t(1;19)(q23;p13): a Pediatric Oncology Group study. *Blood* (1990) **76**: 117–22.

18. Uckun FM, Sensel MG, Sather HN *et al.* Clinical significance of translocation t(1;19) in childhood acute lymphoblastic leukemia in the context of contemporary therapies: a report from the Children's Cancer Group. *J Clin Oncol* (1998) **16**: 527–35.

19. Shurtleff SA, Buijs A, Behm FG *et al.* TEL/AML1 fusion resulting from a cryptic t(12;21) is the most common genetic lesion in pediatric ALL and defines a subgroup of patients with an excellent prognosis. *Leukemia* (1995) **9**: 1985–9.

20. Rubnitz JE, Shuster JJ, Land VJ *et al.* Case–control study suggests a favorable impact of TEL rearrangement in patients with B-lineage acute lymphoblastic leukemia treated with antimetabolite-based therapy: a Pediatric Oncology Group study. *Blood* (1997) **89**: 1143–6.

21. Raimondi SC, Shurtleff SA, Downing JR *et al.* 12p abnormalities and the TEL gene (ETV6) in childhood acute lymphoblastic leukemia. *Blood* (1997) **90**: 4559–66.

22. Trueworthy R, Shuster J, Look T *et al.* Ploidy of lymphoblasts is the strongest predictor of treatment outcome in B-progenitor cell acute lymphoblastic leukemia of childhood: a Pediatric Oncology Group study. *J Clin Oncol* (1992) **10**: 606–13.

23. Heerema NA, Sather HN, Sensel MG *et al.* Prognostic impact of trisomies of chromosomes 10, 17, and 5 among children with acute lymphoblastic leukemia and high hyperdiploidy (>50 chromosomes). *J Clin Oncol* (2000) **18**: 1876–87.

24. Harris MB, Shuster JJ, Carroll A *et al.* Trisomy of leukemic cell chromosomes 4 and 10 identifies children with B-progenitor cell acute lymphoblastic leukemia with a very low risk of treatment failure: a Pediatric Oncology Group study. *Blood* (1992) **79**: 3316–24.

25. Cave H, van der Werff ten Bosch J, Suciu S *et al.* Clinical significance of minimal residual disease in childhood acute lymphoblastic leukemia. European Organization for Research and Treatment of Cancer – Childhood Leukemia Cooperative Group. *N Engl J Med* (1998) **339**: 591–8.

26. Campana D, Pui CH. Detection of minimal residual disease in acute leukemia: methodologic advances and clinical significance. *Blood* (1995) **85**: 1416–34.

27. Evans WE, Crom WR, Abromowitch M *et al.* Clinical pharmacodynamics of high-dose methotrexate in acute lymphocytic leukemia. Identification of a relation between concentration and effect. *New Engl J Med* (1986) **314**: 471–7.

28. Koren G, Farrazini G, Sulh H *et al.* Systemic exposure to mercaptopurine as a prognostic factor in acute lymphocytic leukemia in children. *New Engl J Med* (1990) **323**: 17–21.

29. Graham ML, Shuster JJ, Kamen BA *et al.* Changes in red blood cell methotrexate pharmacology and their impact on outcome when

cytarabine is infused with methotrexate in the treatment of acute lymphocytic leukemia in children: a Pediatric Oncology Group study. *Clin Cancer Res* (1996) **2**: 331–7.

30. Evans WE, Relling MV. Pharmacogenomics: translating functional genomics into rational therapeutics. *Science* (1999) **286**: 487–91.

31. Raney RB, Anderson JR, Barr FG *et al*. Rhabdomyosarcoma and undifferentiated sarcoma in the first two decades of life: a selective review of intergroup Rhabdomyosarcoma Study Group experience and rationale for intergroup rhabdomyosarcoma study V. *J Ped Hematol/Oncol* (2001) **23**: 215–20.

32. Smith MD, Ho P, Ungerleider R *et al*. The conduct of Phase I trials in children with cancer. *J Clin Oncol* (1998) **16**: 966–78.

33. Simon R. Optimal two-stage designs for phase II clinical trials. *Contr Clin Trials* (1989) **10**: 1–10.

34. Shuster JJ. Optimal two-stage designs for single arm Phase II cancer trials. *J. Pharm. Statist* (2002) **12**: 39–51.

35. Makuch R, Simon R. Sample size considerations for non-randomized comparitive studies. *J Chron Dis* (1980) **33**: 175–81.

36. Chang M, Shuster J, Kepner J. Group sequential designs for phase II trials. *Contr Clin Trials* (1999) **20**: 353–64.

37. McWilliams N, Hayesm F, Green A *et al*. Cyclophosphamide/doxorubicin vs. cisplatin/teniposide in the treatment of children older than 12 months of age with disseminated neuroblastoma: a Pediatric Oncology Group randomized Phase II study. *Med Pediat Oncol* (1995) **24**: 176–80.

38. Mehta C. *EaST (Early Stopping in Clinical Trials)*. Cambridge, MA: Cytel Software Corp. (1992).

39. Weitman S, Ochoa S, Sullivan J *et al*. Pediatric Phase II cancer chemotherapy trials: a Pediatric Oncology Group study. *J Ped Hematol/Oncol* (1997) **19**: 187–91.

40. Armitage P. Controversies and achievements in clinical trials. *Contr Clin Trials* (1984) **5**: 67–72.

41. Sposto R, Sather H. Determining the duration of comparative clinical trials while allowing for cure. *J Chronic Dis* (1985) **38**: 683–90.

42. O'Brien PC, Fleming TR. A multiple testing procedure for clinical trials. *Biometrics* (1979) **35**: 549–56.

43. Shuster J. Power and sample size for phase III clinical trials of survival. Chapter 7. In: Crowley J, ed., *Handbook of Statistics in Clinical Oncology*. New York: Marcel Dekker (2001).

44. Jonsen AR. Research involving children: recommendations of the National Commission for the Protection of Human Subjects of Biomedical and Behavioral Research. *Pediatrics* (1978) **62**(2): 131–6.

45. Leikin SL. Minors' assent or dissent to medical treatment. *J Pediat* (1983) **102**(2): 169–76.

46. Shalala D. Protecting research subjects – what must be done. *N Engl J Med* (2000) **343**(11): 808–10.

47. Shuster J *et al*. Ethical issues in cooperative cancer therapy trials from a statistical viewpoint, II. Specific issues. *Am J Ped Hematol/Oncol* (1985) **7**(1): 64–70.

48. Hirschfeld S *et al*. Pediatric oncology: regulatory initiatives. *The Oncologist* (2002) **5**: 441–4.

49. Lipshultz SE, Lipsitz SR, Mone SM, Goorin AM *et al*. Female sex and higher drug dose as risk factors for late cardiotoxic effects of doxorubicin therapy for childhood cancer. *New Engl J Med* (1995) **332**(26): 1738–43.

50. Link MP, Goorin AM, Miser AW, Green AA, Pratt CB, Belasco JB, Pritchard J *et al*. The effect of adjuvant chemotherapy on relapse-free survival in patients with osteosarcoma of the extremity. *New Engl J Med* (1986) **314**: 1600–6.

51. Smith M. The impact of doxorubicin dose intensity on survival of patients with Ewing's sarcoma. *J Clin Oncol* (1991) **9**: 889–91.

52. Grier HE, Krailo MD, Tarbell NJ *et al*. The addition of ifosfamide and etoposide to standard chemotherapy in Ewing's sarcoma/primitive neuroectodermal tumor of bone: a Children's Cancer Group/Pediatric Oncology Group study. *New Engl J Med* (2003) **348**: 694–701.

53. D'Angio G, Breslow N, Beckwith B, Evans A, Baum E, DeLorimier A *et al*. Treatment of Wilms' tumor: Results of the Third National Wilms' Tumor Study. *Cancer* (1989) **64**: 349–60.

54. D'Angio G, Evans A, Breslow N, Beckwith B, Bishop H, Feigl P *et al*. The treatment of Wilms' tumor: Results of the National Wilms' Tumor Study. *Cancer* (1976) **38**: 633–46.

55. Maurer H, Beltangady M, Gehan E *et al*. The intergoup rhabdomyosarcoma study – 1. *Cancer* (1988) **61**: 1215.

56. Link M, Donaldson S, Berard C, Shuster J, Murphy SB. Results of treatment of childhood localized non-Hodgkin's lymphoma with combination chemotherapy with or without radiotherapy. *New Engl J Med* (1990) **322**: 1169–74.

57. Matthay KK, Villablanca JG, Seeger RC, Stram DO, Harris RE, Ramsay NK, Swift P *et al*. Treatment of high-risk neuroblastoma with intensive chemotherapy, radiotherapy, autologous bone marrow transplantation, and 13-*cis* retinoic acid. *New Engl J Med* (1999) **341**: 1165–73.

58. Smith M, Arthur D, Camitta B, Carroll AJ, Crist W, Gaynon P, Gelber R, Heerema N, Link M, Murphy SB *et al*. Uniform approach to

risk classification and treatment assignment for
children with acute lymphoblastic leukemia. *J Clin
Oncol* (1996) **14**(1): 18–24.

59. Baker KS, Anderson JR, Link MP, Grier HE *et al*.
    Benefit of intensified therapy for patients with

local or regional embryonal rhabdomyosarcoma:
results from the Intergroup Rhabdomyosarcoma
study IV. *J Clin Oncol* (2000) **18**: 2427–34.

60. Castleberry R. Biology and treatment of neurob-
    lastoma. *Ped Clin North Am* (1997) **44**: 919–37.

8

Gastrointestinal Cancers

DAN SARGENT, RICH GOLDBERG AND PAUL LIMBURG

Mayo Clinic, Rochester, MN 55905, USA

INTRODUCTION

Cancers of the gastrointestinal tract account for approximately 20% of all new cancer cases in the United States, and the same proportion of cancer-related deaths. In this discussion we will use a broad definition of GI cancer, including any cancer of a digestive organ. In this definition we include cancers of the oesophagus, gastro-oesophageal junction, stomach, pancreas, gallbladder, bile duct, liver, small and large intestine, rectum and anus. Incident cancers of the oesophagus, stomach, pancreas, liver, large intestine and rectum all exceed 10 000 a year in the United States. In addition to the high prevalence and the large number of cancer sites within the GI tract, the prognosis of patients with GI cancers varies greatly. For example, patients with cancers of the large intestine, when discovered early in the course of disease, have 5-year survival rates exceeding 90%. In contrast, the prognosis for patients with pancreatic cancer is very poor, with a 5-year survival rate of less than 5% across all stages.

Incidence rates for GI cancers show a similar diversity. In the past 50 years, the incidence rates for liver and gastric cancers in the US have fallen substantially. For example, in 1930, gastric cancer was the most common cancer diagnosis. By 1994, gastric cancer had fallen to 12th in incidence among cancers. In contrast, the rates of colon and rectal cancer have remained very stable. Incidence rates for GI cancers also vary greatly worldwide: gastric cancer is tenfold more prevalent in Asia than in the US.

One common feature in all GI cancers is the prognostic importance of staging. The TNM system has been widely adopted to describe the patient's disease status at the time of detection, and has great relevance to the choice of therapy and eventual outcome in all GI cancers. The importance of early detection is clear, and some GI cancers are sufficiently frequent and amenable to detection to allow cost-effective screening.

In this chapter we will review, for the major sites of the GI tract, the important clinical trials that have been conducted. Whenever possible, we will highlight the methodological and design issues of these trials, in an effort to provide insight into their results. We will describe, through this review, how the current standard treatments in each disease site have evolved, as well as presenting some of the most pressing issues for future research.

Textbook of Clinical Trials. Edited by D. Machin, S. Day and S. Green
© 2004 John Wiley & Sons, Ltd ISBN: 0-471-98787-5

OESOPHAGEAL CANCER

Oesophageal cancer is an area where controversy as to the appropriate and optimal therapy exists in almost every aspect. In patients with localised disease (stage 1–3), the roles of surgery, radiotherapy and chemotherapy, alone or in combination, have all been both advocated and questioned. In advanced disease, it seems clear that chemotherapy regimes have provided some degree of progress, albeit limited.

LOCALISED DISEASE

In the past two decades, a large number of randomised clinical trials, involving thousands of patients, have investigated the contributions of radiotherapy or chemotherapy, both alone and in combination, in the pre-operative and post-operative settings or as definitive therapy without surgery. Pre-operative radiotherapy, as a single modality, has been shown in two relatively small randomised trials to provide no additional benefit compared to surgery. These two trials, reported by Launois et al.[1] and Gignoux et al.,[2] randomised 124 and 208 patients, respectively. Chemotherapy as a single modality added to surgery was investigated in 440 patients by Kelsen et al.[3] and shown to have no advantage over surgery alone. The larger sample size of this study lends credence to this result. The two modalities have also been compared to each other as single agents,[4] and no difference in patient outcomes were observed. Based on these results it seems clear that single modality therapy has limited if any impact on patient outcome.

Recently, interest has focused on combined radiochemotherapy regimens in the pre-operative setting. The results in this regard have been conflicting. Four studies have been conducted, three with negative results and one with a positive conclusion. Bosset et al.[5] randomised 297 patients to pre-operative chemoradiation followed by surgery versus surgery alone, and found no evidence of a difference in overall survival (a relative risk for survival between the two arms of 1.0), though they did observe an advantage in disease-free survival in the treated group. In smaller trials, Le Prise et al.[6] and Urba et al.[7] reached the same conclusion based on 86 and 100 randomised patients, respectively. In contrast, Walsh et al.,[8] in a trial of 113 patients, found a striking survival advantage for the combined modality pre-operative approach, with a median survival of 16 months in the multimodality arm compared to 11 months in the surgery alone arm ($p = 0.01$). However, the Walsh study has been criticised for several factors, including the small sample size, poorer than expected survival for the surgery alone control group, and the fact that the study was stopped early at an unplanned interim analysis. In an effort to resolve this controversy, a large multicentre randomised trial was mounted in the US, with an accrual goal of 500 patients. Unfortunately, accrual to the trial was very slow, and the trial was closed early, far short of its accrual goal. Currently, the combined modality pre-operative approach has been widely adopted, despite the conflicting evidence of benefit.

Additional controversy exists in this setting as to whether surgery itself is beneficial. The Radiation Therapy Oncology Group (RTOG) has conducted two randomised trials that have not included surgery as part of the treatment. Herskovic et al.[9] randomised 129 patients to radiation alone versus combined chemoradiotherapy. The study was stopped early (planned sample size of 150 patients) when the first planned interim analysis showed a significant survival advantage to the combined modality group. The RTOG then followed that study with a study comparing two doses of radiotherapy, both combined with chemotherapy.[10] This study was also stopped early, in this case due to a lack of any additional benefit in the high-dose radiation arm. No trials to date have compared a surgical approach to a non-surgical approach, such a trial would scientifically be highly desirable but the practical feasibility of such a trial is questionable.

Based on these results, it is clear that there is no consensus as to a 'standard of care' for patients with localised oesophageal cancer, and that there is a great need for additional clinical trials. Historically, trials in this setting have tended to be small and underpowered for detecting moderate effects on outcome. Larger, more definitive trials should be conducted.

ADVANCED DISEASE

Trials in advanced oesophageal cancer have been plentiful, though attention in this setting has focused more on Phase II trials than randomised Phase III trials. A multitude of agents have been investigated, alone and in combination. It is clear that progress has been made; over the last 20 years median survival for advanced oesophageal cancer has increased from 3 months to 6–9 months or greater. The emphasis on Phase II trials, in an attempt to find a promising new approach, is certainly appropriate given the modest results available from current chemotherapies.

GASTRIC CANCER

While the incidence of gastric cancer has declined in the United States over several decades, 21 600 new diagnoses and 12 400 deaths were still expected in 2002.[11] The nearly 40% cure rate that these numbers imply likely results from a better natural history than oesophageal or pancreatic cancer, early detection via endoscopy, improvements in surgery, and the post-operative use of chemotherapy with radiation for patients with resected disease. While gastric cancer is unusual among GI primary sites because of the large number of antineoplastic agents that show some activity (as measured by tumour response rate), in the advanced disease setting even the most active combination chemotherapy regimens result in remissions that generally last for only a few months and median survivals of less than one year.

LOCALISED DISEASE

The ideal operation for gastric cancer, including the issues of limited versus total gastrectomy and extended versus more limited lymph node dissection, has been a matter of controversy. Trials done in the 1980s and 1990s have led to the conclusion that the most important surgical principle is achievement, when possible, of a pathologically negative resection (an R_0 resection). However, patients have improved post-operative quality of life if some of the stomach is retained, and most surgeons resect only as much of the stomach as is needed to achieve pathologically free margins. The rich lymphatic networks of the stomach can sometimes result in apparently clear margins, yet residual intralymphatic disease may be present in 'skip areas'. This has implications regarding post-operative treatment, and suggests a potential role for adjuvant radiation to the tumour bed and regional structures.

Many surgeons, particularly those in Japan, advocate extended lymph node dissections as a means to improve outcome due to the central location of the stomach with many lymph node-bearing areas at risk for metastatic spread. In a landmark study the Dutch Gastric Cancer Group employed a single Japanese surgeon to train participating Dutch surgeons to perform the classical Japanese extended lymphadenectomy.[12] These investigators randomised 711 eligible patients to resection of the primary tumour with clear gastric margins and either standard (D1) or extended lymphadenectomy (D2). Three-year survival rates were 56% and 58% respectively for the two cohorts, suggesting no advantage to more aggressive surgery. The British Medical Research Council conducted a similar, albeit smaller (400 patients) trial that confirmed this finding.[13]

The adjuvant therapy of gastric cancer, mainly using 5-FU based regimens, has been a matter of investigation for many years. Many randomised trials of chemotherapy versus surgery alone have been reported and these individual trials have generally been negative. A meta-analysis of 21 randomised controlled trials conducted worldwide, that included 3962 patients with 1840 allocated to surgery alone and 2122 allocated to adjuvant chemotherapy, did show a modest potential benefit for treatment.[14] The odds ratio (OR) in favour of chemotherapy was 0.84 overall, but the principal benefit was confined to patients enrolled in trials done in Asia ($n = 888$ patients, OR 0.58) as opposed to Western patients

($n = 3074$, OR 0.96). This finding lends some support to the possibility of a geographically or ethnicity based difference in the natural history of this disease, a finding supported by some epidemiologic evidence. Studies of post-operative radiation versus surgery alone have not shown any advantages, although interpretation of the limited data addressing this issue is problematic.

Adjuvant radiation and chemotherapy used in combination has recently been shown to be advantageous in North American patients. In a 603 patient study, patients were randomised to either surgery alone or to surgery followed by combined modality therapy.[15] In the treatment arm patients were given 5-FU plus leucovorin before and after 4500 cGY to the gastric bed (with radiosensitising 5-FU + leucovorin administered for four consecutive days at the beginning and three days near the end of the radiation). Adjuvant chemoradiotherapy led to a significant median survival advantage of 36 compared to 27 months ($p = 0.005$) and a reduction in local regional relapse rate to 67% compared to 82%. In addition to these outcome improvements, two important patterns of care findings were noted. The trial recommended but did not demand at least a D1 resection and noted that a D2 resection was preferred. However, when operative reports were analysed, only 10% of patients had D2 resections, 36% D1 resections, with the balance having less aggressive surgery. Secondly, pretreatment radiation field review by a single radiation oncologist indicated that 35% of submitted treatment plans contained major or minor deviations from the protocol, indicating a need for education of surgeons and radiation oncologists as to the preferred procedures in these settings. Some readers have raised the possibility that the chemotherapy and radiation were beneficial mainly because of suboptimal surgery in this cohort of patients.

ADVANCED DISEASE

Palliative therapy does make a meaningful difference to many patients with advanced disease in gastric cancer, whose median survival with supportive care alone is around three months. One or more agents from virtually all classes of chemotherapy drugs have demonstrable activity, and median survivals approaching one year have been reported with several combination chemotherapy regimens. One example representative of modern Phase III trials randomised patients to epirubicin, cisplatin and 5-FU (ECF) versus 5-FU, doxorubicin and methotrexate (FAMtx).[16] The overall response rate was 45% compared to 21% ($p = 0.0002$) and the overall survival was 8.9 months compared to 5.7 months ($p = 0.0009$) for ECF over FAMtx. Despite the intensive nature of these two regimens, and other combinations tested to date, the beneficial effects in terms of improved patient longevity have been modest. Earlier detection, improvements in the management of local regional disease, and the testing of new agents seem to provide the best avenues towards better outcomes.

PANCREATIC CANCER

Pancreas cancer has a very poor prognosis. It affects approximately 27 000 new patients each year in the US, and is fatal in approximately 95% of cases. As in all GI cancers, therapy includes surgery, radiotherapy and chemotherapy, depending on the disease stage.

LOCALISED DISEASE

In the setting of resectable or locally advanced disease, both radiotherapy and chemotherapy, and the combination, have been tested extensively. Studies conducted prior to the mid-1990s tended to be small and underpowered, which has led to a variety of conflicting results.

In locally advanced disease, the Gastrointestinal Tumor Study Group (GITSG) randomised 227 patients to three arms: radiotherapy alone, or radiotherapy at two different dose levels given with chemotherapy (5-FU).[17] Accrual to the radiotherapy alone arm was stopped early due to poor results. Two studies have investigated the need for chemoradiotherapy versus chemotherapy alone, with conflicting results. Klaassen *et al.*,[18] in a two-arm randomised study of 191 patients, found no advantage for combined therapy versus chemotherapy alone, while GITSG[19] reported that overall survival was improved with the addition of radiation to chemotherapy in a two-arm study of 43 patients. The small sample sizes of all these trials make definitive conclusions difficult, but there is little evidence to support a role for radiation alone in this setting.

In the setting of a complete surgical resection, several small randomised studies have suggested a benefit to post-operative chemotherapy or chemoradiotherapy. None of these trials enrolled greater than 114 patients, limiting the ability to draw conclusions. The recent report by Neoptolemos *et al.*[20] provided much more conclusive evidence in this regard. In this study, 541 eligible patients were randomised to receive post-operative chemotherapy (6 months of post-surgical treatment), chemoradiotherapy (a 10-day course of radiotherapy accompanied by chemotherapy), both or neither (the design was not a true 2×2 factorial because clinicians were allowed to choose to participate in either one or both randomisations). In this study, there was no benefit to the chemoradiotherapy, while a clear benefit was observed for the chemotherapy group compared to the no treatment group (median survivals of 19.7 versus 14.0 months). Interestingly, the authors of that study did not conclude that a no treatment arm was inappropriate for future trials, in fact they are currently sponsoring a three-arm trial in 990 patients of two different chemotherapy approaches (5-FU with folinic acid or gemcitabine) versus surgery alone. This trial has been criticised for including patients with involved margins after surgery and also primaries arising in the ampulla and bile ducts.

ADVANCED DISEASE

Chemotherapy has been considered the standard of care in the US for advanced pancreatic cancer, despite the lack of any randomised trial demonstrating a survival benefit for chemotherapy versus no treatment. The use of chemotherapy was justified by the occasional tumour response that was observed. Single agent therapy with 5-FU has been used as the control arm for multiple randomised trials, with the assumption that 5-FU was at worst a toxic placebo, thus if a new experimental regimen were shown superior to 5-FU, it would indeed have improved efficacy when compared to no treatment. Burris *et al.*[21] reported a Phase III randomised trial with 126 patients that showed an improved overall survival for gemcitabine compared to 5-FU alone (median survivals of 5.7 versus 4.4 months respectively, $p = 0.003$). The Burris trial established gemcitabine as a new standard of care in this setting. Ongoing and future trials will likely use gemcitabine as a base, comparing gemcitabine alone to a multi-drug chemotherapy regimen including gemcitabine.

A recently completed trial in pancreatic cancer can be used to illustrate the need for careful consideration of an agent prior to Phase III testing. Due in large part to the dismal prognosis and limited treatment options available for patients with pancreatic cancer, pressure has been applied to rapidly introduce novel agents into Phase III trials. The goal is to seek to speed the process of testing a new agent by avoiding the Phase II stage of testing. Such was the case in a randomised Phase III trial reported by Moore *et al.*,[22] where a novel agent (a matrix metalloproteinase inhibitor (MMPI)) was tested against gemcitabine in 277 patients. In this trial the MMPI had significantly inferior outcome compared to gemcitabine. The trial was carefully and appropriately designed to allow early stopping if the results were extreme, which in this case they were. A Phase II trial may have identified the lack of efficacy of this agent prior to its large-scale testing.

COLORECTAL CANCER

Colorectal cancer is the most common malignancy in the GI tract. Not surprisingly, it is also the GI cancer that has been the most extensively investigated in clinical trials.

Likely as the direct result of these intensive research efforts, considerable progress has been made in many facets of colorectal cancer, including chemoprevention, early detection and treatment.

CHEMOPREVENTION

Cancer chemoprevention can be defined as the use of nutritional or pharmaceutical agents to prevent, inhibit or reverse carcinogenesis at a pre-invasive stage of disease. Candidate agents are often identified through a combination of epidemiological and laboratory-based research. Since most subjects enrolled onto chemoprevention trials are generally healthy (except for their increased cancer risk), minimal toxicity represents an important criterion for selecting candidate agents. Colorectal adenomas are commonly employed as intermediate endpoint biomarkers to facilitate more rapid completion of colorectal cancer chemoprevention trials. To date, several colorectal cancer chemoprevention agents have been investigated, including fibre, antioxidant vitamins, calcium and nonsteroidal anti-inflammatory drugs (NSAIDs). Selective cyclooxygenase-2 enzyme inhibitors, which may have a better safety profile than traditional NSAIDs, have received considerable attention in this context as well. Further discussion regarding the current status of these agents is provided below.

Dietary fibre represents a heterogeneous mixture of complex materials derived primarily from plant cell walls. Extensive observational data collected over more than three decades suggest that fibre might help to prevent colorectal neoplasia by diluting or adsorbing faecal carcinogens, reducing colonic transit time, altering bile acid metabolism, or increasing short-chain fatty acid production. However, high fibre interventions have not been associated with a reduced risk for recurrent colorectal adenomas in five clinical trials.[23–27] In fact, one small randomised study observed a higher adenoma recurrence rate among subjects in the active fibre intervention group.[25] It remains possible that administration of dietary fibre at an earlier point in tumourigenesis (for example, prior to first adenoma formation) might have a more appreciable anti-carcinogenic

effect. Nonetheless, the existing data do not support a major role for this agent in colorectal cancer chemoprevention.

Antioxidant vitamins such as the retinoids, carotenoids, ascorbic acid and alpha-tocopherol may prevent carcinogen formation by neutralising free radicals within the intestinal lumen. Although somewhat inconsistent, the preponderance of data from case–control and cohort studies support an inverse association between antioxidant vitamin intake and colorectal cancer risk. Four colorectal cancer chemoprevention trials have investigated antioxidant vitamins at different doses and in various combinations. One relatively small study found that recurrent adenomas were less common among subjects treated with vitamin A (30 000 IU per day), vitamin C (1 g per day) and vitamin E (70 mg per day) over a mean intervention period of 17.8 months.[28] Another three-year chemoprevention trial reported a 69% reduction in the number of recurrent colorectal polyps among subjects randomised to receive multiple antioxidants (beta-carotene, selenium, vitamin C, vitamin E) plus calcium versus placebo compounds.[29] Conversely, two larger trials of vitamin C and vitamin E yielded unremarkable results.[30,31] Thus, definitive evidence for a protective benefit from antioxidant vitamins on colorectal cancer risk remains to be demonstrated.

Calcium may serve as a colorectal cancer chemoprevention agent through at least two mechanisms: functionally removing toxic bile acids from the faecal stream and decreasing cellular proliferation in the large bowel mucosa. Data compiled from 24 observational studies yielded a summary risk estimate of 0.86 (95% CI = 0.74–0.98) for colorectal cancer among subjects with high versus low calcium intakes.[32] In addition to encouraging data from the relatively small clinical trial of multiple antioxidants plus calcium mentioned above,[29] the Calcium Polyp Prevention Study found that treatment with calcium carbonate at 3 g per day for 4 years was associated with a statistically significant 15% reduction in recurrent colorectal adenoma risk, as compared to placebo.[33] Further data regarding the chemopreventive potential of calcium (and vitamin D) are being collected from the large Women's Health Initiative Clinical Trial,[34] which should help to clarify whether or not application of this agent to average-risk subjects has measurable value.

NSAIDs are a structurally diverse class of pharmaceutical agents that appear to reduce proliferation, delay cell cycle progression and induce apoptosis in epithelially-lined tissues. Extensive data from rodent models suggest that NSAID administration can reduce gastrointestinal tumour incidence and/or multiplicity by up to 80%. In human populations, regular NSAID use has been associated with decreased colorectal cancer risk in numerous observational studies. Despite a consistent demonstration of probable benefit, NSAIDs have not been rigorously evaluated in colorectal cancer chemoprevention trials until recently. The Physicians' Health Study ($n = 22\,071$ subjects), which was a randomised, double-blind, placebo-controlled trial of aspirin 325 mg every other day to prevent cardiovascular disease, did analyse colorectal cancer incidence rates as a secondary endpoint. After a mean follow-up period of 5 years, no statistically significant difference was observed between the active and placebo groups (RR = 1.15; 95% CI = 0.80–1.65).[35] Extension of the follow-up period to 12 years did not appreciably alter the risk estimate (RR = 1.03; 95% CI = 0.83–1.28).[36] However, certain limitations of the Physicians' Health Study trial design, such as the relatively low aspirin dose and lack of uniform colorectal cancer surveillance guidelines, may have hindered its ability to detect a protective association.

The chemopreventive effects of traditional NSAIDs are thought to result primarily from inhibition of cyclooxygenase-2 (COX-2). Selective COX-2 inhibitors like celecoxib and rofecoxib are therefore being aggressively pursued as potential colorectal cancer prevention agents. In the first trial to be reported, celecoxib 400 mg twice per day was associated with statistically significant reductions in both the mean number and total burden of colorectal polyps among subjects with familial adenomatous polyposis.[37] Additional COX-2 inhibitor trials are ongoing to confirm the initial findings and to evaluate the effect of these agents on sporadic colorectal cancer risk.

A number of other candidate agents, including oestrogen compounds, ursodeoxycholic acid, difluoromethylornithine and Bowman–Birk inhibitor, have shown promising results in cell culture experiments, animal model systems and/or observational studies. Further data regarding these (and other) potential colorectal cancer chemopreventive agents are anticipated in the near future as new Phase I, II and III clinical trials are organised and completed.

EARLY DETECTION

Due to a variety of factors, colorectal cancers are very amenable to early detection. First, the biology of colorectal carcinogenesis is becoming increasingly well understood, as evidenced by continued expansion of knowledge regarding the molecular events associated with different stages in the adenoma–carcinoma sequence. This relatively slow process typically requires several years to progress from normal mucosa to advanced neoplasia, which affords a clear opportunity for detecting lesions at an asymptomatic stage. Second, there are a variety of possible screening methods that range from non-invasive stool tests or imaging studies to invasive endoscopic evaluations. Third, due to the high incidence of colon cancer, such screening may be cost-effective in terms of screening costs versus years of life saved. Fourth, the high incidence of colon cancer provides a motivation for many individuals to seek out screening. Based on these and other considerations, several randomised trials of various screening methods have been conducted.

With respect to faecal occult blood testing, three large clinical trials have shown that regular screening may reduce colorectal cancer mortality by 13–33%.[38–40] In two trials from Europe, subjects ($n = 61\,933$ and $n = 150\,251$) were randomised to undergo screening every other year versus usual care. In the Minnesota Colon Cancer

Study, subjects ($n = 46\,551$) were randomised to annual screening, biennial screening or usual care. Follow-up in these studies ranged from 11–18 years. Interestingly, only one trial found that programmatic screening was associated with a statistically significant reduction in colorectal cancer incidence.[40] These data suggest that pre-invasive adenomas (arguably the most relevant screening target) are poorly detected by faecal occult blood testing. Thus, despite the inclusion of faecal occult blood testing in widely endorsed colorectal cancer screening guidelines,[41,42] further pursuit of more sensitive and specific stool biomarkers is needed.

Direct examination of the distal colorectum by flexible sigmoidoscopy represents another option for colorectal cancer screening. However, this procedure is at least moderately invasive and may be associated with transient discomfort. As such, adherence to recommendations for initial and repeat flexible sigmoidoscopies was recently evaluated in the Prostate, Lung, Colorectal and Ovarian (PLCO) Cancer Screening Trial. Among subjects randomised to the screening intervention arm ($n = 17\,713$), 83% completed the baseline flexible sigmoidoscopy. Additionally, 87% of subjects who were eligible for repeat testing after three years complied with the follow-up evaluation.[43] At present, the effects of flexible sigmoidoscopy screening on colorectal cancer incidence in the PLCO trial cohort remain unknown. An even larger flexible sigmoidoscopy screening trial is underway at 14 centres in the United Kingdom and Wales ($n = 170\,432$ randomised subjects).[44] When available, data from these two trials should be highly informative regarding the utility of flexible sigmoidoscopy screening to reduce colorectal cancer incidence rates in the general population.

Colonoscopy is currently the gold standard for structural evaluation of the large intestine. Cost-effectiveness models suggest that one-time screening colonoscopy between ages 50–54 years may be a rationale colorectal cancer prevention approach.[45] Existing early detection guidelines support a slightly more conservative strategy (i.e. colonoscopy every 10 years, in the absence of symptoms or other known risk factors). However, screening colonoscopy has not yet been investigated in a randomised clinical trial, with the exception of one ongoing feasibility study.[46] Two novel methods of colorectal cancer screening, CT colonography and DNA-based stool assays, are currently being tested in population-based clinical trials as well. Results from these studies are anticipated in the near future and may necessitate further modification of current early detection algorithms.

TREATMENT: COLON CANCER

Localised Disease

Surgery is the primary modality for the treatment of localised colon cancer. Depending on disease stage, surgery alone produces 5-year survival rates of 50% to greater than 90%. As opposed to gastric and rectal cancer, however, the surgical technique for colon cancer resection has been the subject of limited investigation in randomised clinical trials. One large surgical trial recently completed accrual of approximately 900 patients. In this study, patients were randomised to either the standard 'open' colectomy or a 'minimally invasive' laparoscopically assisted colectomy.[47] The trial's primary endpoint was cancer recurrence, and it was designed to demonstrate equivalence of the two approaches. The trial also included extensive quality of life and cost-effectiveness assessments.

The value of adjuvant treatment for patients with stage 3 colon cancer (cancer able to be completely resected, but with positive lymph nodes in the resection specimen) is well accepted. The first trial conducted with a positive result was conducted by the North Central Treatment group, initiated in 1978.[48] This was a three-arm trial, with a sample size of approximately 135 patients per arm, comparing no post-surgical treatment to adjuvant treatment with either levamisole alone or 5-FU plus levamisole. The initial results of this trial indicated a moderate but statistically significant benefit for the 5-FU plus levamisole arm compared to control. Given the novelty of this result, in a decision that likely would never be made in the current day, the investigative team decided to embark on a larger, confirmatory trial prior to the release of the results to the oncology community. This confirmatory trial, known as Intergroup trial 0035, enrolled over 1200 patients to the same three arms as the initial trial. Intergroup 0035 clearly demonstrated improved overall survival in patients treated with adjuvant 5-FU and levamisole.[49] These findings lead in part to the 1990 consensus statement from the National Cancer Institute that patients with stage 3 colon cancer who are unable to enter a clinical trial should be offered adjuvant treatment with 5-FU plus levamisole unless there are contraindications.[50]

A number of clinical trials were in progress at the time of the publication of the beneficial results from the use of adjuvant 5-FU plus levamisole. Several of these trials included a no post-surgical treatment control arm, and thus these trials were closed prior to reaching their accrual goals due to ethical reasons. Included in this list of trials that were closed prematurely were five Phase III randomised trials testing 5-FU plus leucovorin versus no post-surgical treatment control. The results from three of these trials were pooled for analysis;[51] the other two were reported separately.[52,53] In each of these analyses, adjuvant 5-FU plus leucovorin showed a survival advantage compared to control. In subsequent studies, throughout the 1990s, various investigative groups conducted trials comparing various different schedules and combinations of 5-FU combined with either leucovorin or levamisole. None of these trials demonstrated a statistically significant improvement in survival between study arms, although through such trials it did become clear that 6 months of 5-FU plus leucovorin was at least as effective as 12 months of 5-FU plus levamisole.[54,55] As a result, the current standard of care in the United States (as of 2002) for stage 3 colon cancer is 6 months of 5-FU plus leucovorin.

In the discussion in the preceding paragraph, all of the regimens discussed were based on the delivery of 5-FU as a short-term bolus infusion. Based on promising results in the advanced disease setting (as discussed below), multiple clinical trials have been conducted using regimens based on a long-term infusion with 5-FU. Intergroup trial 0153 directly compared a bolus to an infusional 5-FU based regimen in a randomised Phase III trial of 1078 patients (terminated early at an interim analysis–original planned sample size of 1800 patients).[56] In this trial no difference in efficacy was observed between the arms, although the toxicity profile did differ substantially. Based on these results, two recent Phase III randomised trials in the United States have used control arms of 6 months of bolus 5-FU plus leucovorin. However in Europe, regimens using short-term 24–48 hour 5-FU infusions are more popular.

Future efforts in the adjuvant treatment of stage 3 colon cancer will likely be directed in two areas – first, to improving the treatment options available, and second, and relatedly, to tailoring therapy to the individual patient. In the treatment area, for the time being, new studies will randomise patients to treatments based on adding a new treatment to a 5-FU and leucovorin regimen. For example, the two recent large Phase III trials in the United States compared 5-FU and leucovorin to either a 5-FU, leucovorin and irinotecan (trial C89803) or 5-FU, leucovorin and oxaliplatin (trial C-06). In somewhat of a leap of faith, the trial currently being planned by the US Gastrointestinal Intergroup will compare 5-FU, leucovorin and irinotecan to 5-FU, leucovorin and oxaliplatin. This leap is necessitated by the new realities of conducting trials in the adjuvant colon setting – namely, that patient outcome has been sufficiently improved that significant follow-up is required in order to obtain sufficient events to power a study. Both the C89803 and C-06 trials will require a minimum of three years of follow-up prior to any formal analysis. The options for conducting a follow-up study are thus to wait at least three years, or to push ahead, assuming that at least one of the experimental regimens will prove superior to the current standard. A discussion of the second area, tailoring therapy to the individual patient, will be deferred until the next section.

One additional insight into the conduct of clinical trials in GI cancers may be gained by examining the steady increase in the sample sizes that has occurred in stage 3 colon clinical trials over the past two decades. In trials conduced in the early 1980s, sample sizes of 100–200 per arm were typical,[48,52] with some exceptions (such as the NSABP C-01 trial, with approximately 380 patients per arm).[57] With such a sample size, the study provided adequate power to detect only a relatively large effect. Fortunately, 5-FU, when combined with either levamisole or leucovorin, did provide a rather large effect, with a reduction in the hazard of death by approximately 25%.[58] However, the likelihood of a subsequent treatment advance by such a magnitude is unlikely, and smaller advances may indeed be clinically relevant. Therefore, more modern trials in stage 3 disease have included sample sizes of 1600 (trial C89803), 2400 (trial C-06) and 4900 patients for a four-arm trial (the QUASAR trial).[54] As therapy continues to improve, the sample size necessary to detect further incremental advances will continue to grow. One possible strategy for practically conducting such large trials is discussed in the next section.

As opposed to the adjuvant treatment of stage 3 disease, the benefit of adjuvant treatment for stage 2 (node negative) disease is unclear. In many previous trials, patients with stage 2 disease have been pooled together with stage 3 patients. The sample size for such trials has typically been based on an analysis pooling the data from both patient groups. For a variety of reasons, patients with stage 3 disease have typically constituted a majority of the enrollment to such trials, thus each individual trial has been underpowered to detect a moderate benefit of treatment in stage 2 patients. Due to the limited sample size in each trial, two attempts have been made to pool data from several trials in order to gain a sufficient sample size to draw a definitive conclusion regarding the value of adjuvant therapy in stage 2 disease. However, the two analyses have reported differing conclusions. One analysis, reported by

Mamounas et al.,[59] pooled data from four randomised trials conducted by the NSABP. In none of these four trials was there a direct randomised comparison between treatment and control. In their analysis, the authors estimated the magnitude of the difference in outcome between the two study arms in each of the four studies. They then compared whether this difference in outcome differed by patient stage. The authors concluded that the treatment effect within each study was similar between stage 2 and stage 3 patients, and since it had been previously demonstrated that treatment is beneficial in stage 3 patients, they concluded that treatment is also beneficial in stage 2 patients.

The second investigation[60] used a more direct approach. In this analysis, the study team pooled the data from stage 2 patients who had participated in five randomised trials of 5-FU plus leucovorin versus control. They found no statistically significant benefit of treatment, based on a pooled sample size of just over 1000 patients. Due to the excellent outcome of stage 2 patients, with an approximately 80% 5-year survival in untreated patients, even this pooled sample size had poor power to detect a small but possibly important improvement in patient outcome (only 60% power to detect an 85% 5-year survival in treated patients). Thus, the benefit of 5-FU based adjuvant therapy in stage 2 disease remains unclear, and further pooled analyses will likely be necessary. A large randomised trial of a monoclonal antibody in the setting of stage 2 disease has recently completed accrual of over 1700 patients (trial C9581); the results of this trial should help clarify the appropriate treatment for patients with stage 2 disease.

Advanced Disease

It is likely that more clinical trials have been conducted in advanced colon cancer than in any other GI disease site. This is due to the high incidence of the cancer, and the fact that it is to at least some degree sensitive to chemotherapeutic agents. Trials in advanced colon cancer typically include patients with advanced rectal cancer, as the response to chemotherapy has not been shown to depend on the precise site of the patient's disease within the colorectum.

The drug 5-FU has been the mainstay of treatment for colorectal cancer for over 40 years. From 1950–1990, a multitude of trials were conducted in an effort to improve the efficacy of 5-FU based regimens, by changing methods of administration, combining it with various supplemental agents (such as leucovorin or levamisole), or changing the dose and schedule. Regarding the timing of administration, the clear result of multiple studies is that, among regimens where 5-FU is delivered as a bolus injection, the particulars of the administration have a definite impact on toxicity, some impact on tumour response, but little impact on patient survival. The addition of leucovorin to 5-FU has been demonstrated in a meta-analysis to provide increased efficacy in terms of response rate compared to 5-FU alone.[61] In another meta-analysis, a schedule where the 5-FU is delivered by a continuous infusion has been shown to provide an advantage in both toxicity and overall survival compared to bolus schedules.[62,63] However, the improvement in median survival was modest at 0.8 months, thus many practitioners (at least in the United States) have continued to administer the bolus 5-FU based regimens based on perceived benefits of patient and physician convenience.

After 40 years of testing variations on a 5-FU theme, two more recent developments have added excitement to the advanced colorectal cancer clinical trials arena. The first is the introduction of oral 5-FU based regimens. The oral method of delivery offers clear benefits in terms of patient preference. However, an oral approach would not likely be accepted if it did not provide at least equivalent efficacy to an IV approach. Therefore, two large equivalence trials have been conducted comparing an oral to an IV regimen. These two trials, one reported by Hoff et al.[64] and the other by van Cutsem et al.,[65] enrolled 605 and 602 patients respectively, and were formally designed to test the equivalence of the oral regimen to the IV approach. In both cases, formal equivalence was declared.

At almost the same time as the introduction of oral 5-FU based agents for advanced colorectal cancer, new chemotherapeutic agents have been added to 5-FU with promising results. Based on results with the agent irinotecan in patients who had failed a 5-FU based regimen,[66,67] trials with irinotecan were performed in the setting of patients with previously untreated advanced disease. As reported by Saltz et al.[68] and Douillard et al.,[69] irinotecan, when added to 5-FU and leucovorin, resulted in improved time to progression and overall survival when compared to 5-FU and leucovorin alone in first-line treatment of advanced disease. These two relatively large trials (683 and 387 patients, respectively) established a new standard of care in this setting. In the Saltz trial irinotecan was added to a bolus 5-FU schedule, while the Douillard trial added irinotecan to an infusional 5-FU regimen, thus the optimal method in which to give 5-FU with the new agent remained unclear. Recently, the drug oxaliplatin has shown promising activity when combined with 5-FU and leucovorin in several studies,[70,71] with reported median survivals equaling or exceeding 18 months.

The proven efficacy of irinotecan as second-line therapy in patients who fail 5-FU based therapy has complicated the design of first-line advanced disease trials. Traditionally, overall survival has been used as the primary endpoint for such studies, and extending the patient's longevity remains the ultimate goal. However, given that there are second- and even third-line therapies with proven benefit, the relative merits of overall survival as the primary outcome for a trial warrant a reconsideration. Consider the design used in the Saltz trial,[68] where irinotecan plus 5-FU and leucovorin was compared to 5-FU and leucovorin. In this trial, patients who progressed on the 5-FU and leucovorin arm were able to receive irinotecan off study, as it was approved for the second-line indication. The availability of this effective second-line agent provided at least the theoretical possibility that the two primary study arms could show no difference in terms of overall survival, even though irinotecan was beneficial to patients on both arms of the study. For this reason, time to tumour progression was specified as the primary endpoint for the trial. In retrospect, the addition of irinotecan as a component of the initial treatment resulted in both improved time to progression and overall survival, making the result clear. However, these factors must be taken into consideration for future trials, where at minimum data on the use of second- and third-line therapy should be collected.

TREATMENT: RECTAL CANCER

Rectal cancer is second to colon cancer among GI malignancies in the number of new cases per year. When the initial diagnosis for rectal cancer is as advanced disease, i.e. not surgically completely resectable, its primary treatment is in the same manner as for advanced colon cancer. However, the optimal adjuvant treatment for rectal cancer is the issue of considerable study. Questions abound as to the importance of surgical technique, the value of radiation therapy, the optimal chemotherapy regimen and the timing of therapy, either pre- or post-resection.

Surgery/Adjuvant Therapy

Prior to 1990, external beam radiotherapy in the post-operative setting was considered by many as the standard of care in the United States, based primarily on an observed benefit in lowering the risk of local recurrence. In particular, radiation as a single agent added to surgery had never been shown to improve overall survival compared to surgery alone. In a randomised study of 204 patients, Krook et al.[72] demonstrated a benefit in overall survival of post-operative combined therapy with radiation and 5-FU and semustine compared to radiation alone. The 1990 NIH consensus statement concluded that 'Combined postoperative chemotherapy and radiation therapy improves local control and survival in stage II and III patients and is recommended'.[50] In a subsequent study conducted by the US GI Intergroup, two questions were asked in a 2×2 factorial design: is semustine necessary, and can therapy

be optimised by using continuous infusion 5-FU based therapy as opposed to bolus. All patients in this study received radiation. This study of 680 patients concluded that (1) semustine is not necessary, and (2) infusional 5-FU based therapy during the radiotherapy provides a survival advantage compared to bolus therapy.[73]

Two studies conducted by the National Surgical Breast and Bowel Project (NSABP) have questioned the value of radiation in the post-operative setting. In the Krook and O'Connell studies mentioned above, all patients received radiation, and the studies focused on the relative benefit of different chemotherapy regimens. In contrast, NSABP study R-01 tested three arms in a randomised manner in 574 patients: no post-surgical treatment, post-operative radiation and post-operative chemotherapy. A survival benefit was observed for the chemotherapy arm compared to the no treatment arm, but this advantage was not observed in the radiation alone arm.[74] The NSABP followed this study with a two-arm randomised trial of 741 patients comparing chemotherapy alone to chemotherapy plus radiation.[75] The results of this trial showed no improvement in overall survival for the combined modality arm, although there was a statistically significant improvement in the rate of local recurrence associated with radiation. Despite these two consistent results, radiation continues to be commonly used in the post-operative treatment of stage 2 and 3 rectal cancer.

Increasingly, practitioners are turning to delivering radiotherapy for rectal cancer in the pre-operative setting. There are several theoretical advantages to the pre-operative approach. Perhaps most importantly, from the patient's perspective, pre-operative therapy may shrink the tumour sufficiently to allow a sphincter-sparing resection. Pre-operative radiotherapy has been shown to improve outcome compared to no treatment in a large randomised trial of the Swedish Rectal Cancer Trial group. This trial randomised 1168 patients to a two-arm trial of a short course (25 Gy in 1 week) of pre-operative radiation compared to no pre-operative treatment, and showed a statistically significant improvement in both local recurrence rate and overall survival.[76] In the United States, the standard pre-operative regimen is to deliver the 5-week post-operative course of 50.4 Gy pre-operatively. The efficacy of this approach has never been established in a randomised trial. A comparison of these two pre-operative approaches is clearly warranted.

Regardless of the specifics of the pre-operative approach, a burning question concerns whether the pre- or post-operative approach provides the best outcome. Two randomised trials have been attempted in the United States, and both were closed early far short of their accrual goals due to poor accrual. However, an ongoing trial in Europe has been more successful, with accrual of over 600 patients to one of the two approaches.[77] The 50.4 Gy long course radiation is being used in both arms, and both arms are receiving the same chemotherapy regimen in combination with the radiation.

In addition to the controversies present in chemotherapy and radiation therapy, there is considerable interest in the optimal surgical management of this disease. In particular, the surgical approach of total mesorectal excision (TME) has been promoted as an important surgical advance. Based on case-series and other historical data, proponents of TME have claimed significant reductions in local recurrence rates and improved overall survival compared to standard surgery.[78] However, TME has never been tested against non-TME surgery in a randomised trial, and such a trial is unlikely to ever be conducted. In a large randomised trial of 1861 patients conducted by the Dutch Colorectal Cancer Group, pre-operative radiation was shown to reduce the rate of local recurrence compared to no radiation when all patients received TME surgery.[79] In this early report, with a median follow-up of 2 years in living patients, there was no improvement in overall survival for patients receiving radiation.

In summary, it is clear that rectal cancer is an area where randomised clinical trials have made several important contributions to improving patient outcomes. Post-operative chemotherapy and chemoradiotherapy, and pre-operative radiation therapy have been shown to reduce the local recurrence rate and improve overall survival based on large randomised trials. It is also clear that considerable work remains to define the optimal timings and combinations of the different treatment modalities.

SELECTED METHODOLOGIC ISSUES WITH EXAMPLES

The number and variety of large Phase III randomised trials that have been conducted in GI cancers brings to light a number of clinical trials methodology issues that have direct relevance to the conduct and conclusions that can be drawn from such trials. In this section we will highlight three such issues: subgroup analysis, the study of prognostic and predictive factors, and monitoring of clinical trials for safety.

SUBGROUP ANALYSIS

Studies are often conducted in multiple possible heterogeneous groups of patients in order to achieve a necessary sample size, or to complete a trial more quickly. The conduct subgroup analyses, that is, to examine the result of a trial separately in different groups of randomised patients, is extremely important. In fact, such analyses can help demonstrate the robustness of a result: if a study finding can be shown to be consistent in different patient groups, such as patients of different ages, or patients enrolled from different countries, then the overall result cannot be explained by an extreme result in one subset of patients. Additionally, subgroup analyses are important in generating hypotheses for future study. However, caution must be exercised when examining the results of subset analyses, particularly if they were not pre-specified in advance.

One example of a subgroup analysis of great controversy in the setting of GI cancers is whether post-surgical adjuvant treatment is beneficial for patients with stage 2 colon cancer, as discussed previously. Historically, most trials in adjuvant colon cancer have included patients with both stage 2 and 3 disease. The majority of patients in such trials have been stage 3 patients, and subset analyses within these trials have consistently shown 5-FU based chemotherapy to be beneficial in this group. However, because the majority of patients in such trials have not been stage 2, and because the prognosis for the stage 2 patients is overall more favourable, with fewer patient deaths and thus less statistical power, the individual studies have not shown consistent results in the subset of B2 patients. As mentioned above, two pooled analyse have been conducted, with conflicting results. Both analyses are to be commended for obtaining and using the individual patient data from each of the included trials, and for having very complete follow-up for the studies used. However, both analyses could be criticised for other methodologic issues. The first, by the NSABP investigators,[59] pooled data from multiple trials with different treatment arms, none of which compared directly a no treatment arm to what would be considered a standard treatment by current standards. The second, by the IMPACT investigators,[60] did pool results from randomised trials of no post-surgical treatment to therapy with 5-FU and leucovorin, the current US standard of care. However, these investigators did not include data from two large trials testing 5-FU and levamisole versus control, which despite having the 5-FU modulated by a different agent did indeed test a very similar question, with 5-FU and levamisole shown in large randomised trials to give results indistinguishable from 5-FU and leucovorin. Additionally, the IMPACT investigators used a less powerful analysis than might be possible. The original trials included in the IMPACT analysis included patients with both stage 2 and 3 cancers. In these trials, treatment was proven beneficial overall. Therefore, the most relevant question is whether the effect of treatment differed between the stage 2 patients and the stage 3 patients. This question could be tested by obtaining all of the data from the trials, examining the degree of benefit overall, and then testing for a stage by treatment interaction. This is the most statistically powerful method for testing the

treatment benefit in both subgroups of patients; the absence of a significant interaction implies that there is no evidence that the benefit of treatment differs by patient subgroup.

Two adjuvant rectal trials conducted by the NSABP, trials R-01[74] and R-02,[75] can be used to demonstrate a different feature of subgroup analyses. The first trial, R-01, demonstrated a significant benefit in terms of overall survival for the addition of chemotherapy following resection compared to no post-surgical treatment. However, in subgroup analyses, this benefit seemed to be limited to the male patients, which could not be explained. The NSABP is to be commended for treating this finding as hypothesis generating, and testing the hypothesis in their next study R-02. In study R-02, the randomisation scheme differed for men and women, with females being randomised to two arms and males to four arms. The results of R-02 did not demonstrate the need for different treatment for the two genders, which put the issue to rest after being tested as appropriate in a randomised trial. This experience demonstrates the value of confirming a finding that results from a subgroup analysis prior to accepting the result into clinical practice.

TUMOUR MARKER STUDIES

A second area of considerable interest and debate in the GI cancer community regards the use of putative prognostic and predictive markers to guide the choice of therapy for an individual patient. Hundreds if not thousands of studies have been done on markers based on immunohistochemistry, flow cytometry, chromosomal markers such as allelic loss and microsatellite instability, pathologic features, and many others. Unfortunately, few if any of these markers have made their way into clinical practice. The reasons for this lack of progress are many,[80] we will focus here on three that are directly related to the later stages of clinical trials: analyses confined to patient subgroups, inadequate sample size and improper design.

In any report investigating tumour markers based on patients from clinical trials, the rate of sample collection is an important issue. In the case of retrospective trials conducted on tissue obtained from a clinical trial, often tissue is available on only a subset of the patients who entered the initial trial. In these retrospective marker studies, comparisons are frequently made between characteristics such as baseline demographics and/or tumour stage for the patients whose tumours were used in the marker study and those whose tissues were not used. However, even if the characteristics for the patients who were used in the analysis and those who were not appear similar, the results of such studies could still be biased. Such an example has been described by Pajak et al.,[81] who reported on a study originally conducted by Grignon et al.[82] In their study, in patients with advanced prostate adenocarcinoma, Grignon et al. studied the relationship between tumour p53 status and prognosis in 129 of 456 patients entered onto a trial conducted by the Radiation Therapy Oncology Group (RTOG study 86-10). When reanalysed by Pajak et al., it was shown that the distribution of treatment received and combined Gleason Score of patients who had p53 assessed was identical to those who did not have p53 assessed. However, the survival of those patients who had a p53 determination performed on their tumour, and were thus included in the study, was significantly worse than those not included in the study.

This example demonstrates the possible pitfalls of performing marker studies on patient subsets. Despite such examples, the approach of collecting a set of patients with tissue available, testing a possible prognostic or predictive marker, and reporting the results continues to be the method by which most markers are examined. The reasons for this are many: expediency, ethical issues of mandatory tissue submission, and policies of informed consent and institutional review boards. It does raise the issue of whether for future prospective studies, tissue submission should be mandatory prior to patient entry on a therapeutic clinical trial. Such a discussion raises ethical and legal issues that are beyond the scope of this work, but such discussions are ongoing for

several Phase III trials that are in development in the US.

SAFETY MONITORING

As a final clinical trials methodologic issue, we consider the process of monitoring patient safety in clinical trials. Clinical trials have been conducted for many years, and detailed and effective methods have been developed for ensuring the safety of participants. One of the fundamental tenants of clinical trials is the progression of an agent or regimen through a series of trials, starting in small, typically single-centre Phase I studies, on to somewhat larger, possibly multi-centre Phase II trials, then on to Phase III trials. The sequential nature of such trials, among other features, allows for considerable experience with an agent or drug combination prior to a large, multi-centre trial. The recent pressure towards developing and testing agents more rapidly, although beneficial in many ways, does challenge this established mechanism for establishing the safety of an agent. More Phase I/II, Phase II/III, or even Phase I/III trials are being conducted, the result of which is that agents or combinations are being pushed into the multi-centre setting more rapidly that in the past. This warrants an examination of why caution is warranted as agents are taken from Phase I testing to larger trials.

Phase I trials have a successful history as the first step in testing new cancer therapies. However, several factors must be considered as a new agent or combination of agents is taken from a Phase I trial to a Phase II or Phase III trial. These factors relate to possible differences between patients entered onto Phase I trials and those entered on later trials. First, Phase I trials often include patients with any type of solid tumour. This speeds the completion of the trial, and is justified because in many cases the tolerability of an agent is not related to the location of the patient's primary tumour. However, in some instances the tolerability of an agent may differ in patients with different tumour types. Second, Phase I trials are frequently conducted at highly specialised cancer centres, where medical personnel experienced with detailed monitoring and rapid intervention reduce the consequences of and future risk for toxicity whenever possible. In contrast, Phase II and III trials are often conducted in the community setting, where the clinical staff may be using a new agent or combination of agents for the first time.

A final reason for caution is that patients are enrolled onto Phase I trials only after failing all standard therapies. This has several implications. Patients enrolled on Phase I trials have typically been previously exposed to cytotoxic agents, thus they may be physically or emotionally more robust and tolerate a new therapy better than a patient in the first-line setting. Additionally, only patients that have tolerated their initial therapy acceptably are likely to choose enrollment, or be considered candidates, for a Phase I trial. A final issue with respect to patients who have been previously treated is that patients and their physicians may have a sense of the rate of disease progression such that patients with the most virulent disease are often not even considered for enrollment in a Phase I trial.

In part due to the combination of these various factors, study sponsors, including the National Cancer Institute, have developed sophisticated systems to aid in the timely identification of toxicity problems in ongoing studies. Despite these systems, gaps remain. For example for agents that are commercially available, expedited reporting of severe but expected events may not be required. If such an event were occurring at a greater frequency than expected, and expedited reporting was not required, a multi-centre trial may not detect such an incidence for weeks or months due to the nature of the process of data collection, editing, entry and analysis. This has led some groups to propose supplements to the standard systems to collect data on all severe events in a timely manner.[83]

Even when data is reported in a timely manner, care must be taken in interpreting the data received. As an example, consider the experience in two large Phase III randomised trials reported on by Rothenberg et al.[84] The Rothenberg et al.

report was prompted by the finding of an unexpected number of early deaths on two GI cancer trials, one in advanced colorectal cancer and the other in adjuvant cancer. In one of the trials in the review, 23 patients were reported to have died within 60 days of initiation of therapy. When these 23 events were reported to the group operations office for this trial, only 10 were deemed to have been related to treatment. However, upon independent review, 16 of the 23 events were deemed treatment-related or treatment-induced.

Several conclusions can be drawn regarding toxicity in clinical trials. First, as the pace of drug development continues to quicken, it is likely that there will continue to be agents pushed into large trials prior to full and extensive Phase I and II testing. Second, effective systems must be established to monitor toxicity in trials of all phases. Third, an independent assessment of the attribution of an event may be beneficial, as local investigators may be hesitant to attribute a poor event to a treatment. In addition, new metrics (such as 60-day all-cause mortality[85]) and new terminology (such as treatment-induced, treatment-exacerbated and treatment-unrelated deaths[84]) may be helpful in standardising the reporting of adverse events in clinical trials.

CASE STUDY: 5-FU PLUS LEUCOVORIN IN COLON CANCER

As is clear, the history of clinical trials in GI cancer is long and has been very successful. As an example illustrating several facets of both the past history of GI clinical trials and issues that will likely be faced again in future studies, here we present a case study of the development, establishment and replacement of what was once the US standard of care for advanced colorectal cancer and, as of 2002, remains the standard for adjuvant stage 3 colon cancer, the 'Mayo Clinic' bolus regimen of 5-FU and leucovorin delivered for 5 consecutive days every 4 or 5 weeks.

The activity of fluorinated pyrimidines in the treatment of GI cancers has been reviewed extensively. 5-Fluorouracil (5-FU) is the most ubiquitous of the fluorinated pyrimidines, which at least in part exert their antineoplastic effect by inhibiting the activity of the enzyme thymidylate synthase (TS), which in turn interferes with DNA synthesis in dividing cells. Often agents designed to improve the efficacy of fluorinated pyrimidines are combined with these agents in an effort to preferentially sensitise tumour cells relative to host cells to the agent(s). Leucovorin is an agent commonly used in such a setting. The Mayo regimen of 5-FU and leucovorin is thus a combination of an active chemotherapy agent, 5-FU, with a 'biochemical modulator' leucovorin.

Prior to the early 1980s, 5-FU was primarily administered as a single agent. Administered in this fashion, it was associated with limited activity and moderate toxicity. Response rates for metastatic colorectal cancer were low, in the neighbourhood of 10%, and these responses were short-lived, lasting on average a few months.[61]

Based on pre-clinical laboratory studies,[86–88] the addition of leucovorin to cell culture with one of the metabolites of 5-FU, fluorodeoxuridylate monophosphate (FdUMP), resulted in enhanced binding to and inhibition of TS as compared to the binding when FdUMP was used alone. This improved inhibition of thymidylate synthase resulted in inhibited DNA synthesis and resulted in enhanced tumour shrinkage. Depending on the model systems, optimal concentration of leucovorin ranged from leucovorin 1–20 mmol/L.[89–93] These studies supported the use of leucovorin doses ranging from 10 to 600 mg/m^2 in clinical trials where leucovorin was added to 5-FU in an effort to improve on 5-FU's single agent activity. While such laboratory studies provided basic information on the modulation of 5-FU using leucovorin, the applicability of these results to humans with colorectal cancer was unclear. Based on clinical experience, individuals with colorectal cancer clearly exhibit significant heterogeneity in their response to treatment. The sequence of administration of 5-FU and leucovorin, the optimal concentration of leucovorin, and the appropriate interval of 5-FU and leucovorin administration all were variables to be studied to explore the efficacy of 5-FU and leucovorin in inhibiting tumour growth.

Early investigators studying the biochemical modulation of 5-FU with leucovorin in the treatment of colorectal and gastric cancers included Machover and colleagues.[94,95] The Machover regimen consisted of administering high-dose leucovorin at 200 mg/m^2/d prior to 5-FU at a dose of 370 mg/m^2/d, with both drugs given consecutively for 5 days. With this dose of leucovorin, the blood level is approximately 10–20 μmol/L.[96] In large part to lower the cost of the regimen (leucovorin was very expensive at the time), the 'Mayo' regimen was devised to use the identical 5-FU schedule to the Machover regimen, but to use low-dose leucovorin at a dose of 20 mg/m^2/d, which resulted in blood levels of 1–2 μmol/L.

This regimen was first tested as part of a randomised Phase II study in advanced unresectable colorectal cancer.[97] Three of the treatment arms are relevant for this discussion: (1) 5-FU as a single agent administered at a dose of 500 mg/m^2/d by IV bolus for 5 consecutive days every 5 weeks; (2) the Machover regimen repeated at 4 weeks, 8 weeks and every 5 weeks thereafter; and (3) the Mayo regimen repeated at the same frequency as the Machover regimen. In this trial, provision was made in the protocol to escalate the 5-FU dose on any treatment arm if there was no observed myelosuppression or significant non-haematologic toxicity during the previous treatment course. When the toxicity was analysed after treatment of the first 100 patients, the starting dose of 5-FU for the Mayo regimen was increased to 425 mg/m^2/d in order to produce definite but tolerable toxicity that was of similar magnitude between the six treatment arms.[98] The original combination of low-dose leucovorin with 370 mg/m^2/d of 5-FU for 5 consecutive days was empiric; no formal Phase I trial of this regimen had ever been performed. In the 208 eligible patients entered on the three study arms of interest, the overall response rates were 10% for 5-FU alone, 26% for the Machover regimen, and 43% for the Mayo regimen. Both leucovorin regimens demonstrated significant improvement in response rate and overall survival compared to 5-FU alone.

Concurrent to the previously mentioned study, investigators at the Roswell Park Memorial Cancer Institute (RPMI) began testing a regimen of leucovorin 500 mg/m^2/d with 5-FU 600 mg/m^2/d given for 6 consecutive weeks followed by a 2-week rest period.[99] In a small study, the RPMI regimen was shown to significantly improve the tumour response rate compared to single agent 5-FU. Shortly thereafter, the RPMI and Mayo regimens were compared in a randomised trial of 366 patients.[100] In this trial, the objective response rates and overall survival was similar between the two arms. The toxicity profile of the two regimens did differ, but no clear winner was identified. Based largely on cost considerations, investigators from the Mayo Clinic and the North Central Cancer Treatment group chose to pursue the Mayo regimen for future testing.

The activity seen with the combination of leucovorin and 5-FU in the advanced disease setting naturally led to the evaluation of several of these regimens in the adjuvant treatment of patients with stage 2 and 3 colon cancer. In a study that was suspended after accrual of 317 patients (based on the results of a large trial that demonstrated 5-FU plus levamisole was an effective treatment in this setting[49]), patients with resected stage 2 or 3 colon cancer were randomised to the Mayo 5-FU plus leucovorin regimen for 6 months or to a no treatment control arm.[53] The 5-year survival for treated patients was 74%, compared to 63% in the control group ($p = 0.02$). This result established the efficacy of the Mayo 5-FU plus leucovorin regimen in the adjuvant setting.

Following this small study, a large trial was conducted to test four different combinations of 5-FU with leucovorin and/or levamisole in patients with stage 2 and 3 colon cancer.

The regimens included the Mayo 5-FU plus leucovorin regimen for 6 months, 5-FU plus levamisole for 12 months, 5-FU with high-dose leucovorin (the RPMI regimen) for 8 months, or 5-FU plus leucovorin plus levamisole for 12 months. In this study of 3759 patients, results

were similar between the Mayo and RPMI 5-FU plus leucovorin programmes, and the 5-FU plus both leucovorin and levamisole regimen.[55] Based on the essentially identical activity profiles of these regimens, the choice between the two 5-FU and leucovorin regimens (Mayo and RPMI) has been based on issues related to schedule (some patients preferred weekly therapy over five consecutive days of treatment), cost (at the time of these studies leucovorin was expensive), toxicity profile and clinician's preference.

From the late 1980s until the year 2000, the Mayo regimen of 5-FU and leucovorin was regarded as the standard of care for advanced colon cancer. As discussed previously, in the late 1990s and early 2000s, several randomised trials were conducted in both the US and Europe in which infusion-based 5-FU regimens or regimens that combine 5-FU with CPT-11 or oxaliplatin have demonstrated improved patient outcomes compared to those seen with the Mayo regimen. In addition, the oral agent capecitabine has been approved as an alternative to IV 5-FU in advanced disease. Thus it appears that in the advanced disease setting, the Mayo 5-FU + leucovorin regimen has been replaced as the standard of care, indeed a welcome advance. In the adjuvant setting, no randomised trial has been completed that demonstrates improved overall survival for a multiple drug combination, or equivalence for an oral regimen, although trials in both areas have completed accrual and are awaiting results. Increased toxicity has clearly been demonstrated for multiple drug combinations in the adjuvant setting,[84] demonstrating the value of waiting for the results from these definitive trials before adopting a promising new therapy as a standard of care in the community.

REFERENCES

1. Launois B, Delarue D, Campion JP, Kerbaol M. Preoperative radiotherapy for carcinoma of the esophagus. *Surg, Gynecol Obstet* (1981) **153**: 690–2.
2. Gignoux M, Roussel A, Paillot B, Gillet M, Schlag P, Favre J-P, Dalesio O, Buyse M,

Duez N. The value of preoperative radiotherapy in esophageal cancer: results of a study of the E.O.R.T.C. *World J Surg* (1987) **11**: 426–32.

3. Kelsen DP, Ginsberg R, Pajak TF, Sheahan DG, Gunderson L, Mortimer J, Estes N, Haller DG, Ajani J, Kocha W, Minsky BD, Roth JA. Chemotherapy followed by surgery compared with surgery alone for localized esophageal cancer. *New Engl J Med* (1998) **339**: 1979–84.

4. Kelsen DP, Minsky BD, Smith M, Beitler J, Niedzwiecki D, Chapman D, Bains M, Burt M, Heelan R, Hilaris B. Preoperative therapy for esophageal cancer: a randomized comparison of chemotherapy versus radiation therapy. *J Clin Oncol* (1990) **8**: 1352–61.

5. Bosset J-F, Gignoux M, Triboulet J-P, Tiret E, Mantion G, Elias D, Lozach P, Ollier J-C, Pavy J-J, Mercier M, Sahmoud T. Chemoradiotherapy followed by surgery compared with surgery alone in squamous-cell cancer of the esophagus. *New Engl J Med* (1997) **337**: 161–7.

6. Le Prise E, Etienne PL, Meunier B, Maddern G, Hassel MB, Gedouin D, Boutin D, Campion JP, Launois B. A randomized study of chemotherapy, radiation therapy, and surgery versus surgery for localized squamous cell carcinoma of the esophagus. *Cancer* (1994) **73**: 1779–84.

7. Urba SG, Orringer MB, Turrisi A, Iannettoni M, Forastiere A, Strawderman M. Randomized trial of preoperative chemoradiation versus surgery alone in patients with locoregional esophageal carcinoma. *J Clin Oncol* (2001) **19**: 305–13.

8. Walsh TN, Noonan N, Hollywood D, Kelly A, Keeling N, Hennessy TPJ. A comparison of multimodal therapy and surgery for esophageal adenocarcinoma. *New Engl J Med* (1996) **335**: 462–7.

9. Herskovic A, Martz K, Al-Sarraf M, Leichman L, Brindle J, Vaitkevicius V, Cooper J, Byhardt R, Davis L, Emami B. Combined chemotherapy and radiotherapy compared with radiotherapy alone in patients with cancer of the esophagus. *New Engl J Med* (1992) **326**: 1593–8.

10. Minsky BD, Berkey B, Kelsen DK, Ginsberg R, Pisansky T, Martenson J, Komaki R, Okawara G, Rosenthal, S. Preliminary results of intergroup INT 0123 randomized trial of combined modality therapy (CMT) for esophageal cancer: standard vs. high dose radiation therapy. *Proc Am Soc Clin Oncol* (2000) **19**: 239a (abstr. 927).

11. Jemal A, Thomas A, Murray T, Thun M. Cancer statistics, 2000. *CA: a Cancer J Clin* (2002) **52**: 23–47.

12. Bonenkamp JJ, Hermans J, Sasako M, van de Velde JH. Extended lymph node dissection for gastric cancer. *New Engl J Med* (1999) **340**: 908–14.

13. Cuschieri A, Weeden S, Fielding J, Bancewicz J, Craven J, Joypaul V, Sydes M, Fayers P. Patient survival after D1 and D2 resections for gastric cancer: long-term results of the MRC randomized surgical trial. Surgical Cooperative Group. *Br J Cancer* (1999) **79**: 1522–30.

14. Janunger KG, Hafstrom L, Nygren P, Glimelius B. A systematic overview of chemotherapy effects in gastric cancer. *Acta Oncol* (2001) **40**: 309–26.

15. Macdonald JS, Smalley SR, Benedetti J, Hundahl SA, Estes NC, Haller DG, Ajani JA, Gunderson LL, Jessup JM, Martenson JA. Chemoradiotherapy after surgery compared with surgery alone for adenocarcinoma of the stomach or gastroesophageal junction. *New Engl J Med* (2001) **345**: 725–30.

16. Webb A, Cunningham D, Scarffe JH, Harper P, Norman A, Joffe JK, Hughes M, Mansi J, Findlay M, Hill A, Oates J, Nicolson M, Hickish T, O'Brien M, Iveson T, Watson M, Underhill C, Wardley A, Meehan M. Randomized trial comparing epirubicin, cisplatin, and fluorouracil versus fluorouracil, doxorubicin, and methotrexate in advanced esophagogastric cancer. *J Clin Oncol* (1997) **15**: 261–7.

17. Moertel CG, Frytak S, Hahn RG, O'Connell MJ, Reitemeier RJ, Rubin J, Schutt AJ, Weiland LH, Childs DS, Holbrook MA, Lavin PT, Livstone E, Spiro H, Knowlton A, Kalser M, Barkin J, Lessner H, Mann-Kaplan R, Ramming K, Douglas HO, Thomas P, Nave H, Bateman J, Lokich J, Chaffey J, Corson JM, Zamcheck N, Noval JW. Therapy of locally unresectable pancreatic carcinoma: a randomized comparison of high dose (6000 Rads) radiation alone, moderate dose radiation (4000 Rads +5−fluorouracil), and high dose radiation +5−fluorouracil. *Cancer* (1981) **48**: 1705–10.

18. Klaassen DJ, MacIntyre JM, Catton GE, Engstrom PF, Moertel CG. Treatment of locally unresectable cancer of the stomach and pancreas: a randomized comparison of 5-fluorouracil alone with radiation plus concurrent and maintenance 5-fluouorouracil – an Eastern Cooperative Oncology Group Study. *J Clin Oncol* (1985) **3**: 373–8.

19. Gastrointestinal Tumor Study Group. Treatment of locally unresectable carcinoma of the pancreas: comparison of combined-modality therapy (chemotherapy plus radiotherapy) to chemotherapy alone. *J Natl Cancer Inst* (1988) **80**: 751–5.

20. Neoptolemos JP, Dunn JA, Stocken DD, Almond J, Link K, Beger H, Bassi C, Falconi M, Pederzoli P, Dervenis C, Fernandez-Cruz L, Lacaine F, Pap A, Spooner D, Kerr DJ, Friess H, Buchler MW, Members of the European Study

Group for Pancreatic Cancer. Adjuvant chemoradiotherapy and chemotherapy in resectable pancreatic cancer: a randomised controlled trial. *Lancet* (2001) **358**: 1576–85.

21. Burris HA, Moore MJ, Andersen J, Green MR, Rothenberg ML, Modiano MR, Cripps MC, Portenoy RK, Storniolo AM, Tarassoff P, Nelson R, Dorr FA, Stephens CD, Von Hoff DD. Improvements in survival and clinical benefit with gemcitabine as first-line therapy for patients with advanced pancreas cancer: a randomized trial. *J Clin Oncol* (1997) **15**: 2403–13.

22. Moore MJ, Hamm J, Eisenberg P, Dagenais M, Hagan K, Fields A, Greenberg B, Schwartz B, Ottaway J, Zee B, Seymour L. A comparison between gemcitabine (GEM) and the matrix metalloproteinase (MMP) inhibitor BAY12-9566 (9566) in patients (pts) with advanced pancreatic cancer. *Proc Am Soc Clin Oncol* (2000) **19**: 240a (abstr. 930).

23. McKeown-Eyssen GE, Bright-See E, Bruce WR, Jazmaji V, Cohen LB, Pappas SC, Saibil FG. A randomized trial of a low fat high fibre diet in the recurrence of colorectal polyps. Toronto Polyp Prevention Group. *J Clin Epidemiol* (1994) **47**: 525–36.

24. MacLennan R, Macrae F, Bain C, Battistutta D, Chapuis P, Gratten H, Lambert J, Newland RC, Ngu M, Russell A. Randomized trial of intake of fat, fiber, and beta carotene to prevent colorectal adenomas. The Australian Polyp Prevention Project. *J Natl Cancer Inst* (1995) **87**: 1760–6.

25. Bonithon-Kopp C, Kronborg O, Giacosa A, Rath U, Faivre J. Calcium and fibre supplementation in prevention of colorectal adenoma recurrence: a randomised intervention trial. European Cancer Prevention Organisation Study Group. *Lancet* (2000) **356**: 1300–6.

26. Alberts DS, Martinez ME, Roe DJ, Guillen-Rodriguez JM, Marshall JR, van Leeuwen JB, Reid ME, Ritenbaugh C, Vargas PA, Bhattacharyya AB, Earnest DL, Sampliner RE. Lack of effect of a high-fiber cereal supplement on the recurrence of colorectal adenomas. Phoenix Colon Cancer Prevention Physicians' Network. *New Engl J Med* (2000) **342**: 1156–62.

27. Schatzkin A, Lanza E, Corle D, Lance P, Iber F, Caan B, Shike M, Weissfeld J, Burt R, Cooper MR, Kikendall JW, Cahill J. Lack of effect of a low-fat, high-fiber diet on the recurrence of colorectal adenomas. Polyp Prevention Trial Study Group. *New Engl J Med* (2000) **342**: 1149–55.

28. Ponz de Leon M, Roncucci L. Chemoprevention of colorectal tumors: role of lactulose and of other agents. *Scand J Gastroenterol Suppl* (1997) **222**: 72–5.

29. Hofstad B, Almendingen K, Vatn M, Andersen SN, Owen RW, Larsen S, Osnes M. Growth and recurrence of colorectal polyps: a double-blind 3-year intervention with calcium and antioxidants. *Digestion* (1998) **59**: 148–56.

30. McKeown-Eyssen G, Holloway C, Jazmaji V, Bright-See E, Dion P, Bruce WR. A randomized trial of vitamins C and E in the prevention of recurrence of colorectal polyps. *Cancer Res* (1988) **48**: 4701–5.

31. Greenberg ER, Baron JA, Tosteson TD, Freeman DH Jr, Beck GJ, Bond JH, Colacchio TA, Coller JA, Frankl HD, Haile RW. A clinical trial of antioxidant vitamins to prevent colorectal adenoma. Polyp Prevention Study Group. *New Engl J Med* (1994) **331**: 141–7.

32. Bergsma-Kadijk JA, van't Veer P, Kampman E, Burema J. Calcium does not protect against colorectal neoplasia. *Epidemiology* (1996) **7**: 590–7.

33. Baron JA, Beach M, Mandel JS, van Stolk RU, Haile RW, Sandler RS, Rothstein R, Summers RW, Snover DC, Beck GJ, Bond JH, Greenberg ER. Calcium supplements for the prevention of colorectal adenomas. Calcium Polyp Prevention Study Group. *New Engl J Med* (1999) **340**: 101–7.

34. The Women's Health Initiative Study Group. Design of the women's health initiative clinical trial and observational study. *Contr Clin Trials* (1998) **19**: 61–109.

35. Gann PH, Manson JE, Glynn RJ, Buring JE, Hennekens CH. Low-dose aspirin and incidence of colorectal tumors in a randomized trial. *J Natl Cancer Inst* (1993) **85**: 1220–4.

36. Sturmer T, Glynn RJ, Lee IM, Manson JE, Buring JE, Hennekens CH. Aspirin use and colorectal cancer: post-trial follow-up data from the Physicians' Health Study. *Ann Int Med* (1998) **128**: 713–20.

37. Steinbach G, Lynch PM, Phillips RK, Wallace MH, Hawk E, Gordon GB, Wakabayashi N, Saunders B, Shen Y, Fujimura T, Su LK, Levin B. The effect of celecoxib, a cyclooxygenase-2 inhibitor, in familial adenomatous polyposis. *New Engl J Med* (2000) **342**: 1946–52.

38. Jorgensen OD, Kronborg O, Fenger C. A randomised study of screening for colorectal cancer using faecal occult blood testing: results after 13 years and seven biennial screening rounds. *Gut* (2002) **50**: 29–32.

39. Scholefield JH, Moss S, Sufi F, Mangham CM, Hardcastle JD. Effect of faecal occult blood screening on mortality from colorectal cancer: results from a randomised controlled trial. *Gut* (2002) **50**: 840–4.

40. Mandel JS, Church TR, Bond JH, Ederer F, Geisser MS, Mongin SJ, Snover DC, Schuman LM. The effect of fecal occult-blood screening on the incidence of colorectal cancer. *New Engl J Med* (2000) **343**: 1603–7.

41. Winawer SJ, Fletcher RH, Miller L, Godlee F, Stolar MH, Mulrow CD, Woolf SH, Glick SN, Ganiats TG, Bond JH, Rosen L, Zapka JG, Olsen SJ, Giardiello FM, Sisk JE, Van Antwerp R, Brown-Davis C, Marciniak DA, Mayer RJ. Colorectal cancer screening: clinical guidelines and rationale. *Gastroenterology* (1997) **112**: 594–642.

42. Smith RA, Cokkinides V, von Eschenbach AC, Levin B, Cohen C, Runowicz CD, Sener S, Saslow D, Eyre HJ. American Cancer Society guidelines for the early detection of cancer. *CA: a Cancer J Clin* (2002) **52**: 8–22.

43. Weissfeld JL, Ling BS, Schoen RE, Bresalier RS, Riley T, Prorok PC. Adherence to repeat screening flexible sigmoidoscopy in the Prostate, Lung, Colorectal, and Ovarian (PLCO) Cancer Screening Trial. *Cancer* (2002) **94**: 2569–76.

44. UK Flexible Sigmoidoscopy Screening Trial Investigators. Single flexible sigmoidoscopy screening to prevent colorectal cancer: baseline findings of a UK multicentre randomised trial. *Lancet* (2002) **359**: 1291–300.

45. Ness RM, Holmes AM, Klein R, Dittus R. Cost-utility of one-time colonoscopic screening for colorectal cancer at various ages. *Am J Gastroenterol* (2000) **95**: 1800–11.

46. Winawer SJ, Zauber AG, Church TR, Mandelson M, Feld A, Bond JH. National Colonoscopy Study (NCS) preliminary findings: a randomized clinical trial of general population screening colonoscopy. *Gastroenterology* (2002) T1560.

47. Stocchi L, Nelson H. Laparoscopic colectomy for colon cancer: trial update. *J Surg Oncol* (1998) **68**: 255–67.

48. Laurie JA, Moertel CG, Fleming TR, Wieand HS, Leigh JE, Rubin J, McCormack GW, Gerstner JB, Krook JE, Mailliard J, Twito DI, Morton RF, Tschetter LK, Barlow JF. Surgical adjuvant therapy of large-bowel carcinoma: an evaluation of levamisole and the combination of levamisole and fluorouracil. *J Clin Oncol* (1989) **7**: 1447–56.

49. Moertel CG, Fleming TR, Macdonald JS, Haller DG, Laurie JA, Goodman PJ, Ungerleider JS, Emerson WA, Tormey DC, Glick JH, Veeder MH, Mailliard JA. Levamisole and fluorouracil for adjuvant therapy of resected colon carcinoma. *New Engl J Med* (1990) **322**: 352–8.

50. NIH Consensus Conference. Adjuvant therapy for patients with colon and rectal cancer. *J Am Med Assoc* (1990) **264**: 1444–50.

51. International Multicentre Pooled Analysis of Colon Cancer Trials (IMPACT) Investigators. Efficacy of adjuvant fluorouracil and folinic acid in colon cancer. *Lancet* (1995) **345**: 939–44.

52. Francini G, Petrioli R, Lorenzini L, Mancini S, Armenio S, Tanzini G, Marsili S, Aquino A, Marzocca G, Civitelli S, Mariani L, De Sando D, Bovenga S, Lorenz M. Folinic acid and 5-fluorouracil as adjuvant chemotherapy in colon cancer. *Gastroenterology* (1994) **106**: 899–906.

53. O'Connell MJ, Mailliard JA, Kahn MJ, Macdonald JS, Haller DG, Mayer RJ, Wieand HS. Controlled trial of fluorouracil and low-dose leucovorin given for 6 months as postoperative adjuvant therapy for colon cancer. *J Clin Oncol* (1997) **15**: 246–50.

54. QUASAR Collaborative Group. Comparison of fluorouracil with additional levamisole, higher-dose folinic acid, or both, as adjuvant chemotherapy for colorectal cancer: a randomised trial. *Lancet* (2000) **355**: 1588–96.

55. Haller DG, Catalano PJ, Macdonald JS. Fluorouracil (FU), leucovorin (LV) and levamisole (LEV) adjuvant therapy for colon cancer: five-year final report of INT-0089. *Proc Am Soc Clin Oncol* (1998) **17**: 256a (abstr. 982).

56. Poplin E, Benedetti N, Estes D, Haller DG, Mayer R, Goldberg R, Macdonald J. Phase III randomized trial of bolus 5-FU/leucovorin/levamisole versus 5-FU continuous/infusion/levamisole as adjuvant therapy for high risk colon cancer (SWOG 9415/INT-0153). *Proc Am Soc Clin Oncol* (2000) **19**: 240a.

57. Wolmark N, Fisher B, Rockette H. Postoperative adjuvant chemotherapy or BCG for colon cancer: results from NSABP protocol C-01. *J Natl Cancer Inst* (1988) **80**: 30–6.

58. Sargent DJ, Goldberg RM, Jacobson SD, Macdonald JS, Labianca R, Haller DG, Shepherd LE, Seitz JF, Francini G. A pooled analysis of adjuvant chemotherapy for resected colon cancer in elderly patients. *New Engl J Med* (2001) **345**: 1091–7.

59. Mamounas E, Wieand S, Wolmark N, Bear HD, Atkins JN, Song K, Jones J, Rockette H. Comparative efficacy of adjuvant chemotherapy in patients with Dukes' B versus Dukes' C colon cancer: results from four National Surgical Adjuvant Breast and Bowel Project Adjuvant Studies (C-01, C-02, C-03, and C-04). *J Clin Oncol* (1999) **17**: 1349–55.

60. International Multicentre Pooled Analysis of B2 Colon Cancer Trials (IMPACT B2) Investigators. Efficacy of adjuvant fluorouracil and folinic acid in B2 colon cancer. *J Clin Oncol* (1999) **17**: 1356–63.

61. Advanced Colorectal Cancer Meta-analysis Project. Modulation of fluorouracil by leucovorin in patients with advanced colorectal cancer: evidence in terms of response rate. *J Clin Oncol* (1992) **10**: 896–903.

62. Meta-Analysis Group in Cancer. Efficacy of intravenous continuous infusion of fluorouracil compared with bolus administration in advanced colorectal cancer. *J Clin Oncol* (1998) **16**: 301–8.

63. Meta-Analysis Group in Cancer. Toxicity of fluorouracil in patients with advanced colorectal cancer: effect of administration schedule and prognostic factors. *J Clin Oncol* (1998) **16**: 3537–41.

64. Hoff PM, Ansari R, Batist G. Comparison of oral capecitabine versus intravenous fluorouracil plus leucovorin as first-line treatment in 605 patients with metastatic colorectal cancer: results of a randomized phase III study. *J Clin Oncol* (2001) **19**: 2282–92.

65. Van Cutsem E, Twelves C, Cassidy J. Oral capecitabine compared with intravenous fluorouracil plus leucovorin in patients with metastatic colorectal cancer: results of a large phase III study. *J Clin Oncol* (2001) **19**: 4097–106.

66. Rougier P, Van Cutsem E, Bajetta E. Randomised trial of irinotecan versus fluorouracil by continuous infusion after fluorouracil failure in patients with metastatic colorectal cancer. *Lancet* (1998) **352**: 1407–12.

67. Cunningham D, Pyrhonen S, James RD. Randomised trial of irinotecan plus supportive care versus supportive care alone after fluorouracil failure for patients with metastatic colorectal cancer. *Lancet* (1998) **352**: 1413–18.

68. Saltz LB, Cox JV, Blanke C, Rosen LS, Fehrenbacher L, Moore MJ, Maroun JA, Ackland SP, Locker PK, Pirotta N, Elfring GL, Miller LL. Irinotecan plus fluorouracil and leucovorin for metastatic colorectal cancer. *New Engl J Med* (2000) **343**: 905–14.

69. Douillard JY, Cunningham D, Roth AD, Navarro M, James RD, Karasek P, Jandik P, Iveson R, Carmichael J, Alakl M, Gruia G, Awad L, Rougier P. Irinotecan combined with fluorouracil compared with fluorouracil alone as first-line treatment for metastatic colorectal cancer: a multicentre randomised trial. *Lancet* (2000) **355**: 1041–7.

70. De Gramont A, Figer A, Seymour M, Homerin M, Hmissi A, Cassidy J, Boni C, Cortes-Funes H, Cervantes A, Freyer G, Papamichael D, Le Bail N, Louvet C, Hendler D, de Braud F, Wilson C, Morvan F, Bonetti A. Leucovorin and fluorouracil with or without oxaliplatin as first-line treatment in advanced colorectal cancer. *J Clin Oncol* (2000) **18**: 2938–47.

71. Goldberg RM, Morton RF, Sargent DJ, Fuchs C, Ramanathan S, Williamson S, Findlay B, NCCTG, CALGB, ECOG, SWOG, NCIC. N9741 oxaliplatin (Oxal) or CPT-11 + 5-fluorouracil (5FU)/leucovorin (LV) or oxal + CPT-11 in advanced colorectal cancer (CRC). Initial toxicity and response data from a GI intergroup study. *Proc Am Soc Clin Oncol* (2002) **21**: 128a.

72. Krook JE, Moertel CG, Gunderson LL, Wieand HS, Collins RT, Beart RW, Kubista TP, Poon MA, Meyers WC, Mailliard JA, Twito DI, Morton RF, Veeder MH, Witzig TE, Cha S, Vidyarthi SC. Effective surgical adjuvant therapy for high-risk rectal carcinoma. *New Engl J Med* (1991) **324**: 709–15.

73. O'Connell MJ, Martenson JA, Wieand HS, Krook JE, Macdonald JS, Haller DG, Mayer RJ, Gunderson LL, Rich TA. Improving adjuvant therapy for rectal cancer by combining protracted-infusion fluorouracil with radiation therapy after curative surgery. *New Engl J Med* (1994) **331**: 502–7.

74. Fisher B, Wolmark N, Rockette H, Redmond C, Deutsch M, Wickerham DL. Postoperative adjuvant chemotherapy or radiation therapy for rectal cancer: results from NSABP Protocol R-01. *J Natl Cancer Inst* (1988) **80**: 21–9.

75. Wolmark N, Wieand HS, Hyams DM, Colangelo L, Dimitrov NV, Romond EH, Wexler M, Prager D, Cruz AB Jr, Gordon PH, Petrelli NJ, Deutsch M, Mamounas E, Wickerham DL, Fisher ER, Rockette H, Fisher B. Randomized trial of postoperative adjuvant chemotherapy with or without radiotherapy for carcinoma of the rectum: National Surgical Adjuvant Breast and Bowel Project Protocol R-02. *J Natl Cancer Inst* (2000) **92**: 388–96.

76. Swedish Rectal Cancer Trial. Improved survival with preoperative radiotherapy in resectable rectal cancer. *New Engl J Med* (1997) **336**: 980–7.

77. Sauer R, Fietkau R, Wittekind C, Martus P, Rodel C, Hohenberger W, Jatzko G, Sabitzer H, Karstens JH, Becker H, Hess C, Raab R. Adjuvant versus neoadjuvant radiochemotherapy for locally advanced rectal cancer. A progress report of a phase-III randomized trial (protocol CAO/ARO/AIO-94). *Strahlenther Onkol* (2001) **177**: 173–8.

78. Enker WE, Thaler HT, Cranor ML, Polyak T. Total mesorectal excision in the operative treatment of carcinoma of the rectum. *J Am Coll Surg* (1995) **181**: 335–46.

79. Kapiteijn E, Marijnen CAM, Nagtegaal ID, Putter H, Steup WH, Wiggers T, Rutten HJT, Pahlman L, Glimelius B, Han J, van Krieken HJM, Leer JWH, van de Velde JH. Preoperative radiotherapy combined with total mesorectal excision for resectable rectal cancer. *New Engl J Med* (2001) **345**: 638–46.

80. Hammond MEH, Taube SE. Issues and barriers to development of clinically useful tumor markers: a development pathway proposal. *Semin Oncol* (2002) **29**: 213–21.

81. Pajak TF, Clark GM, Sargent DJ, McShane LM, Hammond MEH. Statistical issues in tumor marker studies. *Arch Pathol Lab Med* (2000) **124**: 1011–15.

82. Grignon D, Caplan R, Sarkar F. p53 status and prognosis of locally advanced prostatic adenocarcinoma. *J Natl Cancer Inst* (1997) **89**: 158–65.

83. Sargent DJ, Goldberg RM, Mahoney MR, Hillman DW, McKeough T, Hamilton SF, Darcy JM, Anderson VL, Krook JE, O'Connell MJ. Rapid reporting and review of an increased incidence of a known adverse event. *J Natl Cancer Inst* (2000) **92**: 1011–13.

84. Rothenberg ML, Meropol NJ, Poplin EA, Van Cutsem E, Wadler S. Mortality associated with irinotecan plus bolus fluorouracil/leucovorin: summary findings of an independent panel. *J Clin Oncol* (2001) **19**: 3801–7.

85. Goldberg RM, Sargent DJ, Morton RF, Mahoney MR, Krook JE, O'Connell MJ. Sensing toxicity and adjusting ongoing clinical trials protocols to enhance patient safety: the history and performance of the NCCTG 'Real Time Toxicity Monitoring Program'. *J Clin Oncol* (2002) **20**: 4591–6.

86. Ullman B, Lee M, Martin DW Jr, Santi DV. Cytotoxicity of 5-fluoro-2-deoxyuridine: requirement for reduced folate co-factors and antagonism by methotrexate. *Proc Natl Acad Sci* (1978) **75**: 980–3.

87. Evans RM, Laskin JD, Hakala MT. Effect of excess folates and deoxyinosine on the activity and site of action of 5-fluorouracil. *Cancer Res* (1981) **41**: 3288–95.

88. Waxman S, Bruckner H. The enhancement of 5-fluorouracil antimetabolic activity by leucovorin, menadione, and alpha-tocopherol. *Eur J Cancer Clin Oncol* (1982) **18**: 685–92.

89. Keyomarsi K, Moran RG. Folinic augmentation of the effects of fluoropyrimidines on murine and human leukemic cells. *Cancer Res* (1986) **46**: 5229–35.

90. Houghton JA, Williams LG, Loftin SK. Relationship between the dose rate of [6RS] leucovorin administration, plasma concentrations of reduced folates, and pools of 5,10 methylenetetrahydrafolates and tetrahydrafolates in human colon adenocarcinoma xenografts. *Cancer Res* (1990) **50**: 3493–502.

91. Houghton JA, Williams LG, Loftin SK. Factors that influence the therapeutic activity of 5-fluorouracil [6RS] leucovorin combinations in colon adenocarcinoma xenografts. *Cancer Chemother Pharmacol* (1992) **30**: 423–32.

92. Houghton JA, Williams LG, Cheshire PJ. Influence of the dose of [6RS] leucovorin on reduced folate pools and 5-fluorouracil-mediated thymidylate synthase inhibition in human colon adenocarcinoma xenografts. *Cancer Res* (1990) **50**: 3940–6.

93. Cao S, Frank C, Rustum YM. Role of fluoropyrimidine scheduling and (6R,S) leucovorin dose in a preclinical animal model of colorectal carcinoma. *J Natl Cancer Inst* (1996) **88**: 430–6.

94. Machover D, Goldschmidt E, Chollet P. Treatment of advanced colorectal and gastric adenocarcinomas with 5-fluorouracil and high-dose folinic acid. *J Clin Oncol* (1986) **4**: 685–96.

95. Machover D, Schwartenberg L, Goldschmidt E. Treatment of advanced colorectal and gastric adenocarcinomas with 5-FU combined with high-dose folinic acid: a pilot study. *Cancer Treat Rep* (1982) **66**: 1803–7.

96. Rustum YM, Trave F, Zakrzewski SF. Biochemical and pharmacologic basis for potentiation of 5-fluorouracil action by leucovorin. *NCI Monogr* (1987) **5**: 165–70.

97. Poon MA, O'Connell MJ, Moertel CG. Biochemical modulation of fluorouracil: evidence of significant improvement in survival and quality of life in patients with advanced colorectal carcinoma. *J Clin Oncol* (1989) **7**: 1407–18.

98. O'Connell MJ. A phase III trial of 5-fluorouracil and leucovorin in the treatment of advanced colorectal cancer: a Mayo Clinic/North Central Cancer Treatment Group study. *Cancer* (1989) **63**: 1026–30.

99. Petrelli N, Herrara L, Rustum Y. A prospective randomized trial of 5-fluorouracil vs. 5-fluorouracil and high dose leucovorin +5–fluorouracil and methotrexate in previously untreated patients with advanced colorectal carcinoma. *J Clin Oncol* (1987) **5**: 1559–65.

100. Buroker TR, O'Connell MJ, Wieand HS. Randomized comparison of two schedules of fluorouracil and leucovorin in the treatment of advanced colorectal cancer. *J Clin Oncol* (1994) **12**: 14–20.

9

Haematologic Cancers

CHARLES A. SCHIFFER[1] AND STEPHEN L. GEORGE[2]

[1]Karmanos Cancer Institute, Wayne State University School of Medicine, Detroit, MI 48201, USA
[2]Department of Biostatistics and Bioinformatics, Duke University Medical Centre, Durham, NC 27710, USA

INTRODUCTION

The story of therapeutic research for acute myeloid leukaemia (AML) is one of mixed success. AML has been studied extensively both in the clinic and in the laboratory, in part because of the accessibility of cells for *in vitro* testing, and has served as a model for the elucidation of many of the principles of anti-neoplastic therapy and translational research in infectious disease and transfusion medicine supportive care. Complete remission after initial therapy is achieved in about two-thirds of patients, a significant fraction of whom can be cured with additional post-remission treatment. Unfortunately, however, the great majority of patients eventually relapse and succumb to complications of the disease and its treatment. The incidence of AML spans the entire age spectrum but is most common in adults greater than 60 years of age and the prognosis is particularly poor in these individuals.

Large numbers of randomised trials have been performed in patients with AML including comparative evaluations of different doses and types of chemotherapeutic agents, the use of haematopoietic growth factors, stem cell transplantation in first remission and modulation of various mechanisms of intrinsic drug resistance.[1-7] Some of these trials have, in fact, changed the standard care of the disease but most have unfortunately been negative in that the newer approaches failed to improve remission rates and overall survival. Intensive treatment regimens have improved outcome in younger patients, but clinical trials in patients 60 years and older by the Cancer and Leukemia Group B (CALGB) and others have shown remarkably consistent poor results, with complete remission (CR) rates of around 50%, and only 10% of patients surviving four years.[1,8,9] Indeed, it is arguable that the prognosis of older patients with AML has not changed in the last 15 years. Therefore, it is imperative that new therapies are evaluated in as efficient a fashion as possible. There are a number of issues which can serve as impediments to new drug development, some of which are idiosyncratic to AML. This chapter will review some of these problems and suggest and discuss some of the statistical issues in trial design.

Textbook of Clinical Trials. Edited by D. Machin, S. Day and S. Green
© 2004 John Wiley & Sons, Ltd   ISBN: 0-471-98787-5

BACKGROUND

AML occurs as a consequence of an acquired mutation in a haematopoietic stem cell which results in a failure of normal maturation and differentiation of myeloid cells and an accumulation of juvenile leukaemia cells or 'blasts'. By mechanisms which are not well understood, the expansion of this malignant clone suppresses normal blood cell formation and patients usually present with symptoms related to absence of normal blood cells including weakness and fatigue due to anaemia, infection because of decreased number of normal white blood cells, and bleeding because of marked decreases in the number of platelets. Because this is a systemic disease, initial treatment is with chemotherapy, generally including an anthracycline and cytarabine (ara-c), administered for three and seven days respectively. This induces a period of low blood counts for three to four weeks at which time the patient is at risk for bleeding and infection and invariably requires transfusions of red blood cells, platelets and the use of systemic antibiotics. Should therapy be successful, a complete remission is obtained which is defined as normal blood counts and bone marrow with no evidence of leukaemia.[10] It is known that small amounts of leukaemia remain, which cannot be detected morphologically with the microscope, because without further therapy, leukaemia invariably relapses, generally within six months. Remission rates are approximately 75% in younger patients but are only 50% in older patients (greater than 60 years of age).

There have been major improvements in infectious disease and transfusion supportive care so that, today, the major cause of initial treatment failure is drug-resistant leukaemia (i.e. persistence of leukaemia after treatment). Randomised trials comparing different types of anthracyclines, different doses and schedules of administration of ara-c, and the use of growth factors for supportive care, have not improved these induction results. With appropriate post-remission therapy, approximately 35% of patients less than 50 years of age remain disease-free after three years, with almost all of these patients being functionally

cured of their leukaemia; however, less than 10% of patients greater than 60 years of age remain in long-term remission.[1,6,8,9] Multiple randomised trials evaluating high-dose therapy with either autologous or allogeneic stem cell rescue have produced results similar to those achieved with chemotherapy alone, although the causes of treatment failure vary somewhat, with lower rates of relapse with transplant approaches offset by higher treatment associated mortality.[6] In addition, transplant approaches are generally suitable only for younger patients.

AML is also an extremely heterogeneous disorder biologically. Multiple subtypes can be identified by cytogenetic or molecular studies of the leukaemia cells. Some of these subtypes (predominantly found in younger patients) have an excellent prognosis with cure rates of approximately 60%, whereas other subtypes, generally characterised by chromosome loss and duplication, have almost no patients cured with chemotherapy alone.[11] The latter is much more common in older patients, particularly those in whom AML developed as a progression of a prior bone marrow disorder either of a myeloproliferative nature or more commonly following a myelodysplastic syndrome.

Cytogenetic and molecular characterisation of the type of AML can be critical as evidenced by the remarkable results achieved in recent years in acute progranulocytic leukaemia (APL), a subgroup representing about 10% of patients with AML, predominantly in younger adults and children.[12] All patients with APL have a balanced translocation between chromosomes 15 and 17, resulting in a mutation of the gene coding for the retinoic acid nuclear receptor. By complex mechanisms, this confers unique sensitivity to an oral retinoid, all-trans retinoic acid (ATRA), which has appreciably fewer side effects than traditional chemotherapy. A series of randomised trials have elucidated the optimal means of combining ATRA with chemotherapy such that more than 70% of patients with this previously devastating leukaemia can be cured.[13] Interestingly, APL also has a unique sensitivity to arsenical compounds. It is hoped that similar strategies with different compounds can be discovered for other AML variants with discrete activating mutations, as has recently also been achieved in patients with chronic myeloid leukaemia (CML) with the use of the tyrosine kinase inhibitor imatinib mesylate (STI571), which specifically targets the abnormal enzyme produced by the bcr/abl mutation characteristic of CML.[14]

Some studies have suggested differential responsiveness of AML subtypes to different types of chemotherapy. In particular, patients with more favourable balanced translocations seem to benefit from high-dose ara-c-based consolidation therapy. In contrast, patients with poor prognosis chromosomal changes do not benefit from these more intensive chemotherapeutic approaches,[15] although a fraction may be cured with the graft versus leukaemia effect induced by allogeneic stem cell transplantation. Stem cell transplant is currently not a possibility for older patients. Because of this, many treatment cooperative groups have devised different therapeutic approaches for older and younger patients, with manipulations of stem cell transplantation being evaluated in the latter group.

IMPROVING THERAPY FOR OLDER PATIENTS WITH AML

Rates of complete remission are much lower and remission duration more abbreviated in patients greater than the age of 60 years as a consequence of more intrinsic drug resistance and more baseline organ dysfunction than are encountered in younger individuals. New therapeutic approaches should focus both on increasing remission rates as well as on prolonging remission and enhancing the cure fraction of such patients. Many AML studies have focused on older patients because of the large numbers of such patients available for studies as well as the feeling that the overall results of therapy are so poor that it would be possible to identify truly active agents very rapidly because differences with historical or randomised controls would be obvious.

However, there are a number of both practical and biologic issues complicating the conduct of such trials:

- Evaluation of post-remission manipulations is made more difficult by the low complete response rate, so that less than 50% of patients initially entered on trial are eligible for post-remission treatment. In addition, many such patients are not candidates for intensive therapy because of compromised organ function from toxicities encountered during induction, and because many older patients do not recover fully normal blood counts even after a significant anti-leukaemic response during induction.
- In addition, many older individuals decline post-remission treatment, preferring to spend their remaining time outside of the hospital, as far from aggressive medical ministrations as possible.

Thus, randomised studies of new therapies introduced post-remission need larger numbers of patients to account for this drop-off in patients as the study progresses. This represents a major issue since only a small fraction of such patients are captured for clinical trials.

Furthermore:

- AML in older individuals is extremely heterogeneous. Some therapies might be appropriate only for certain AML subtypes and positive effects can be missed when tested in the overall AML population. This may be particularly true for newer targeted therapies.
- A focus on patients with highly resistant disease represents a particularly high hurdle for new therapies and treatments. Modest, but nonetheless important, benefits which could be of value to other patient groups could be missed by studying only patients in very poor prognostic groups.

These problems are particularly relevant, because there is no shortage of new agents which could and should be evaluated in AML. In addition to a continued supply of cytotoxic drugs, there will be large numbers of anti-angiogenesis compounds, immune modulators, signal transduction inhibitors (either with specific or more generic enzymatic targets), as well as new and less acutely toxic approaches to stem cell transplant. Many of the non-cytotoxic therapeutic approaches also have the allure of oral treatment with potentially much less toxicity.

If an agent can be safely added to the usual dose of conventional therapy, it might be most efficient to utilise the new therapy in both induction and consolidation, thereby perhaps maximising the chance to detect anti-leukaemic activity. Possible study designs for trials of new post-remission therapies are shown in Table 9.1, where conventional therapy might refer to a few courses of low-dose ara-c which results in a median remission duration of approximately eight months and less than 10% long-term disease-free survival.[9] This is slightly better than observation without treatment which produces very few if any long-term disease-free survivors and shorter CR durations. The choice among the various randomised approaches might be influenced by the unique features of the agent being tested. Also, given the very poor results observed with standard therapy, it could be argued that a straightforward Phase II trial in which the new agent is evaluated alone could have merit, although the usual problems with historical controls and patient selection would be issues. However, a number of anti-cancer agents have been approved by the FDA in recent years under an accelerated approval mechanism, based on Phase II data alone which showed benefit in patients with resistant disease and otherwise few therapeutic options.

STATISTICAL ISSUES IN DESIGN AND ANALYSIS

Because of the nature of AML and its treatment, several statistical issues in the design and analysis of clinical trials need special attention. Four of these are discussed: factorial designs, outcome measures, competing risks and statistical modelling.

FACTORIAL DESIGNS

The treatment phases for AML are conventionally divided into an initial phase of induction therapy and, for those achieving a complete remission during this phase, a post-remission or maintenance therapy phase. The post-remission phase is sometimes further divided into earlier consolidation therapy and later maintenance therapy, but for our purposes here, two phases are sufficient. It is natural to design studies to compare therapies in each of these two phases, leading to factorial designs, in which patients are randomly assigned to one of two or more induction therapies (the first factor) and then to one of two or more maintenance therapies (the second factor). With two possible treatment assignments in each phase, this is a 2×2 factorial design, a common and well-known statistical design. Much has been written about this design applied in the clinical trials setting.[16] The twist in the current situation is that the second randomisation is applicable only for patients who respond to the induction therapy. As noted above, in the case of older AML patients, only about 50% of all patients entered on study may respond and, thus, be eligible and medically suitable for the second randomisation.

It is typical to separate the objectives of such studies into a comparison of induction regimens with respect to response rates and, separately, a comparison of maintenance regimens with respect to the length of remission, disease-free survival or overall survival. For example,

Table 9.1. Possible study designs evaluating new agents in post-remission therapy

---

Phase II studies
New agent alone

Randomised Phase III studies
Observation vs. new agent
Conventional vs. new agent
Conventional vs. conventional + new agent
Conventional followed by observation vs. new agent
New agent in both induction and consolidation

CALGB 8923 was a randomised clinical trial of this type involving AML patients at least 60 years old.[2,9] The induction phase involved a randomisation between GM-CSF, a haematopoietic growth factor, and placebo following initial chemotherapy. The hypothesis was that the GM-CSF would reduce infectious complications and perhaps increase the response rate. Responding patients were to be randomised to receive one of two post-remission regimens, cytarabine alone or a combination of cytarabine and mitoxantrone. Overall, 388 participants were randomised to the induction therapies; 205 (53%) achieved a CR, but only 169 (44%) were randomised in the post-remission phase.

One of the problems with the usual approach to these designs is that there is no direct estimation or testing of the four possible treatment policies implied in the design. The policies are defined by selecting one of two induction therapies followed by one of two post-remission therapies, if a response is obtained and the patient consents to continue. One paper deals directly with this issue, making efficient use of data from all patients.[17] There are also methodologic issues about when the randomisation to the post-remission therapy should be done. For example, if both randomisations are done at the time of study entry with a planned intent to treat analysis, then the inevitable (and anticipated) large patient drop-out can substantially complicate evaluation of the second therapeutic manoeuvre.

OUTCOME MEASURES

There are various choices for outcome measures in clinical trials involving AML patients. The primary ones are:

- Response rate – the proportion of patients who achieve an initial clinical response to the induction therapy is referred to as the response rate. In older AML patients, as in all leukaemia patients, the critical category is the complete response (CR) rate, although partial responses are sometimes included in Phase II trials where attention is focused on identifying activity of an agent, no matter how small. Achievement of a complete response is *sine qua non* for long-term control of disease. However, the CR rate is a very imperfect surrogate for more meaningful clinical outcome measures described below, and has been defined differently by different leukaemia treatment groups, and should never be used as a substitute for them, especially in Phase III clinical trials. The primary role for the CR rate is as a measure of clinical activity in Phase II trials.

- Event-free survival (EFS) – this is the time from the start of study until a failure to respond, relapse (for those achieving a CR) or death, whichever occurs first. This outcome measure is a good measure of the overall control of disease from the start of therapy and combines the effects of induction and post-remission therapies. In a Phase III trial, all randomised patients contribute to any analysis of EFS under the usual intent-to-treat approach.[18] Standard techniques for time-to-event data (survival methods) are used in design and analysis for EFS, and for the other time-to-event endpoints defined next.[19]

- Disease-free [or relapse-free] survival (DFS) – this is a standard outcome measure in trials of adjuvant therapy for solid tumours, but in AML trials, DFS refers to the survival time spent free of disease. Thus, DFS is applicable only to patients who achieve a CR. It is defined as the time from achieving a CR to relapse or death, whichever occurs first. Since patients who fail to achieve a CR are excluded, this measure is unsuitable as an overall assessment of therapy. However, it is useful for comparing two or more post-remission therapies as long as it is recognised that the distribution of DFS is not representative of the result to be expected for all patients.

- Length of remission (LR) – the length of remission is ordinarily defined as the time from achieving CR to the time of relapse, with deaths in remission counted as censored observations. This measure suffers from the same problems as DFS and, in addition, the usual

Kaplan–Meier estimation is no longer valid (see discussion below on competing risks).

- Overall survival (OS) – the time from the start of study to death is an obviously critical outcome measure for any generally fatal disease like AML in older adults. It has the virtue of being unambiguously defined and captures a result of obvious significance. However, there are often difficulties in interpretation, particularly if multiple therapies are given, or if patients cross over to the alternative therapy after relapse. Nevertheless, the importance of overall survival is so fundamental that it should always be analysed, even if it is not used as the primary outcome measure.

- Other outcome measures – there are some other measures occasionally used in AML studies, particularly measures of quality of life (QOL).[20] Some attempt to measure survival or related time to event measures adjusted for quality of life. For example, the Q-TWiST method discounts survival time spent with an unacceptable level of adverse symptoms due to treatment.[21] Such methods attempt to quantify the generally accepted notion that simply prolonging survival is not a sufficient objective. Improved quality of life is equally important.

COMPETING RISKS

For some purposes in designing and analysing trials of therapy for older AML patients, it is informative to use the techniques of competing risks analysis.[22] That is, rather than using a composite measure such as EFS, one can break this measure into its constituent parts by considering the time to each outcome separately. The term 'competing risks' refers to various risks of failure, each competing with the others. This terminology originally arose in the context of analysing various causes of death, but it is applicable more generally. The fundamental problem from a statistical perspective is that the risks cannot be assumed to be operating independently from each other. Thus, methods which assume such independence, such as the Kaplan–Meier life table analysis,

which treats other risks as independent censoring mechanisms, are inherently flawed. One way to properly account for the dependence is through the use of the cumulative incidence curve, a topic that has been extensively explored in recent years.[23]

STATISTICAL MODELS

Statistical models are heavily used in AML trials. The usual time-to-event measures (EFS, DFS, OS) are often handled non-parametrically in the primary analysis (e.g., Kaplan–Meier estimates, logrank tests, etc.), but the semi-parametric proportional hazards regression model is surely the most commonly used method to adjust for covariates in the analysis.[19] In addition, because of the nature of AML, increasing interest is being focused on so-called cure models, in which it is hypothesised that an unknown fraction (c) of patients are cured (or at least will have long-term control of disease) and the rest ($1 - c$) are not.[24] Interest then focuses on estimating c, comparing the cure rates of various treatments, identifying factors predictive of c, and identifying prognostic factors for the time-to-failure in the patients not cured. In older patients with AML, this model has not been used as much due to the obviously low value of c, but it has been important in other leukaemias.

SUMMARY

Acute myeloid leukaemia in the older patient is a common and important disease which is relatively resistant to current therapies. Careful consideration of the particular characteristics of this disorder is required when designing clinical trials. There will be a large number of compounds available for evaluation in upcoming years and it is desirable that such studies be conducted using the most efficient and informative designs to rapidly identify therapies which lengthen survival and increase the fraction of patients who are cured.

REFERENCES

1. Mayer RJ, Davis RB, Schiffer CA, Berg DT, Powell BL, Schulman P, Omura GA, Moore JO, McIntyre OR, Frei E. 3. Intensive postremission chemotherapy in adults with acute myeloid leukemia. Cancer and Leukemia Group B. *N Engl J Med* (1994) **331**: 896–903.

2. Stone RM, Berg DT, George SL, Dodge RK, Paciucci PA, Schulman P, Lee EJ, Moore JO, Powell BL, Schiffer CA. Granulocyte-macrophage colony-stimulating factor after initial chemotherapy for elderly patients with primary acute myelogenous leukemia. *N Engl J Med* (1995) **332**: 1671–7.

3. Rowe JM, Andersen JW, Mazza JJ, Bennett JM, Paietta E, Hayes FA, Oette D, Cassileth PA, Stadtmauer EA, Wiernik PH. A randomized placebo-controlled phase III study of granulocyte-macrophage colony-stimulating factor in adult patients (> 55 to 70 years of age) with acute myelogenous leukemia: a study of the Eastern Cooperative Oncology Group (E1490). *Blood* (1995) **86**: 457–62.

4. Lowenberg B, Suciu S, Archimbaud E, Ossenkoppele G, Verhoef GE, Vellenga E, Wijermans P, Berneman Z, Dekker AW, Stryckmans P, Schouten H, Jehn U, Muus P, Sonneveld P, Dardenne M, Zittoun R. Use of recombinant GM-CSF during and after remission induction chemotherapy in patients aged 61 years and older with acute myeloid leukemia: final report of AML-11, a phase III randomized study of the Leukemia Cooperative Group of European Organisation for the Research and Treatment of Cancer and the Dutch Belgian Hemato-Oncology Cooperative Group. *Blood* (1997) **90**: 2952–61.

5. Godwin JE, Kopecky KJ, Head DR, Willman CL, Leith CP, Hynes HE, Balcerzak SP, Appelbaum FR. A double-blind placebo-controlled trial of granulocyte colony-stimulating factor in elderly patients with previously untreated acute myeloid leukemia: a Southwest oncology group study (9031). *Blood* (1998) **91**: 3607–15.

6. Cassileth PA, Harrington DP, Appelbaum FR, Lazarus HM, Rowe JM, Paietta E, Willman C, Hurd DD, Bennett JM, Blume KG, Head DR, Wiernik PH. Chemotherapy compared with autologous or allogeneic bone marrow transplantation in the management of acute myeloid leukemia in first remission. *N Engl J Med* (1998) **339**: 1649–56.

7. Baer MR, George SL, Dodge RK, O'Loughlin KL, Minderman H, Caligiuri MA, Powell BL, Kolitz JE, Schiffer CA, Bloomfield CD, Larson RA. Phase III study of the multidrug resistance modulator PSC-833 in previously untreated patients 60 years of age and older with acute myeloid leukemia: Cancer and Leukemia Group B study 9720. *Blood* (2002) **100**: 1224–32.

8. Schiffer CA, Dodge R, Larson RA. Long-term follow-up of Cancer and Leukemia Group B studies in acute myeloid leukemia. *Cancer* (1997) **80**: 2210–14.

9. Stone RM, Berg DT, George SL, Dodge RK, Paciucci PA, Schulman PP, Lee EJ, Moore JO, Powell BL, Baer MR, Bloomfield CD, Schiffer CA. Postremission therapy in older patients with de novo acute myeloid leukemia: a randomized trial comparing mitoxantrone and intermediate-dose cytarabine with standard-dose cytarabine. *Blood* (2001) **98**: 548–53.

10. Cheson BD, Cassileth PA, Head DR, Schiffer CA, Bennett JM, Bloomfield CD, Brunning R, Gale RP, Grever MR, Keating MJ. Report of the National Cancer Institute-sponsored workshop on definitions of diagnosis and response in acute myeloid leukemia. *J Clin Oncol* (1990) **8**: 813–19.

11. Byrd JC, Mrozek K, Dodge RK, Carroll AJ, Edwards CG, Arthur DC, Pettenati MJ, Patil SR, Rao KW, Watson MS, Koduru PR, Moore JO, Stone RM, Mayer RJ, Feldman EJ, Davey FR, Schiffer CA, Larson RA, Bloomfield CD, Cancer and Leukemia Group. Pretreatment cytogenetic abnormalities are predictive of induction success, cumulative incidence of relapse, and overall survival in adult patients with de novo acute myeloid leukemia: results from Cancer and Leukemia Group B (CALGB 8461). *Blood* (2002) **100**: 4325–36.

12. Tallman MS, Andersen JW, Schiffer CA, Appelbaum FR, Feusner JH, Woods WG, Ogden A, Weinstein H, Shepherd L, Willman C, Bloomfield CD, Rowe JM, Wiernik PH. All-trans retinoic acid in acute promyelocytic leukemia: long-term outcome and prognostic factor analysis from the North American Intergroup protocol. *Blood* (2002) **100**: 4298–302.

13. Fenaux P, Chastang C, Chevret S, Sanz M, Dombret H, Archimbaud E, Fey M, Rayon C, Huguet F, Sotto JJ, Gardin C. A randomized comparison of all transretinoic acid (ATRA) followed by chemotherapy and ATRA plus chemotherapy and the role of maintenance therapy in newly diagnosed acute promyelocytic leukemia. The European APL Group. *Blood* (1999) **94**: 1192–200.

14. Druker BJ, Sawyers CL, Kantarjian H, Resta DJ, Reese SF, Ford JM, Capdeville R, Talpaz M. Activity of a specific inhibitor of the BCR-ABL tyrosine kinase in the blast crisis of

chronic myeloid leukemia and acute lymphoblastic leukemia with the Philadelphia chromosome. *N Engl J Med* (2001) **344**: 1038–42.

15. Bloomfield CD, Lawrence D, Byrd JC, Carroll A, Pettenati MJ, Tantravahi R, Patil SR, Davey FR, Berg DT, Schiffer CA, Arthur DC, Mayer RJ. Frequency of prolonged remission duration after high-dose cytarabine intensification in acute myeloid leukemia varies by cytogenetic subtype. *Cancer Res* (1998) **58**: 4173–9.

16. Peterson B, George SL. Sample size requirements and length of study for testing interaction in a $2 \times k$ factorial design when time-to-failure is the outcome. *Contr Clin Trials* (1993) **14**: 511–22.

17. Lunceford JK, Davidian M, Tsiatis AA. Estimation of survival distributions of treatment policies in two-stage randomization designs in clinical trials. *Biometrics* (2002) **58**: 48–57.

18. Lachin JM. Statistical considerations in the intent-to-treat principle. *Contr Clin Trials* (2000) **21**: 167–89.

19. Hosmer DW, Lemeshow S. *Applied Survival Analysis*. New York: John Wiley & Sons (1999).

20. Chow SC, Ki FY. Statistical issues in quality-of-life assessment. *J Biopharm Stat* (1996) **6**: 37–48.

21. Gelber RD, Goldhirsch A, Cole BF, Wieand HS, Schroeder G, Krook JE. A quality-adjusted time without symptoms or toxicity (Q-TWiST) analysis of adjuvant radiation therapy and chemotherapy for resectable rectal cancer. *J Natl Cancer Inst* (1996) **88**: 1039–45.

22. Gooley TA, Leisenring W, Crowley J, Storer BE. Estimation of failure probabilities in the presence of competing risks: new representations of old estimators. *Stat Med* (1999) **18**: 695–706.

23. Klein JP, Rizzo JD, Zhang MJ, Keiding N. Statistical methods for the analysis and presentation of the results of bone marrow transplants. Part I: unadjusted analysis. *Bone Marrow Transpl* (2001) **28**: 909–15.

24. Ghitany ME, Maller R, Zhou S. Estimating the proportion of immunes in censored samples: a simulation study. *Stat Med* (1995) **14**: 39–49.

10

Melanoma

P.-Y. LIU[1] AND VERNON K. SONDAK[2]

[1]Fred Hutchinson Cancer Research Centre, Seattle, WA 98109 1024, USA
[2]University of Michigan Comprehensive Cancer Centre, Ann Arbor, MI 48109 0932, USA

INTRODUCTION

Randomised Phase III clinical trials are the gold standard for medical decision making, particularly in terms of adjuvant therapies where a modest incremental benefit is sought. However, there is sometimes marked disagreement among clinicians in their interpretation of Phase III trial results. Nowhere is this more evident than in the arena of adjuvant therapy of resected 'high-risk' melanoma. In this chapter, we will review the results of several key randomised trials and attempt to reconcile at times conflicting clinical interpretations.

BACKGROUND

A basic familiarity with malignant melanoma is required in order to understand the statistical and clinical issues presented herein.

The prognosis of localised cutaneous melanoma is based on several well-defined factors. Patho-logic analysis of the primary tumour can predict the likelihood of regional and distant metastasis and death from melanoma. Clinically localised melanomas are grouped into three prognostic categories based on the thickness of the primary tumour as measured by the pathologist using a micrometer built into the microscope eye-piece (Breslow's thickness). Melanomas less than 1.0 mm in thickness have an overall excellent prognosis with relatively minimal intervention and are considered 'low-risk' lesions. Melanomas between 1.0 and 3.9 mm are considered to be intermediate risk, while melanomas 4.0 mm or greater are considered 'high-risk' tumours. The presence of ulceration of the primary tumour increases the risk of metastasis and death within any given thickness category.[1]

The thickness is highly predictive of the risk of regional lymph node metastasis, with nodal involvement in $<5\%$ of melanomas that are <1.0 mm versus $>30\%$ in melanomas ≥ 4.0 mm. Intermediate-thickness melanomas have an inter-mediate risk of nodal spread, on the order of 20%. The prognostic significance of the presence of nodal metastasis far outweighs the significance of tumour thickness: a thin or intermediate-thickness melanoma with nodal metastases generally has

Textbook of Clinical Trials. Edited by D. Machin, S. Day and S. Green
© 2004 John Wiley & Sons, Ltd ISBN: 0-471-98787-5

a worse prognosis than a thick melanoma with negative nodes. Once nodal metastasis has been documented, the number of involved nodes is the strongest predictor of subsequent outcome, along with the manner of detection of the metastasis. Melanoma in clinically enlarged nodes portends a worse prognosis than melanoma in clinically normal nodes.[1]

The mainstay of treatment for localised or regionally metastatic melanoma is surgery. Adequate wide excision of the primary tumour site (generally taking a margin of 1 to 2 cm of normal skin around the visible edge of the melanoma or biopsy scar) is highly efficacious in controlling disease at the primary site.[2,3]

Three main options are available for staging regional nodes in patients with cutaneous melanoma: clinical staging, surgical staging by complete (elective) lymph node dissection, and surgical staging by sentinel lymph node biopsy.

CLINICAL STAGING

Physical examination is the mainstay of clinical staging of the regional nodes. Any palpable lymph nodes that are ≥ 1 cm in maximum diameter or very hard or fixed to adjacent structures must be considered highly suspicious for metastatic involvement. Unfortunately, both the specificity and sensitivity of physical examination for detecting melanoma nodal metastases are low. In muscular or obese patients, even relatively large lymph node metastases can be missed on physical examination. Lymph nodes may be enlarged after a biopsy procedure due to reactive hyperplasia without containing metastasis. Most importantly, metastatic involvement of normal-sized lymph nodes cannot be identified by physical examination.

Radiologic studies–computed tomography (CT) and positron emission tomography (PET)–are also available to clinically stage the regional nodes. CT shares many of the deficiencies of physical examination: enlarged nodes may not be malignant, and normal-sized nodes harbouring metastases will be deemed normal. PET is more sensitive than CT for differentiating melanoma-containing

from reactive nodes, but is still not able to identify microscopic foci of melanoma in normal nodes.[4] Currently, neither PET nor CT are routinely recommended for clinical staging.

For patients with low-risk melanomas, i.e., those that are <1 mm in Breslow's depth and have no evidence of ulceration or significant regression, clinical staging by physical examination is standard practice. Currently, surgical staging is used in the majority of patients with higher-risk lesions. For any patient with clinically evident nodal involvement, a complete therapeutic lymph node dissection is associated with cure in about 20% to 40% of patients.

SURGICAL STAGING BY COMPLETE (ELECTIVE) LYMPH NODE DISSECTION

Elective removal of clinically normal regional nodes identifies evidence of metastasis about 20% of the time, and is clearly a more accurate determinant of nodal status than clinical staging. Retrospective reviews suggested a survival advantage for elective node dissection compared to clinical staging with subsequent therapeutic node dissection at the time of nodal recurrence.[5] To date, however, no prospective study has demonstrated an overall survival advantage for elective node dissection.[3,6] Although the lack of a demonstrated benefit is not the same as the demonstration of no benefit, elective dissection of clinically normal nodes is not considered standard practice for cutaneous melanoma at the present time. It is clear, however, that elective node dissection results in durable regional disease control in the vast majority of patients, and failures within the dissected nodal basin are quite uncommon.

SURGICAL STAGING BY SENTINEL LYMPH NODE BIOPSY

Sentinel lymph node biopsy is based on the concept that lymphatic fluid from an area of skin drains specifically to an initial node or nodes ('sentinel nodes') prior to disseminating to other nodes in the same or nearby basins. Morton *et al.* described a reliable method for identification and removal of the sentinel node draining the site of a cutaneous melanoma.[7] They showed conclusively that the pathologic status of the sentinel node accurately determines whether melanoma cells have metastasised to that specific lymph node basin.[8] An important aspect of sentinel node biopsy is a detailed histologic examination of the sentinel lymph nodes. Generally, this examination is more thorough than is practical to perform on the larger number of nodes obtained during elective node dissection. This more detailed pathologic analysis, combined with the ability to identify sentinel nodes that are outside the defined boundaries of a regional basin, makes sentinel node biopsy the most sensitive and specific test for nodal metastasis currently available. The prognostic value of sentinel node status has been demonstrated in multiple studies. In published multivariate analyses, histologic status of the sentinel nodes is the most powerful predictor of disease-specific survival.[9] Overall, 5-year disease-specific survival is >80% for patients with negative sentinel nodes, compared to about 50% for patients with one or more positive sentinel nodes. Importantly, patients with positive sentinel nodes go on to elective complete lymph node dissection. Among patients with negative sentinel nodes, only 4% or fewer ultimately experience a clinically evident relapse within the nodal basin. Thus, sentinel node biopsy matches the excellent regional control achieved by elective node dissection while subjecting fewer patients to the morbidity of the complete node dissection procedure.

ADJUVANT THERAPY FOR MELANOMA

The development of effective adjuvant therapy has been a long-standing goal of melanoma researchers, and the subject of over 100 randomised clinical trials involving a host of different agents.[10] Adjuvant therapy is the systemic or regional administration of drugs or radiation to patients after apparently successful surgery, in an effort to minimise the risk of subsequent recurrence. Although many patients are cured by surgery, some benefit from adjuvant treatment while others will relapse regardless of adjunctive measures. Currently there are no predictive methods to distinguish one group of patients from another, therefore it is necessary to treat all patients in hopes of gaining an incremental benefit for a select few. Hence, in addition to the overall level of efficacy, clinicians evaluate toxicity, convenience, cost-effectiveness and the prospects of post-relapse salvage therapy when deciding whether to employ adjuvant therapy. Virtually all of these factors can be determined accurately only in randomised trials.

In 1995, high-dose interferon-α2b (IFN-α2b) was approved by the United States Food and Drug Administration, based on the positive results of a single, randomised Phase III clinical trial, E1684. The FDA's decision was considered controversial at the time. Subsequent randomised trials involving the same basic interferon regimen have not only failed to put this controversy to rest, but have in fact enhanced it.

ADJUVANT INTERFERON CLINICAL TRIALS

E1684

Eastern Cooperative Oncology Group (ECOG) trial E1684, with 280 eligible patients with thick primary ($\geq$4.00 mm) or node-positive melanoma who were randomly assigned after surgery to observation or post-operative adjuvant treatment with IFN-α2b for one year, demonstrated statistically-significant improvements in relapse-free and overall survival for patients randomised to the interferon arm. IFN-α2b therapy increased the median relapse-free survival by 9 months (1.72 years for IFN-α2b patients versus 0.98 years for observation patients) and produced a relative 42% improvement in the 5-year relapse-free survival rate (37% for IFN-α2b patients versus 26% for observation patients). In addition, IFN-α2b therapy significantly increased median overall survival by 1 year (3.82 years for IFN-α2b patients versus 2.78 years for observation patients) and produced a 24% relative improvement in the 5-year overall survival rate (46% for IFN-α2b patients versus 37% for observation patients).[11]

Side effects were common and frequently severe, but even when adjusted for time with toxicity, the results favoured adjuvant IFN-α2b therapy.[12]

E1690

A subsequent Intergroup adjuvant therapy trial, E1690, also compared the high-dose IFN-α2b to observation after complete resection of all known disease.[13] This was a three-arm trial involving 608 eligible patients. The eligibility criteria were the same as for E1684, except for the fact that elective node dissection was not required for patients entered onto E1690 with thick primary melanomas and clinically negative nodes. Results of this trial confirmed the relapse-free survival advantage seen in E1684 but with no survival advantage observed.

E1694

In light of the discordant survival results in E1684 and E1690, the initial results of another Intergroup trial, E1694, have received intense scrutiny. This trial compared one year of high-dose interferon not to an observation control as in the two earlier studies, but rather to two years of a ganglioside vaccine called GMK. This was the largest of the three trials, with 774 eligible patients between two study arms. For the first time, staging of the lymph nodes by sentinel node biopsy was performed in a significant fraction of patients. Gangliosides are carbohydrate antigens found on the surface of melanoma cells, as well as normal cells of neural crest origin and tumour cells of other types. A pilot randomised trial suggested a relapse-free survival benefit in patients who were treated with purified ganglioside GM2 (the specific ganglioside in the GMK vaccine) plus BCG compared to those treated with BCG alone.[14] In May 2000, the E1694 trial's independent Data Safety Monitoring Committee concluded that the high-dose interferon arm was associated with highly significantly improved relapse-free and overall survival, and mandated that the study results be disclosed early.[15]

CLINICAL CONSIDERATIONS

RELAPSE-FREE SURVIVAL VERSUS OVERALL SURVIVAL

It has been the authors' experience that clinicians tend to view clinical trial results as dichotomous, that is, 'positive' or 'negative'. Moreover, particularly for adjuvant therapy trials, the acceptance of a clinical trial as 'positive' is often restricted to trials demonstrating a statistically significant benefit in overall survival. From this perspective, there seems to be an obvious discrepancy among the two observation-controlled trials: E1684 demonstrated seemingly striking benefits from the high-dose interferon regimen in both relapse-free and overall survival, whereas E1690 validated only the relapse-free survival benefit with no survival difference. However, the importance of relapse-free survival may be worth closer examination in the current setting.

Statistically it is commonly known that, compared to overall survival, disease relapse is a less objective endpoint because it depends on the definition of relapse as well as the frequency and method of detection. Defining relapse is less of an issue in the adjuvant setting since patients enter the study with no detectable disease and thereafter any new disease found is considered a relapse. In a well-conducted clinical trial the interval and method of disease assessment are specified in the protocol and generally complied with by trialists, thereby rendering relapse-free survival a more reliable endpoint than in other situations. From the purely clinical viewpoint, patients have made clear that they are willing to accept even toxic adjuvant therapies that provide improvements in relapse-free survival, even if they do not result in any prolongation of overall survival. This observation has been directly validated in melanoma patients,[16] and represents the perception that time spent without signs or symptoms of recurrent cancer is inherently of value even in the absence of prolongation of total lifespan. In addition, relapse-free survival often represents a truer reflection of the biologic activity of an adjuvant therapy since randomised trials rarely include rigorous controls on post-relapse salvage therapy. The confounding effect of such treatment on overall survival is unknown and not assessable.

RECONCILING THE STUDY RESULTS BASED ON CLINICAL CONSIDERATIONS

Two of the three randomised Phase III trials of high-dose interferon, E1684 and E1690, demonstrate a relapse-free survival advantage. The third trial, E1694, also shows a relapse-free survival benefit but with GMK vaccine and not observation as the control treatment. The implication of this design difference is discussed in detail below. Nevertheless, many consider there is uniformity of evidence that high-dose interferon has biologic activity in at least delaying relapse after surgical therapy. This fact alone, combined with the lack of proven alternatives, is enough for many patients to choose interferon therapy in the absence of consensus regarding the overall survival benefit.

Crossover to interferon therapy upon relapse might have partially affected the outcome of at least one study. The original trial, E1684, was unlikely to have been affected by crossover for two reasons. Surgical staging of the regional nodes by complete (elective or therapeutic) node dissection was required. Hence, few patients were likely to experience regional relapse or other resectable recurrence, where secondary resection and delayed adjuvant interferon could be employed. Most relapses occurred in non-resectable distant sites. In recent medical practice, interferon is rarely employed for the treatment of measurable metastatic disease.

In contrast, the E1690 trial required only clinical staging of the regional nodes, and surgery was not required for patients with thick primary tumours and clinically negative nodes. Among all relapsed patients ($n = 114$ in the high-dose interferon arm and $n = 121$ in the observation control arm), 54% on high-dose interferon and 45% on observation experienced regional recurrence only. Retrospective data collection indicated more patients relapsing on the observation arm received subsequent interferon-α-containing regimens (31% vs. 15%) and/or biochemotherapy (17% vs. 6%).

While there is some evidence of differential post-relapse treatment received, concluding that the lack of interferon survival benefit observed in E1690 is due to these differences is not justified. Making this conclusion presupposes survival efficacy from these salvage therapies, which cannot be substantiated with currently available data. In addition, comparing outcomes by post-relapse treatment groups provides little useful information because patients were not randomised to salvage treatment strategies upon relapse. As is inherent in observational data, unknown patient selection factors cannot be accounted for by analysis techniques and their impact can easily remain even after adjusting for known prognostic factors. Therefore, although available data appear compatible with the notion that initial observation after surgery followed by high-dose interferon in case of resectable relapse presents an alternative strategy to routine use of adjuvant high-dose interferon, this study offers no proof for the conjecture. The conservative conclusion is that salvage treatment difference is a possible confounding factor that limits the confidence regarding the lack of overall survival benefit of high-dose interferon from study E1690.

STATISTICAL CONSIDERATIONS

Although clinical factors clearly impact on the interpretation of the three trials, our main goal is to examine the statistical aspects of these trials to determine the extent to which they actually present 'conflicting' information. We focus first on E1684 and E1690.

STATISTICAL TESTS EMPLOYED AND PRESENTATION OF RESULTS

One source of confusion could be due to the fact that one-sided p-values were presented for E1684 but two-sided p-values were presented for E1690. Since all comparisons involved were one-sided in nature (i.e., is high-dose interferon superior to observation after surgery), we use all one-sided p-values (p_1) in this discussion. In addition, all hazard ratios are expressed as observation arm versus treatment arm ratios. Thus, a hazard ratio >1 indicates an excess of hazard in the observation arm, or treatment advantage.

Another possible source of confusion could be the fact that, in E1684, statistically significant p-values for relapse-free and overall survival differences by the stratified logrank test (adjusted for disease burden and presentation at initial diagnosis versus recurrent nodal disease status) were reported (Table 2 of Ref. 11). But when Cox regression analysis was performed, further adjusting for age, time from diagnosis to randomisation and ulceration status of the primary tumour, a significant interferon over observation benefit was presented only for those with nodal disease (Table 4 of Ref. 11). The hazard ratio was 1.64 for relapse-free survival and 1.49 for overall survival with $p_1 = 0.01$ in both cases. However, these hazard ratios (presented in their reciprocals as interferon over observation ratios, 0.61 and 0.67, in actuality) were labelled 'Treatment with IFN' without reference to the positive nodal disease subset. An interaction term between the interferon treatment and the thick primary, no nodal disease patient category was actually included in the Cox models and the results were presented in the same table with the label 'CS1/PS1 + IFN'. The hazard ratios were 0.36 and 0.34 respectively for relapse-free survival and overall survival. These interaction hazard ratios translated into observation over interferon hazard ratios of 0.60 and 0.50 for relapse-free and overall survival in patients with thick primary tumours and pathologically negative nodes, reflecting the occurrence that interferon-treated patients fared worse than the observation patients in this subset. For the readers who did not appreciate these details of the Cox modelling, the hazard ratios for the nodal disease subset could have been over-interpreted as the Cox model treatment effects for the study as a whole, which were not presented in the original publication. Such misinterpretation might have

contributed to an exaggerated impression of the overall survival benefit from E1684.

TRIAL SIZE, OVERALL RESULTS AND OTHER ASPECTS

To interpret the combined results E1684 and E1690, it is useful to compare the study parameters and overall results. Tables 10.1–10.3 are extracted mainly from Ref. 13. Since there was not a low-dose interferon arm in E1684, only the high-dose interferon and observation arms of E1690 are included in the tables. Due to the limitations of data availability, all randomised patients regardless of eligibility determination are presented for consistency.

The tables indicate that when E1690 results became available, the study had 50% more patients than E1684, reflecting wider participation from the US Melanoma Intergroup. The patient enrollment periods were non-overlapping. Although the updated data for E1684 had longer follow-up at the time of E1690 publication, more

Table 10.1. E1684 and E1690 study characteristics

Study	E1684	E1690*
Participating groups	ECOG	ECOG, SWOG, CALGB, MDACC
Patient accrual period	1984–1990	1991–1995
N (all randomised)	286	427
Median follow-up (years)	6.9	4.3
Event count: RFS	197	241
Event count: OS	175	190

*High-dose interferon and observation arms only.

Table 10.2. E1684 and E1690 patient disease stage distribution

Disease stage	T4 N0	T1-4 N+ (occult)	T1-4 N+ (overt)	N+ Recurrent
E1684	11%	12%	14%	63%
E1690	26%	11%	12%	50%

Table 10.3. E1684 and E1690 results

Study	Hazard ratio	95% CI	p-Value*
Relapse-free survival			
E1684**	1.43	(1.08, 1.89)	0.002
E1690	1.28	(1.0, 1.65)	0.03
Overall survival			
E1684**	1.32	(0.98, 1.77)	0.03
E1690	1.0	(0.75, 1.33)	0.50

*One-sided p-value by stratified logrank test.
**Ref. 21.

events were analysed for E1690 from the larger sample size and the fact that few events occurred after 5 years. The main known patient characteristic difference was in the distribution of disease stage. There were more node-negative patients (26% vs. 11%) and fewer recurrent disease patients (63% vs. 50%) in E1690, representing a somewhat more favourable prognosis. It may be worth pointing out that, among those with nodal disease, there did not appear to be survival differences between newly diagnosed and recurrent disease patients. The more favourable relapse and survival experiences of the observation patients in E1690 compared to those in E1684 (5-year relapse-free survival of 35% vs. 26% and overall survival of 54% vs. 37%) remain largely unexplained by known factors. Regarding the treatment outcome, the magnitude of the interferon benefit was smaller in E1690 than in E1684 for both relapse-free survival (hazard ratio 1.43 vs. 1.28) and overall survival (hazard ratio 1.32 vs. 1.00). The larger event counts in E1690 resulted in narrower confidence intervals. As offered by the authors as one plausible conclusion,[13] the combined evidence from these two trials seems to indicate that, for node positive and thick primary, node-negative melanoma patients, treatment of high-dose interferon prolongs relapse-free survival. Survival benefit, if it exists, may be more limited.

It is worth pointing out that E1690 was designed with not one but two primary comparisons, comparing high-dose interferon and low-dose interferon to observation (but not to each other) with a one-sided p-value of 0.0125 for each comparison to maintain an overall one-sided type I error rate of 0.025 for the study. When the results were presented, however, one-sided p-values less than 0.025 were treated as statistically significant for each comparison, representing a study-wide, one-sided type I error rate of 0.05 or a two-sided error rate of 0.10. Also, per design the study was sized so that the power for each individual comparison was 0.83. In other words, the type II error rate for each comparison was 0.17 for an approximate study-wide type II error rate of 0.34. Should the true magnitude of benefit from both interferon regimens be the same, the power to detect both effects in the same study was close to 0.66. With the inflated type I error rate in the end, the overall power would increase somewhat but would likely remain less than adequate for detecting reasonable effects from both treatment arms. Hence, the question about the low-dose interferon regimen's treatment effect was essentially unanswered in this study, yet clinicians seem to have uniformly concluded that low-dose interferon is inactive in E1690.

WHAT DOES E1694 TELL US?

E1694 was designed to detect a GMK vaccine benefit over interferon as the contemporary treatment standard. As is often practiced with superiority designs, the trial would be stopped at planned interim analyses if the hypothesised vaccine benefit could be definitively ruled out. This provision was incorporated in the study design in the following manner. Instead of the typical, highly stringent interim p-value requirements, the GMK vaccine needed only to be inferior to interferon at a fixed, one-sided p-value of 0.05 for relapse-free survival in order to consider study termination at interim analyses. Such evidence might not establish the vaccine inferiority but would certainly rule out its superiority.

Considering the substantially more favourable vaccine toxicity profile, a more appropriate trial design might have sought to demonstrate the equivalence of the two agents in their efficacy rather than the superiority of the vaccine. In fact the Data and Safety Monitoring Committee in this case seemed to have followed the equivalence principle and disclosed the study results only when there was decisive evidence that the GMK vaccine was inferior to high-dose interferon in both relapse-free survival ($p_1 = 0.0015$) and overall survival ($p_1 = 0.009$).[15] Because no observation control arm was incorporated in the study design, the clinical interpretation of E1694 in this respect is subject to debate. Obviously, if it were known that the GMK vaccine had some level of clinical efficacy, the finding that high-dose interferon was significantly better in both disease-free and overall survival would be of great clinical significance and would substantiate the benefits identified in the initial E1684 trial. Without this knowledge, some have maintained the possibility of a deleterious vaccine effect and insisted that the study cannot be used to give information on the non-design comparison of interferon versus observation.

Unfortunately, no credible evidence exists that the GMK vaccine is either beneficial or deleterious. It is likely that the GMK vaccine acted essentially as placebo and the study provided further validation that high-dose interferon was efficacious over no treatment in both relapse-free and overall survival. But we do not know this for certain. As the dramatic survival difference between E1684 and E1690 observation patients amply illustrates,[13] comparison of patient outcomes in the GMK vaccine arm to historical controls in the other two trials offers few clues to the efficacy of the vaccine.

Data were presented that, among the vaccine-treated patients, those displaying antibody responses had a trend towards favourable outcomes Ref. 17. Even assuming that the analyses corrected for the inherent responder versus non-responder bias,[20] the results still cannot be used to establish a causal relationship between vaccine response and favourable outcome. As pointed out in numerous publications, response to treatment could simply serve as a selection mechanism wherein responders represented a better prognosis group. One may contend that it is difficult to reconcile a trend in favour of antibody responders with speculations of a deleterious effect of the vaccine resulting from production of 'blocking' antibodies. However, it is known that effects of prognostic factors such as disease stage can easily overwhelm any treatment effects.

DID ANY SUBSET OF PATIENTS BENEFIT MORE FROM INTERFERON?

The predominant subcategories of high-risk melanoma patients are those having thick primary tumours with clinically or pathologically negative nodes and those having documented involvement of the nodes. Among the node-positive patients, subsets include those with 1, 2 to 3 and ≥ 4 nodes; patients with clinically evident versus microscopic nodal involvement; and patients found to have nodal involvement at the time of initial presentation versus those developing recurrent disease in the nodes.

The initial findings of E1684 indicated that the subset of patients with thick primary tumours and pathologically negative nodes had no benefit, and perhaps even a detrimental effect, from adjuvant interferon.[11] The veracity of this finding was called into question from the outset, because of the small number of node-negative patients (a total of 31 out of 280 eligible patients, or 11%) and an imbalance in a major prognostic factor (ulceration of the primary tumour) biasing the results in favour of the observation arm. In contrast, subset analysis of the results of trial E1690 found that the relapse-free survival benefit for patients with thick primary tumours and clinically negative nodes (making up 25% of the eligible patient population) was identical to that for the study population as a whole.[13] Subset analysis of E1694 showed the greatest interferon over vaccine benefit for the subset of thick, node-negative patients.[15]

Indeed, in each of the three clinical trials, subset analysis indicated a different group as obtaining the most benefit from high-dose interferon: the subset with one single positive node in E1684; the subset with two to three positive nodes in E1690; and the node-negative subset in E1694. The authors properly suggested that, taken together, there was no indication of preferential treatment effect in any one subset.[15] These results exemplify the lack of reliability of subset results, a phenomenon previously discussed in regard to other melanoma clinical trials.[18] Without appropriate study size for adequate power within subsets, and control for inflated type errors stemming from multiple testing, *post hoc* subset analyses suffer both high false-positive and high false-negative rates.

CONCLUSIONS

Three randomised trials evaluating high-dose interferon, involving over 1600 patients, have been conducted, yet its treatment benefit remains controversial. The combined evidence indicates that, for high-risk melanoma patients, treatment of high-dose interferon prolongs relapse-free survival. Survival benefit is less certain. There is no credible evidence to suggest that interferon exerts a differential effect in different subsets of 'high-risk' patients.

There are many reasons why high-dose interferon has not been uniformly embraced by physicians and patients around the world, even though it is the only adjuvant therapy yet shown to have any sustained impact on relapse-free survival. When the three trials are looked at in the light of statistical principles, what seem to be glaring differences are more plausibly regarded as understandable variations reflecting trial design and analysis, combined with the fluctuations inherent in human clinical trials conducted over time in similar yet subtly different patient populations.

While it is easy to conclude that further research is necessary to determine if high-dose interferon α-2b improves overall survival, there is in fact little chance that definitive further research will take place. Only one current clinical trial, the Sunbelt Melanoma Trial, is comparing one year of high-dose interferon to a control group. This study includes only patients with a single positive sentinel node identified at the time of initial presentation.[19] As such, it is comprised

of a far more homogeneous patient population than any prior clinical trial, potentially enhancing the scientific validity. Of note, this group now constitutes by far the largest fraction of 'high-risk' melanoma patients being seen and treated in the United States today, yet less than 10% of participants in the three prior trials combined were from this category. Unfortunately, this trial is likely to be small compared to the most recent Intergroup trials and, regardless of the results, it will not directly address the role of interferon in all of the other high-risk categories.

It is now nearly 20 years since the design of clinical trial E1684, and 8 years since the FDA's approval of high-dose interferon-α for the adjuvant therapy of high-risk melanoma, and we may never fully know to what extent this toxic and inconvenient regimen improves overall survival. The implications of that statement are profound, and the burden they place on clinical trialists is clear: design and analyse our trials carefully to have the greatest probability of a clear and unambiguous result.

REFERENCES

1. Balch CM, Soong SJ, Gershenwald JE, *et al.* Prognostic factors analysis of 17,600 melanoma patients: validation of the American Joint Committee on Cancer melanoma staging system. *J Clin Oncol* (2001) **19**: 3622–34.
2. Veronesi U, Cascinelli N. Narrow excision (1-cm margin): a safe procedure for thin cutaneous melanoma. *Arch Surg* (1991) **126**: 438–41.
3. Balch CM, Soong S, Ross MI, *et al.* Long-term results of a multi-institutional randomized trial comparing prognostic factors and surgical results for intermediate thickness melanomas (1.0 to 4.0 mm). Intergroup Melanoma Surgical Trial. *Ann Surg Oncol* (2000) **7**: 87–97.
4. Wagner JD, Schauwecker D, Davidson D, *et al.* Prospective study of fluorodeoxyglucose-positron emission tomography imaging of lymph node basins in melanoma patients undergoing sentinel node biopsy. *J Clin Oncol* (1999) **17**: 1508–15.
5. Balch CM. The role of elective lymph node dissection in melanoma: rationale, results, and controversies. *J Clin Oncol* (1988) **6**: 163–72.
6. Cascinelli N, Morabito A, Santinami M, MacKie RM, Belli F. Immediate or delayed dissection

of regional nodes in patients with melanoma of the trunk: a randomised trial. WHO Melanoma Programme. *Lancet* (1998) **351**(9105): 793–6.

7. Morton D, Wen D, Wong J, *et al*. Technical details of intraoperative lymphatic mapping for early stage melanoma. *Arch Surg* (1992) **127**: 392–9.

8. Morton DL, Thompson JF, Essner R, *et al*. Validation of the accuracy of intraoperative lymphatic mapping and sentinel lymphadenectomy for early-stage melanoma: a multicenter trial. Multicenter Selective Lymphadenectomy Trial Group. *Ann Surg* (1999) **230**: 453–65.

9. Gershenwald JE, Thompson W, Mansfield PF, *et al*. Multi-institutional melanoma lymphatic mapping experience: the prognostic value of sentinel lymph node status in 612 stage I or II melanoma patients. *J Clin Oncol* (1999) **17**: 976–83.

10. Sondak VK, Wolfe JA. Adjuvant therapy for melanoma. *Curr Opin Oncol* (1997) **9**: 189–204.

11. Kirkwood JM, Strawderman MH, Ernstoff MS, *et al*. Interferon alfa-2b adjuvant therapy of high-risk resected cutaneous melanoma: the Eastern Cooperative Oncology Group trial EST 1684. *J Clin Oncol* (1996) **14**: 7–17.

12. Cole BF, Gelber RD, Kirkwood JM, *et al*. Quality-of-life – adjusted survival analysis of interferon alfa-2b adjuvant treatment of high-risk resected cutaneous melanoma: an Eastern Cooperative Oncology Group study. *J Clin Oncol* (1996) **14**: 2666–73.

13. Kirkwood JM, Ibrahim JG, Sondak VK, *et al*. High- and low-dose interferon alfa-2b in high-risk melanoma: first analysis of Intergroup trial E1690/S9111/C9190. *J Clin Oncol* (2000) **18**: 2444–54.

14. Livingston PO, Wong GYC, Adluri S, *et al*. Improved survival in stage III melanoma patients with GM2 antibodies: a randomized trial of adjuvant vaccination with GM2 ganglioside. *J Clin Oncol* (1994) **12**: 1036–44.

15. Kirkwood JM, Ibrahim JG, Sosman JA, *et al*. High-dose interferon alfa-2b significantly prolongs relapse-free and overall survival compared with the GM2-KLH/QS-21 vaccine in patients with resected stage IIB–III melanoma: results of Intergroup trial E1694/S9512/C509801. *J Clin Oncol* (2001) **19**: 2370–80.

16. Kilbridge KL, Weeks JC, Sober AJ, *et al*. Patient preferences for adjuvant interferon alfa-2b treatment. *J Clin Oncol* (2001) **19**: 812–23.

17. Kirkwood JM, Ibrahim J, Lawson DH, *et al*. High-dose interferon alfa-2b does not diminish antibody response to GM2 vaccination in patients with resected melanoma: results of the multicenter Eastern Cooperative Oncology Group phase II trial E2696. *J Clin Oncol* (2001) **19**: 1430–6.

18. Sondak VK. Multi-institutional melanoma vaccine trial [Letter]. *Ann Surg Oncol* (1996) **3**: 588–9.

19. McMasters KM, Sondak VK, Lotze MT, Ross MI. Recent advances in melanoma staging and therapy. *Ann Surg Oncol* (1999) **6**: 467–75.

20. Anderson JR, Cain KC, Gelber RD. Analysis of survival by tumor response. *J Clin Oncol* (1983) **1**: 710–19.

21. Kirkwood JM, Manola J, Ibrahim J, *et al*. A pooled analysis of ECOG and Intergroup trials of adjuvant high-dose interferon for melanoma. Accepted for publication in Clinical Cancer Research (2004).

11

Respiratory Cancers

JOAN H. SCHILLER[1] AND KYUNGMANN KIM[2]

Departments of [1]Medicine and [2]Biostatistics and Medical Informatics, University of Wisconsin, Madison, WI 53792, USA

INTRODUCTION

Carcinoma of the lung and bronchus is estimated to account for almost 13% of all new cancer cases, but to be responsible for about 157 200 deaths in the United States in 2003.[1] This represents more than 28% of all deaths due to cancer, exceeding the number of deaths due to the next four leading cancers, colon, breast, prostate and pancreas, all combined.

The incidence of the disease continues to rise, particularly in women and blacks, and thus is likely to present a significant public health problem for years to come. Cigarette smoking is attributed as the cause of 80% to 90% of lung cancer cases, with the risk for lung cancer among smokers being 20 to 30 times that among non-smokers. Other risk factors include exposure to asbestos and radon. Asbestos exposure, known to cause malignant mesothelioma, increases the risk for lung cancer, especially among smokers. There are limited data on molecular and genetic profile as a risk factor, and familial predisposition to lung cancer. Diet's role in lung cancer is even less obvious.

Despite the significant reduction in smoking, especially among the male population since the late 1970s, the incidence of lung cancer is still rising because of long latency and a steady increase in smoking among the female population.

With the litigation and subsequent settlement between the tobacco industry and the state governments in the US, the marketing effort of the US tobacco industry has shifted to the emerging markets in Asia and Eastern Europe. As a consequence, the smoking-related public health problem is predicted to pose a serious threat to the national security in a country such as China, in which smoking has increased dramatically in recent years.

The best investment for prevention of smoking-related cancer incidence and death, as well as other diseases such as cardiovascular and other pulmonary diseases, appears to be in smoking cessation and prevention of taking up the smoking habit among teenagers and females.

CLASSIFICATIONS

Lung cancer consists of four major histological types: adenocarcinoma, squamous cell carcinoma, large-cell carcinoma and small-cell carcinoma. Because of the unique biological features of small-cell lung cancer (SCLC), its staging and treatment

Textbook of Clinical Trials. Edited by D. Machin, S. Day and S. Green
© 2004 John Wiley & Sons, Ltd   ISBN: 0-471-98787-5

differ radically from the other three types of lung cancer, which are collectively called non-small-cell lung cancer (NSCLC).

Besides histological classification, lung cancer is also classified according to the Tumour, Node and Metastasis (TNM) staging and the International Staging Classification. The TNM staging system is applied primarily to NSCLC and consists of three components, each according to primary tumour (T), nodal involvement (N) and distant metastasis (M) as summarised in Table 11.1. The International Staging Classification summarised in Table 11.2 is based on the TNM staging.[2] It is this classification that forms the basis for management and treatment of patients with NSCLC.

A staging system entirely different from that for NSCLC is used for patients with small-cell carcinoma of the lung. Small-cell lung cancer is clinically categorised into two stages: limited and extensive. Limited-stage SCLC is defined as tumours confined to one hemithorax and its regional lymph nodes that can be encompassed in a tolerable irradiation field. Extensive-stage SCLC is defined as any extent of disease beyond that classification.

Table 11.1. TNM staging

Primary tumour (T)

TX   Tumour proven by the presence of malignant cells in bronchopulmonary secretions but not visualised
        roentgenographically or bronchoscopically, or any tumour that cannot be assessed as in a retreatment
        staging
T0   No evidence of primary tumour
Tis   Carcinoma *in situ*
T1   A tumour that is 3.0 cm or less in greatest dimension, surrounded by lung or visceral pleura, and without
        evidence of invasion proximal to a lobar bronchus at bronchoscopy
T2   A tumour more than 3.0 cm in greatest dimension, or a tumour of any size that either invades the visceral
        pleura or has associated atelectasis or obstructive pneumonitis extending to the hilar region. At
        bronchoscopy, the proximal extent of demonstrable tumour must be within a lobar bronchus or at least
        2.0 cm distal to the carina. Any associated atelectasis or obstructive pneumonitis must involve less than
        an entire lung
T3   A tumour of any size with direct extension into the chest wall (including superior sulcus tumours),
        diaphragm, or the mediastinal pleura or pericardium without involving the heart, great vessels, trachea,
        oesophagus or vertebral body, or a tumour in the main bronchus within 2 cm of the carina without
        involving the carina
T4   A tumour of any size with invasion of the mediastinum or involving the heart, great vessels, trachea,
        oesophagus, vertebral body for carina or presence of malignant pleural effusion; a satellite nodule
        within the same lobe

Nodal involvement (N)

NX   Regional lymph nodes cannot be assessed
N0   No demonstrable metastasis to regional lymph nodes
N1   Metastasis to lymph nodes in the peribronchial or the ipsilateral hilar region, or both, including direct
        extension
N2   Metastasis to ipsilateral mediastinal lymph nodes and subcarinal lymph nodes
N3   Metastasis to contralateral mediastinal lymph nodes, contralateral hilar lymph nodes, ipsilateral or
        contralateral scalene or supraclavicular lymph nodes

Distant metastasis (M)

M0   No distant metastasis
M1   Distant metastasis, including pulmonary nodule not in the same lobe as the primary tumour

Table 11.2. International Staging Classification for lung cancer

Stage	TNM subset	Five-year survival (%)	
		Clinical stage	Pathological stage
IA	T1, N0, M0	61	67
IB	T2, N0, M0	38	57
IIA	T1, N1, M0	34	55
IIB	T2, N1, M0; T3, N0, M0	24	39
IIIA	T3, N1, M0; T1–3, N2, M0	9	25
IIIB	T4, any N, M0; any T, N3, M0	13	23
IV	Any T, any N, M1	1	–

INCIDENCE

In the year 2002, 1 284 900 new cases of invasive cancer were expected in the United States, excluding carcinoma *in situ* of any site except the urinary bladder and also excluding basal and squamous cell cancers of the skin. Lung cancer is estimated to account for 13% (169 400 cases) of all new cancer cases, 14% (90 200) in males and 12% (79 200) in females.

The annual age-adjusted incidence rate of lung cancer in the male population has been in a steady decline since its peak in the early 1980s. However, that in the female population appears to be still increasing, although the rate of increase has slowed in the late 1990s.

PROGNOSIS

Prognosis for patients diagnosed with lung cancer is dismal, with less than 15% surviving longer than 5 years from the time of diagnosis, and it is highly dependent on stage of the disease as indicated in Table 11.2.

SALIENT FEATURES OF SMALL-CELL LUNG CANCER

Small-cell lung cancer, which makes up a quarter to a third of all lung cancer at diagnosis, differs from NSCLC in a number of important ways.

First, it has a more rapid clinical course and natural history, with the rapid development of metastases, symptoms and eventually death. Left untreated, the median survival time is typically 12–15 weeks for patients with local disease and 6–9 weeks for those with advanced disease. Second, it exhibits features of neuroendocrine differentiation in many patients, which may be distinguishable histopathologically and is associated with paraneoplastic syndromes. Third, unlike NSCLC, SCLC is exquisitely sensitive to both chemotherapy and radiotherapy, although resistant disease often develops.

Due to sensitivity of patients with SCLC to chemotherapy, it can pose challenges in design of clinical trials for drug development as will be discussed in some detail.

CLINICAL TRIALS IN LUNG CANCER

Clinical trials have resulted in significant seminal trials which have led to changes in the management of these patients. Those seminal studies in screening, chemoprevention and treatment are outlined.

SCREENING AND EARLY DETECTION

Three US randomised screening studies failed to detect an impact of screening high-risk patients with chest radiographs or sputum cytology on mortality, although earlier stage cancers were detected in the screened groups.[3–5] These studies have been criticised for a number of potential methodological and statistical problems, such as over-diagnosis and analysing data by survival rather than mortality.[6]

Recently, several clinical studies have demonstrated that early stage lung cancers can be detected with the use of spiral CT that would not have been detected by routine chest X-ray.[7] Spiral CT is a CT scan which does not evaluate the mediastinum and thus does not use contrast or require the presence of a radiologist, employs low doses of radiation and can be completed within one patient 'breath'. Because it can be done rapidly and does not require a radiologist to be present, it is being used in some centres to screen for lung cancers in high-risk populations. However, it has not been determined whether there is a survival benefit with this technique.[6,7] Given the availability of this scanning technique in the community, it is imperative that clinical trials be completed to determine if the early detection of small tumours results in improved survival that is not a result of lead time or length bias.

TREATMENT: NON-SMALL-CELL LUNG CANCER

Treatment of NSCLC is dependent primarily on stage of disease at the time of diagnosis and stage, in turn, is dependent upon the size of the tumour (T), location of nodal involvement (N), if any, and presence or absence of distant metastases (M). The current TNM staging classification is shown in Table 11.1 and the stage grouping in Table 11.2.

Stage I Disease

A lobectomy is the treatment of choice for stage I NSCLC, with cure rates of 60–80% reported. Within stage I, patients with T2, N0 disease do not fare as well as those with T1, N0 cancers. In approximately 20% of patients with medical contraindications to surgery but with adequate pulmonary function, high-dose radiotherapy will result in cure. No role of adjuvant chemotherapy for stage I NSCLC has been identified.

Chemoprevention: Patients with a resected stage I NSCLC are at high risk of approximately 1% per year for the development of second lung cancers, prompting a number of ongoing clinical trials looking at the role of chemoprevention. Surprisingly, several randomised studies have demonstrated that the use of vitamin A or one of its derivatives at best, does not prevent lung cancer in smokers and at worst, may increase the risk of developing it.[8–10] Preliminary studies have suggested that selenium may reduce the incidence of lung cancer and total cancer mortality. In a multi-centre, double-blind, randomised, placebo-controlled trial, 1312 patients were randomised to receive either selenium or placebo.

The selenium group had fewer total carcinomas, including lung cancer with a relative risk of 0.54 and a 95% confidence interval of (0.30 to 0.98) ($p = 0.04$).[11] This has formed the basis for an intergroup chemoprevention trial which is now ongoing.

Stage II and 'Non-Bulky' IIIA Disease

Treatment of locally advanced NSCLC is one of the most controversial issues in the management of lung cancer. Treatment options include surgery for less-advanced disease, or radiotherapy, either of which has been given with or without chemotherapy for control of micrometastases. Interpretation of the results of clinical trials involving patients with locally advanced disease has been clouded by a number of issues, including changing diagnostic techniques, different staging systems and heterogeneous patient populations that may have disease that ranges from 'non-bulky' stage IIIA (clinical N1 nodes, with N2 nodes discovered only at the time of surgery or mediastinoscopy), to 'bulky' N2 nodes (enlarged adenopathy clearly visible on chest X-ray films, or multiple nodal level involvement), to clearly inoperable stage IIIB disease.

Post-operative Thoracic Radiotherapy: The treatment for stage II and selected IIIA NSCLC patients is surgical resection. However, many of these patients will relapse, prompting numerous trials evaluating the role of post-operative radiotherapy or chemotherapy. A meta-analysis examining the role of post-operative radiotherapy (PORT) found that patients randomised to receive PORT actually had an inferior survival to those randomised to observation alone.[12] In a meta-analysis of 2128 patients in nine clinical trials of post-operative radiotherapy, a 7% survival decrement from radiation was identified. However, this particular analysis included a number of trials from the 1960s and 1970s when staging was highly inaccurate and relatively outmoded radiation therapy technologies were utilised. In addition, several of the trials included in this report aggressively treated patients with no evidence of nodal involvement or those with early nodal involvement only, a group that by today's standards would not be subjected to post-operative radiation therapy. More recent studies looking at the role of PORT have concluded that PORT does not prolong survival, but does enhance local control. The most comprehensive randomised trial in this regard was performed by the Lung Cancer Study Group and it demonstrated major improvement in intrathoracic disease control.[13] For those patients receiving thoracic radiotherapy, the intrathoracic failure rate was only 3%, compared to 43% for patients not receiving post-operative radiotherapy, although no significant survival advantage was identified.

Adjuvant Chemotherapy: Given the propensity of these resected patients to relapse with distant disease, adjuvant post-operative chemotherapy has been of significant interest. A meta-analysis published in 1995 found a small improvement in survival with post-operative adjuvant chemotherapy that borderlined on statistical significance ($p = 0.08$),[14] leading some clinicians to conclude that adjuvant chemotherapy was of benefit. However, a randomised intergroup study has been completed in which patients were randomised to receive either radiotherapy plus chemotherapy (cisplatin and etoposide for four cycles) or radiotherapy alone. The median and long-term survival of the two arms was nearly identical.[15] Once again, the fact that the meta-analysis included older studies, in which chemotherapy regimens, staging and other clinical characteristics were different, may account for this discrepancy. Although the role of neoadjuvant chemotherapy is under investigation, it cannot be routinely recommended until the results of randomised clinical trials confirm clinical benefit.

Pre-operative Chemotherapy plus Surgery: There have been two small randomised studies involving surgery with or without pre-operative chemotherapy which popularised this approach. Both involved 60 patients and both report response rates of 35–62% following induction chemotherapy. Both have also reported prolonged survival, prompting early closure of both trials. In the European trial, the median survival time was 26 months for patients receiving pre-operative chemotherapy plus surgery, compared to 8 months for patients treated with surgery alone.[16] In the MD Anderson trial, the median survival of the 32 patients randomised to the surgery-alone group was 11 months compared to 64 months in the 28 patients randomised to the combined-modality arm.[17] Of note, however, is the fact that updated results of the MD Anderson trial, while still statistically significant, showed a narrowing of the survival curves, with a median survival of 14 months and 21 months for the surgery alone and combined modality arms, respectively.[18]

A larger trial has recently been reported.[19] Three hundred and fifty-five patients with stage I, II or IIIA disease were randomised to three cycles of chemotherapy followed by surgery or to surgery alone. Median survival (37 months vs. 26 months) and 2-year survival (52% vs. 59%) were not statistically different between the two groups. However, a subset analysis in which patients who died within 150 days of perioperative problems were excluded revealed a 0.77 reduction in risk which was statistically significant ($p = 0.03$). Other subset analysis looked at outcome by patient stage and found that the patients with N0/N1 disease who received chemo/surgery had a hazard ratio of 0.68, compared to patients with N2 disease, where the hazard ratio was 1.04.

Despite the results of the Depierre trial, many clinicians continue to use pre-operative chemotherapy for patients with stage IIIA disease. An intergroup study evaluating chemo/RT vs. chemo/RT surgery has recently been completed; these results are eagerly awaited.

Locally Advanced 'Bulky' Stage IIIA/IIIB Disease

The optimal treatment for bulky stage IIIA and stage IIIB disease is also controversial. Current investigational efforts are directed at identifying the optimal combined-modality approach, involving treatments directed at local control of the disease, i.e., surgery or radiotherapy, and micrometastatic disease, i.e., chemotherapy. Possibilities include radiotherapy only, preoperative chemotherapy, or chemotherapy plus radiotherapy.

Chemotherapy plus Radiation Therapy: Chemotherapy plus radiotherapy is the treatment of choice for patients with bulky or inoperable stage III disease. Two randomised studies have demonstrated an improvement in median and long-term survival with chemotherapy followed by radiation therapy versus radiotherapy alone.[20,21] More recently, two randomised trials have shown that concurrent chemoradiotherapy results in prolonged survival, albeit at the expense of enhanced toxicity, compared to sequential treatment.[22,23] Other active areas of investigation include choice of chemotherapy, fractionation and treatment fields.

Recently, weekly, low-dose 'sensitising' chemotherapy plus radiation therapy has become popular, primarily due to lower toxicities when administered with radiotherapy than 'standard' dose chemotherapy.[24] However, this schedule has never been looked at in a formal phase III setting, so its relative efficacy compared to standard dose chemotherapy has not been rigorously assessed.

Stage IV Disease

Several meta-analyses have demonstrated that chemotherapy improves survival in patients with metastatic NSCLC (approximately 10% 1-year survival untreated vs. 35–40% 1-year survival with treatment),[25,26] particularly if the chemotherapy is platin-based.[14] In the past 10 years, numerous different cytotoxic drugs have become available for the treatment of lung cancer patients. These include, among others, vinorelbine, the taxanes (docetaxel and paclitaxel), gemcitabine and the topoisomerase I inhibitors (irinotecan and topotecan). Randomised studies have shown that these agents improve survival when combined with cisplatin, as compared to cisplatin alone,[27,28] or the other agent alone.[29,30] However, there is probably little difference in outcome between agents when combined with cisplatin, although there are clear differences in toxicity and cost.[31,32]

Second-Line Chemotherapy

Docetaxel was recently approved for the second-line treatment of NSCLC, based upon two clinical trials. One trial compared two doses of docetaxel with best supportive care, and found an improvement in median and long-term survival, despite a low response rate of 7%.[33] The other trial compared docetaxel to either vinorelbine or ifosfamide (the treatment physician was allowed to choose) and found an improvement in long-term, although not median survival.[34]

'Targeted' Therapy

Given the overall poor results with standard cytotoxic therapies and the number of advances that have been made recently in our understanding of the biology of cancer, a strong interest has emerged in targeting pathways unique to neoplastic cells. One such example is the epidermal growth factor receptor (EGFr), which has been found to be expressed in the majority of patients with lung cancer. Based upon two phase II trials in previously treated NSCLC patients, in which response rates of 10–20% were found,[35,36] two phase III trials were initiated comparing chemotherapy plus an EGFr inhibitor, ZD1839, with chemotherapy in untreated NSCLC. Somewhat surprisingly, no benefit was observed in these trials.[37,38] These unexpected findings have resulted in clinical researchers, statisticians and the pharmaceutical industry re-aiming the principles of study design.

TREATMENT: SMALL-CELL LUNG CANCER

Small-cell lung cancer differs from NSCLC in a number of important ways: (1) it has a more rapid clinical course and natural history, with the rapid development of metastases, symptoms and death; (2) it exhibits features of neuroendocrine differentiation in many patients which may be distinguishable histopathologically and is associated with paraneoplastic syndromes; and (3) unlike NSCLC, SCLC is exquisitely sensitive to both chemotherapy and radiotherapy, although resistant disease often develops. Because of the rapid development of distant disease and its extreme sensitivity to the cytotoxic effects of chemotherapy, this mode of therapy forms the backbone of treatment for this disease.

First-Line Therapy

A number of combination chemotherapeutic regimens are available for SCLC. With these chemotherapy regimens, overall response rates of 75–90% and complete response rates of 50% for localised disease can be anticipated. For extensive-stage disease, overall response rates of about 75% with complete response rates of 25% are common. Despite these high response rates, however, the median survival time remains about 14 months for limited-stage disease and 7–9 months for extensive-stage disease. Less than 5% of extensive-stage patients have long-term survival of greater than 2 years.

A phase III randomised trial has been reported in abstract form, in which patients with SCLC were randomised to the control arm of etoposide and cisplatin, versus cisplatin and the topoisomerase I inhibitor, irinotecan.[39] Median survival and 1-year survival was 420 days and 60% in the cisplatin/irinotecan arm and 300 days and 40% in the cisplatin/etoposide arm. If ongoing phase III studies confirm these results, cisplatin/irinotecan would become the first combination of chemotherapy to improve survival over cisplatin/etoposide in SCLC patients in decades.

Second-Line Therapy

No curative regimens for patients with recurrent disease have been identified. Topotecan has a 20–40% response rate in patients with 'sensitive' SCLC, those patients who relapsed two or more months after their first-line therapy, with a median survival of 22–27 weeks. For patients with 'refractory' disease which progressed through or within 3 months of completion of first-line therapy, the response rate in

phase II studies is only between 3% and 11%. Median survival is about 20 weeks.[40] Results of a randomised trial comparing topotecan with CAV (cyclophosphamide, adriamycin and vincristine) as second-line therapy revealed no difference in response rates, duration of response, or survival between the two groups.[41]

Chemotherapy plus Chest Irradiation

Numerous studies have been done with chemotherapy and thoracic radiotherapy for patients with limited-stage SCLC. Conflicting results have been attributed to differences in chemotherapy regimens and different schedules integrating chemotherapy and thoracic radiation, concurrent, sequential and 'sandwich' approaches. Two recent meta-analyses concluded that thoracic radiation does result in a small but significant improvement in survival and major control of the disease in the chest, although no conclusions could be made regarding the optimal sequencing of chemotherapy and thoracic radiation.[25,42]

Fractionation of Radiotherapy: For limited-stage SCLC, thoracic radiotherapy has been known to improve survival, but the best ways of integrating chemotherapy and thoracic radiotherapy are uncertain. In order to settle this question, a phase III randomised clinical trial was conducted in which 417 patients with limited SCLC were randomised to receive a total of 45 Gy of radiotherapy, either twice-daily over a 3-week period or once-daily over a 5-week period, concurrently with four 21-day cycles of cisplatin plus etoposide.[43] Twice-daily radiotherapy improved median survival as compared with once-daily radiotherapy (23 months vs. 19 months, $p = 0.04$). However, grade 3 or 4 oesophagitis was significantly more frequent with twice-daily than with once-daily fractionation (32% vs. 16%, $p < 0.001$).

Prophylactic Cranial Irradiation

Numerous trials have demonstrated that prophylactic brain irradiation (PCI) does not enhance survival, but does decrease the risk of brain metastases without a decrease in mental function.[44] However, a recent meta-analysis demonstrated a small but statistically and clinically significant improvement in survival with PCI.[45]

METHODOLOGIC ISSUES

With the traditional cytoreductive and cytotoxic chemotherapy, both as single agents and in combination, there are well-established and accepted designs for phases I, II and III clinical trials. In general these designs are based on the paradigm that with the increased myelosuppression, tumour cells are more likely to be killed, leading to shrinkage of tumours, and that there is a monotonically increasing dose–response and dose–toxicity relationship. It is also assumed that tumour shrinkage will eventually lead to clinical benefit such as prolonged survival or improved quality of life. In essence, tumour shrinkage has served as a surrogate for clinical benefit.

PHASE I CLINICAL TRIALS

In typical phase I clinical trials with acute dose-limiting toxicities as the primary endpoint, a standard dose-escalation scheme with a cohort of fixed number of patients treated at each dose level is used to estimate the so-called maximum tolerated dose (MTD) or safe dose[46,47] to be used in subsequent phase II studies. However, the choice of the initial dose and dose levels have been rather *ad hoc*. Worse yet, the standard dose-escalation design does not provide a well-defined basis for estimation of the MTD and is known to have several shortcomings such as slow dose escalation at the beginning and underestimation of the targeted dose-limiting toxicity.[48] Most critically, the standard design does not provide an estimate of the probability of toxicity at the recommended dose level. Nevertheless this standard dose-escalation design for phase I clinical trials has served a useful function in this setting.

In order to avoid slow dose-escalation and underestimation, a number of variations on the standard methods have been proposed.[49,50] These methods typically include initial dose-escalation in a single patient and a later switch-over to standard dose-escalation at the earliest indication of dose-limiting toxicity, and may also include intra-patient dose-escalation.[50]

In order to address the failure of the standard dose-escalation designs to provide an estimate of the probability of toxicity at the recommended dose level, several new approaches have been proposed, including the continual reassessment method.[51] This method is primarily based on Bayesian statistical modelling of the dose–toxicity relationship with a targeted toxicity probability for the MTD. With radiotherapy concerned with late-onset toxicities as the primary endpoint, the standard dose-escalation design for phase I clinical trials is inadequate because of the long-term follow-up required for late-onset toxicities associated with radiotherapy. With late-onset toxicities, the continual reassessment method has been extended by statistical models for the distribution for time to toxicity and by pooling toxicity information across patients receiving the same dose level.[52]

PHASE II CLINICAL TRIALS

In phase II clinical trials with cytotoxic chemotherapy, multi-stage designs with objective tumour response defined as shrinkage of tumour by more than 50% as the primary endpoint are widely used.[53–55] These are essentially sequential designs in the sense that a decision to treat additional patients for establishment of clinical efficacy is predicated by the observed clinical efficacy or safety with the patients from the previous stages. This is primarily to avoid treating patients with seemingly ineffective therapy.

Typically these designs are based on tests of statistical hypotheses with specific minimally acceptable and maximally unacceptable tumour response rates associated with type I and II error probabilities. Given these design parameters available from historical data, there are many candidate designs. In order to select a design, one may use either the minimax or the optimality criterion.[56] Subject to type I and II error probabilities, the minimax designs minimised the maximum sample size required, while the optimal designs minimised the expected sample size under the null hypothesis that the true response rate is less than or equal to the maximally unacceptable response rate. Oftentimes they are very disparate, causing confusions to those not so statistically sophisticated. A graphical search method may be used to search for what appears to be a compromise between the minimax and the optimal designs with more desirable practical features such as having much smaller maximum sample size than the optimal design and much smaller expected sample size than the minimax design.[57]

PHASE III CLINICAL TRIALS

Overall survival typically being the ultimate criterion for evaluation of the efficacy of cancer treatment in phase III clinical trials, a traditional randomised, controlled design with time to death due to all causes as the primary endpoint has become recognised as a golden standard for establishment of standard therapies in cancer. However, depending on the disease setting, other endpoints such as time to disease progression, time to treatment failure, etc. may be appropriate as a surrogate endpoint despite the problems associated with the surrogate endpoint.[58]

It has been argued that the traditional way of moving to phase III trials based on the results of phase II trials perhaps was the cause of failure of many experimental therapies including the recent failure of experimental therapies including novel targeted therapies such as matrix metalloproteinase inhibitors and epidermal growth factor receptor inhibitors.[59] One approach is to combine phase II and III trials into two-stage designs involving selection and testing based on acceptable primary endpoints or in combination with auxiliary endpoints for phase III trials.[60,61] A sequential Bayesian phase II/III design has been proposed for a non-small-cell lung cancer involving an adjuvant adenovirus for p53.[62] In this Bayesian design, local control of unresectable stage II or III NSCLC and overall survival are

considered simultaneously in a parametric mixture model.

SMALL-CELL LUNG CANCER

As was noted earlier, small-cell lung cancer is known to be biologically distinct from other histologic subtypes of lung cancer in both laboratory and clinical studies. It is the most chemosensitive type of lung cancer and as a consequence it poses some difficulties in development of investigational cytotoxic drugs. For example, there is ethical concern for testing investigational cytotoxic drugs in previously untreated small-cell lung cancer patients.

As a result of these observations, it has been suggested that different phase II designs be used depending on whether patients had been previously treated with cytotoxic drugs or have relapsed following treatment with cytotoxic drugs.[63] Also depending on whether patients are refractory to or have relapsed during previous treatment, different values for minimally acceptable and maximally unacceptable response rates should be used in phase II clinical trials. Different considerations should be given to elderly patients or patients with poor prognosis as well.

TARGETED THERAPY AND CYTOSTATIC DRUGS

Advances in molecular biology and cancer genetics coupled with biotechnology are bringing forth a number of new novel agents which appear to target molecular pathways such as cancer initiation, angiogenesis, invasion or metastasis. Examples include antiangiogenesis agents, epidermal growth factor receptor inhibitors, protein kinase inhibitors, matrix metalloproteinase inhibitors and other so-called molecular targeted therapies. These new agents are not expected to shrink tumours. Instead they are expected to inhibit tumour growth or prevent metastasis as they have demonstrated in a number of animal models. With the emergence of these different classes of agents with entirely different mode of action and expected therapeutic effects, the traditional designs for phase I, II and III clinical trials appear no longer adequate.[64–66]

With these cytostatic agents, it is unclear whether there is a clear dose–toxicity and dose–response relationship to help guide us in determining the most appropriate dose for phase II and III clinical trials. Indeed the paradigm for dose-escalation designs for cytotoxic agents for phase I clinical trials appears no longer relevant as acute toxicities may not be meaningful with such agents.

This obviously calls for new methods for estimating a safe, but effective dose in phase I clinical trials. In such a setting with cytostatic drugs, it was suggested that a biological endpoint other than toxicity be used in phase I trials to define the dose for subsequent phase II trials.[64] For phase II preliminary efficacy screening trials, single-arm designs can be used in which comparisons are made with historical control data. Sequentially measured times to disease progression within each patient who have failed previous treatment may be used in phase II designs where statistical hypotheses regarding a hazard ratio of times to disease progression before and after treatment with cytostatic drugs can be tested.[65] Considering the heterogeneity of cancer, one may wish to distinguish antiproliferative activity attributable to cytostatic drugs from less aggressive disease in phase II screening trials. In that setting, one may use a randomised discontinuation design in which all patients are treated initially with the cytostatic drug and only those whose disease is stable are randomised in a double-blind fashion to the same cytostatic drug, active vs. placebo.[66]

As illustrated above, these new classes of drugs will challenge the existing paradigm for design, conduct and analysis of phase I, II and III clinical trials in cancer. These challenges are certainly not unique to lung cancer clinical trials. Clinical investigators and statisticians need to work more closely to address these challenges in developing most efficient and relevant clinical trial designs to help advance the care of patients with lung cancer.

REFERENCES

1. Jemal A, Murray T, Samuels A, Ghafoor A, Ward E, Thun MJ. Cancer statistics, 2003. *CA Cancer J Clin* (2003) **53**: 5–26.
2. Mountain CF. Revisions in the international system for staging of lung cancer. *Chest* (1997) **111**: 1710–17.
3. Frost JK, Ball WC, Levin M, Tockman MS, Baker RR, Carter D, Eggelston JC, Erozan YS, Gupta PK, Khouri NF, Marsh BR, Stitik FP. Early lung cancer detection: results of the initial (prevalence) radiologic and cytologic screening in the Johns Hopkins study. *Am Rev Respir Dis* (1984) **130**: 549–54.
4. Flehinger BJ, Melamed MR, Zaman MB, Heelan RT, Perchick WB, Martini N. Early lung cancer detection: results of the initial (prevalence) radiologic and cytologic screening in the Memorial Sloan–Kettering study. *Am Rev Respir Dis* (1984) **130**: 555–60.
5. Fontana RS, Sanderson DR, Taylor WF, Woolner LB, Miller WE, Muhm JR, Uhlenhopp MA. Early lung cancer detection: results of the initial (prevalence) radiologic and cytologic screening in the Mayo Clinic Study. *Am Rev Respir Dis* (1984) **130**: 561–5.
6. Patz EF, Goodman PC, Bepler G. Screening for lung cancer. *N Engl J Med* (2000) **343**: 1627–33.
7. Henschke CI, Naidich DP, Yankelevitz DF, McGuinness G, McCauley DI, Smith JP, Libby DM, Pasmantier MW, Vazquez M, Koizumi J, Flieder D, Altorki NK, Miettinen OS. Early Lung Cancer Action Project: initial findings on repeat screening. *Cancer* (2001) **92**: 153–9.
8. van Zandwijk N, Dalesio O, Pastorino U, de Vries N, van Tinteren H. Euroscan, a randomized trial of vitamin A and N-acetylcysteine in patients with head & neck cancer or lung cancer. *J Natl Cancer Inst* (2000) **92**: 977–86.
9. Omenn GS, Goodman GE, Thornquist MD, Balmes J, Cullen MR, Glass A, Keogh JP, Meyskens FL, Valanis B, Williams JH, Barnhart S, Hammar S. Effects of a combination of beta carotene and vitamin A on lung cancer and cardiovascular disease. *N Engl J Med* (1996) **334**: 1150–5.
10. The Alpha-Tocopherol, Beta Carotene Cancer Prevention Study Group. The effect of vitamin E and beta carotene on the incidence of lung cancer and other cancers in male smokers. *N Engl J Med* (1994) **330**: 1029–35.
11. Clark LC, Combs GF, Turnbull BW, Slate EH, Chalker DK, Chow J, Davis LS, Glover RA, Graham GF, Gross EG, Krongrad A, Lesher JL, Park HK, Sanders BB, Smith CL, Taylor JR. Effects of

selenium supplementation for cancer prevention in patients with carcinoma of the skin: a randomized controlled trial. *J Am Med Assoc* (1996) **276**: 1957–63.

12. PORT Meta-analysis Trialists Group. Postoperative radiotherapy in non-small-cell lung cancer: systematic review and meta-analysis of individual patient data from nine randomised controlled trials. *Lancet* (1998) **352**: 257–63.

13. The Lung Cancer Study Group. Effects of postoperative mediastinal radiation on completely resected stage II and stage III epidermoid cancer of the lung. *N Engl J Med* (1986) **315**: 1377–81.

14. Non-small Cell Lung Cancer Collaborative Group. Chemotherapy in non-small cell lung cancer: a meta-analysis using updated data on individual patients from 52 randomised clinical trials. *Br Med J* (1995) **311**: 899–909.

15. Keller SM, Adak S, Wagner H, Herskovic A, Komaki R, Brooks BJ, Perry MC, Livingston RB, Johnson DH for the Eastern Cooperative Oncology Group. A randomized trial of postoperative adjuvant therapy in patients with completely resected stage II or IIIA non-small cell lung cancer. *N Engl J Med* (2000) **343**: 1217–22.

16. Rosell R, Gomez-Codina J, Camps C, Maestre J, Padille J, Canto A, Mate JL, Li S, Roig J, Olazabal A, Canela M, Ariza A, Skacel Z, Morera-Prat J, Abad A. A randomized trial comparing preoperative chemotherapy plus surgery with surgery alone in patients with non-small-cell lung cancer. *N Engl J Med* (1994) **330**: 153–8.

17. Roth JA, Fossella F, Komaki R, Ryan MB, Putnam JB, Lee JS, Dhingra H, DeCaro L, Chasen M, McGavran M, Atkinson EN, Hong WK. A randomized trial comparing perioperative chemotherapy and surgery with surgery alone in resectable stage IIIA non-small-cell lung cancer. *J Natl Cancer Inst* (1994) **86**: 673–80.

18. Roth JA, Atkinson EN, Fossella F, Komaki R, Ryan MB, Putnam JB, Lee JS, Dhingra H, DeCaro L, Chasen M, Hong WK. Long-term follow-up of patients enrolled in a randomized trial comparing perioperative chemotherapy and surgery alone in resectable stage IIIA non-small-cell lung cancer. *Lung Cancer* (1998) **21**: 1–6.

19. Depierre A, Milleron B, Moro-Sibilot, Chevret S, Quoix E, Lebeau B, Braun D, Breton J-L, Lemarie E, Gouva S, Paillot N, Brechot J-M, Janicot H, Lebas F-X, Terrioux P, Clavier J, Foucher P, Monchatre M, Coetmeur D, Level M-C, Leclerc P, Blanchon F, Rodier J-M, Thiberville L, Villeneuve A, Westeel V, Chastang C. Preoperative chemotherapy followed by surgery compared with primary surgery in resectable stage I (except T1N0), II, and IIIa non-small cell lung cancer. *J Clin Oncol* (2002) **20**: 247–53.

20. Dillman RO, Herndon J, Seagren SL, Eaton WL, Green MR. Improved survival in stage III non-small cell lung cancer: seven-year follow-up of cancer and leukemia group B (CALGB) 8433. *J Natl Cancer Inst* (1996) **88**: 1210–15.

21. Sause W, Kolesar P, Taylor S, Johnson D, Livingston R, Komaki R, Emami E, Curran W, Byhardt R, Fisher B. Final results of phase III trial in regionally advanced unresectable non-small cell lung cancer: Radiation Therapy Oncology Group (RTOG) 88-08 and Eastern Cooperative Oncology Group (ECOG) 4588. *Chest* (2000) **117**: 358–64.

22. Furuse K, Fukuoka M, Kawahara M, Nishikawa H, Takada Y, Kudoh S, Katagami N, Ariyoshi Y. Phase III study of concurrent versus sequential thoracic radiotherapy in combination with mitomycin, vindesine, and cisplatin in unresectable stage III non-small-cell lung cancer. *J Clin Oncol* (1999) **17**: 2692–9.

23. Curran W, Scott C, Langer C, Komaki R, Lee J, Hauser S, Movsas B, Wasserman T, Russell A, Byhardt R, Sause W, Cox J. Phase III comparison of sequential vs. concurrent chemoradiation for patients with unresected stage III non-small cell lung cancer (NSCLC): initial report of the Radiation Therapy Oncology Group (RTOG) 9410. *Proc Am Soc Clin Oncol* (2000) **18**: 484a.

24. Choy H, Akerley W, Safran H, Graziano S, Chung C, Williams T, Cole B, Kennedy T. Multiinstitutional phase II trial of paclitaxel, carboplatin, and concurrent radiation therapy for locally advanced non-small-cell lung cancer. *J Clin Oncol* (1998) **16**: 3316–22.

25. Soquet PJ, Chauvin F, Boissel JP, Cellerino R, Cormier Y, Ganz PA, Kaasa S, Pater JL, Quoix E, Rapp E, Tunarello D, Williams J, Woods BL, Bernard JP. Polychemotherapy in advanced non-small cell lung cancer: a meta-analysis. *Lancet* (1993) **342**: 19–21.

26. Marino P, Pampallona S, Preatoni A, Cantoni A, Inveinezzi F. Chemotherapy vs. supportive care in advanced non-small cell lung cancer: results of a meta-analysis of the literature. *Chest* (1994) **106**: 861–5.

27. Sandler A, Nemunaitis J, Denham C, von Pawel J, Cormier Y, Gatzemeier U, Mattson K, Manegold C, Palmer M, Gregor A, Nguyen B, Niyikiza C, Einhorn L. Phase III trial of gemcitabine plus cisplatin versus cisplatin alone in patients with locally advanced or metastatic non-small cell lung cancer. *J Clin Oncol* (2000) **18**: 122–30.

28. Wozniak AJ, Crowley JJ, Balcerzak SP, Weiss GR, Spiridonidis CH, Baker LH, Albain KS, Kelly K, Taylor SA, Gandara DR, Livingston RB. Randomized trial comparing cisplatin with cisplatin plus vinorelbine in the treatment of advanced

non-small-cell lung cancer: a Southwest Oncology Group study. *J Clin Oncol* (1998) **16**: 2459–65.

29. Lilenbaum RC, Herndon J, List M, Desch C, Watson D, Holland J, Weeks JC, Green MR. Single agent (SA) versus combination chemotherapy (CC) in advanced non-small cell lung cancer: a CALGB randomized trial of efficacy, quality of life (QoL), and cost effectiveness. *Proc Am Soc Clin Oncol* (2002) **20**: 1a.

30. Sederholm C. Gemcitabine (G) compared with gemcitabine plus carboplatin (GC) in advanced non-small cell lung cancer (NSCLC): a phase III study by the Swedish Lung Cancer Study Group (SLUSG). *Proc Am Soc Clin Oncol* (2002) **20**: 1162a.

31. Kelly KJ, Crowley J, Bunn PA, Presant CA, Grevstad PK, Moinpour CM, Ramsey SD, Wozniak AJ, Weiss GR, Moore DF, Israel VK, Livingston RB, Gandara DR. Randomized phase III trial of paclitaxel plus carboplatin versus vinorelbine plus cisplatin in the treatment of patients with advanced non-small-cell lung cancer: a Southwest Oncology Group trial. *J Clin Oncol* (2001) **19**: 3210–18.

32. Schiller JH, Harrington D, Belani CP, Langer C, Sandler A, Krook J, Zhu Z, Johnson DH for the Eastern Cooperative Oncology Group. Comparison of four chemotherapy regimens for advanced non-small cell lung cancer. *N Engl J Med* (2002) **346**: 92–8.

33. Shepherd F, Dancey J, Ramlau R, Mattson K, Gralla R, O'Rourke M, Levitan N, Gressot L, Vincent M, Burkes R, Coughlin S, Kim Y, Berille J. Prospective randomized trial of docetaxel versus best supportive care in patients with non-small cell lung cancer previously treated with platinum-based chemotherapy. *J Clin Oncol* (2000) **18**: 2095–103.

34. Fossella FV, DeVore R, Kerr RN, Crawford J, Natale RR, Dunphy F, Kalman L, Miller V, Lee JS, Moore M, Gandara D, Karp D, Vokes E, Kris M, Kim Y, Gamza F, Hammershaimb L. Randomized phase III trial of docetaxel versus vinorelbine or ifosfamide in patients with advanced non-small cell lung cancer previously treated with platinum-containing chemotherapy regimens. *J Clin Oncol* (2000) **18**: 2354–62.

35. Fukuoka M, Yano S, Giaccone G, Tamura T, Nakagawa K, Douillard J-Y, Nishiwaki Y, Vansteenkiste JF, Kudo S, Averbuch S, Macleod A, Feyereislova A, Baselga J. Final results from a phase II trial of zd1839 ('Iressa') for patients with advanced non-small cell lung cancer (IDEAL 1). *Proc Am Soc Clin Oncol* (2002) **20**: 298a.

36. Kris MG, Natale RB, Herbst RS, Lynch TJ, Prager D, Belani CP, Schiller JH, Kelly K, Spiridonidis C, Albain KS, Brahmer JR, Sandler A,

Crawford J, Lutzker SG, Lilenbaum R, Helms L, Wolf M, Averbuch S, Ochs J, Kay A. A phase II trial of zd1839 ('Iressa') in advanced non-small cell lung cancer patients who had failed platinum- and docetaxel-based regiments (IDEAL 2). *Proc Am Soc Clin Oncol* (2002) **20**: 292a.

37. Johnson D, Herbst R, Giaccone G, Schiller J, Natale R, Miller V, Wolf M, Holton A, Averbuch S, Grous J. Zd1839 ('Iressa') in combination with paclitaxel and carboplatin in chemotherapy-naive patients with advanced non-small-cell lung cancer: results from a phase III clinical trial (Intact2). *Ann Oncol* (2002) **13**(Suppl 5): 127–8.

38. Giaccone G, Johnson DH, Manegold C, Scagliotti GV, Rosell R, Wolf M, Rennie P, Ochs J, Averbuch S, Fandi A. A phase III clinical trial of zd1839 ('Iressa') in combination with gemcitabine and cisplatin in chemotherapy-naive patients with advanced non-small-cell lung cancer (Intact 1). *Ann Oncol* (2002) **13**(Suppl 5): 2.

39. Giaccone G, Johnson DH, Manegold C, Scagliotti GV, Rosell R, Wolf M, Rennie P, Ochs J, Averbuch S, Fandi A. Irinotecan plus cisplatin compared with etoposide plus cisplatin for extensive small cell lung cancer. *N Engl J Med* (2002) **346**: 85–91.

40. Schiller J, Kim K, Hutson P, DeVore R, Glick J, Stewart J, Johnson D. Phase II study of topotecan in patients with extensive-stage small cell carcinoma of the lung: an Eastern Cooperative Oncology Group trial (E1592). *J Clin Oncol* (1996) **14**: 2345–52.

41. von Pawel J, Schiller J, Sheperd F, Kleisbauer J, Chrysson N, Steward D, Fields S, Clark P, Palmer M, Depierre A, Carmichael J, Krebs J, Ross G, Gralla R. Topotecan versus CAV for the treatment of recurrent small cell lung cancer. *J Clin Oncol* (1999) **17**: 658–67.

42. Pignon J, Arriagada R, Ihde D, Johnson D, Perry M, Souhami R, Brodin O, Joss R, Kies M, Lebeau B, Onoshi T, Osterlind K, Tattersall M, Wagner H. A meta-analysis of thoracic radio therapy for small-cell lung cancer. *N Engl J Med* (1992) **327**: 618–24.

43. Turrisi AT, Kim K, Blum R, Sause WT, Livingston RB, Komaki R, Wagner H, Aisner S, Johnson DH. Twice-daily compared with once-daily thoracic radiotherapy in limited small-cell lung cancer treated with concurrently with cisplatin and etoposide. *N Engl J Med* (1999) **340**: 265–71.

44. Arriagada R, Le Chevalier T, Borie F, Riviere A, Chomy P, Monnet I, Tardivon A, Viader F, Tarayre M, Benhamou S. Prophylactic cranial irradiation for patients with small-cell lung cancer in complete remission. *J Natl Cancer Inst* (1995) **87**: 183–90.

45. Auperin A, Arriagada R, Pignon J, Pechoux C, Gregor A, Stephens R, Kristjansen P, Johnson B, Ueoka H, Wagner H, Aisner J. Prophylactic cranial irradiation for patients with small cell lung cancer in complete remission. *N Engl J Med* (1999) **341**: 476–84.

46. Schneiderman MA. Mouse to man: statistical problems in bringing a drug to clinical trial. *Proc Fifth Berkeley Symp Math Stat Prob* (1967) **4**: 855–66.

47. Geller NR. Design of phase I and II clinical trials in cancer: a statistician's view. *Cancer Invest* (1984) **2**: 483–91.

48. Storer B, DeMets DL. Current phase I/II designs: are they adequate? *J Clin Res Drug Dev* (1987) **1**: 21–30.

49. Storer B. Design and analysis of phase I clinical trials. *Biometrics* (1989) **45**: 925–37.

50. Simon R, Freidlin B, Rubinstein L, Arbuck SG, Collins J, Christian MC. Accelerated titration designs for phase I clinical trials in oncology. *J Natl Cancer Inst* (1997) **89**: 1138–47.

51. O'Quigley J, Pepe M, Fisher L. Continual reassessment method: a practical design for phase I clinical trials in cancer. *Biometrics* (1990) **46**: 33–48.

52. Cheung YK, Chappell R. Sequential designs for phase I clinical trials with late-onset toxicities. *Biometrics* (2000) **56**: 1177–82.

53. Gehan E. The determination of the number of patients required in a preliminary and a follow-up trial of a new chemotherapeutic agent. *J Chronic Dis* (1961) **13**: 346–53.

54. Lee YJ, Staquet M, Simon R, Catane R, Muggia F. Two-stage plans for patient accrual in phase II cancer clinical trials. *Cancer Treat Rep* (1979) **63**: 721–61.

55. Fleming TR. One-sample multiple testing procedures for phase II trials. *Biometrics* (1982) **38**: 143–51.

56. Simon R. Optimal two-stage designs for phase II clinical trials. *Contr Clin Trials* (1989) **10**: 1–10.

57. Jung SH, Carey M, Kim K. Graphical search for two-stage designs for phase II clinical trials. *Contr Clin Trials* (2001) **22**: 367–72.

58. Fleming TR. DeMets DL. Surrogate endpoints in clinical trials: are we being misled? *Ann Int Med* (1996) **125**: 605–13.

59. Scher HI, Heller G. Picking the winners in a sea of plenty? *Clin Cancer Res* (2002) **8**: 400–404.

60. Thall PF, Simon R, Ellenberg SS. Two-stage selection and testing designs for comparative clinical trials. *Biometrika* (1988) **75**: 303–10.

61. Schaid DJ, Wieand S. Therneau TM. Optimal two-stage screening designs for survival comparisons. *Biometrika* (1990) **77**: 507–13.

62. Inoue LYT, Thall PF, Berry DA. Seamlessly expanding a randomized phase II trial to phase III. *Biometrics* (2002) **58**: 823–31.

63. Moore TD, Korn EL. Phase II trial design considerations for small-cell lung cancer. *J Natl Cancer Inst* (1992) **8**: 150–4.

64. Korn EL, Arbuck SG, Pluda JM, Simon R, Kaplan RS, Christian MC. Clinical trials designs for cytostatic agents: are new approaches needed? *J Clin Oncol* (2001) **19**: 265–72.

65. Mick R, Crowley JJ, Carroll RJ. Phase II clinical trial design for noncytotoxic anticancer agents for which time to disease progression is the primary endpoint. *Proc Am Assoc Clin Res* (1999) **59**: 228a.

66. Rosner GL, Stadler W, Ratain MJ. Randomized discontinuation design: application to cytostatic antineoplastic agents. *J Clin Oncol* (2002) **20**: 4478–84.

CARDIOVASCULAR

12

Cardiovascular

LAWRENCE FRIEDMAN AND ELEANOR SCHRON

National Heart, Lung, and Blood Institute, Bethesda, MD 20892 2482, USA

INTRODUCTION

Most of the principles in developing, managing and analysing clinical trials in cardiovascular diseases are the same as for other conditions. There are some special aspects, however, that we will review here, and then provide examples for in the subsequent sections.

A major point that influences many of the clinical trials is that in developed countries, and unfortunately more and more in developing nations, cardiovascular disease is common. Atherosclerosis and hypertension are the primary causes of cardiovascular disease in adults, although there are many contributing factors to these (often termed risk factors). Although clinical trials have been conducted in other causes of cardiovascular disease, including congenital conditions, there are far fewer trials in these areas. Therefore, because in developed countries most heart disease, stroke and peripheral vascular diseases are due to atherosclerosis and hypertension, and because most of the cardiovascular disease clinical trials have been conducted in developed countries, this chapter will emphasise those.

Because cardiovascular diseases are common, small treatment benefits may yield important

public benefits, particularly if the treatment is simple and inexpensive, such as aspirin. Again because the condition is common, when there are potential treatments that are simple to administer, trials may be conducted in communities outside of academic health centres, with their special expertise and facilities.

Another important consideration is that atherosclerotic and hypertensive cardiovascular diseases are chronic conditions, often taking decades to develop and lasting many years after being first diagnosed. Clinical trials, therefore, may be initiated well before the development of risk factors (sometimes called primordial prevention), after the development of risk factors, but before the occurrence of organ damage (primary prevention), or after organ damage has occurred (secondary prevention). Some interventions are potentially useful in all three settings, but others, particularly expensive or invasive approaches, may be best suited for secondary prevention. The relative importance of risk factors and clinical findings may also differ, affecting the likely impact of the interventions. After a heart attack, for example, how well the surviving myocardium functions in pumping blood may be more important in determining longevity than cholesterol

Textbook of Clinical Trials.   Edited by D. Machin, S. Day and S. Green
© 2004 John Wiley & Sons, Ltd   ISBN: 0-471-98787-5

level (though the latter has been clearly shown to affect recurrent infarctions and death). Often, treatments for atherosclerotic or hypertensive cardiovascular diseases do not cure the underlying conditions. Rather, they may reduce the likelihood of having clinical sequelae or control the serious consequences of disease.

As noted, the common causes of cardiovascular diseases (atherosclerosis and hypertension) are multifactorial in origin. Atherosclerosis may be influenced by cholesterol level, blood pressure, cigarette smoking, obesity, physical activity, inflammatory processes, diabetes, age and genetics, plus other factors. Hypertension may be influenced by things such as diet (intake of salt and various nutrients), obesity, physical activity, stress or emotion, and genetics. With regard to genetic influences, it is not thought that the common cardiovascular diseases or their risk factors are influenced by single genes. Rather, there are likely to be many genes that interact with environmental conditions to effect most common cardiovascular diseases. Because of the multiple risk factors, clinical trial interventions that alter individual factors might yield only modest reductions in clinical outcomes such as myocardial infarction or death from cardiovascular causes. Antihypertensive drugs, though, that lower blood pressure regardless of the reason for the hypertension, have been shown to give impressive reductions in stroke,[1] much of which is due to hypertension. On the other hand, treating hypertension has led to only modest reductions in heart disease, probably because the other risk factors for heart disease were unchanged. The multifactorial nature of much cardiovascular disease has led some to design trials that have attempted to intervene on several factors simultaneously.

Whether as part of a clinical trial, or because of usual clinical care, many participants in cardiovascular disease clinical trials are on multiple interventions. This can affect adherence to study protocol and may lead to various drug interactions.

We typically think of cardiovascular disease as affecting the heart, as in coronary heart disease, or the brain, as in stroke, but other parts of the body, such as the kidneys or the legs (as in intermittent claudication), may be affected. Even within a single organ such as the heart, the presentation of cardiovascular disease may take various forms, such as angina pectoris, myocardial infarction, cardiac arrhythmias of different sorts, heart failure and sudden death. The interventions studied in clinical trials may be directed at any of those, though some interventions, such as blood pressure lowering drugs, may affect more than one outcome.

One issue in designing and interpreting the results of cardiovascular disease trials is choice of the outcome. As noted, interventions may affect only one aspect of the disease. Therefore, investigators would prefer to use as the outcome of interest only that most likely to be modified by the treatment. But for outcomes such as cause-specific mortality, that is not easy. Even a rather broad outcome such as death due to cardiovascular disease has limitations, because many deaths are unwitnessed and autopsies much less common than in the past. When finer splits are used, such as death due to arrhythmia or myocardial infarction, the difficulties mount.[2] Similar problems exist for non-fatal events, such as myocardial infarction. In the Framingham Heart Study, more than 25% of myocardial infarctions were 'silent', that is, occurred without symptoms and were only recognised on electrocardiographic examination.[3] Extra efforts need to be made to identify these, as they convey considerable risk of death, even though they are asymptomatic.

Because many of the cardiovascular disease conditions are common, there is rarely a shortage of people with the condition of interest for most clinical trials. Particularly with multicentre, in fact, multinational, trials, there are adequate numbers of potential participants so that studies using clinical outcomes are feasible. It is usually not necessary to resort to trials with surrogate endpoints on account of participant unavailability. However, when a trial seeks special subtypes of cardiovascular disease, subject availability becomes more of an issue. It is still usually unnecessary to conduct trials with surrogate endpoints, but extra efforts do have to be made to identify and enroll the participants. Connected with this, many physicians sub-specialise in particular types of cardiovascular disease. Involving the kind of physician most likely to have knowledge of and access to the relevant patient population is therefore essential.[4]

The large size of many cardiovascular clinical trials means that stratification to ensure balance among key baseline factors is usually unnecessary, with the notable exception of site, in multicentre trials. Site is almost always a stratification variable. Beyond that, investigators should stratify on at most a very few variables. For example, for studies of heart failure, we often stratify by left ventricular ejection fraction; for studies of arrhythmia, we might stratify by type of arrhythmia and ejection fraction; for primary prevention trials, we might stratify by age and sex; and for trials of blood pressure lowering, we would stratify by prior use of antihypertensive drugs.

One feature of trials in cardiovascular disease that always needs to be considered is the dramatic reduction in mortality from heart disease and stroke over the past few decades in most developed countries.[5] As a result of a combination of improved prevention and much better medical care, death rates in developed countries have decreased to a level that makes mortality outcome studies less feasible. From a public health and a patient standpoint, this is certainly a happy state to be in, but it means that clinical trials must be designed with the expectation that the event rates may be considerably less than expected. The trials need either to be much larger, or else the outcome needs to be a combination of death and other clinical events.

The remainder of this chapter will consider issues in specific trials. It is divided into trials of drugs or biologics, trials of devices and surgical procedures, and trials of lifestyle or other non-pharmacologic interventions. For fuller discussions of various cardiovascular disease clinical trials, see the book, *Clinical Trials in Cardiovascular Disease.*[6]

TRIALS OF PHARMACOLOGIC AGENTS

Pharmaceutical agents are the most common interventions tested in clinical trials of cardiovascular disease. Most trials of drugs are similar in structure and design to trials in any other field of medicine. A few points, however, should be made. Because, as noted above, most cardiovascular disease takes decades to develop, there is a long period when people have few if any symptoms. The likely existence of atherosclerosis, for example, is usually determined by the presence of risk factors, such as hypertension, hyperlipidaemia or family history, advanced age in people who have the typical lifestyle of most Western countries, and the use of sophisticated imaging methods. Prevention of the sequelae of atherosclerosis is therefore quite feasible. Because participants in trials of primary prevention are asymptomatic, several principles apply. First, serious or troublesome adverse events due to interventions in people who are generally healthy are unacceptable and not tolerated by the participants. Therefore, only drugs that are well-characterised (and are presumably safe and well-tolerated) are generally studied in prevention trials. Second, the rate of clinical events is likely to be low. Unless the trials use surrogate outcomes, they need to be very large (thousands and sometimes tens of thousands of participants) and long (often five years or more). Third, people who are asymptomatic and consequently notice no obvious benefit from treatment may have trouble adhering to the regimen, especially in a long trial. Therefore, a considerable 'drop-out' rate must be built into the sample estimate, increasing the size of the trial even more.

Among the first large clinical trials in cardiovascular disease were trials of lipid lowering. The Coronary Drug Project, which began in the 1960s, tested five interventions (clofibrate, nicotinic acid, dextrothyroxine, and two doses of equine estrogen) against a placebo in men with a history of a myocardial infarction.[7,8] These early efforts at lipid modification were only modestly successful. The interventions had major adverse events and three were stopped before the scheduled end of the trial. In addition to the adverse events, the amount of lipid lowering was relatively small, in general, so the lack of improvement in mortality, the primary outcome, was perhaps not surprising. Nicotinic acid was shown to reduce non-fatal reinfarction, however, and post-trial follow-up disclosed a significant reduction in mortality.[9] A key finding in the Coronary Drug Project was that the mortality rate in the control group was only two-thirds of that predicted when the study was started. This probably reflected selection of better risk participants, but improved care may also have played a role. This phenomenon is one that many cardiovascular trials conducted since the Coronary Drug Project have had to take into account in the sample size estimates.

The next large lipid-lowering trial was the Lipid Research Clinics Coronary Primary Prevention Trial.[10] This trial compared cholestryramine resin versus placebo to see if there would be a difference in the primary outcome of coronary heart disease death or non-fatal myocardial infarction in 3806 men free of prior evidence of heart disease, but with hyperlipoproteinaemia. There were 155 events in the intervention group and 187 in the placebo group (one-sided $p < 0.05$). This study was one of the first to show benefits from lipid lowering, even though some questioned the significance of the results, given the one-sided test.

More definitive outcomes from cholesterol lowering had to wait for the development of agents that were more effective in lowering lipids and, importantly, better tolerated. The clinical trials of hydroxymethylglutaryl coenzyme A (HMG-CoA) reductase inhibitors ('statins') were primarily conducted in the 1990s. Trials such as the Scandinavian Simvastatin Survival Study (4S),[11] the Cholesterol and Recurrent Events (CARE) trial[12] and the MRC/BHF Heart Protection Study[13] have clearly demonstrated that cholesterol lowering in both people with known heart disease and in those at high risk, but without evidence of heart disease, leads to impressive reductions in all-cause mortality and in coronary heart disease events.

The 4S trial compared simvastatin against placebo in 4444 participants with known coronary heart disease and elevated serum cholesterol. The intervention lowered low-density lipoprotein cholesterol by 35% and mortality by 30%.[11] The CARE trial compared pravastatin against placebo in 4159 post-myocardial infarction patients. The baseline serum cholesterol level was somewhat lower in this trial than in the 4S trial. As in 4S, there was greater than a 30% reduction in low-density lipoprotein cholesterol and a 24% relative benefit in the primary outcome of coronary heart disease death plus non-fatal myocardial infarction.[12] The MRC/BHF Heart Protection Study extended these finding to those who had coronary heart disease or were otherwise at high risk, regardless of the baseline cholesterol level.[13]

As a result of these and other trials of cholesterol lowering and trials of blood pressure reduction, new evidence-based guidelines for treatment of risk factors such as hyperlipidaemia and hypertension have been developed and widely disseminated. Therefore, regardless of whether the trial is one of primary prevention or in people with known end-organ damage, the control group must be adequately treated. This means that the event rate in the control group will be less than it has been in past years, making it even more difficult to detect benefit from a new intervention.

An example of a recent trial designed to mimic clinical practice illustrates some of these issues. The Antihypertensive and Lipid-Lowering Treatment to Prevent Heart Attack Trial, or ALLHAT, compared treatment, in a blinded fashion, beginning with three different antihypertensive agents against the control, which was thiazide diuretic treatment, in more than 40 000 people aged 55 or over who had hypertension and at least one other risk factor. Thus, the hypertension component of ALLHAT used an 'active control' arm. The primary outcome of this component was fatal coronary heart disease or non-fatal myocardial infarction. ALLHAT also included a lipid-lowering agent in over 10 000 of the enrolled participants in a factorial design. The primary outcome for the lipid component was all-cause mortality; this part of ALLHAT was an open, or non-blinded study.[14-16]

One of the antihypertensive agents, an alpha-adrenergic blocker, was stopped early because although there was little difference in the primary outcome, there was a significant increase in heart failure in the alpha-adrenergic blocker arm, compared with the diuretic arm. The other two antihypertensive treatments, a calcium channel blocker and an angiotensin-converting enzyme inhibitor, continued to the scheduled end of the trial. There were no differences between either of these arms and the active control thiazide diuretic arm for the primary outcome. There were some differences in secondary outcomes, with the diuretic being superior to the other agents for heart failure, for example. The blood pressure component of ALLHAT showed that in an active control trial, a very large sample size needed to be used to achieve adequate power, even when the primary outcome was a combination of events. Also contributing to the need for a large sample was the fact that about 30% of the participants who had a follow-up visit at five years had discontinued the study drug.

With respect to the lipid component, there was no significant difference in total mortality, despite the fact that many other studies have shown benefit from lipid-lowering treatments.[17] One explanation may be that there was only a modest difference in low-density lipoprotein cholesterol between the two groups. Almost 30% of the control group participants were receiving non-study lipid-lowering therapy by the end of the trial. The non-blinded design probably helped foster that. The public campaigns aimed at getting people to reduce their cholesterol levels undoubtedly played a role. Also, people who were thought to require lipid-lowering therapy and those already on such therapy were not eligible to be enrolled. Because only those already entered in ALLHAT for the hypertension component were candidates for the lipid-lowering component, the originally expected number of about 20000 enrollees turned out to be 10355, further limiting the study power.

Rates of death in people who have had a myocardial infarction used to be quite high. Modern therapy has reduced those rates remarkably. Thus, trials using mortality alone as an endpoint may no longer be feasible even in survivors of a heart attack, unless a very high risk group is studied. This has led to increased use of combination endpoints, such as cardiovascular mortality plus non-fatal myocardial infarction. The Heart Outcomes Prevention Evaluation (HOPE) study compared the angiotensin-converting enzyme inhibitor ramipril against placebo in 9297 people with either known vascular disease or diabetes plus another risk factor. The primary outcome was myocardial infarction, stroke or death from cardiovascular causes. Thus, even though this was a high-risk sample, and the sample size was considerable, it was necessary to have a combination endpoint to achieve adequate power. There was a highly significant and clinically impressive reduction in the primary outcome from ramipril.[18]

A similar study is the Prevention of Events with Angiotensin-Converting Enzyme Inhibitor Therapy, or PEACE.[19] This trial is not yet completed, but it too compares an angiotensin-converting enzyme inhibitor (trandolapril) against standard therapy in over 8000 people with documented coronary heart disease and a left ventricular ejection fraction of at least 40%. The reason for the ejection fraction criterion is that angiotensin-converting enzyme inhibitors have been shown to be beneficial in those with heart failure or low ejection fraction. This eligibility criterion, however, also means that the event rate is lower than if those with impaired ejection fraction were included. So in order to have adequate power, even in this relatively large study, a combination of events is necessary as the primary outcome. Originally, the sample size was set at 14000, and the primary outcome was cardiovascular death and non-fatal myocardial infarction. Early in the trial, primarily for feasibility reasons, the sample size was reduced to 8100 and the primary outcome expanded to include the need for coronary revascularisation procedures. Procedures such as need for revascularisation are often included as part of the endpoint. This can be appropriate, but is subject to considerable bias if the trial is not blinded, which PEACE is.

Antihypertensive agents and lipid-lowering drugs have generally been approved by drug regulatory agencies on the basis of their effects on blood pressure and cholesterol, rather than on their effects on clinical outcomes. The clinical outcomes, however, are so important that many trials have successfully tested their effects on death, myocardial infarction and stroke.[11–16,18,20]

Cardiac ventricular arrhythmias are known to correlate with total and sudden death. Therefore, for years, it was thought that drugs that reduced cardiac arrhythmias should be approved on the basis of their antiarrhythmic effect, on the assumption that they would be clinically beneficial. However, when the trials were done that looked at clinical outcomes, it was seen that arrhythmia suppression was not a good surrogate for mortality.

The Cardiac Arrhythmia Suppression Trial (CAST) tested whether suppression of ventricular arrhythmias by any of three antiarrhythmic drugs would reduce the incidence of sudden cardiac death. In the first part of this trial, over 1700 patients whose ventricular arrhythmias were suppressed by encainide, flecainide or moricizine were randomly assigned to the drug that was most effective in suppressing the arrhythmia or matching placebo. However, two of the drugs, encainide and flecainide, were soon seen to significantly increase both sudden death and all-cause mortality and they were discontinued early in the study.[21] The study was continued with moricizine as the only antiarrhythmic drug. This too was stopped ahead of schedule because of adverse trends in mortality.[22] As a result of CAST, the use of surrogate outcomes in many clinical trials has been seriously questioned.

Another feature of many drug trials in cardiovascular disease is that a 'stepped care' approach is used. This is common in trials of blood pressure lowering. Because a single drug is often either insufficiently effective or not well tolerated by the participant,

use of second, third and even fourth choice drugs is built into the protocol. For example, in the Systolic Hypertension in the Elderly program,[20] a multicentre, randomised, double-blind, placebo-controlled, community-based trial, 4736 participants with isolated systolic hypertension were randomised to receive either chlorthalidone, 12.5 mg daily, or matching placebo. The goal systolic blood pressure differed for each participant depending upon initial systolic blood pressure. If the blood pressure remained above the goal at two consecutive monthly visits, the dose was increased to 25 mg of chlorthalidone or matching placebo daily. If the participants were still above the goal at two consecutive visits, 25 mg of atenolol daily or matching placebo was added. In participants who still did not reach the goal systolic blood pressure, the dose was increased to 50 mg of atenolol or matching placebo. If atenolol was contraindicated, 0.05 to 0.1 mg of reserpine or matching placebo daily was substituted. Blood pressure above *a priori* established escape levels, despite maximal stepped-care therapy or corresponding placebo, was an indication for prescribing open-label active drug therapy.[20]

Some trials of pharmaceutical agents compare strategies, rather than drugs. Recently, the Atrial Fibrillation Follow-up Investigation of Rhythm Management (AFFIRM) evaluated which of two approaches for treating patients with atrial fibrillation was better.[23,24] Participants had to have atrial fibrillation, be over age 65 (or under 65 and at high risk for stroke) and the enrolling physician had to deem it appropriate to treat patients as part of the assigned strategy for up to five years. AFFIRM included 4060 people, enrolled at over 200 sites in Canada and the United States, who were randomised to either rhythm or rate control strategies for managing their atrial fibrillation. Investigators could select from various options on an approved menu of pharmacologic and non-pharmacologic therapies. Cardioversion and antiarrhythmic drugs were used to maintain sinus rhythm (called 'rhythm control'). Agents such as digitalis, calcium channel blockers and β-blockers, or ablation of the atrioventricular junction and pacemaker implantation, were used to control the ventricular response rate from the atrial fibrillation (called 'rate control'). The trial showed that there was no significant difference in the primary outcome (all-cause mortality), though there was a trend favouring the rate control group, and there were fewer adverse effects in the rate control group.

TRIALS OF DEVICES AND SURGICAL PROCEDURES

Devices and surgical procedures are commonly used in patients with heart disease. Examples of devices are replacements for heart valves, stents that help keep coronary vessels that have been opened patent, cardiac pacemakers and cardiac defibrillators. Examples of surgical procedures are corrections of congenital abnormalities, coronary artery bypass grafts (CABG) and aneurysm resection. Trials of various surgical procedures are usually surgery versus medical treatment or surgery versus device implantation. Examples are coronary artery bypass graft procedures in patients with ischaemia that are compared against use of thrombolytic agents or against implantation of coronary artery stents, or coronary bypass graft procedures in patients with stable angina pectoris that have been compared against best medical therapy. Less often, there are trials comparing one surgical procedure against another. Devices may be compared against surgery, as noted, or against medical care, or sometimes, against another device.

Obviously, as with all clinical trials, the questions in these kinds of trials need to be important and the answer relevant, the study needs to be appropriately designed and carried out, and the data must be properly analysed. In addition, there are certain features of such studies that need to be considered. First, there is an unavoidable integration of the intervention being employed and the technique with which it is done. The skill of the investigator is far more important than in, for example, drug trials. Unless the investigator has considerable surgical competence or experience in implanting a device, an intervention might be claimed to be not beneficial, or even harmful, when in the hands of a more skilled operator it would be beneficial. This was seen in the Department of Veterans Affairs trial comparing surgical and medical management of angina pectoris.[25] Thirteen hospitals participated in this trial. Three of the hospitals had surgical mortality considerably greater than the other 10. The results comparing surgery against medical care were favourable for surgery among patients at high risk of death from their disease, even when all 13 hospitals were included in the analysis. However, for lower risk patients, only the comparison involving the 10 hospitals with better surgical results showed benefit from surgery. These data may reflect normal variation, but they raise the issue of requiring a certain level of experience from the surgeons before they participate in a trial.

The issue of skill of the operators who insert a device also needs to be emphasised. Most recent clinical trials of device implantation require that the operators have experience with a certain minimum number of devices before being allowed to participate in the trial. This does not guarantee that only highly skilled operators will be involved, but it means that the trial is a better test of how the device will perform in close to optimal circumstances. An example is the experience required of investigators and the establishment of minimum standards for the device and lead systems used in the Antiarrhythmics Versus Implantable Defibrillators (AVID) trial.[26]

A second, related issue is how broadly the study results can be generalised if only the most experienced surgeons participate in the trial. After a drug study shows benefit from a new pharmaceutical agent, presumably most practitioners are able to administer the drug in a safe, effective manner. Transferring surgical technique and skill from investigators in the trial to others is less straightforward. Similarly, if a device is shown to be beneficial, and then used more widely by less well-trained operators, the results will not be as positive as in the clinical trial setting.

Trials of both devices and surgical procedures affect the way in which the primary trial outcome is assessed. Because of the invasive nature of the intervention, it is likely, indeed expected, that there will be an early adverse experience associated with the procedure. The trauma involved; the consequences of anaesthesia, particularly if general anaesthesia is used; and the risks of infection will almost inevitably lead to morbidity and perhaps mortality early after the intervention. Therefore, the study needs to be designed such that it lasts long enough for any hoped-for benefit to overcome the early unfavourable experience. Sometimes, the expected benefit does not appear for quite some time. Not only the investigators, but institutional ethics committees and prospective study participants need to understand this implication.

An example is the Program on the Surgical Control of Hyperlipidemia.[27,28] This trial compared partial ileal bypass surgery against medical therapy in patients with a prior myocardial infarction. The goal was to decrease the absorption of lipids, thereby reducing serum cholesterol. For the first two years of the trial, there was little difference in the primary outcome, all-cause mortality, with the surgical group doing slightly worse than the control group. The curves crossed after about three years, and at the scheduled end of the trial, there was a non-significant trend in favour of surgery. The study investigators followed the participants after the formal end of the trial. The trend in favour of surgery continued and five years after the end, the mortality difference was statistically significant.[28]

This study shows that data monitoring committees need to consider how long to wait to see if the benefit appears and counterbalances the known risks. Even though the primary outcome was not sufficiently adverse early in the trial to justify stopping, other factors combined with lack of benefit might have influenced a monitoring committee to do so. For example, in POSCH, there were side effects such as diarrhoea and, more seriously, a higher rate of kidney stones and gallstones.[27] The slight early adverse trend in mortality plus the increased morbidity could have led to a decision to stop the study prematurely.

Changes in surgical technique or modifications in devices while the study is being conducted can cause difficulties in interpreting the results of clinical trials. If, partway through a study, there is an important change in the intervention, depending on the outcome, it may be hard to reach a clear conclusion about the possible benefits of the intervention. In the past, implantable cardioverter defibrillators required a thoracotomy. This carried considerable risk that needed to be considered when inserting the device. Leads that could be inserted transvenously were subsequently developed, reducing the early complication rate. The AVID trial and the Canadian Implantable Defibrillator Study (CIDS) trial, both of which compared implantable cardioverter defibrillators against medical therapy in people resuscitated from cardiac arrest, were in the process of enrolling patients when the switch in practice from primarily using thoracotomy-based defibrillators to transvenous defibrillators occurred.[26,29] Because both types of defibrillator performed similarly, there was no problem in combining the results. This was particularly the case because it was shown significantly in AVID and with a strong trend in CIDS that the defibrillator was more effective in reducing mortality than antiarrhythmic drug therapy. If there were no difference, or if drug therapy turned out to be superior overall, questions about the validity of the trial might have been raised, given the mid-study switches in device use.

Trials of cardiovascular devices involve several other issues that are not common to other kinds of trials. One is the decision during study design as to the primary question. The device is developed to meet certain specifications. These include minimising the possibility of rejection by the patient, reducing the likelihood of development of thrombi and emboli, physical characteristics such as size and weight, and, importantly, does it do what it is designed to do. Does a defibrillator detect and convert life-threatening rhythm disturbances? Does a pacemaker detect and correct severe bradycardia? Can a stent be easily employed and will it retain its structural integrity? These are engineering questions that should be addressed and satisfactorily answered before a clinical trial is conducted. The clinical trial should be designed to answer the questions posed by the clinician. Will the device reduce mortality and/or morbidity, what is the restenosis/occlusion rate, and what are the risks and side effects? The answers to these questions incorporate the structural and functional aspects of the device, the skill of the person inserting the device, and the often unknown biologic interaction between patients and the device.

The fact that only devices designed and fully expected to be mechanically functional are used raises a serious ethical issue. If the device defibrillates, for example, how can it be withheld from someone with known life-threatening cardiac arrhythmias? This was faced in the AVID trial.[30,31] The rationale for the trial was that the balance between expected reduction in death due to arrhythmias versus death from other causes, plus adverse events such as infection, and the possible seriously impaired quality of life, was uncertain.

A key issue is the risk level of the patients being enrolled. If the patients are at truly very high risk of arrhythmic death, even though optimal medical therapy is being used, then it might be inappropriate to randomise them to medical therapy if a possibly useful device or surgical procedure exists. The defibrillator trials that were done showed that in moderately high-risk patients, the use of the defibrillator saved lives with an acceptable number of adverse events. If the risk level is less, however, as might be the case in patients with better left ventricular ejection fraction, the balance between benefit and potential harm might remain unknown, and the use of a defibrillator might not be justified, absent clear demonstration of benefit in a clinical trial.[32,33]

Trials have looked at various ways of identifying patients at sufficiently high risk to see if defibrillators are beneficial, but not at so high risk that it would be unethical to randomise. The Multicentre Automatic Defibrillator Implantation Trial (MADIT) compared use of an implanted defibrillator versus conventional medical therapy in 196 patients with heart failure, a prior myocardial infarction, left ventricular ejection fraction less than or equal to 35%, a documented episode of asymptomatic unsustained ventricular tachycardia, and inducible, non-suppressible ventricular tachyarrhythmia on electrophysiologic testing. In this very high-risk group of patients, the defibrillator led to highly significant reductions in all-cause and cardiac mortality.[34] A subsequent study by the same group of investigators (MADIT II) assessed whether the implantable defibrillator would reduce mortality in patients with a prior myocardial infarction and left ventricular ejection fraction less than or equal to 30%. Electrophysiologic testing was not used to identify high-risk patients. Because the risk of mortality was lower in this study than in the prior study, 742 patients were randomised to receive either the implantable defibrillator or conventional medical therapy. Here too, there was a significant reduction in mortality in the defibrillator group.[35]

One trial of a device that raised considerable questions about ethics was the Randomised Evaluation of Mechanical Assistance for the Treatment of Congestive Heart Failure (REMATCH), which was conducted from 1997 to 2001. This trial compared use of a left ventricular assist device versus medical therapy in 129 patients with end-stage heart failure who were not candidates for cardiac transplantation. The one-year survival was 52% in the group receiving the left ventricular assist device and 25% in the medical therapy group, a highly significant difference. At two years, the rates of survival were 23% and 8%. There were over twice as many serious adverse events (infection, bleeding, device malfunction) in the device group as in the medical arm.[36,37]

Because the expected survival rate in these patients was so low, there were many questions about the ethics of randomisation. It was known that the device was mechanically sound, and worked in the short-term as a bridge to transplantation. The justification for the trial was that long-term benefit, either for survival or quality of life, was unknown. For a more extensive discussion of the design issues and ethics of this kind of trial, using REMATCH as an example, see the report of a conference on mechanical cardiac support.[38]

It is uncommon (and often impractical) for trials of devices or surgical procedures to be blinded. Occasionally, however, this can be done. One such trial was Mode Selection Trial in Sinus Node Dysfunction (MOST).[39] Dual-chamber (atrioventricular) pacing was compared with single-chamber (ventricular) pacing in 2010 patients with clinically important bradycardia. The primary outcome was death or non-fatal stroke. All patients received a dual-chamber device, but in those randomised to single-chamber pacing, only one lead was activated, therefore mode of pacing was randomised rather than type of device. Physician investigators and patients were blinded regarding whether the patient was in the dual- or single-chamber arm; cross-over at the last follow-up was 31.4% for those assigned to ventricular pacing, almost half of these due to pacemaker syndrome. This was in contrast to another study that inserted only single-chamber devices in those randomised to that group and dual-chamber devices only in those randomised to the dual-chamber group. Here the cross-over rate was 2.7%.[40] This latter trial was not blinded, but cross-over from single- to dual-chamber pacing would have required another procedure, accounting for the low cross-over rate.

As with many drug trials, trials of devices can look at either single devices (or upgrades of these devices as they become available) or classes of devices. The AVID[26] trial compared the use of advanced-generation units with tiered therapy capable of antitachycardia pacing, cardioversion and defibrillation, as well as bradycardia pacing, made by more than one company, against any of several drugs (though primarily amiodarone), thus testing whether the strategy of using implantable defibrillators was preferable to a strategy of pharmacologic approach. This kind of trial is more likely to be done by public organisations, such as the National Institutes of Health, than by industry. Industry-supported trials, such as the previously discussed MADIT,[34] almost always compare a single manufacturer's device.

To the extent that the devices in the 'strategy-approach' trial are similarly effective, the results can be more broadly generalised to a class of devices. There is a risk, however, that devices made by one manufacturer will be better than others, blurring the outcome of the trial.

Another feature of device and surgical trials is that unlike most drugs (vaccines being an exception) that need to be administered regularly, devices are implanted and expected to work for a long time, and surgery, unless reversed, can be life-long. Batteries and other components may need to be replaced, but unless there are problems, they last for years. This is generally a strength of such trials. There is less problem with compliance to protocol and long-term follow-up is not only feasible, but desirable. The several coronary artery bypass graft surgery trials assessed outcome 10, and in some cases more than 20 years after the initial procedure.[41]

If a drug trial turns out not to show benefit from the drug, simply stopping administration is usually sufficient. But what if the device or surgery trial turns out not to show benefit? What is the obligation of the investigator, especially if the device or procedure is shown by the trial to be harmful? The Coronary Artery Bypass Graft (CABG) Patch trial[42] compared transthoracic implantation of cardioverter defibrillators against control in patients undergoing CABG surgery. At the end of an average 32 months follow-up, there was no significant mortality difference between the groups. All patients were given the results of the trial and subsequent therapy was individualised. All patients were urged to have electrophysiologic testing to see if they were at high risk of serious arrhythmia, and thus possibly in need of the defibrillator in the future. About 40% of the patients in the intervention group elected to have the device turned off or removed [J.T. Bigger, personal communication].

TRIALS OF BEHAVIOUR CHANGE

Trials of behaviour change are fairly common in heart disease. They include trials aimed at smoking prevention or cessation; diet change for weight loss, blood pressure reduction or cholesterol reduction; and exercise for risk factor reduction and better outcomes in people with a heart attack or heart failure.

These sorts of trials have several aspects that make them different from most other trials. First, there is considerable cross-over or recidivism by the study participants. The interventions are ones that many can either implement on their own or stop because they are difficult to maintain. Second, partly as a consequence of the first, the trials are quite resource intensive on the part of the interventionists. Implantation of devices or surgical procedures require major efforts by the investigator or surgeon, but usually only on a one-time basis. Trials of behaviour change require considerable effort on a continuing basis to help participants stay with a change from what may have been a life-long habit of smoking, eating poorly or sedentary lifestyle. Third, again as a consequence of the first two factors, the study duration is often much shorter than with other types of trials. Getting people to adhere to an exercise programme for months, let alone years, is extraordinarily difficult. And of course volunteers willing to be randomised to exercise or no exercise will have more of an interest in exercise than the general public. Therefore, those allocated to the no-exercise programme group will have more of a tendency to cross-over. Fourth, because of the generally shorter duration of the trials, surrogate outcomes are more often used than in other trials in heart disease. Rather than assessing clinical outcomes such as heart disease or stroke, the behaviour trials will often use weight change, biochemical measures, or attitude or knowledge assessed by questionnaires or interviews. Fifth, standardisation of the intervention and measurement of the degree of compliance are more complicated. Unless highly controlled feeding studies are performed, we have only modestly good ways of assessing overall food and nutrient intake. This is particularly so if maintenance of caloric intake is one of the objectives of the trial, as weight would not be able to serve as a marker of change in diet. Sixth, societal changes

and pressure can affect the trials in major ways. If there are changes in restaurant or workplace smoking regulations during the time of a trial looking at ways to get people to stop smoking, the likely trends in the control group as a result of the new regulations will make detection of benefit from the intervention more difficult.

Examples of successful trials of diet intervention are the Dietary Approaches to Stop Hypertension (DASH) trial[43] and a subsequent trial of the DASH diet with different levels of sodium intake.[44] The first DASH study enrolled 459 adults with systolic blood pressure under 160 mm Hg and diastolic pressure 80 to 95 mm Hg. Participants were randomly allocated to one of three groups: a diet rich in fruits and vegetables; a diet rich in fruits and vegetables plus low-fat dairy products and reduced saturated fat ('combination' diet); or a control diet with fruit, vegetable and fat content similar to that commonly eaten in the United States. At the end of eight weeks, both of the intervention diets reduced blood pressure, with a greater reduction from the diet containing low-fat dairy products. The second DASH study enrolled 412 participants in a factorial design trial. Participants were assigned to either the DASH combination diet or the control diet and to any of three levels of sodium intake. The moderate and low sodium intake diets reduced blood pressure in both the DASH diet and control diet groups. The DASH diet led to lower blood pressure than the control diet at each sodium level.

In the DASH studies, the food was specially prepared and provided to the participants. Whether or not the DASH-type diet can be maintained, over time, in people obtaining their food in the usual way, was studied in PREMIER, a trial of 810 participants whose blood pressure is greater than optimal or who have mild hypertension.[45] Participants were randomised to one of three arms: advice only; comprehensive lifestyle intervention using behavioural approaches; and a combined comprehensive lifestyle intervention plus the DASH diet. The behavioural approaches consisted of 18 counselling sessions. Unlike

DASH, the participants were not provided specially prepared foods. The primary outcome was systolic blood pressure six months after randomisation. At six months, the systolic blood pressure had decreased by 11.1 mm Hg in the combined group, 10.5 mm Hg in the behavioural intervention group, and 6.6 mm Hg in the advice only group. The largest reductions in diastolic blood pressure and in the percentage of people with hypertension were also seen in the combined group, with the behavioural intervention group a close second. Thus, a combination of behavioural approaches and dietary changes can result in meaningful blood pressure reduction. Even so, the DASH diet, unlike in the previous feeding studies,[43,44] did not contribute significantly beyond the comprehensive lifestyle intervention alone. The adoption of the diet in PREMIER was not as intensive as in the feeding studies. Whether the changes observed in PREMIER persist at 18 months is being assessed.[45]

A different kind of behavioural intervention trial was the Enhancing Recovery in Coronary Heart Disease (ENRICHD)[46] study. This trial enrolled 2481 patients at 73 hospitals who had had a myocardial infarction within the previous 28 days. In addition, all participants had depression, low social support, or both. Because depression and poor social support are associated with increased mortality after a heart attack, it was thought that intervening on those factors might lead to improved survival. Those randomised to intervention received counselling; the control group received usual medical care. Both groups received information on heart disease risk factors. Although the intervention decreased depression and improved social support, there was no difference at three years in the primary outcome of death or recurrent myocardial infarction (24.1% vs. 24.2%).[47]

The ENRICHD study raises several issues. First, despite the association between depression and heart disease, treatment of depression may not lead to change in mortality from heart disease. That is, depression may not be a causative factor. Second, the observed improvement in depression and social support may not have been of great

enough magnitude to alter mortality. This is what happened in some of the early trials of cholesterol lowering that failed to show improvement in mortality. The early lipid-lowering drugs were not as effective as the current ones in reducing cholesterol. Third, the measures of depression and social support, particularly when obtained shortly after a major event such as a heart attack, might not reflect true 'baseline'. Fourth, however, even though mortality and recurrent infarction were unchanged, the apparent improvements in depression and social support are not trivial findings. Unlike surrogate outcome variables that have little clinical meaning, these outcomes are clinically important in their own right.

Often, it is more appropriate to conduct behaviour change trials in community settings, with one group of communities compared against another. The changes, in order to be effective, need to be community-wide. An example of efforts to improve response time to symptoms of a heart attack was the Rapid Early Action for Coronary Treatment (REACT) trial. This study involved 10 matched pairs of cities. One group of cities received intervention through the media, community organisations, and professional and patient education in an effort to improve the response time in the event of symptoms of an acute myocardial infarction. The other group of cities served as the control. The primary outcome was time from symptom onset to arrival in the hospital emergency department. REACT showed increased use of the emergency medical system, but no difference between the groups in time to arrival at the hospital.[48]

There have been several trials aimed at changing multiple risk factors for heart disease in community settings.[49–51] These trials showed small differences between the intervention communities and the control communities in selected variables. In general, however, they were not particularly successful in achieving large differences despite intensive education efforts. The reasons are probably multiple. Among them are that the interventions were not delivered in sufficiently persuasive manners and that the control communities showed changes because of national attention to the need to stop smoking, improve diet and get better preventive medical attention.

The less than outstanding results from these community-wide efforts at behaviour change illustrate both the difficulties in achieving behaviour change and the problems in community, as opposed to individual, interventions.

SUMMARY

There are certain features that need to be considered in cardiovascular disease trials, whether they are primary prevention or secondary prevention. Those features include the chronic nature of the common cardiovascular diseases, the multiple risk factors responsible for those diseases, and the fact that huge numbers of people develop cardiovascular disease of one form or another. In this chapter, we have reviewed these and other factors, and described selected trials of drugs, devices and surgical procedures, and behavioural interventions that exemplify these features. Overall, however, trials of cardiovascular diseases are designed, conducted and analysed in ways similar to trials of other conditions.

Future trials may include targeting and 'optimising' interventions based on genotype and the use of new diagnostic and imaging techniques, potentially yielding better characterisation of the disease or condition pathology.

REFERENCES

1. Chobanian AV, Bakris GL, Black HR, Cushman WC, Green LA, Izzo JL, *et al.* Seventh report of the Joint National Committee on prevention, detection, evaluation, and treatment of high blood pressure. *Hypertension* (2003) **42**: 1206–52.
2. Greene HL, Richardson DW, Barker AH, Roden DM, Capone RJ, Echt DS, *et al.* Classification of deaths after myocardial infarction as arrhythmic or nonarrhythmic (the Cardiac Arrhythmia Pilot Study). *Am J Cardiol* (1989) **63**: 1–6.
3. Kannel WB. Silent myocardial ischemia and infarction: insights from the Framingham Study. *Cardiol Clin* (1986) **4**: 583–91.
4. Bardy GH, Lee KL, Mark DB, Poole JE, Fishbein DP, Singh SN, *et al.* The Sudden Cardiac Death-Heart Failure Trial (SCD-HeFT). In:

Woosley RL, Singh SN, eds, *Arrhythmia Treatment and Therapy*. New York: Marcel Dekker (2000) 323–42.
5. National Institutes of Health and National Heart, Lung and Blood Institute. *Morbidity & Mortality: 2002 Chart Book on Cardiovascular, Lung, and Blood Diseases*. U.S. Department of Health and Human Services, Public Health Service, National Institutes of Health (2002).
6. *Clinical Trials in Cardiovascular Disease. A Companion to Braunwald's Heart Disease*. Philadelphia: W.B. Saunders (1999).
7. Canner PL, Klimt CR. The Coronary Drug Project. Experimental design features. *Contr Clin Trials* (1983) **4**: 313–32.
8. The Coronary Drug Project Research Group. Clofibrate and niacin in coronary heart disease. *JAMA* (1975) **231**: 360–81.
9. Canner PL, Berge KG, Wenger NK, Stamler J, Friedman L, Prineas RJ, *et al.* Fifteen year mortality in Coronary Drug Project patients: long-term benefit with niacin. *J Am Coll Cardiol* (1986) **8**: 1245–55.
10. Lipid Research Clinics Coronary Primary Prevention Trial. The Lipid Research Clinics Coronary Primary Prevention Trial results. I. Reduction in incidence of coronary heart disease. *JAMA* (1984) **251**: 351–64.
11. The Scandinavian Simvastatin Survival Study. Randomised trial of cholesterol lowering in 4444 patients with coronary heart disease: the Scandinavian Simvastatin Survival Study (4S). *Lancet* (1994) **344**: 1383–9.
12. Sacks FM, Pfeffer MA, Moye LA, Rouleau JL, Rutherford JD, Cole TG, *et al.* The effect of pravastatin on coronary events after myocardial infarction in patients with average cholesterol levels. Cholesterol and Recurrent Events Trial investigators. *N Engl J Med* (1996) **335**: 1001–9.
13. MRC/BHF Heart Protection Study of cholesterol lowering with simvastatin in 20,536 high-risk individuals: a randomised placebo-controlled trial. *Lancet* (2002) **360**: 7–22.
14. ALLHAT Collaborative Research Group. Major cardiovascular events in hypertensive patients randomized to doxazosin vs chlorthalidone: the antihypertensive and lipid-lowering treatment to prevent heart attack trial (ALLHAT). *JAMA* (2000) **283**: 1967–75.
15. The ALLHAT Officers and Coordinators for the ALLHAT Collaborative Research Group. Major outcomes in moderately hypercholesterolemic, hypertensive patients randomized to pravastatin vs usual care. The Antihypertensive and Lipid-Lowering Treatment to Prevent Heart Attack Trial (ALLHAT-LLT). *JAMA* (2002) **288**: 2998–3007.

16. The ALLHAT Officers and Coordinators for the ALLHAT Collaborative Research Group. Major outcomes in high-risk hypertensive patients randomized to angiotensin-converting enzyme inhibitor or calcium channel blocker vs diuretic. The Antihypertensive and Lipid-Lowering Treatment to Prevent Heart Attack Trial (ALLHAT). *JAMA* (2002) **288**: 2981–97.

17. National Institutes of Health and National Heart, Lung and Blood Institute. Third Report of the National Cholesterol Education Program (NCEP) Expert Panel on Detection, Evaluation, and Treatment of High Blood Cholesterol in Adults (Adult Treatment Panel III). U.S. Department of Health and Human Services, Public Health Service (2001).

18. Yusuf S, Sleight P, Pogue J, Bosch J, Davies R, Dagenais G. Effects of an angiotensin-converting-enzyme inhibitor, ramipril, on cardiovascular events in high-risk patients. The Heart Outcomes Prevention Evaluation Study Investigators. *N Engl J Med* (2000) **342**: 145–53.

19. Pfeffer MA, Domanski M, Rosenberg Y, Verter J, Geller N, Albert P, *et al*. Prevention of events with angiotensin-converting enzyme inhibition (the PEACE study design). Prevention of Events with Angiotensin-Converting Enzyme Inhibition. *Am J Cardiol* (1998) **82**: 25H–30H.

20. SHEP Cooperative Research Group. Prevention of stroke by antihypertensive drug treatment in older persons with isolated systolic hypertension. Final results of the Systolic Hypertension in the Elderly Program (SHEP). *JAMA* (1991) **265**: 3255–64.

21. Echt DS, Liebson PR, Mitchell LB, Peters RW, Obias-Manno D, Barker AH, *et al*. Mortality and morbidity in patients receiving encainide, flecainide, or placebo. The Cardiac Arrhythmia Suppression Trial. *N Engl J Med* (1991) **324**: 781–8.

22. The Cardiac Arrhythmia Suppression Trial II Investigators. Effect of the antiarrhythmic agent moricizine on survival after myocardial infarction. *N Engl J Med* (1992) **327**: 227–33.

23. The Planning and Steering Committee of the AFFIRM Study for the NHLBI AFFIRM Investigators. Atrial Fibrillation Follow-up Investigation of Rhythm Management – the AFFIRM study design. *Am J Cardiol.* (1997) **79**: 1198–202.

24. The Atrial Fibrillation Follow-up Investigation of Rhythm Management (AFFIRM) Investigators. A comparison of rate control and rhythm control in patients with atrial fibrillation. *N Engl J Med* (2002) **347**: 1825–33.

25. Detre K, Peduzzi P, Murphy M, Hultgren H, Thomsen J, Oberman A, *et al*. Effect of bypass surgery on survival in patients in low- and high-risk subgroups delineated by the use of simple clinical variables. *Circulation* (1981) **63**: 1329–38.

26. The AVID Investigators. Antiarrhythmics Versus Implantable Defibrillators (AVID) – rationale, design, and methods. *Am J Cardiol* (1995) **75**: 470–5.

27. Buchwald H, Varco RL, Matts JP, Long JM, Fitch LL, Campbell GS, *et al*. Effect of partial ileal bypass surgery on mortality and morbidity from coronary heart disease in patients with hypercholesterolemia. Report of the Program on the Surgical Control of Hyperlipidemia (POSCH). *N Engl J Med* (1990) **323**(14): 946–55.

28. Buchwald H, Varco RL, Boen JR, Williams SE, Hansen BJ, Campos CT, *et al*. Effective lipid modification by partial ileal bypass reduced long-term coronary heart disease mortality and morbidity: five-year posttrial follow-up report from the POSCH. Program on the Surgical Control of the Hyperlipidemias. *Arch Intern Med* (1998) **158**: 1253–61.

29. Connolly SJ, Gent M, Roberts RS, Dorian P, Roy D, Sheldon RS, *et al*. Canadian implantable defibrillator study (CIDS): a randomized trial of the implantable cardioverter defibrillator against amiodarone. *Circulation* (2000) **101**: 1297–302.

30. Epstein AE. AVID necessity. *PACE Pacing Clin Electrophysiol* (1993) **16**: 1773–5.

31. Fogoros RN. An AVID dissent. *PACE Pacing Clin Electrophysiol* (1994) **17**: 1707–11.

32. The AVID Investigators. A comparison of antiarrhythmic-drug therapy with implantable defibrillators in patients resuscitated from near-fatal ventricular arrhythmias. *N Engl J Med* (1997) **337**: 1576–83.

33. Domanski MJ, Epstein A, Hallstrom A, Saksena S, Zipes DP. Survival of antiarrhythmic or implantable cardioverter defibrillator treated patients with varying degrees of left ventricular dysfunction who survived malignant ventricular arrhythmias. *J Cardiovasc Electrophysiol* (2002) **13**: 580–3.

34. Moss AJ. Background, outcome, and clinical implications of the Multicentre Automatic Defibrillator Implantation Trial (MADIT). *Am J Cardiol* (1997) **80**: 28F–32F.

35. Moss AJ, Zareba W, Hall WJ, Klein H, Wilber DJ, Cannom DS, *et al*. Prophylactic implantation of a defibrillator in patients with myocardial infarction and reduced ejection fraction. *N Engl J Med* (2002) **346**: 877–83.

36. Rose EA, Moskowitz AJ, Packer M, Sollano JA, Williams DL, Tierney AR, *et al*. The REMATCH trial: rationale, design, and end points. Randomised Evaluation of Mechanical Assistance for the Treatment of Congestive Heart Failure. *Ann Thorac Surg* (1999) **67**: 723–30.

37. Rose EA, Gelijns AC, Moskowitz AJ, Heitjan DF, Stevenson LW, Dembitsky W, *et al*. Long-term mechanical left ventricular assistance for end-stage heart failure. *N Engl J Med* (2001) **345**: 1435–43.

38. Stevenson LW, Kormos RL, Bourge RC, Gelijns A, Griffith BP, Hershberger RE, *et al*. Mechanical cardiac support 2000: current applications and future trial design, June 15–16, 2000, Bethesda, Maryland. *J Am Coll Cardiol* (2001) **37**: 340–70.

39. Lamas GA, Lee KL, Sweeney MO, Silverman R, Leon A, Yee R, *et al*. Ventricular pacing or dual-chamber pacing for sinus-node dysfunction. *N Engl J Med* (2002) **346**: 1854–62.

40. Connolly SJ, Kerr CR, Gent M, Roberts RS, Yusuf S, Gillis AM, *et al*. Effects of physiologic pacing versus ventricular pacing on the risk of stroke and death due to cardiovascular causes. Canadian Trial of Physiologic Pacing Investigators. *N Engl J Med* (2000) **342**: 1385–91.

41. Yusuf S, Zucker D, Peduzzi P, Fisher LD, Takaro T, Kennedy JW, *et al*. Effect of coronary artery bypass graft surgery on survival: overview of 10-year results from randomised trials by the Coronary Artery Bypass Graft Surgery Trialists Collaboration. *Lancet* (1994) **344**: 563–70.

42. Bigger JT Jr. Prophylactic use of implanted cardiac defibrillators in patients at high risk for ventricular arrhythmias after coronary-artery bypass graft surgery. Coronary Artery Bypass Graft (CABG) Patch Trial Investigators. *N Engl J Med* (1997) **337**: 1569–75.

43. Appel LJ, Moore TJ, Obarzanek E, Vollmer WM, Svetkey LP, Sacks FM, *et al*. A clinical trial of the effects of dietary patterns on blood pressure. DASH Collaborative Research Group. *N Engl J Med* (1997) **336**: 1117–24.

44. Sacks FM, Svetkey LP, Vollmer WM, Appel LJ, Bray GA, Harsha D, *et al*. Effects on blood pressure of reduced dietary sodium and the Dietary Approaches to Stop Hypertension (DASH) diet. *N Engl J Med* (2001) **344**: 3–10.

45. Writing Group of the PREMIER Collaborative Research Group. Effects of comprehensive lifestyle modification on blood pressure control. Main results of the PREMIER clinical trial. *JAMA* (2003) **289**: 2083–93.

46. The ENRICHD Investigators. Enhancing recovery in coronary heart disease (ENRICHD) study intervention: rationale and design. *Psychosom Med* (2001) **63**: 747–55.

47. Writing Committee for the ENRICHD Investigators. Effects of treating depression and low perceived social support on clinical events after myocardial infarction. The Enchancing Recovery in Coronary Heart Disease Patients (ENRICHD) randomized trial. *JAMA* (2003) **289**: 3106–16.

48. Luepker RV, Raczynski JM, Osganian S, Goldberg RJ, Finnegan JR Jr, Hedges JR, *et al*. Effect of a community intervention on patient delay and emergency medical service use in acute coronary heart disease: the Rapid Early Action for Coronary Treatment (REACT) trial. *JAMA* (2000) **284**: 60–7.

49. Farquhar JW, Fortmann SP, Flora JA, Taylor CB, Haskell WL, Williams PT, *et al*. Effects of communitywide education on cardiovascular disease risk factors. The Stanford Five-City Project. *JAMA* (1990) **264**: 359–65.

50. Luepker RV, Murray DM, Jacobs DR, Mittelmark MB, Bracht N, Carlaw R, *et al*. Community education for cardiovascular disease prevention: risk factor changes in the Minnesota Heart Health Program. *Am J Public Health* (1994) **84**: 1383–93.

51. Carleton RA, Lasater TM, Assaf AR, Feldman HA, McKinlay S, Pawtucket Heart Health Program Writing Group. The Pawtucket Heart Health Program: community changes in cardiovascular risk factors and projected disease risk. *Am J Public Health* (1995) **85**: 777–85.

DENTISTRY AND MAXILLO-FACIAL

13

Dentistry and Maxillo-facial

MAY C.M. WONG, COLMAN MCGRATH AND EDWARD C.M. LO

Dental Public Health, Faculty of Dentistry, The University of Hong Kong, Hong Kong

INTRODUCTION

SCOPE OF THE CHAPTER

Dentistry is concerned with the prevention and treatment of diseases and disorders of the teeth, gums (periodontium) and oral cavity. The two most common oral diseases are dental caries (tooth decay) and periodontal (gum) diseases. Data from the Global Oral Health Databank of the World Health Organization (http://www. whocollab.od.mah.se/index.html) reports that at least half of the children and nearly all of the adults in most countries throughout the world have been affected by dental caries. In addition, findings from epidemiological surveys throughout the world have reported that less than 10% of their adult population have no periodontal disease (completely healthy gums). One of the more life-threatening diseases of the oral cavity is oral cancer, primarily cancer involving the oral mucosa (lining of the oral cavity). The prevalence of oral cancer varies from country to country, in most countries it accounts for less than 1% of the total cancer incidence whereas in the Indian subcontinent it can account for 30–50% of the total cancer incidence.[1]

Aside from oral diseases there are a number of conditions or disorders of the oral cavity that are of concern. Malalignment and malocclusion of teeth (crooked teeth) is prevalent and severe in many countries and most report a growing demand for orthodontic treatment to correct the malocclusion. In the US, it is estimated that around half of the population are in need of some kind of orthodontic treatment to improve their occlusion.[2] Another problem has been the need for replacement of missing teeth; congenitally absent or lost because of caries or periodontal disease. Removable prosthesis (dentures or false teeth) and fixed prosthesis (bridges) as well as implants (screw in teeth) have been used to address these problems.

As the scope of dentistry is very wide, it would not be possible to include all kinds of clinical trials in dental research in this chapter. Instead, the discussion here will focus on the more common oral diseases and conditions. First, the disease aetiology and measurements of dental caries and periodontal disease will be presented. Second, clinical trials methods used in dentistry will then be outlined and illustrated with examples. Third, the designs of clinical trials conducted in the areas of dental

Textbook of Clinical Trials.   Edited by D. Machin, S. Day and S. Green
© 2004 John Wiley & Sons, Ltd   ISBN: 0-471-98787-5

caries, oral rehabilitation, periodontal disease and orthodontics will be discussed. Fourth, the current issues of evidence-based dentistry and hierarchical data analysis will also be discussed. Last, the impact of clinical trials on dental practice will be summarised.

DISEASE AETIOLOGY AND MEASUREMENTS

Evidence from animal and epidemiological studies shows that dental caries arise from demineralisation of tooth hard tissue due to organic acids produced by plaque bacteria on the tooth surface.[3] Frequent intake of fermentable carbohydrates, especially sugars, has been shown to be related to the development of dental caries.[4] The most common measure used in clinical trials to quantify the severity of dental caries is to count the number of decayed, filled and missing (due to caries) teeth or tooth surfaces, the DMFT or DMFS index.[5] The current treatment approach for dental caries emphasises prevention of the disease by strengthening the tooth, such as the use of fluorides and fissure sealants, modification of the diet, such as the use of sugar substitutes, and appropriate health behaviours. Cavities produced by the caries process can be filled by various direct and indirect restorative materials.

Periodontal disease is characterised by the inflammatory response of the gums and its sequel to the toxic substances produced by the plaque bacteria.[6] The current treatment approach for periodontal disease emphasises primary and secondary prevention of the disease through the removal of plaque by mechanical and chemical means, e.g. toothbrushing and the use of mouthrinses. There are also various surgical and non-surgical ways to treat the periodontal pockets that are formed in more advanced periodontal disease states. Many indices have been used in clinical trials to quantify the amount of plaque on the tooth surfaces, ranging from a simple dichotomous scale of presence or absence of visible plaque[7] to recording the thickness of the plaque at the gum margin[8] or the area of tooth surface covered by plaque.[9] Gingivitis is usually measured by the presence or absence of bleeding after gentle probing[7] or in an ordinal scale using various

clinical signs.[10] For more advanced periodontal disease, usually the depth of the periodontal pocket and/or the attachment loss are measured in millimetres using marked probes.

Following the developments in medical research, patient-based outcomes measures have also been developed and employed in dental research. These have focused primarily on the concept of patient satisfaction and health-related quality of life measures. A number of questionnaires have been developed recently to measure the oral health-related quality of life of people, for example, the Oral Health Impact Profile (OHIP) and the General Oral Health Assessment Index (GOHAI).[11] Some of these have been used in clinical studies to assess the outcome of dental treatment,[12,13] to supplement the clinical assessments.

CLINICAL TRIALS METHODS

In dental research, the clinical trials methods used mainly follow those developed and adopted in medical research. The basic design principles and considerations are very similar, thus the following discussion on clinical trials methods can be kept short and precise for general areas, with specific areas unique in dentistry discussed in more detail. A few references on clinical trial methodology and some from the dental literature are recommended for general reading.[14–17]

RANDOMISED CONTROLLED TRIALS

As with the developments in medical research, randomised controlled trials (RCTs) have become the gold standard in conducting clinical trials in dentistry. The key features of RCTs are treatment modalities being assigned randomly to the subjects and the existence of a control group. The controls can either be concurrent controls as in parallel studies or self-controls as in crossover studies. The treatment received in the control group can be placebo or standard treatment. In the perfect setting, RCTs should also be double-blinded which requires that both the subjects and the examiners/observers involved in the trials are not aware of the assignment of the treatment modalities to the subjects, thus reducing any biases in the comparison of the groups besides randomisation.

Informed consent, ethical consideration, data monitoring and pre-study sample size calculation are also important issues in conducting RCTs. Subjects should be informed about the research protocols, their roles as participants in the studies, the different treatment modalities, the possibility of any side-effects or risks arising from receiving the treatments, and their rights of discontinuing participation. After the explanation of the above details to the subjects, the subjects should be given ample opportunity and time to ask any questions and to discuss the trial with family and friends. Written consent is normally required, however under special circumstances, verbal consent may be employed.[18] It is good practice that clinical trials only be conducted after approval from local ethical committees in order to protect human rights.

Data monitoring is especially important in large-scale, multicentre RCTs and usually a data monitoring committee is established to monitor the data collected during the study. The committee needs to monitor the data for patient safety and statistical significance, while keeping their findings confidential to prevent the introduction of bias.[15]

PARALLEL AND CROSSOVER STUDY DESIGNS

In the parallel study design, concurrent groups of subjects are involved in the study and the comparison of the different modalities is the comparison of between-subject variation. When the number of treatment modalities increases, the corresponding sample size required in order to achieve a particular level of power and significance needs to be increased greatly. Crossover study design is a self-controlled study design, subjects serve as their own controls. Thus, the comparison of the different modalities is the comparison of within-subject variation. The use of the

subjects as their own controls prevents confounding by many characteristics that may influence the outcome. In a crossover study each subject is given the different treatments (or treatment and placebo) under comparison, one after another. Each subject is his/her own control. The sequence of assignment is generally randomised, so that this is in effect a type of RCT. A 'washing-out period' may be required between treatments, to permit the effects of the previous treatment to disappear. However, since subjects who participate in clinical trials with crossover design need to receive all treatment regimens and undergo 'washing-out periods' between treatments, it can make the investigation periods of the clinical trials very long and not feasible.[19]

Crossover trials are frequently employed in oral hygiene studies where treatment effects are reversible. An example is a single-blind, short-term crossover clinical trial where the plaque removal performance of three commercially available manual toothbrushes was compared.[20] A sample of 25 dental hygiene students participated (age 19 to 42 years old). The participants were instructed to refrain from toothbrushing or flossing for 24 hours before the trial. A pre-brushing plaque index using disclosing solution was performed on each participant. One of the three test brushes was then randomly assigned to each participant, and they were allowed to brush for 90 seconds without the aid of a mirror. A post-brushing plaque index was then performed on each participant. This procedure was repeated twice more at 2-week intervals so that each participant was tested with all three toothbrushes.

Crossover design will not be applicable if the treatment has protracted 'carry-over' effect, i.e. the effect of the treatment is not reversible. In this situation, either parallel or split-mouth design should be adopted. For example in the case of dental caries, since most carious lesions occur in the pit and fissure on the occlusal surfaces of the posterior teeth, the effectiveness of sealing these pits and fissures in order to prevent dental caries is studied. In studies for comparing the effectiveness of fissure sealant compared to non-sealed teeth or sealant with different active ingredients to prevent caries, crossover design is not applicable as once the teeth are sealed, the process is not reversible. Thus for these studies, either parallel design or split-mouth design would be used. In the setting of parallel design, subjects are assigned to different concurrent test groups; while in the setting of split-mouth design, different teeth of the same group of subjects are assigned to different test groups at the same study period.[21]

SPLIT-MOUTH DESIGN

Split-mouth design is one of the self-controlled study designs, that is unique in dentistry. This design is characterised by subdividing the mouth of the subjects into homogeneous within-patient experimental units such as quadrants (upper left, upper right, lower left and lower right sides of the mouth), sextants (upper left posterior, upper anterior, upper right posterior, lower left posterior, lower anterior and lower right posterior), contralateral (left and right) or ipsilateral (upper and lower) quadrants or sextants or a symmetrical combination of these. With these within-patient experimental units, a range of two to six different treatment modalities can be randomly assigned to the experimental units.[22] The number of treatment modalities usually equals the number of within-patient experimental units. For instance, in a study where two treatment modalities are compared, the within-patient experimental units would usually be the left or right sides of the mouth. In a study where four treatment modalities are compared, the within-patient experimental units could be the four quadrants of the mouth. The split-mouth design has been the principal research tool in periodontal clinical trials to compare different treatment modalities. In the periodontal literature, at least 11 different types of split-mouth design have been described.[22]

The major advantage of using the split-mouth design, like the crossover design, is that subjects serve as their own controls, thus this design may be more efficient than designs with between-subject comparisons. However, in contrast to the crossover design, since the subjects are receiving all the treatment modalities at the different parts of the mouth concurrently, the study period of the investigation could be shorter. The study period could then be of the same duration as if the parallel design was used, but the number of subjects used could be reduced. In an investigation of the efficiency of split-mouth design compared to whole-mouth design (with the use of parallel study design), it was concluded that when disease characteristics are symmetrically distributed over the within-patient experimental units, the split-mouth design could provide moderate to large gains in relative efficiency. For periodontal disease, division of the mouth into two experimental units, either left and right or upper and lower sides, provided the greatest symmetry of the disease characteristics.[22]

Besides the distribution of the disease, one should also consider the carry-across effects arising from the split-mouth designs. Carry-across effects occur where treatment performed in one experimental unit can affect the treatment response in other experimental units of the mouth. These effects cannot be estimated from split-mouth data, thus unless prior knowledge indicates that no carry-across effects exist, reported estimates of treatment efficacy are potentially biased. Thus, researchers should weigh the potential gain in precision against a potential decrease in validity when using split-mouth designs in clinical trials.[23] In a study to compare the effectiveness of two electric toothbrushes in plaque removal, a split-mouth design was used in which either the first (upper right) and third (lower left) quadrants or the second (upper left) and fourth (lower right) quadrants of 84 subjects were brushed with one or the other toothbrush in a random assignment.[24] In this situation, since the distribution of plaque inside the mouth is symmetrical, and the use of different toothbrushes in brushing different parts of the mouth should not affect the other parts, i.e. no carry-across effect, the use of a split-mouth design should be appropriate. In studies to compare the effectiveness of fluoride toothpaste in preventing dental caries, split-mouth design is not advisable as the fluorides from the toothpaste could go freely within the mouth, i.e. with a carry-over effect. For these studies, parallel design should be more appropriate.

BLINDING

In order to achieve double-blinding, the subjects and examiners/observers should not be able to tell which treatment modalities have been assigned to the subjects. This can be done, for example, in a mouthrinse study comparing the test mouthrinse with placebo; the placebo mouthrinse is made with the same appearance and taste as the test mouthrinse, so that the subjects would not be able to distinguish the two by sight and they are not told which mouthrinse they have been assigned. On the other hand, the examiners/observers are also not able to reach the information for the assignment of the mouthrinse to the subjects.[25] However, in many other situations, we can only blind the examiners/observers but not the subjects (single-blinding). In the study we mentioned above concerning the comparison of the effectiveness of three electric toothbrushes in plaque removal, it is inevitable that the subjects will know which toothbrush they were using, thus in this situation, the best that one can achieve is to blind the investigator from knowing which toothbrushes have been assigned to which quadrants of the subjects.[24] There are situations where even single-blinding is not feasible. In a study comparing the performance of two dental filling materials, amalgam (metal) versus resin-modified glass ionomer cement (tooth colour), it would be very difficult to blind the investigator as one can distinguish the two by their appearance.[26] In conducting clinical trials, one should use the maximum degree of blindness that is possible. In studying the prevalence of caries and fluorosis of children from a water-fluoridated site and a nearby non-fluoridated site, children were transported to a common examination site so as to blind the investigators from knowing the residence of the children.[27] Instead of having the investigators examining the children at the sites and then recognising the fluoride content in the water, this method of transporting the children to a common examination site demonstrates an innovative way for researchers to maximise the degree of blindness.

CLINICAL TRIALS IN DENTISTRY

CARIES PREVENTION AND TREATMENT STUDIES

The aims for these prevention studies are to investigate the effectiveness of different ways of preventing dental caries. These include different methods of strengthening the teeth (such as the use of fluorides in different forms), modification of diet (such as the use of sugar substitutes), or modification of health behaviours (such as tooth brushing techniques and habits, oral education programmes). The target populations for these studies are mainly children, the elderly and special needs groups. Most of the clinical trials are phase I or phase II types. For those studies investigating the effectiveness of different forms of fluorides (in the form of toothpaste, topical fluorides, sealant), randomisation of the assignment of groups with different regimes (including the control group) can be done at the individual level with parallel design. In a study to compare the effectiveness of two toothpastes with different concentration of fluoride to arrest root carious lesions, 201 subjects with at least one root carious lesion were recruited from dental school patients. They were randomly assigned to use either Prevident 5000 Plus (5000 ppm F) or Colgate Winterfresh Gel (1100 ppm F), both containing sodium fluoride in the same silica base. Measurements of lesion hardness, area, distance from the gingival margin, cavitation and plaque were recorded at baseline and 3 months later by a single examiner.[28]

For those studies involving the modification of diet and behaviour, field studies were used more often because randomisation of the assignment of groups with different regimes would be easier to achieve at the school or community level. In a 3-year community intervention trial to determine the caries preventive effect of sugar-substituted chewing gum among Lithuanian school children, a total of 602 children, aged 9–14 years, from five secondary schools in Kaunas, Lithuania were recruited. Baseline clinical and radiographic caries examinations were given. The schools were randomly allocated to receive one of the five interventions: sorbitol/carbamide gum; sorbitol gum; xylitol gum; control gum; and no gum. Children in the four active intervention groups were asked to chew at least five pieces of gum per day, preferably after meals. The children were re-examined clinically after 1, 2 and 3 years, and radiographically after 3 years.[29]

In both the above examples, parallel design was adopted. However, studies like the comparison of two different fissure sealant materials could be carried out using the split-mouth design. In a study to compare the retention and the caries preventive effect of a glass ionomer developed for fissure sealing (Fuji III) and a chemically polymerised resin-based fissure sealant (Delton), 179 7-year-old children with at least one pair of permanent first molars that were caries-free or only had incipient lesions were recruited from schools. A split-mouth design was adopted by assigning the two sealing materials randomly to the contralateral teeth. Follow-up examinations for sealant retention were done after 6 months, 1 year, 2 years and 3 years.[30]

In order to determine the level of fluoride that should be used (dose finding), some studies have focused on comparing the effectiveness of different concentrations of fluorides in caries prevention. For example, in a randomised, double-blind study comparing the anti-caries effectiveness of sodium fluoride dentifrices containing 1700 ppm, 2200 ppm and 2800 ppm fluoride ion relative to an 1100 ppm fluoride ion control, a population of 5439 schoolchildren, aged 6–15 years, was recruited from an urban central Ohio area with a low fluoride content water supply (<0.3 ppm). Subjects were stratified according to gender, age and baseline DMFS scores derived from the visual–tactile baseline examination. Random allocation of the four treatment groups was done: 0.243% sodium fluoride (1100 ppm fluoride ion), 0.376% sodium fluoride (1700 ppm fluoride ion), 0.486% sodium fluoride (2200 ppm fluoride ion)

and 0.619% sodium fluoride (2800 ppm fluoride ion). All products were formulated with the same fluoride-compatible silica abrasive. Subjects were examined by visual–tactile and radiographic examination at baseline and after 1, 2 and 3 years of using the sodium fluoride dentifrices.[31]

The aims of the caries treatment studies were to investigate the performance of the different materials or different approaches used to fill up the decayed cavities in the mouth in terms of bond strength and retention of the materials. As the treatments being delivered cannot be reversed, thus crossover design is not applicable for these studies. Among these studies, the use of split-mouth design was more common. In a study to compare the clinical performance of two glass ionomer cements, ChemFlex (Dentsply DeTrey) and Fuji IX GP (GC), when used with the atraumatic restorative treatment (ART) approach in China, 89 schoolchildren aged between 6 and 14 years who had bilateral matched pairs of carious posterior teeth were included. A split-mouth design was used in which the two materials were randomly placed on contralateral sides. The performance of the restorations was assessed directly and also indirectly from die-stone replicas at baseline and after 6, 12 and 24 months.[32]

ORAL REHABILITATION STUDIES

One concern of oral rehabilitation studies is to compare a range of treatment modalities to replace missing teeth including removable and fixed dental prostheses, and the use of implants. Depending on the treatment modalities, parallel, split-mouth and crossover designs have been applied in these studies. In a 5-year parallel study to compare implant-retained mandibular overdentures (IRO) with complete dentures (CD), 61 and 60 patients were randomly assigned to the IRO and CD groups. The clinical aspects and patient satisfaction were measured.[33]

In a split-mouth study, sandblasted and acid-etched (SLA) implants (recently introduced to reduce the healing period between surgery and prosthesis) were compared to titanium plasma-sprayed (TPS) implants under loaded conditions 1 year after placement. Thirty-two healthy patients with comparable bilateral edentulous sites and no discrepancies in the opposing dentition were recruited. The surgical procedure was performed by the same operator and was identical for all the test and control sites. Abutment connection was carried out at 35 Ncm 6 weeks post-surgery for test sites and 12 weeks for the controls by the same dentist who was blinded to the type of surface of the implant. Provisional restoration was fabricated and a new tightening was performed after 6 weeks. Similar gold–ceramic restorations were cemented on the same type of solid abutments on both sites. Clinical measures and radiographic changes were recorded by the same operator who was blinded to the type of surface of the implant, 1 year post-surgery.[34]

In a study to compare two designs of maxillary implant overdentures, a crossover trial was designed to measure differences in patient satisfaction with maxillary long-bar implant overdentures with and without palatal coverage opposed by a fixed mandibular implant-supported prosthesis. A mandibular fixed prosthesis was inserted in 13 total edentulous participants, who were then divided into two groups. One group ($n = 7$) received maxillary long-bar overdentures with palate, then long-bar overdentures without palate. The other group ($n = 6$) received the same treatments in the reverse order. For each overdentures design, mastication tests and patient satisfaction were assessed 2 months after the fitting of the overdenture to allow adaptation.[35]

Besides clinical outcomes, very often patient-based outcomes such as patient satisfaction and quality of life measures were also measured in these oral rehabilitation studies. As in the above quoted example, patients were asked to rate (1) their general satisfaction with the upper prosthesis; (2) satisfaction on the physical functions of the prosthesis such as retention, stability, comfort, ease of cleaning, etc.; and (3) satisfaction on the psychosocial functions such as a esthetics, self-confidence, etc.

using both the Visual Analogue Scale and the Category Scale.[35] In another study, an oral-specific quality of life measure, the Oral Health Impact Profile,[36] was used to measure the impact of the clinical intervention on quality of life. Three groups of subjects were compared, edentulous/edentate subjects who requested and received complete implant-stabilised oral prostheses (IG, $n = 26$), edentulous/edentate subjects who requested implants but received conventional dentures (CDG1, $n = 22$), and edentulous subjects who had new conventional complete dentures (CDG2, $n = 35$).[13] OHIP is one of the most comprehensive instruments available in evaluating oral health-related quality of life.

TRIALS RELATED TO PERIODONTAL DISEASE

In order to prevent periodontal disease, plaque removal and prevention of calculus deposit was one of the key concerns. Thus ways to improve toothbrushing (mechanical means to remove plaque) or the use of mouthrinse or toothpaste with active ingredients like chlorhexidine and pyrophosphate ion (chemical means to remove plaque and to prevent calculus deposition) were investigated. Two main streams of therapy existed: non-surgical and surgical therapy. The aims for these studies were to investigate the effectiveness of the treatment modalities in reducing the depth of the periodontal pocket or improving periodontal attachment level.

Similar to the caries research, different study designs in RCT have been applied to periodontal research; one particular design issue that has been discussed more in periodontal research compared to other areas in dental research is the consideration of therapeutic equivalence. This is important because clinical trials for testing superiority and for testing equivalency should have different designs and there has been a tendency by the clinicians in periodontal research to confuse the difference between the two.[37] Clinical trials whose purposes are to show equivalence of two or more treatments have traditionally utilised methods for demonstrating superiority. Thus if no statistical differences are found, this only demonstrates that the treatments are not superior to the others, they may not be equivalent.[19] The sample size requirements for both equivalence and superiority studies investigating products used in periodontal regeneration have been investigated. It was found that since equivalence clinical trials require much smaller differences between groups, thus much larger sample sizes are required.[38]

ORTHODONTIC STUDIES

In orthodontic studies, two main concerns are the effectiveness of early orthodontic treatment for Class II malocclusion and the value of maxillary arch expansion for the treatment of posterior crossbite. Relatively speaking, fewer RCTs are done in this research area. Some researchers have argued that even though RCT has become the gold standard of conducting medical research, it could only apply to a very narrow spectrum of orthodontic questions. One quoted example is 'it would be nearly impossible to enroll fully-informed subjects into any study whose alternatives are of markedly different morbidity: extraction versus non-extraction or orthodontics versus surgery'.[39] Three confusions (or inertia) have been summarised in explaining why the move to conduct RCTs in orthodontic research has been slow. First, there is a remarkable level of non-acceptance that the highest level of evidence is derived from RCTs and retrospective investigation is regarded as more useful. Second, there is the argument that it is not ethical to subject patients to a random allocation of treatments if it is already known that one of the treatments is superior. Third, there is a feeling that RCTs are very large and difficult to manage and then they are expensive and a large amount of funding is required.[40] O'Brien has provided solutions to the above confusions: (1) one should accept that RCTs derive the highest level of evidence and retrospective investigation still has a great value in generating questions for RCTs; (2) one should not simply believe that most treatments are superior to another without being tested in an unbiased manner, thus it is actually unethical to provide treatment that has not been properly evaluated; (3) careful planning and

monitoring of the trials are all that is needed for conducting RCTs. He has also urged journal editors to promote the publication of RCTs. Hopefully, there should be a paradigm shift in conducting RCTs in orthodontic research in future years.

CURRENT ISSUES

EVIDENCE-BASED DENTISTRY

One of the major implications of conducting clinical trials is to provide scientific evidence for the clinicians when they are making clinical decisions. Evidence-based medicine was defined as 'the conscientious, explicit and judicious use of current best evidence in making decisions about the care of individual patients'.[41] Dental researchers started addressing the issues of evidence-based dentistry (EBD) in the 1990s and a series of articles has been published to address the concepts of EBD, the misunderstandings of EBD, the barriers to EBD and the processes of finding, evaluating and applying the evidence.[42-48] Various studies making use of the EBD approach have been applied to different areas in dental research and the journal *Evidence-Based Dentistry* has also been published since November 1998.

Systematic literature review is the foundation of the EBD approach. It differs from narrative review as in the latter case the authors or experts do not use standardised ways to retrieve articles and summarise information. Thus different writers may arrive at different conclusions for the same question. In systematic review, standards in finding, evaluating and synthesising evidence are reported and thus the conclusion is more reliable.

The Cochrane Collaboration is an international organisation that 'has developed in response to Archie Cochrane's call for systematic, up-to-date reviews of all relevant RCTs of health care' (http://www.cochrane.org). In an influential book, Cochrane[49] drew attention to the importance of organising critical summaries of all relevant RCTs by specialty or subspecialty areas of health care, so that people can make more informed decisions. The first 'Cochrane Centre' was opened and funded in the UK in October 1992, to facilitate systematic reviews of randomised controlled trials across all areas of health care. Currently, there are 15 Cochrane Centres around the world. However, the Cochrane Centres are not directly responsible for preparing and maintaining systematic reviews. This is the responsibility of international collaborative review groups, which also maintain registers of systematic reviews currently being prepared or planned, so that unnecessary duplication of effort can be minimised and collaboration promoted. Currently there are about 50 review groups covering all of the important areas of health care and dentistry included in the Cochrane Oral Health Group (http://www.cochrane-oral.man.ac.uk). The principal output of the collaboration is the Cochrane Reviews which are published electronically in successive issues of *The Cochrane Database of Systematic Reviews*. Ten Cochrane Reviews have been finished in the Cochrane Oral Health Group, including: fluoride gels for preventing dental caries in children and adolescents; guided tissue regeneration for periodontal infra-bony defects; interventions for preventing oral mucositis or oral candidiasis for patients with cancer receiving chemotherapy; interventions for treating burning mouth syndrome, oral mucositis, oral leukoplakia, oral candidiasis and oral lichen planus; orthodontic treatment for posterior crossbites; and potassium nitrate toothpaste for dentine hypersensitivity. Twenty-seven protocols are registered currently to review various fluoride products in preventing caries, various regimes of interventions for replacing missing teeth, and various orthodontic treatments protocols, etc.

HIERARCHICAL AND MULTILEVEL DATA ANALYSIS

Hierarchical data (or clustered data) is common in dental research, as people may have up to 32 teeth and taking measurements from multiple teeth of the same individual is very typical in the data collection of clinical trials in dentistry. For example, in caries prevention studies, the individual teeth of the subjects will be examined and in periodontal research, usually six sites of each tooth will be examined; all these measurements are possibly correlated or clustered. More examples have been given by Macfarlane and Worthington[50] and Gilthorpe et al.[51] With these correlated or clustered data, conventional statistical methods, which assume observations being independent, are not appropriate for the analysis. Thus special statistical analysis is required when data have a hierarchical structure. Analysing data without recognising the hierarchical structure and treating the observations as independent will lead to a spurious increase in the sample size, and corresponding spurious significant relationship.[52] For example in periodontal research, one might take up to six site measurements for each tooth and with 28 teeth (not including the wisdom teeth) for an individual, the total number of observations for one individual could then be 168. Thus it is easy to have thousands of observations with only 20 subjects. In a study, the total number of sites assessed was 2236 distributed on 559 teeth in 22 subjects.[53] One way to overcome this problem is to aggregate the raw observations to the highest level of the data structure, for example, site/teeth level measurements can be aggregated to the level of an individual subject like the DMFT/DMFS index, mean probing pocket depth, etc. Thus one measurement was taken from each individual and conventional statistical analysis could then be applied. However, aggregation has several drawbacks, the most obvious of which is the loss of detailed information. Therefore, the aggregated measure differentiates poorly both trait and severity of the measures made at the disaggregated level. Furthermore, aggregation is of little value when the focus of interest lies at a lower level of the data hierarchy, for example sites with periodontal pockets.[54]

'Multilevel modelling' (MLM)[55] or equivalently 'hierarchical linear modelling'[56] is a class of techniques developed to analyse hierarchical data. It was first adopted to analyse educational data. These techniques are the modified version of statistical methods available for the analysis of single-level data structures (e.g. multiple regression, logistic regression, log-linear modelling) for the analysis of data with hierarchical structure. One could carry out the multilevel data analysis through the use of software specially written for MLM, like MLwiN (http://multilevel.ioe.ac.uk), or one could write up macros in other statistical softwares like SAS, S-plus.[57] In carrying out MLM, one should specify the number of levels in the model and then the variables incorporated at each of the levels. Back to the example of the periodontal study in which the number of sites assessed was 2236 distributed on 559 teeth in 22 subjects.[53] One of the analyses performed by the researchers was a multilevel analysis on the factors affecting the change in probing pocket depth at the sites over the course of the treatment. A three-level model was built with site as level 1, tooth as level 2 and subject as level 3. At the site level, 12 variables were constructed (e.g. presence of plaque at the site, treatment received at the site); at the tooth level, three variables were included (e.g. tooth type) and at the subject level, 19 variables were constructed (e.g. age, gender, smoking habit). The above analysis was performed using the software MLn (the non-Windows[TM] version of MLwiN). With the use of MLM, it is then possible to investigate the change in probing pocket depth at the site with the consideration of the effects from the site itself, the tooth that it belongs to and the subject overall. In order to evaluate whether a three-level model is necessary, one should test the 'null model' that no independent variables were included and then check the significance of the variance at each level and fit the model accordingly. Several other studies using multilevel modelling in analysing caries, periodontal and orthodontics data have also been published.[54,57−59]

IMPACT OF TRIALS ON DENTAL PRACTICE

DIET AND DENTAL CARIES

Evidence of the role of diet, particularly sugars, in relation to dental caries has largely been collated from animal experiences or *in vitro* studies. Human studies have largely been of the observational type: world-wide epidemiological studies, 'before and after' studies, and studies among people with both high and low sugar consumption. Very few interventional studies on human subjects have been conducted,[4,60] and are unlikely to be undertaken in the future given the difficulties of placing groups of people on rigid dietary regimes for long periods of time and because of ethical issues. The main conclusion of studies relating to sugar and dental caries has been that (1) consumption of sugar, even at high levels, is associated with only a small increase in caries increment if the sugar is taken up to four times a day and none between meals; (2) consumption of sugar both between meals and at meals is associated with a marked increase in caries increment.[61,62] These conclusions have shaped key dental education messages of oral health promotion campaigns relating to diet and dental health around the world and also formed the basis of dentist−patient dental health education relating to diet and dental caries.[63] Other trials have provided evidence of variations in caries incidence with different types of sugars, notably, the low caries rate associated with the use of sugar alcohols like xylitol.[60] This has led to more widespread use of non-carcinogenic sugar alternatives in drinks and foodstuffs.[64] However, this may be attributed more to their low caloric value than their low cariogenicity.

WATER FLUORIDATION

Evidence of the effectiveness of water fluoridation has largely been based on cross-sectional and ecological studies, 'before and after' studies, and fewer cohort or case−control studies. No randomised controlled trials have been reported in the dental literature. Systematic reviews of the effectiveness of water fluoridation have concluded that it is an effective, efficient and safe method of preventing dental caries and possibly promotes equity in oral health in society.[65] The studies have examined the relationship between dental caries experience and the fluoride content of the water supply and have shown clearly the association between increased fluoride concentration in the drinking water and decreased dental caries experience in the population. However, the studies have suggested that there is little benefit where water fluoride concentrations exceed 1 ppm. These findings have resulted in the implementation of water fluoridation in many industrialised and developing countries where central water supplies have made it feasible to do so. It remains a key World Health Organization goal for oral health.

However, a number of studies relate to the negative influences of water fluoridation on dental and general health, primarily on the effects of water fluoridation in producing dental fluorosis (tooth mottling) among the population.[66] Fluoride at a concentration of 1 ppm is likely to produce a small increase in dental mottling. However, in the most part such mottling is unlikely to be of aesthetic concern. Despite strong evidence of the effectiveness and safety of water fluoridation some communities have ceased to fluoridate their water supplies because of legal issues, social acceptance and concern about the additional benefits of fluoridated water where other sources of fluoride are readily accessible.

ALTERNATIVES TO WATER FLUORIDATION

A wide range of alternative methods for administering systemic fluoride have been suggested in the literature, particularly milk fluoridation and salt fluoridation.[67] Extensive literature describing the study of fluoride compounds administered with calcium-rich food, as well as clinical trials and laboratory experiments with fluoridated milk, have demonstrated the effectiveness of milk fluoridation in caries prevention.[68] However, the criticism of decreased bioavailability of the fluoride, the cost and administrative burden involved, and conflicting evidence of efficacy has resulted in few community milk fluoridation programmes.

Salt fluoridation has also been advocated as an alternative to water fluoridation. Evidence of the effectiveness of salt fluoridation has largely come from test and control community studies in several different countries.[69] Despite the fact

that salt fluoridation offers the consumer a choice to use fluoride supplements or not, there are only a handful of countries where it is widely available and consumed. Concerns about the appropriate dosage (a minimum of 200 mg/l F is recommended) and safety for general health may impede its widespread implementation.[70]

Fluoride supplements in the form of tablets to drops have long been considered an alternative to water fluoridation. Although the effectiveness of fluoride supplements was endorsed by many small clinical studies, closer examination of the experimental conditions of these, their methods and the analysis of their results undermined confidence in their findings. More modern, well-conducted clinical trials of supplements suggest that today, in children also exposed to fluoride from other sources such as toothpaste, the marginal effect of fluoride supplements is very small and there is substantial risk of fluorosis if supplements are used by young children.[71] This has resulted in changes to recommended fluoride dosage schedules and deferment of the age commencing the use of supplements, implemented in many countries. Overall, poor compliance and potential risks of fluorosis make fluoride supplements a poor public health measure and they are infrequently prescribed in dental practice.[72]

FLUORIDATED TOOTHPASTE

The daily use of fluoride toothpaste is a highly effective method of delivering fluoride to the tooth surface and has proved to be a major aid to caries prevention.[73] The concentration of fluoride at 1000 ppm F has been suggested as a safe and effective means of preventing caries.[74] Although evidence suggests that toothpastes with higher fluoride concentrations are more effective in preventing dental caries, because of safety concerns dentifrices exceeding 1500 ppm F are only sold by prescription in many countries.[75] However, for children trials have suggested that a lower concentration of fluoride in dentifrices (250–500 ppm F) be used and that only a minimum amount (less than 5 mm) should be placed on the brush to minimise risk.[76] Some trials have suggested that combining more than one fluoride agent is more effective than using one source of fluoride agent in preventing dental caries. However, different formulations of toothpaste appear to have similar effectiveness.[77] To some extent the use of dentifrice has removed the need for professionally applied fluoride agents, except in special circumstances.

OTHER FORMS OF TOPICAL FLUORIDE

Many forms of professionally applied fluoride have been studied, including solutions, gels or foams of sodium fluoride, stannous fluoride, organic amine fluoride, acidulated phosphate fluoride and non-aqueous fluoride varnishes in an alcoholic solution of natural resins and difluorosilane agents covered by a polyurethane coating. All of these professionally applied topical agents have anti-caries benefits, although the benefits and ease of application vary.[78] However, a recent systematic review of the periodic scientific literature undertaken to determine the strength of the evidence for the efficacy of professional caries preventive methods applied to high-risk individuals, and the efficacy of professionally applied methods to arrest or reverse non-cavitated carious lesions, concluded that the strength of the evidence was judged to be fair for fluoride varnishes and insufficient for all other methods.[79] In dental practice professionally applied fluoride is infrequently employed owing to more widespread use of other fluoride sources, reports of inconclusive evidence and because of health care reimbursement for such preventive procedures.

FISSURE SEALANTS

Most carious lesions occur in the pit and fissure on the occlusal surface of posterior teeth. Over the years clinical trials have demonstrated the effectiveness of sealing these fissures and pits in preventing dental caries.[21] Light-curing and auto-polymerising sealants are equally effective. However, the cost-effectiveness of fissure sealants in clinical trials remains questionable.[80] Thus, fissure sealants should be employed on

clinical grounds, on patients with special needs, a history of extensive caries in the primary detention or caries involving one or more molars.[81] It is important that they are reviewed at regular intervals.

TREATMENT OF CARIES LESIONS

A key focus of research has been the performance of direct posterior restorations (fillings), the longevity and reasons for failure of direct resin-based composite (RBC), amalgam and glass ionomer cement (GIC) restorations in stress-bearing posterior cavities. Predominantly studies have been either of the longitudinal or retrospective cross-sectional type, with few controlled clinical studies. GIC perform significantly worse compared with amalgam and RBC.[82] However, reasons for placement and replacement of direct restorations in dental practice relates to many factors, and aesthetic and safety concerns have resulted in an increased use of RBC or GIC restorations in posterior teeth.[83] The handling and fluoride leaching properties of GIC have made them popular in general practice.[84]

REPLACEMENT OF MISSING TEETH

A range of treatment modalities to replace missing teeth have been studied, including removable and fixed dental prostheses and the use of implants. Increasingly these studies have incorporated patients' perceptions of outcomes. Evidence has largely been collated from longitudinal or case–control studies with relatively few RCTs. Implant-retained overdentures are reported to be superior to complete dentures.[33] In addition, implants are useful in the treatment of partial edentulism. However, the widespread use of implants in practice has been limited by a number of factors including health care cover and costs, operator experience and appropriateness for individual cases.

Another contentious issue has been the use of resin-bonded bridges (RBBs) which provide a greater degree of conservation of tooth structure of abutments compared with designs of conventional fixed prostheses in the treatment of partial edentulism.[85] A key concern has been the longevity of RBBs, however studies suggest that with appropriate case selection, preparation design and cementation they are a viable treatment option compared to conventional bridges. Increasingly RBBs are being employed in dental practice in the treatment of short edentulous spaces.

TRIALS RELATING TO PERIODONTAL DISEASE

A key focus of periodontal trials has been the need for plaque control to prevent periodontal diseases and for the maintenance of periodontal health.[86] Primarily studies have focused on mechanical methods of plaque control. Studies have shown that the most important plaque control method is toothbrushing; precise technique is less important than the result, which is removal of plaque without causing damage to the teeth or gums.[87] It is widely promoted to establish toothbrushing practice as a daily routine from childhood.

Additional methods of mechanical plaque control include interdental cleaning aids such as dental floss. While such aids have been shown to be effective in plaque control with minimum damage if used correctly, they are generally prescribed depending on the individual's periodontal health and their ability to use them appropriately.[88]

Chemical antimicrobial agents may be a useful adjunct measure to managing periodontal health. In particular the use of chlorhexidene in the chemical control of plaques has widely been advocated, particularly in acute phases and in preventing post-surgical infection.[89] However, with the long-term use of chlorhexidene there is a tendency for it to stain (extrinsic) teeth. In more recent times the addition of antimicrobial agents to dentifrices to aid plaque control has become commonplace.[90] The use of chemical agents in the removal of plaque, while effective, is not recommended over the use of mechanical agents.[91]

In the treatment of periodontal disease many trials have concluded that non-surgical periodontal therapy is more appropriate than surgical periodontal therapy, and that surgical therapy should only be considered when sites fail to respond to non-surgical methods despite adequate oral hygiene.[92] State-funded and third-party payers of oral health care usually require detailed justification for surgical periodontal care.

ORTHODONTICS

While there has been considerable growth in the practice of orthodontics there is a dearth of evidence-based research, particularly RCTs.[40] A contentious issue has been the timing of orthodontics and the need for early orthodontic intervention. The evidence relating to early orthodontic treatment is inconclusive, with the result that many clinicians decide, on a case-by-case basis, when to provide orthodontic treatment.[93] Another key concern has been the value of maxillary arch expansion for the treatment of posterior crossbite. A Cochrane Review on the subject was unable to propose recommendations based on inadequate trials.[94] Lack of evidence relating to the value of orthognathic surgery versus orthodontic camouflage in the treatment of mandibular deficiency, and also as to the need for extraction of teeth for orthodontic purposes, has resulted in clinicians deciding on a case-by-case basis without any clinical guidelines.[95]

CONCLUSION

Currently the lack of high-quality research within dentistry, namely the lack of RCTs, has impeded the identification of best dental practice and the implementation of evidence-based practice within dentistry. There is however widespread recognition of these problems and concerted efforts to undertake more collaborative high-quality research that can inform policies and guidelines to be implemented in dental practice.

REFERENCES

1. Stjernsward J, Stanley K, Eddy D, Tsechkovski M, Sobin L, Koza I, Notaney KH. National cancer

control programs and setting priorities. *Cancer Detect Prevent* (1986) **9**: 113–24.

2. Proffit WR, Fields HW, Morav LJ. Prevalence of malocclusion and orthodontic treatment need in the United States: estimates from the NHANES III survey. *Int J Adult Orthodont Orthognat Surg* (1998) **13**: 97–106.

3. Bowden GHW, Edwardsson S. Oral ecology and dental caries. In: Thylstrup A, Fejerskov O, eds, *Textbook of Clinical Cariology*. Copenhagen: Munksgaard (1994) 45–70.

4. Gustafsson BE, Quensel CE, Lanke LKS. The Vipeholm dental caries study. The effect of different levels of carbohydrate intake on caries activity in 436 individuals observed for five years (Sweden). *Acta Odontol Scand* (1954) **11**: 232–64.

5. World Health Organization. *Oral Health Surveys: Basic Methods*, 4th edn. Geneva: WHO (1997).

6. Zambon JJ. Periodontal diseases: microbial factors. *Ann Periodontol* (1996) **1**: 879–925.

7. Ainamo J, Bay I. Problems and proposals for recording gingivitis and plaque. *Int Dental J* (1975) **25**: 229–35.

8. Silness J, Loe H. Periodontal disease in pregnancy. II. Correlation between oral hygiene and periodontal condition. *Acta Odontol Scand* (1964) **22**: 112–35.

9. Turesky S, Gilmore ND, Glickman I. Reduced plaque formation by the chloromethyl analogue of Victamine C. *J Periodontol* (1970) **41**: 41–3.

10. Loe H, Silness J. Periodontal disease in pregnancy. I. Prevalence and severity. *Acta Odontol Scand* (1963) **21**: 533–51.

11. Slade GD, ed. *Measuring Oral Health and Quality of Life*. Chapel Hill: University of North Carolina (1997).

12. Dolan TA. The sensitivity of the geriatric oral health assessment index to dental care. *J Dental Educ* (1997) **61**: 37–46.

13. Allen PF, McMillan AS, Locker D. An assessment of sensitivity to change of the Oral Health Impact Profile in a clinical trial. *Commun Dent Oral Epidemiol* (2001) **29**: 175–82.

14. Pocock SJ. *Clinical Trials: A Practical Approach*. Chichester, UK: John Wiley & Sons (1983).

15. Dennison DK. Components of a randomized clinical trial. *J Periodont Res* (1997) **32**: 430–8.

16. Koch GG, Paquette DW. Design principles and statistical considerations in periodontal clinical trials. *Ann Periodontol* (1997) **2**: 42–63.

17. Friedman LM, Furberg CD, DeMets DL. *Fundamentals of Clinical Trials*, 3rd edn. Mosby: Springer (1998).

18. Lau G. Ethics. In: Kalberg J, Tsang K, eds, *Introduction to Clinical Trials*. Hong Kong: The University of Hong Kong (1998) 73–112.

19. Burns DR, Elswick RK Jr. Equivalence testing with dental clinical trials. *J Dental Res* (2001) **80**: 1513–17.

20. McDaniel TF, Miller DL, Jones RM, Davis MS, Russell CM. Effects of toothbrush design and brushing proficiency on plaque removal. *Compend Contin Educ Dent* (1997) **18**: 572–7.

21. Morphis TL, Toumba KJ, Lygidakis NA. Fluoride pit and fissure sealants: a review. *Int J Paediat Dent* (2000) **10**: 90–8.

22. Hujoel PP, Loesche WJ. Efficiency of split-mouth designs. *J Clin Periodontol* (1990) **17**: 722–8.

23. Hujoel PP, DeRouen TA. Validity issues in split-mouth trials. *J Clin Periodontol* (1992) **19**: 625–7.

24. Dörfer CE, Berbig B, von Bethlenfalvy ER, Staehle HJ, Pioch T. A clinical study to compare the efficacy of 2 electric toothbrushes in plaque removal. *J Clin Periodontol* (2001) **28**: 987–94.

25. Corbet EF, Tam JO, Zee KY, Wong MC, Lo EC, Mombelli AW, Lang NP. Therapeutic effects of supervised chlorhexidine mouthrinses on untreated gingivitis. *Oral Dis* (1997) **3**: 9–18.

26. Donly KJ, Segura A, Kanellis M, Erickson RL. Clinical performance and caries inhibition of resin-modified glass ionomer cement and amalgam restorations. *J Am Dental Assoc* (1999) **130**: 1459–66.

27. Stephen KW, Macpherson LM, Gilmour WH, Stuart RA, Merrett MC. A blind caries and fluorosis prevalence study of school-children in naturally fluoridated and nonfluoridated townships of Morayshire, Scotland. *Commun Dent Oral Epidemiol* (2002) **30**: 70–9.

28. Lynch E, Baysan A, Ellwood R, Davies R, Petersson L, Borsboom P. Effectiveness of two fluoride dentifrices to arrest root carious lesions. *Am J Dent* (2000) **13**: 218–20.

29. Machiulskiene V, Nyvad B, Baelum V. Caries preventive effect of sugar-substituted chewing gum. *Commun Dent Oral Epidemiol* (2001) **29**: 278–88.

30. Poulsen S, Beiruti N, Sadat N. A comparison of retention and the effect on caries of fissure sealing with a glass-ionomer and a resin-based sealant. *Commun Dent Oral Epidemiol* (2001) **29**: 298–301.

31. Biesbrock AR, Gerlach RW, Bollmer BW, Faller RV, Jacobs SA, Bartizek RD. Relative anti-caries efficacy of 1100, 1700, 2200, and 2800 ppm fluoride ion in a sodium fluoride dentifrice over 1 year. *Commun Dent Oral Epidemiol* (2001) **29**: 382–9.

32. Lo EC, Luo Y, Fan MW, Wei SH. Clinical investigation of two glass-ionomer restoratives used with the atraumatic restorative treatment approach in China: two-years results. *Caries Res* (2001) **35**: 458–63.

33. Meijer HJ, Raghoebar GM, Van't Hof MA, Geertman ME, Van Oort RP. Implant-retained mandibular overdentures compared with complete dentures; a 5-years' follow-up study of clinical aspects and patient satisfaction. *Clin Oral Implant Res* (1999) **10**: 238–44.

34. Roccuzzo M, Bunino M, Prioglio F, Bianchi SD. Early loading of sandblasted and acid-etched (SLA) implants: a prospective split-mouth comparative study. *Clin Oral Implant Res* (2001) **12**: 572–8.

35. de Albuquerque RF Jr, Lund JP, Tang L, Larivee J, de Grandmont P, Gauthier G, Feine JS. Within-subject comparison of maxillary long-bar implant-retained prostheses with and without palatal coverage: patient-based outcomes. *Clin Oral Implant Res* (2000) **11**: 555–65.

36. Slade GD, Spencer AJ. Development and evaluation of the Oral Health Impact Profile. *Commun Dental Health* (1994) **11**: 3–11.

37. Duke SP, Garrett S. Equivalence in periodontal trials: a description for the clinician. *J Periodontol* (1998) **69**: 650–4.

38. Gunsolley JC, Elswick RK, Davenport JM. Equivalence and superiority testing in regeneration clinical trials. *J Periodontol* (1998) **69**: 521–7.

39. Johnston LE Jr. Let them eat cake: the struggle between form and substance in orthodontic clinical investigation. *Clin Orthodont Res* (1998) **1**: 88–93.

40. O'Brien K. Editorial: Is evidence-based orthodontics a pipedream? *J Orthodont* (2001) **28**: 313.

41. Sackett DL, Rosenberg WM, Gary JA, Haynes RB, Richardson WS. Evidence based medicine: what it is and what it isn't. *Br Med J* (1996) **312**: 71–2.

42. Sutherland SE. The building blocks of evidence-based dentistry. *J Can Dental Assoc* (2000) **66**: 241–4.

43. Sutherland SE. Evidence-based dentistry: Part I. Getting started. *J Can Dental Assoc* (2001) **67**: 204–6.

44. Sutherland SE. Evidence-based dentistry: Part II. Searching for answers to clinical questions: how to use MEDLINE. *J Can Dental Assoc* (2001) **67**: 277–80.

45. Sutherland SE. Evidence-based dentistry: Part IV. Research design and levels of evidence. *J Can Dental Assoc* (2001) **67**: 375–8.

46. Sutherland SE. Evidence-based dentistry: Part V. Critical appraisal of the dental literature: papers about therapy. *J Can Dental Assoc* (2001) **67**: 442–5.

47. Sutherland SE. Evidence-based dentistry: Part VI. Critical appraisal of the dental literature: papers about diagnosis, etiology and prognosis. *J Can Dental Assoc* (2001) **67**: 582–5.

48. Sutherland SE, Walker S. Evidence-based dentistry: Part III. Searching for answers to clinical questions: finding evidence on the Internet. *J Can Dental Assoc* (2001) **67**: 320–3.

49. Crochane AL. *Effectiveness and Efficiency. Random Reflections on Health Services*. London: Nuffield Provincial Hospital Trust (1972).

50. Macfarlane TV, Worthington HV. Some aspects of data analysis in dentistry. *Commun Dental Health* (1999) **16**: 216–19.

51. Gilthorpe MS, Maddick IH, Petrie A. Introduction to multilevel modelling in dental research. *Commun Dental Health* (2000) **17**: 222–6.

52. Altman DG, Bland JM. Units of analysis. *Br Med J* (1997) **314**: 1874.

53. Axtelius B, Söderfeldt B, Attström R. A multilevel analysis of factors affecting pocket probing depth in patients responding differently to periodontal treatment. *J Clin Periodontol* (1999) **26**: 67–76.

54. Gilthorpe MS, Griffiths GS, Maddick IH, Zamzuri AT. The application of multilevel modelling to periodontal research. *Commun Dental Health* (2000) **17**: 227–35.

55. Goldstein H. *Multilevel Statistical Models*, 2nd edn. London: Edward Arnold (1995).

56. Bryk AS, Raudenbush S. *Hierarchical Linear Models: Applications and Data Analysis Methods*. Newbury Park: Sage Publications (1992).

57. Hannigan A, O'Mullane DM, Barry D, Schäfer F, Robers AJ. A re-analysis of a caries clinical trial by survival analysis. *J Dental Res* (2001) **80**: 427–31.

58. Albandar JM, Goldstein H. Multi-level statistical models in studies of periodontal diseases. *J Periodontol* (1992) **63**: 690–5.

59. Gilthorpe MS, Cunningham SJ. The application of multilevel, multivariate modelling to orthodontic research data. *Commun Dental Health* (2000) **17**: 236–42.

60. Scheinin A, Makinen KK. Turku sugar studies. An overview. *Acta Odontol Scand* (1976) **34**: 405–8.

61. Rugg-Gunn AJ. Nutrition, diet and dental public health. *Commun Dental Health* (1993) **10**: 47–56.

62. Sheiham A. Dietary effects on dental diseases. *Public Health Nutr* (2001) **4**: 569–91.

63. Duggal MS, van Loveren C. Dental considerations for dietary counselling. *Int Dental J* (2001) **51**: 408–12.

64. Linke HA. Sugar alcohols and dental health. *World Rev Nutr Diet* (1986) **47**: 134–62.

65. Tresaure ET, Chestnutt IG, Whiting P, McDonagh M, Kleijnen J. The York review—a systematic review of public water fluoridation. *Br Dental J* (2002) **192**: 495–7.

66. McDonagh MS, Whiting PF, Wilson PM, Sutton AJ, Chestnutt I, Cooper J, Misso K, Bradley M, Treasure E, Kleijnen J. Systematic review of water fluoridation. *Br Med J* (2000) **321**: 855–9.

67. O'Mullane DM. Systemic fluorides. *Adv Dental Res* (1994) **8**: 181–4.

68. Marino R. Should we use milk fluoridation? A review. *Bull Pan Am Health Org* (1995) **29**: 287–98.

69. Stephen KW. Fluoride prospects for the new millennium – community and individual patient aspects. *Acta Odontol Scand* (1999) **57**: 352–5.

70. Bergmann KE, Bergmann RL. Salt fluoridation and general health. *Adv Dental Res* (1995) **9**: 138–43.

71. Riordan PJ. Fluoride supplements for young children: an analysis of the literature focusing on benefits and risks. *Commun Dental Oral Epidemiol* (1999) **27**: 72–83.

72. Burt BA. The case for eliminating the use of dietary fluoride supplements for young children. *J Public Health Dent* (1999) **59**: 269–74.

73. Clarkson JJ, McLoughlin J. Role of fluoride in oral health promotion. *Int Dental J* (2000) **50**: 119–28.

74. Stephen KW. Dentifrices: recent clinical findings and implications for use. *Int Dental J* (1993) **43**: 549–53.

75. Ripa LW. Clinical studies of high-potency fluoride dentifrices: a review. *J Am Dental Assoc* (1989) **118**: 85–91.

76. Warren JJ, Levy SM. A review of fluoride dentifrice related to dental fluorosis. *Paediat Dent* (1999) **21**: 265–71.

77. Holloway PJ, Worthington HV. Sodium fluoride or sodium monofluorophosphate? A critical view of a meta-analysis on their relative effectiveness in dentifrices. *Am J Dent* (1993) **6**: S55–8.

78. Newbrun E. Topical fluorides in caries prevention and management: a North American perspective. *J Dental Educ* (2001) **65**: 1078–83.

79. Bader JD, Shugars DA, Bonito AJ. A systematic review of selected caries prevention and management methods. *Commun Dent Oral Epidemiol* (2001) **29**: 399–411.

80. Deery C. The economic evaluation of pit and fissure sealants. *Int J Paediat Dent* (1999) **9**: 235–41.

81. Smallridge J. UK National Clinical Guidelines in Paediatric Dentistry. Management of the stained fissure in the first permanent molar. *Int J Paediat Dent* (2000) **10**: 79–83.

82. Hickel R, Manhart J, Gracia-Godoy F. Clinical results and new developments of direct posterior restorations. *Am J Dent* (2000) **13**: 41D–54D.

83. Wilson NH, Burke FJ, Mjor IA. Reasons for placement and replacement of restorations of direct restorative materials by a selected group of practitioners in the United Kingdom. *Quintess Int* (1997) **28**: 245–8.

84. Yip HK, Smales RJ. Glass ionomer cements used as fissure sealants with the atraumatic restorative treatment (ART) approach: review of literature. *Int Dent J* (2002) **52**: 67–70.

85. Botelho M. Resin-bonded prostheses: the current state of development. *Quintess Int* (1999) **30**: 525–34.

86. Loe H. Oral hygiene in the prevention of caries and periodontal disease. *Int Dental J* (2000) **50**: 129–39.

87. Westfelt E. Rationale of mechanical plaque control. *J Clin Periodontol* (1996) **23**: 263–7.

88. Iacono VJ, Aldrege WA, Luckus H, Schwartzstein S. Modern supragingival plaque control. *Int Dental J* (1998) **48**: 290–7.

89. Jones CG. Chlorhexidine: is it still the gold standard? *Periodontology* (2000) **15**: 55–62.

90. Sheen S, Pontefract H, Moran J. The benefits of toothpaste – real or imagined? The effectiveness of toothpaste in the control of plaque, gingivitis, periodontitis, calculus and oral malodour. *Dental Update* (2001) **28**: 144–7.

91. Sheiham A. Is the chemical prevention of gingivitis necessary to prevent severe periodontitis? *Periodontology 2000* (1997) **15**: 15–24.

92. Greenstein G. Nonsurgical periodontal therapy in 2000: a literature review. *J Am Dental Assoc* (2000) **131**: 1580–92.

93. Kluemper GT, Beeman CS, Hicks EP. Early orthodontic treatment: what are the imperatives? *J Am Dental Assoc* (2000) **131**: 613–20.

94. Harrison JE, Ashby D. Orthodontic treatment for posterior crossbites. *Cochrane Database System Rev* (2001) **1**: CD000979.

95. Berg R. Orthodontic treatment – yes or no? A difficult decision in some cases. *J Orofacial Orthopaed* (2001) **62**: 410–21.

DERMATOLOGY

14

Dermatology

LUIGI NALDI[1] AND COSETTA MINELLI[2]

[1]Department of Dermatology, Ospedali Riuniti di Bergamo, Bergamo, Italy
[2]Unit of Clinical Epidemiology, Pharmacology Research Institute, M.Negri-Villa Camozzi, Ranica, Italy

WHAT IS DERMATOLOGY?

Dermatology deals with disorders affecting the skin and associated specialised structures such as hair and nails. The skin is a biological barrier between ourselves and the outside world consisting of a stratified epithelium, an underlying connective tissue, i.e., dermis, and a fatty layer usually designed as 'subcutaneous'. The skin is not a simple inert covering of the body but a sensitive dynamic boundary. It offers protection against infections, ultraviolet radiation and trauma. It is essential for controlling water and heat loss and contributes to the synthesis of substances such as vitamin D. The skin is also an important organ of social and sexual contact. Body perception, which is deeply rooted within the culture of any given social group, is largely affected by the appearance of the skin and its associated structures.

Extensive disorders affecting the skin may disrupt its homeostatic functions resulting in a properly speaking 'skin failure', needing intensive care with hydration, maintenance of caloric balance and temperature. However, this is a rare event occurring with conditions such as extensive bullous disorders or exfoliative dermatitis. The most usual health consequence of skin disorders is connected with the discomfort of symptoms, such as itching and burning or pain, which frequently accompany skin lesions and interfere with everyday life and sleeping. Moreover, visible lesions may result in a loss of confidence and disrupt social relations. Feelings of stigmatisation and major changes in lifestyle caused by a chronic skin disorder such as psoriasis have been repeatedly documented in population surveys.[1] Additional problems may arise under diverse circumstances: the exudation or loss of substances that interfere locally with the barrier function (and dressing); the shedding of scales whenever excessive desquamation occurs; the need to prevent contact dissemination in the case of transmissible diseases.

A LARGE NUMBER OF DIFFERENT SKIN DISEASES

Unlike most other organs that usually count around 50 to 100 diseases, the skin has a

Textbook of Clinical Trials.   Edited by D. Machin, S. Day and S. Green
© 2004 John Wiley & Sons, Ltd   ISBN: 0-471-98787-5

complement of 1000 to 2000 conditions and over 3000 dermatological categories can be found in the International Classification for Disease version 9 (ICD-9). This is partly justified by the skin being a large and visible organ. Beside disorders primarily affecting the skin, there are cutaneous manifestations with most of the major systemic diseases (e.g., vascular and connective tissue diseases). The classification of skin disorders is far from satisfactory (Table 14.1). Currently, there is a widespread use of symptom-based or purely descriptive terms, such as parapsoriasis or pytiriasis rosea, which reflects our limited understanding of the causes and pathogenetic mechanisms of a large number of skin disorders.

Skin diseases as a whole are very common in the general population. A limited number of prevalence surveys have documented that skin disorders may affect 20–30% of the general population at any one time. The most common diseases are also the most trivial ones. They include such conditions as mild eczematous lesions, mild to moderate acne, benign tumours and angiomatous lesions. More severe skin disorders, which may have an impact in terms of physical disability or even mortality, are rare or very rare. They include, among others, autoimmune bullous diseases, such as pemphigus, severe pustular and erythrodermic psoriasis, generalised eczematous reactions, and such malignant tumours as malignant melanoma and lymphoma. The disease frequency may show variations according to age, sex and geographic area. Eczema is common at any age while acne is decidedly more frequent among male adolescents. Skin tumours are particularly frequent in aged white populations. Infestations and infections such as scabies, pyoderma and dermatophytosis predominate in developing countries and some urban pockets of developed countries. In many cases, skin diseases are minor health problems, which may be trivialised in comparison with other more serious medical conditions. However, as mentioned above, skin manifestations are visible and may cause more distress to the public than more serious medical problems. The issue is complicated by the fact that many skin disorders are not present in the population as a yes or no phenomenon, but as a spectrum of severity. The

Table 14.1. Operational classification of skin diseases

	Anatomical distribution	Morphology	Pathology	Pathogenetic process	Aetiology
Genodermatoses		X			X
Nevi and other development defects		X	X		
Mechanical and thermal injuries					X
Photodermatoses		X		X	
Eczemas		X	X	X	X
Lichenoid disorders		X	X		
Disorders of keratinisation		X	X		
Psoriasis		X	X		
Infections and infestations		X			X
Disorders of skin colour		X			
Bullous eruptions		X	X	X	
Disorders of sebaceous glands	X	X		X	
Disorders of sweat glands	X	X			
Immune-related diseases		X		X	
Urticaria		X		X	X
Vascular disorders		X		X	X
Disorders of hair	X	X	X		
Disorders of nails	X	X	X		
Disorders of subcutaneous fat	X	X	X		
Tumours	X	X	X		

public's perception of what constitutes a 'disease' requiring medical advice may vary according to cultural issues, the social context, resources and time. Minor changes in health policy may have a large health and financial impact simply because a large number of people may be concerned. For example, most of the campaigns conducted to increase the public awareness of skin cancer have led to a large increase in the number of benign skin conditions such as benign melanocytic nevi being evaluated and excised.

Large variations can be documented among different countries in terms of health service organisation for treating skin disorders. A rough indicator of these variations is the density of dermatologists ranging, in Europe, from about 1:20 000 in Italy and France to 1:150 000 in the United Kingdom.

In general, only a fraction of those with skin diseases are expected to seek medical help while an estimated large proportion opt for self-medication. Pharmacists occupy a key role in advising the public on the use of over-the-counter products. Primary care physicians seem to treat the majority of people among those seeking medical advice. Primary care of dermatological problems seems to be imprecisely defined with a large overlap with specialist activity. Most of the dermatologist's workload around the world is concentrated in the outpatient department. In spite of the vast number of dermatological diseases, it has been documented that just a few categories account for about 70% of all dermatological consultations. Brief, more detailed descriptions of the most frequent skin categories are given below while skin cancer is dealt with in another section.

Generally speaking, dermatology requires a low technology clinical practice. Clinical expertise is mainly dependent on the ability to recognise a skin disorder quickly and reliably which, in turn, depends to a large extent on the awareness of a given clinical pattern, based on previous experience and on the exercised eye of a visually literate physician.[2] Complementary diagnostic procedures include skin biopsy, patch testing and immunopathology.

A peculiar aspect of dermatology is the possible option for topical treatment. This treatment modality is ideally suited to localised lesions, the main advantage being the restriction of the effect to the site of application and the limitation of systemic side effects. A topical agent is usually described as a vehicle and an active substance, the vehicles being classified as powder, grease, liquid or combinations such as pastes and creams.

Much traditional topical therapy in dermatology has been developed empirically with so-called magistral formulations. Most of these products seem to rely on physical rather than chemical properties for their effects and it may be an arbitrary decision to appoint one specific ingredient as the 'active' one. Physical effects of topical agents may include detersion, hydration and removal of keratotic scales. The border between pharmacological and cosmetological effects may be imprecisely defined and the term 'cosmeceuticals' is sometimes employed.[3] It should be noted that the evaluation of even the most recent cosmetic products is far from being satisfactory. In addition to pharmacological treatment, a number of non-pharmacological treatment modalities exists including phototherapy or photochemotherapy and minor surgical procedures such as electrodessication and criotherapy. Large variations in treatment modalites for the same condition have been documented, which mainly reflect local traditions and preferences.[4,5]

ACNE

The term acne refers to a group of disorders characterised by abnormalities of the sebaceous glands. Acne vulgaris is the most common condition and is characterised by polymorphous lesions, including comedones (blackheads), inflammatory lesions such as papules or pustules, and scars, affecting the face and less frequently the back and shoulders. A combination of factors are considered as pathogenetic, including the hormonal influence of androgens, seborrhea, abnormalities in the bacterial flora with overgrowth of Propionibacterium Acnei, and plugging of pilosebaceous openings. Mild degrees of acne are extremely common amongst teenagers (more than 80%) and decrease in later life. The prevalence of moderate to severe acne has been estimated at about 14% in 15–24 year-olds, 3% in 25–34 year-olds and about 1% in 35–54 year-olds. It is likely that the vast majority of sufferers of mild acne do not seek medical advice. Around 70% of those affected with acne experience shame and embarrassment because of their acne. Criteria for treatment include clinical severity, as judged by the extension and presence of inflammatory lesions, and the degree of psychological distress from the disease. The aim of treatment is to prevent scarring, limit disease duration and reduce psychological stress. Mild acne is usually treated by topical modalities such as benzoyl peroxide or tretinoin, while moderate severity acne is treated by systemic antibiotics or antiandrogens in women. Oral isotretinoin is used under specialist supervision for severe unresponsive disease. There are a number of published systems for measuring the severity of acne.[6] These vary from sophisticated systems with up to 100 potential grades to simple systems with 4 or 5 grades. A specially designed acne disability index has also been devised to assess the psychological impact of the disease and disability, and has been found to correlate well with severity as measured by an objective grading system, even if a small group experiences disability which is out of proportion with their severity.[7]

ATOPIC DERMATITIS

Typically, this condition is characterised by itching, dry skin and inflammatory lesions especially involving skin creases. Patients suffering from atopic dermatitis may also develop IgE-mediated allergic diseases such as bronchial asthma or allergic rhinitis. An overall cumulative prevalence of between 5% and 20% has been suggested by the age of 11. Around 60–70% of children are clear of significant disease by their mid-teens. Even if genetic factors seem to play a major role, environmental factors such as allergens and irritants are important and there is reasonable evidence to suggest that the prevalence has increased

two to threefold over the last 30 years. There is some evidence that it may be possible to prevent atopic dermatitis in high-risk children born to parents with atopic disease by restricting maternal allergens and reducing house dust mite levels.[8,9] No treatment has been shown to alter the natural history of established eczema and the mainstay of treatment is emollients, which moisturise the skin, and topical steroids.

PSORIASIS

This is a chronic inflammatory disorder characterised by red scaly areas, which tend to affect extensory surfaces of the body and scalp. Its overall prevalence is about 1–3% and males are affected more frequently than females. Several varieties have been described including guttate, pustular and erythrodermic psoriasis. In about 3% of cases it may associate with a peculiar arthritis. Significant disability has been documented with psoriasis. Multifactorial heredity is usually considered for disease causation. This implies interaction between a genetic predisposition and environmental factors. Heritability, a measure that quantifies the overall role of genetic factors, ranges from 0.5 to 0.9. Acute infections, physical trauma, selected medications and psychological stress are usually viewed as triggers. Pustular varieties of psoriasis have been strongly linked with smoking. Sun exposure usually temporarily improves the disease. Altered kinetics of epidermal cells has been repeatedly documented. The lesions are visible and may itch, sting and bleed easily. The aim of treatment is to achieve short-term suppression of symptoms and long-term modulation of disease severity, improving the quality of life with minimal side effects. Topical agents such as vitamin D derivatives, dithranol and steroids can be used for short-term control of the disease. Ultraviolet B phototherapy, psoralen plus ultraviolet A phototherapy (PUVA) and systemic agents such as methotrexate or cyclosporine are employed to control extensive lesions that fail to respond to topical agents. Relapse is common upon withdrawal. Outcomes that matter to the patient include disease suppression and duration of remission, patient satisfaction and autonomy and disease-related quality of life. A number of clinical activity scores have been developed, the most popular being the Psoriasis Area and Severity Index–PASI.[10] There is no documented evidence that such indexes are a reliable proxy for the above-mentioned outcomes. In the long term, a simple measure such as the number of patients reaching complete or nearly complete stable remission appears as the most relevant outcome variable.

LEG ULCERS

Venous and arterial leg ulcers are recognised as the most common chronic wounds in Western populations. A skin ulcer has been defined as a loss of dermis and epidermis produced by sloughing of necrotic tissue. Ulcers persisting for 4 weeks or more have been rather arbitrarily classified as chronic ulcers. Based on population surveys, the point prevalence of leg ulcers ranges from 0.1% to 1.0% and increases with age. Venous ulcers are the end result of superficial or deep venous insufficiency and a venous origin is diagnosed in about 80% of cases. Arterial ulceration may be regarded as a multistep process, starting, in general, with a systemic vascular derangement such as atherosclerosis. The prognosis of leg ulcers is less than satisfactory, with about one-quarter of subjects not healing in over 2 years and the majority of patients having recurrence. In a large-scale clinical study, the healing time varied according to the dimension of the ulcers, their duration and the mobility of the patient. The quality of life of ulcer patients may be severely affected. Social isolation, depression and negative self-image have been associated with ulcers in a high percentage of patients.[11] A number of studies point to the less than satisfactory management of ulcer patients in the community, including the lack of any clinical assessment leading to long periods of ineffective or inappropriate treatment and delays in instituting effective pain-relieving strategies. Ulcer clinics in vascular surgical services in the UK proved to offer advantages over home treatment.[12] The overwhelming rates of recurrence clearly suggest that more attention should be paid to prevention.

SKIN DISORDERS AND CLINICAL TRIAL METHODS: ADAPTING STUDY DESIGN TO SETTING AND DISEASE

As for other disciplines, the last few decades have seen an impressive increase in the number of clinical trials carried out in dermatology. However, there are indications that the upsurge of clinical research has not been paralleled by a refinement in clinical trial methodology and the quality of randomised control trials (RCTs) in dermatology falls well below the usually accepted standards.[13–15] In this section we would like to mention some issues which deserve special attention when designing a randomised clinical trial in this speciality area. There is a need for innovative thinking in dermatology to make clinical research address the important issues and not simply ape the scientific design.

RANDOMISATION

It can be estimated that there are at least a thousand rare or very rare skin conditions where no single randomised trial has been conducted. These conditions are also those which carry a higher burden in terms of physical disability and mortality. The annual incidence rate of many of them is lower than 1 case per 100 000 and frequently less than 1 case per 1 000 000. International collaboration and institutional support is clearly needed. There are no examples of such an effort.

For quite different reasons, there are also common skin conditions where randomised clinical trials have been rarely performed. These conditions include several varieties of eczematous dermatitis (e.g., nummular eczema), psoriasis (e.g., guttate psoriasis) and urticaria (e.g., pressure urticaria), a number of exanthematic reactions (e.g., pytiriasis rosea), rosacea, and common infections such as warts and molluscum contagious. One alleged difficulty with mounting randomised clinical trials in dermatology is the visibility of skin lesions and the consideration that much more than in other areas, patients self-monitor their disease and may have preconceptions and preferences about specific treatment modalities.[16] The decision to treat is usually dictated by subjective issues and personal feelings. As we will consider below, there is a need to educate physicians and the public about the value of randomised trials to assess interventions in dermatology. The need to evaluate the attitudes of patients and to educate should be clearly considered when planning a study and developing modalities to obtain an informed consent from the patient.

Randomised clinical trials are usually designed in dermatology with an expected large effect from the test treatment and most trials do not recruit more than a few dozen patients. In small trials there may be substantial differences in group sizes that will reduce the precision of the estimated differences in treatment effect and hence the efficiency of the study. As a consequence, block randomisation may be preferable. On the other hand, a substantial imbalance may persist in prognostic characteristics, and minimisation can be used to make small groups more similar with respect to major prognostic variables.[17] There is some evidence that the group sizes of clinical trials, apparently based on simple randomisation and published in a number of leading dermatological journals, tend to be much more similar than expected by chance (unpublished data from the European Dermatoepidemiology Network psoriasis project). The cluster around equal sample sizes may be due to publication bias, failure to report blocking, or even to the rectification of an unsatisfactory imbalance by adding extra patients to one treatment.

In many instances, the management of a chronic skin disorder is a multiple step process where different phases can be identified. For example, at least two phases are usually considered when treating psoriasis: a clearance phase, which involves a more intensive treatment approach with the aim of clearing existing psoriasis lesions, and a maintenance phase, with the main aim of preventing disease relapse. The different phases are not necessarily well separated in time. Long-term disease-modifying strategies can be adopted at the same time when a treatment modality for reaching clearance has been started. An example is the treatment of atopic dermatitis by topical steroids and diet. Most randomised clinical trials in dermatology use a simplified approach to evaluating treatment effects and most of them analyse the effect of a single manoeuvre over a limited time span. One as yet not fully explored issue is the potential for combining different treatment approaches in a simultaneous or subsequent order. There are examples of combinations of such treatment modalities as calcipotriol and ultraviolet B radiation in psoriasis treatment, but other rational combinations are not fully explored. A way of addressing the issue is by relying on factorial design. An example of such a design would be a randomised clinical trial of the effect of a low-allergen diet compared with an unrestricted diet in atopic women during pregnancy and breast-feeding on the subsequent development of atopic disorders in children where women are randomised to all the possible combinations of restricted and unrestricted dietetic measures during the periods examined.

BLINDING

There are several reasons for considering blinding as a major bias-reducing procedure in randomised clinical trials of skin disorders. Firstly, it is expected that physicians and patients are subject to strong, though difficult to document, hopes and prejudices about the optimal care of skin disorders. This is reflected, for example, in the large variations of treatment procedures for the same condition which have been repeatedly documented in different areas of dermatology. Secondly, most outcome measures are soft end points involving subjective judgement, which may be influenced to a significant extent by the previous knowledge of the treatment adopted. Thirdly, the visibility of lesions may influence the decision to rely or not on a given treatment to a larger extent as compared with situations where disease variables are not so obvious. On the other hand, there may be problems with blinding which may be difficult or impossible to solve, like with trials comparing complex procedures such as ultraviolet light radiation and drug regimens. An issue which warrants more attention than it is often given in randomised trials is the possibility that certain 'marker variables' occur, together with obvious side effects. These variables, observable during treatment, may in part unblind the trial, even at a subliminal level.[18] This is an issue with the use of topical retinoids and the associated mild cutaneous irritation, which may be noticed but not reported at all as a 'side effect'. It is quite common to find randomised clinical trials where the authors claim blindness in situations where treatment modalities are responsible for frequent and obvious side effects. In 1982, for example, a trial was published examining three different therapeutic strategies for psoriasis: oral etretinate associated with topically applied betamethasone, oral etretinate associated with topically applied placebo, and oral placebo associated with topical betamethasone.[19] Systemic retinoids such as etretinate are responsible for common side effects which are reminiscent of vitamin A overdosage, including dryness of the skin and mucous membranes, while topical steroids commonly produce a transitory blanching effect. It is difficult to accept blindness in the trial when there is no additional information on how blinding was actually assured. It is worth mentioning that the dropout rates showed large variations among the different trial arms because of alleged side effects of treatment.

One way to overcome the problem of an unachievable blindness and avoid the influence of the researcher's subjective judgement is to plan the study so that the clinician who treats the patient is not the same one who judges the effect of the therapy. This way the second clinicians can be blind to the treatment assigned to the patient.

STANDARDISATION OF TREATMENT MODALITIES AND ACCESSORY CARE

Independently of the 'active' intervention administered, accessory non-pharmacological treatment and skin care seem to play a significant role in the outcome of most skin disorders. It is common sense that emollients may improve dry skin and wet soaks may help to dry exudating lesions. As a consequence, accessory care requires careful standardisation. However, while it is relatively easy to ensure that the pharmacological treatment is conducted in an appropriate way (particularly timing and administration route), non-pharmacological accessory care is prone to a larger variability that is affected by social and cultural factors among others. To a greater extent, variability may affect topical treatment as compared with systemic treatment. Topical treatment is usually more cumbersome in comparison with systemic treatment and may well depend on the physician's and patient's consistency. As documented in randomised clinical trials of the retinoid derivative tazarotene in psoriasis, the modalities of application may play a significant role in tolerability and side effects.[20] Once again a well-informed patient as well as an active and supportive clinician are vitally important. The issue of standardisation is also important for assessing compliance when the treatment is self-applied by the patient. If indeed there are limitations with such methods as tablet count for assessing compliance with systemic agents, the limitations are even greater when similar methods are used to monitor the consumption of topical agents in the absence of strict rules to define a 'single dose'. The amount consumed cannot be monitored if patients are not carefully instructed on how to apply the topical agent. The observed compliance behaviour may range from compliant, overusing, erratic using and dropping out.

DIFFERENT STUDY SETTINGS AND DISPARATE DISEASE SEVERITY

We have already mentioned that the contents of primary care for many skin disorders are imprecisely defined as opposed to specialist clinical practice, with possibly large overlapping areas. In addition, it has been noticed that there may be wide variations in terms of severity within any given diagnostic category, with conditions ranging from subclinical manifestations, e.g., psoriatic 'markers', to skin failure, e.g., erythrodermic or generalised pustular psoriasis. Moreover, it should be noticed that for any given disease there might be clinical variants, which may have peculiar prognostic features and responses to treatment, e.g., guttate psoriasis versus plaque psoriasis. As a consequence, it is of the outmost importance that entry criteria in RCTs of skin disorders are defined as precisely as possible. This should include as a major requirement the definition of the study setting, clinical variety, disease severity and duration, previous treatments and concomitant systemic disorders.

It should be noticed that the severity assessment of most skin disorders implies an understanding of the many influences of the disease on the patient's life, including disease-associated discomfort, level of disability and social disruption. Most of these influences are better expressed as a continuum of severity rather than a yes or no phenomenon. On the other hand, there are practical advantages in trying to translate the continuum into a limited number of workable severity categories. The main advantage is a better compliance with the discrete nature of most clinical decisions where thresholds are usually required for implementing interventions (examples of categorical classifications of a severity continuum are tumour staging and arterial hypertension definition). Unfortunately, for many inflammatory skin disorders no reliable severity criteria have been developed. Even when such criteria are available, there is uncertainty about severity thresholds. Consequently, large variations are expected to occur among different RCTs and, in fact, have been documented on several occasions. A rather common attitude in published RCTs is the lack of entry criteria and severity definitions, so that the patient population appears to be recruited in a vacuum.[15,21] One habit which should be discouraged is to include broad diagnostic categories that lack specificity like, for example, the category of 'steroid responsive dermatoses' or 'itching disorders'.

OUTCOME MEASURES

There are obvious analogies between the problems implied in the development of severity criteria and those implied in outcome measures. They both consist of measures that must have the properties of validity and reliability. In addition, outcome measures must be responsive to change, i.e., they must have the ability to identify what may be small but nevertheless clinically important changes. On the other hand, with severity criteria the intent is more to discriminate between individuals. If an instrument is useful to discriminate between severity levels of psoriasis, it does not necessarily mean that it will be able to detect changes which are important as a result of treatment within these categories. The distinction between the two aims (i.e., describing variations between individuals and assessing variations within individuals) is frequently blurred when developing measurement systems for skin disorders. In spite of the fact that, from a clinical point of view, distinguishing between disease severity levels may represent a different issue as compared with assessing clinically important changes in individual patients, the two issues are usually dealt with by relying on identical scale systems in dermatology.

There are indications that many score systems employed in dermatology lack the basic requirements for reliability and validity. Even a simple measure such as the approximate percentage of area involved in a skin disease is prone to wide inter- and intra-observer variations if the evaluation methods are not clearly specified.[22] In spite of their lacking basic requirements, a large number of different scales have been developed for such common disorders as psoriasis or atopic dermatitis (Table 14.2). One example is the 'Psoriasis Area Severity Index' (PASI).[10] This index is obtained by summing up the scores concerning three features of psoriasis, namely the body district affected, the severity of the condition (judged by the degree of erythema, infiltration and desquamation) and

Table 14.2. Measures used in the outcome evaluation of selected skin diseases

Disease	Clinical scales	Disease-specific Quality of Life measures
Acne[6,37,38]	• Lesion counting (papule, pustule and comedone counts) • Plewing and Kligman grading system • Cunliffe score (Leeds technique) • Cook's photonumeric method • American Academy of Dermatology (*AAD*) classification • Allen and Smith photographic method • Fluorescence photography • *GAGS* (Global Acne Grading System)	• *ADI* (Acne Disability Index) • *CADI* (Cardiff Acne Disability Index) • *APSEA* (Assessment of the Psychological and Social Effects of Acne) • *AQL* (Acne Quality of Life) index
Atopic dermatitis[38–40]	• *SCORAD* (severity Scoring of Atopic Dermatitis) • *SASSAD* (Six-Area, Six-Sign Atopic Deramtitis) severity index • *ADASI* (Atopic Dermatitis Area and Severity Index) • *EASI* (Eczema Area and Severity Index) • Rajka and Langerland scoring system • *SSS* (Simple Scoring System) • *BCSS* (Basic Clinical Scoring System) • *ADSI* (Atopic Dermatitis Severity Index) • *SIS* (Skin Intensity Score) • *ADAM* (Assessment Measure for Atopic Dermatitis) • Nottingham Eczema Severity Score	• *EDI* (Eczema Disability Index)
Psoriasis[22,41]	• *Severity scores* based on *individual signs* (involved Body Surface Area, erythema, induration, desquamation) • *PASI* (Psoriasis Area and Severity Index) • *SAPASI* (Self-administered PASI) • *Ultrasound* evaluation of the thickness of psoriasis	• *PDI* (Psoriasis Disability Index) • *PLSI* (Psoriasis Life Stress Inventory)
Leg ulcers[42,43]	• Clinical skin score • *Simple* wound measurements • *Planimetric* wound area measurements	
Dermatological diseases as a class[38,44,45]	• *DIDS* (Dermatology Index of Disease Severity)	• *DLQI* (Dermatology Life Quality Index) • *CDLQI* (Children's Dermatology Life Quality Index) • *IMPACT* (Impact of Skin Disease Scale) • *SKINDEX*

the extension of the disease. The last two are judged according to the body district analysed. Although the PASI score has been widely used, it is largely unsatisfactory.[22] It has never been standardised and there is limited testing for inter- and intra-rater reliability. Validity is another issue. It has never been demonstrated that the weights arbitrarily attributed to each item in the PASI score actually reflect the clinical severity of lesions. PASI is only relying on the dermatologist's judgement of a few clinical features of psoriasis and there is increasing awareness that the patient's judgement is equally important. An additional drawback of PASI is that similar scores can be attributed to varieties of psoriasis which differ clinically and in terms of response to treatment.[23] The 'Self-Administered PASI' (SAPASI), which asks the patient to make the same evaluation as the physician for PASI, does not escape the limitations we have pointed to for PASI as an outcome measure.[24]

To overcome the problems arising from subjective judgement, more 'objective' measures have been repeatedly advocated, such as the use of ultrasound to evaluate the thickness of psoriasis plaques.[23] In fact, any measurement is fully justified only when it represents a good surrogate for clinically important outcomes, such as the patient disability and quality of life.[25]

The notion of responsiveness to change expresses the idea that any measure used in a trial should be sensitive to 'clinically important changes' in response to therapy.[26] A conceptual difficulty arises in specifying what a clinically important change is. With most scales developed in dermatology the issue remains fraught since no 'gold standard' has gained wide acceptance. It should be considered that the 'outcome' of the treatment refers to 'all the possible results that stem from preventive or therapeutic interventions' and consists of several separate dimensions (e.g., discomfort and disability), which may be broken down into components and simple measurable items. Any given measure achieves its value only to the extent to which it serves as a proxy for an outcome component. For example,

if the PASI index accurately quantifies disability or discomfort, then it may be of value as a surrogate outcome measure for psoriasis. What may be a relevant outcome variable is a matter of judgement, based on the knowledge of the disease, the patients' requirements and the values of society. The outcome of skin disorders that affect the quality rather than the quantity of life is expected to be largely culture-dependent. It is our conviction that the development of a 'gold standard' requires a deep understanding of patients' requirements and expectations from treatment. In the lack of reliable scales, trials with the simplest and most objective outcome variables are preferable. Such measures as complete remission or recurrence should be preferred, provided that these categories are clearly defined. Clearly, remission or recurrence are events which occur with a lower frequency as compared with less dramatic variations in disease activity measured by clinical scales. This, in turn, affects the sample size calculation.

There are at least two different choices when analysing outcome measures expressed by any given score system. We might compare the difference between the initial and final scores in the treatment and control groups or, alternatively, ignore the pre-test scores and simply analyse the scores after treatment. There are two important analytical reasons to consider in the use of change scores.[27] The first is that the subtraction of scores before treatment has the effect of removing stable individual differences between subjects, thereby increasing the power of the statistical test. The second reason, which is of relatively minor importance in a randomised trial, is that there may be overall differences between the two groups at the baseline, and the use of change scores can potentially correct for these differences. The usual presentation of score data over time (e.g., PASI score) is to build up a curve based on the mean score values of the treatment and control groups. A common but inappropriate analysis of these curves is to apply two separate sample tests on mean score values at several time points (Figure 14.1). The means may not represent a good descriptor

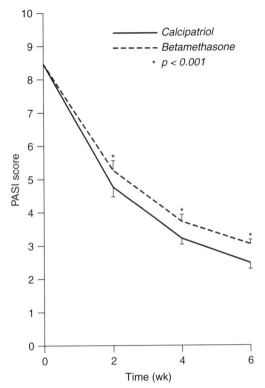

The figure shows a common but unsatisfactory modality of analysing PASI scores collected serially in an RCT. The mean score is calculated at different time points and a graph is presented with lines joining the means at the different time points for the experimental and control group. In the graph, 'errors' bars are attached at each time point and an indicator of statistical significance is placed by each time point to summarise the results of separate significance tests. The curve joining the means may not be a good descriptor of a typical curve for an individual and no account in the analysis is taken of the fact that measurements at different time points are from the same subjects and are likely to be correlated. The number of statistical tests performed and the choice of time points to be tested are additional problematic issues. Further, dividing the results into 'significant' and 'not significant' introduces an artificial dichotomy into serial data.

Source: Reproduced from Kragballe *et al.*,[46] with permission from Elsevier.

Figure 14.1. Problematic analysis of PASI score over time

of a typical curve for an individual and the separate analyses of different time points does not convey information on how individual subjects respond over time. Moreover, this practice can be criticised on statistical grounds because of multiple potentially data-driven statistical tests and because the values over time are not independent and one time point is likely to influence successive time points.[28] It should be noticed that the information from each patient might be diluted when comparing the mean, or better the median, of indexes such as PASI in different treatment groups. In addition, the score of patients who leave the study prematurely and are lost to follow-up cannot be evaluated and the 'intention-to-treat' analysis may be difficult to perform. In this respect, the use of simple clinical variables (e.g., the number of total or partial remissions) could be more informative. A remedy has been proposed for the analysis of serial measurements. In the first stage, a suitable summary of the response in each individual, such as a rate of change or an area under the curve, is identified and calculated. Subsequently, these summary measures are analysed by simple statistical techniques.[28]

In conclusion, the situation of outcome evaluation for many skin disorders could be briefly summarised as follows. (1) Doctor-centrism: considerably more attention has been given to the dermatologists' views on treatment effects than to those of the patients. (2) Biologic reductionism: most of the interest has been concentrated on skin involvement. Only recently have psychological and social factors relevant to outcome been appraised. (3) Process, i.e., what happens along the way, rather than outcome: assessment of involved areas by 'objective' quantitative indexes has been preferred to hazarding definition of synthetic relevant outcomes (e.g., clearing).

PHASE I AND PHASE II STUDIES

The ordered development of treatment modalities according to well-identifiable phases[29] is the exception rather than the rule in dermatology. There are several reasons for this situation. Many treatments are non-pharmacological interventions (e.g., ultraviolet phototherapy) which do not need to comply with the regulatory requirements for drug development, and there are no strict guidelines on how to assess them at an early clinical phase. Secondly, in spite of being so common, the resources allocated to the study of skin disorders are limited as compared with other clinical areas. As a consequence, our understanding of pathomechanisms is limited, as it is the development of disease-specific therapy. Until the causation of the main skin disorders is unravelled, disparate therapies with imprecisely defined biological activities will continue to be available and many treatments will enter the therapeutic arena serendipitously. It was the case of a renal-transplant recipient with psoriasis whose skin lesions cleared with cyclosporine that led to studies demonstrating the efficacy of that drug.[30] Similar considerations can be made for such treatment modalities as topical vitamin D in psoriasis

or the use of minoxidil in androgenetic alopecia. It is widely accepted that a phase I study is one that examines the initial introduction of a drug in human beings with the treatment tested either in normal volunteers or in patients. The main issues are the pharmacokinetics, pharmacodynamics and tolerability of the drug being tested with a focus on assessing inter-patient variability. While problems with systemic drugs in dermatology do not differ from those usually encountered in other speciality areas, some peculiarities exist with the assessment of topical drugs. Penetration within the deep epidermal layers and dermis is a parameter of particular interest since it clearly affects the local activity of the drug itself. On the other hand, pharmacokinetic parameters describing such a penetration are less stringent as compared with systemic drugs. The assessment can be performed on normal or diseased skin. Relevant methods are those which allow measurements of the concentration of the drug in the skin, in a given time, after topical application, while concentration gradients are formed. Such profiles are usually obtained by direct invasive techniques (e.g., skin biopsy) using topically applied radiolabelled drugs. In some instances, a close correlation has been documented between the barrier function of the horny layer, its reservoir function and the resulting penetration into the skin. Penetration into human skin can thus be predicted from drug quantification in horny layer strippings. This allows non-radioactive methods of drug dosage, like high-performance liquid chromatography, to be applied. Indirect measurements such as urinary excretion or blood levels are also analysed as parameters indicative of the systemic adsorption of the drug and possible toxicity. In many instances, it may be of interest to perform penetration studies in the same patient with the drug being applied on the involved versus the uninvolved skin. Whenever the horny layer barrier is disrupted, penetration within the diseased area is usually facilitated. In addition to adsorption, tolerability of a locally applied drug may be of interest. This is usually evaluated by studying local reactions with increasing concentrations of the drug. All the above-mentioned studies are usually conducted on a few healthy subjects or voluntary patients and in an uncontrolled way. Measurement error is a crucial issue, which needs standardisation and careful evaluation at the design level.

For a limited number of topical drugs pharmacodynamic parameters have been developed. An example is the blanching or vasoconstriction assay, which has been employed to screen new topical steroids for clinical efficacy. The bioavailability of steroids from topical formulation has been rather improperly defined as the relative absorption efficiency of a drug, as determined by the release of the steroid from its formulation. Its subsequent penetration through the stratum corneum and viable epidermis into the dermis would produce the characteristic blanching effect. This effect is measured through scores that have a subjective component and need careful standardisation. There have also been some attempts to identify biologic pharmacodynamic markers of some chronic skin disorders like psoriasis to be used at an early stage of drug development.[31] However, these indexes are based on cross-sectional studies and there is still limited information on their modifications with disease activity.

According to the Food and Drug Administration (FDA) regulations, a phase II study is the first controlled clinical study that evaluates the effectiveness of a drug for a given specific therapeutic use in patients. It is also the first study to evaluate the risks of a drug's side effects. Such a study is typically a well-controlled, very closely monitored trial that tests a relatively small, narrowly defined patient population, usually numbering no more than a few hundred patients. If the criterion is the number of patients recruited, then most randomised clinical trials in dermatology would come under this definition.

Study designs that are frequently employed at a preliminary stage in drug development are *within-patient control studies*, i.e., crossover and self-controlled studies or simultaneous within-patient control studies. In dermatology they are also used, albeit improperly, at a more advanced stage. In a survey of more than 350 published RCTs of psoriasis (unpublished data), a self-controlled design accounted for one-third of all the studies examined and was relied on at any stage in drug development. Crossover studies are studies where patients are randomly allocated to study arms, where each arm consists of a sequence of two or more treatments given consecutively. These trials allow the response of a subject to a given treatment A to be contrasted with the same subject's response to treatment B. There are some inconsistencies with the definition of self-controlled studies provided by different authors. We consider as self-controlled studies those clinical trials where patients act simultaneously as their own control. A prerequisite for this kind of study is the existence of pair organs, e.g., eyes, which can be treated by a locally applied drug in the lack of any significant systemic effect. From our definition we exclude either those studies where a single treatment is administered to patients and a 'before–after' comparison is carried out, and the so-called 'N-of-one' RCTs, where different time periods are randomised in a single patient to different treatment.

The main advantage of a within-patient study over a parallel concurrent study is a statistical one. A within-patient study obtains the same statistical power with far fewer patients, while at the same time reducing problems of variability between the populations confronted. Within-patient studies may be useful when studying conditions that are uncommon or show a high degree of patient-to-patient variability. On the other hand, within-patient studies impose restrictions and artificial conditions, which may undermine validity and generalisability of results and may also raise some ethical concern. The washout period of a crossover trial as well as the treatment schemes of a self-controlled design, which entails applying different treatments to various parts of the body, do not seem to be fully justifiable from an ethical point of view. In fact, they don't satisfy the principle of providing the patients enrolled in clinical trials with the best-proven diagnostic and therapeutic method. By necessity these studies are restricted to the evaluation of short-term outcomes. A higher degree of collaboration from

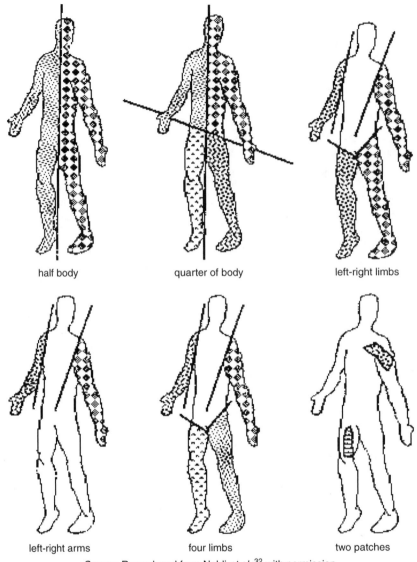

half body   quarter of body   left-right limbs

left-right arms   four limbs   two patches

Source: Reproduced from Naldi *et al.*,[32] with permission.

Figure 14.2. Design of intra-patient comparison in 26 trials concerning dithranol short-contact therapy of psoriasis

the patients is requested as compared with other study designs. Clearly, the impractical treatment modalities in self-controlled studies or washout period in crossover studies may be difficult for the patient to accept. In this kind of study the number of dropouts may be higher when compared to parallel group designs. In a survey of

26 self-controlled trials on short-contact dithranol in psoriasis (Figure 14.2), which had a median number of 16 patients (range 5 to 63), half of the trials experienced dropout.[32] Dropouts may have more pronounced effects in a within-patient study as compared to other study designs because each patient contributes a large proportion of

the total information, and the design is sensitive to departure from the ideal plan. The situation is compounded in self-controlled studies where the dropping out from the study may be caused by observing a difference in treatment effect between the parts in which the patient has been 'split up'. In this case, given that dropouts are related to a difference in treatment effect between interventions, the estimate of the effect of the intervention could be incorrect and falsely equalised. There are several more problems to be considered. Contamination of treated areas and systemic absorption may complicate the interpretation of self-controlled studies, while crossover studies require that the disease lasts long enough to allow the investigator to expose patients to each of the experimental treatments and measure the response. Also the treatment must be one that does not permanently alter the disease or process under study. Carry-over and period effects may clearly compound the analyses.[33] Generalisability is an issue of concern in within-patient controls. Not only entry criteria are usually greatly restricted, e.g., symmetrical lesions, but also outcome measures need to be selected among those reflecting short-term changes in disease activity. Such issues as patient satisfaction and quality of life are obviously beyond the scope of a self-controlled design. It is surprising that self-controlled designs have been the preferred design in situations like topical immunotherapy of alopecia areata or short-contact therapy of psoriasis where patient satisfaction and maintenance of effects over time (e.g., maintenance of the hair restoration to an acceptable extent) are vitally important.

PHASE III TRIALS

From phase III studies we request randomised trials that gather additional information regarding the effectiveness and safety of a treatment, under conditions which are closer to the usual clinical practice as compared with phase II trials. They should study those clinical outcomes that are of major interest to physicians and patients (as opposed to those driven by surrogate end points) and last longer than phase II trials. The distinction between phase II and phase III trials is blurred in dermatology, where most randomised trials are small and, being short-term, employ surrogate measures in well-selected groups of patients. A few points are worth mentioning when discussing the design of phase III studies in the area of dermatology.

PATIENT MOTIVATION AND PREFERENCE

It has already been mentioned that one of the main concerns of patients suffering from a skin disorder is the visibility of lesions and, much more than in other areas, the patient self-monitors his/her disease. Patients' motivations and previous experience are obvious crucial points when entering a trial. Motivations and expectations are likely to influence clinical outcome of all treatments, but they may have a more crucial role in situations where 'soft end points' are of concern as in dermatology. Commonly, more than 20% of the patients entering randomised clinical trials of psoriasis experience improvement on placebo independently of the initial disease extension. Motivations are equally important in pragmatic trials where different packages of management are evaluated, such as in the comparison of a self-administered topical product for psoriasis with hospital-based therapy like phototherapy. Traditionally, motivation is seen as a characteristic of the patient that is assumed not to change with the nature of the intervention. However, it has been argued that it is more realistic to view motivation in terms of the 'fit' between the nature of the treatment and the patient's wishes and perceptions, especially with complex interventions that require the patient's active participation. We have already mentioned that the boundary between disease and non-disease is particularly shady in dermatology. On the other hand, the public is confronted with a great deal of uncontrolled and sometimes misleading or unrealistic messages on how to improve the body's appearance. All in all, there is a need to ensure that patient information and motivations are taken into proper consideration when designing and analysing clinical trials on skin disorders. The issue is not only a matter of 'informed consent'. There is a need to study the influences that determine patients' preferences and to understand how these may affect the outcome of clinical trials. A distinction should be drawn between an informed choice based on factual data–such as a reliable estimate of the risks and benefits of interventions–and attitudes towards treatment based on emotional aspects and preconceptions. In recent years, a number of design variants on the traditional randomised trial have been proposed to take into account patients' preferences. They include the partially randomised patient preference design and the so-called randomised consent or Zelen design.[34] These designs have never gained wide acceptance and none have ever been used in dermatology. The shift from a paternalistic attitude, whereby enrollment decisions are made by doctors, to the choice freely exercised by individual patients is likely to affect the composition of populations in clinical trials. However, when agreement to enrol is based on patients' preferences for individual treatments, as in the Zelen design, the group assembled is unlikely to mirror the target population of all the eligible patients. There is a need to study the influences that determine patients' preferences and understand how these may influence the final outcome of a trial. In a recent survey, Dutch patients affected by psoriasis considered the safety issue and long-term management as more important than fast clearing.[16] It was also important to them to have a vote in the selection of the treatment. It is worth mentioning that the large majority of RCTs in psoriasis are short-term studies dealing with short-term clearance rates that are assessed by the treating physicians. There is room for testing study designs that allow for different preference assessment strategies.

ENTRY CRITERIA

The definition of the study population is of particular importance in dermatology where large variations in disease severity and different clinical subgroups may exist–e.g., plaque versus guttate psoriasis. In addition, there may be problems with variations in disease severity over time. This is commonly observed with chronic inflammatory skin diseases characterised by a relapsing course such as atopic dermatitis or psoriasis. in situations where a variable time-course of the clinical condition is expected, it may be advisable to proceed with sequential evaluations using standardised criteria to judge the stability of the disease over time. Quite surprisingly, information about the stability of the clinical condition is often neglected in clinical trial reports. A review that focused on the selection of patients with psoriasis examined more than 60 clinical trials between 1988 and 1989[21] and documented that information about the stability of the condition was missing in more than 70% of the studies.

Exclusion criteria have the function of selecting the 'more suitable' patients among all possible candidates (e.g., excluding patients in whom the treatment under investigation is contraindicated). This selection also has the aim of reducing factors of variability in the study population, in order to maximise the chance of detecting and quantifying the treatment effect (e.g., excluding patients who are too young or too old). The best way to provide an account of the selection process is a log that lists the included and excluded patients and specifies the reasons for exclusion. This is rarely found in clinical trial reports concerning skin disorders. An example of how far exclusion criteria may operate and limit the possibility of generalising the study results is offered by a clinical trial on the effectiveness of a Chinese herbal extract called 'Dabao' in the treatment of alopecia androgenetica.[35] Among the 3000 patients available to take part in the trial, only 396 were eventually selected to be randomised in the treatment or placebo group. Such exclusion must be a warning when interpreting the actual effectiveness of Dabao on males affected by alopecia androgenetica. It is quite plausible that a similar selection process operates in many RCTs concerning skin disorders.

PLACEBO USE

There are still controversies about the use of placebo in randomised control trials. It is widely accepted that 'in any medical study every patient should be assured of the best proven diagnostic and therapeutic method'. As a consequence, the use of placebo should be proscribed when a 'proven' therapeutic method exists. In spite of these principles, studies which breach the ethical principle are still commonly conducted with the approval of regulatory agencies and institutional review boards. It is widely accepted that placebo-controlled trials have high internal validity, but they may be difficult to apply to clinical practice in situations where alternative interventions of proven efficacy already exist. In these circumstances, the information of clinical value is the effect size of the new intervention as compared with the alternative treatment strategy. The use of placebo may sometimes undermine the validity of the study if the treatment falls short of patients' expectations, resulting in reduced compliance and a large dropout rate. Some years ago a placebo-controlled trial was published on the effect of ebastine, an H_1 receptor antagonist, in chronic urticaria.[36] A number of other non-sedative antihistamine drugs of proven efficacy were available when the trial was conducted. One might argue that it is unethical to deprive the patients in the placebo group of any effective therapy, even if only for a limited time (14 days in this study). As a matter of fact, the authors reported a high number of dropouts due to the lack of effect in the placebo group. A remark on the possible misinterpretation of the results of placebo-controlled trials comes from this study. The authors' conclusion that 'ebastine represents an effective and well tolerated alternative to other non-sedative antihistamine drugs in the treatment of chronic urticaria' is likely to be true but far from proven.

Researchers may have a number of different options for their choice of placebo or comparison intervention in randomised clinical trials but, in practice, many regulatory agencies still consider placebo controls as the 'gold standard'. Placebo controls are usually required for the evaluation of symptom relief or short-term modification of disorders of moderate severity even when an alternative treatment is available. The usual

but questionable claim that justifies this practice from an ethical point of view is that withholding the active therapy does not necessarily affect the long-term prognosis. The above-mentioned issues of symptomatic relief and moderate severity disorders are commonly encountered in dermatology and, in fact, a large number of placebo-controlled RCTs are conducted in this area even when alternative therapies exist. The results of delaying or withholding the treatment may not be straightforward in dermatology. However, there is no question that an extraordinary large number of similar molecules employed for the same clinical indications can be found in this area. These molecules are mostly assessed in placebo-controlled RCTs rather than in comparative RCTs. Examples include topical steroids, oral antihistamines, antifungal drugs and topical antibacterial drugs. More than 200 treatment modalities were identified in a recent survey of published clinical trials of psoriasis with only a few comparative trials. There is a need to establish criteria for the use of placebo in dermatology. They should be developed with the active and informed participation of the public and should be considered by review boards and regulatory agencies. Pragmatic randomised trials contrasting alternative therapeutic regimens are urgently needed to inform clinical decisions.

TIME FRAME FOR EVALUATION AND OUTCOME MEASURES IN CONTEXT

This discussion will focus on chronic inflammatory skin disorders like psoriasis or atopic dermatitis. There is a necessary link between the time frame for evaluation and the measures adopted to assess clinical response; therefore the two issues should be dealt with together. Many chronic inflammatory skin diseases do not necessarily have a progressive deteriorating course, but they may vary in severity over time causing problems that are similar to those encountered with many psychiatric disorders and some rheumatic diseases. Whenever a definite cure is not reasonably attainable, it is common to distinguish between short, intermediate (usually measurable within months) and long-term outcomes. We have already mentioned that clearing the disease in the short term is different from maintaining clearance over time, and long-term results are not simply predictable from short-term outcomes. Most of the score systems available for skin disorders seem to fit best with the clearance issue. On the other hand, it is not easy to define what represents a clinically significant long-term change in the disease status. This is an even more difficult task than defining outcome for other clinical conditions, such as cancer or ischaemic heart diseases, where mortality or major hard clinical end points (e.g., myocardial infarction) are of particular interest. In the long-term, the way the disease is controlled and the treatment side effects are vitally important. It has been documented that compliance with the duration of the treatment is limited and is worst with topical treatments.[16] Measures of the quality of life appear rather attractive. However, what represents an important change for most quality of life measures is imprecisely defined especially if one considers a long-term time frame for evaluation. Clearly, treatment effects can be seen from different perspectives and several dimensions can be taken into account. However, in view of the limitations of the available measures in the long term, simple and cheap outcome measures applicable in all patients seem to be preferable. These may include the number of patients in remission, the number of hospital admissions or ambulatory consultations and major disease flare ups. Dropouts merit special attention. In chronic inflammatory skin diseases that lack hard end points, they may strongly reflect dissatisfaction with treatment. Whatever the outcome measure adopted, dropouts cannot simply be ignored because the patients who do not provide PASI, Disability or Quality of Life scores might be different from those who do. Analysis by randomised group irrespective of subsequent changes is the method recommended for the analysis of clinical trials. This analysis poses special problems when relying on quantitative scores. It is suggested that every effort should be made to ensure that patients have a complete assessment at withdrawal and are followed up. If some categorical outcome variable is also considered, e.g., hospital admission, the relation between the score value at withdrawal and the final outcome may be explored.

OTHER ISSUES

The most precise definition of the profile of an intervention requires a perspective on the risks and benefits, which is wider than the one usually provided by any single RCT. For many chronic skin diseases, efficacy data are derived from short-term RCTs, whereas patients tend to be treated over years. The main issues of safety and long-term effectiveness are usually addressed in the context of observational studies, i.e., phase IV studies. One of the best examples of such a study is the PUVA follow-up study, a cohort study of more than 1400 patients who had received a first course of PUVA-treatment in 1977. These patients are still being followed up and provide information on disease associations and prognostic factors. The study pointed to a dose-related increased risk of non-melanoma skin cancer in PUVA-treated patients. We lack similar studies for many other systemic treatments of psoriasis, including methotrexate, retinoids and cyclosporine. The safety profiles of most systemic antihistamines are also imprecisely defined. Observational studies may represent the most feasible way to study the usefulness of long-term treatment strategies for chronic inflammatory skin diseases, when disease modification rather than symptom control becomes a desired outcome. As has been proposed for some rheumatologic disorders, e.g., rheumatoid arthritis, drug survival, etc. the interval individual patients remain on an agent may offer an indication for long-term acceptability that takes into account adverse effects, lack or loss of effect and patients' preference.

A final mention should be made of those activities that aim at summarising the results of several RCTs on the same issue. There is a large burden of small RCTs[13] addressing disparate clinical questions, as well as a lack of consensus

Table 14.3. List of the systematic reviews on skin conditions already available, or in an advanced stage of development, in the Cochrane Library (*Cochrane Skin Group, August 2000*)

Completed reviews
Surgical treatments for ingrowing toenails
Topical treatments for fungal infections of the skin and nails of the foot
Minocycline for acne vulgaris: efficacy and safety
Interventions for guttate psoriasis
Systemic treatments for metastatic cutaneous melanoma
Antistreptococcal interventions in the treatment of guttate and plaque psoriasis

Reviews undergoing the editorial process
Drug treatments for discoid lupus erythematosus (DLE)
Laser resurfacing for the improvement of facial acne scarring

Protocols under conversion to reviews
Systemic treatments for fungal infections of the skin of the foot
Antihistamines for atopic eczema
Interventions for toxic epidermal necrolysis (TEN)
Complementary therapies for acne
Local treatments for common warts
Interventions for photodamaged skin
Interventions for chronic palmoplantar pustular psoriasis

Source: Reproduced from the Cochrane Library.

on the management of many skin disorders. This creates an increasing emphasis on systematic reviews, and a Cochrane Skin Group has been established within the Cochrane Collaboration in 1997. A list of systematic reviews already available within the Cochrane Library is reported in Table 14.3.

In the light of the increasing role systematic reviews may play with informing clinical practice, special care should be devoted to setting priorities so that the most important questions are addressed first. Otherwise, they would risk amplifying the irrelevant issues. The importance of the involvement of consumers cannot be underestimated. The first analyses from systematic assessment of published RCTs point to some 'peculiarities' of dermatology that have already been discussed in the previous sections, and include among others:

1. The 'moving boundary' between cosmetology and medicine.
2. The need to develop study designs that address questions posed by chronic recurrent diseases.

3. The limitations of available outcome measures that neglect patients' needs and expectations.
4. Problems with external generalisability like the lack of adequate description of the study populations and study settings.
5. The lack of comparative RCTs.
6. The overwhelming role of pharmaceutical industries with defining priorities.

REFERENCES

1. McKenna KE, Stern RS. The outcomes movement and new measures of the severity of psoriasis. *J Am Acad Dermatol* (1996) **34**: 534–8.
2. Webster GF. Is dermatology slipping into its anecdotage? *Arch Dermatol* (1995) **131**: 149–50.
3. Vermeer BJ, Gilchrest BA. Cosmeceuticals – a proposal for rational definition, evaluation, and regulation. *Arch Dermatol* (1996) **132**: 337–40.
4. Peckham PE, Weinstein GD, McCullough JL. The treatment of severe psoriasis: A national survey. *Arch Dermatol* (1987) **123**: 1303–7.
5. Farr PM, Diffey BL. PUVA treatment of psoriasis in the United Kingdom. *Br J Dermatol* (1991) **124**: 365–7.

6. Doshi A, Zaheer A, Stiller MJ. A comparison of current acne grading systems and proposal of a novel system. *Int J Dermatol* (1997) **36**: 416–18.

7. Motley RJ, Finlay AY. Practical use of a disability index in the routine management of acne. *Clin Exp Dermatol* (1992) **17**: 1–3.

8. Zeigher RS, Heller S, Mellon MH, Forsythe AB, Hamburger RN, Schatz M. Effect of combined maternal and infant food-allergen avoidance on development of atopy in early infancy: a randomized study. *J Allerg Clin Immunol* (1989) **84**: 72–89.

9. Arshad SH, Matthews S, Gant C, Hide DW. Effect of allergen avoidance on development of allergic disorders in infancy. *Lancet* (1992) **339**: 1493–7.

10. Frederiksson AJ, Peterssonn DC. Severe psoriasis: oral therapy with a new retinoid. *Dermatologica* (1978) **157**: 238–44.

11. Phillips T, Stanton B, Provan A, Lew R. A study of the impact of leg ulcers on quality of life: financial, social, and psychological implications. *J Am Acad Dermatol* (1994) **31**: 49–53.

12. Moffatt CJ, Franks PJ, Oldroyd M, Bosanquet N, Brown P, Greenhalgh RM, McCollum CN. Community clinics for leg ulcers and impact on healing. *BMJ* (1992) **305**: 1389–92.

13. Williams HC, Seed P. Inadequate size of 'negative' clinical trials in dermatology. *Br J Dermatol* (1993) **128**: 317–26.

14. Lehmann HP, Robinson KA, Andrews JS, Holloway V, Goodman SN. Acne therapy: a methodologic review. *J Am Acad Dermatol* (2000) **47**: 231–40.

15. Naldi L, Svensson A, Diepgen T, Elsner P, Grob JJ, Coenraads PJ, Bavinck JN, Williams H. European Dermato-Epidemiology Network. Randomized clinical trials for psoriasis 1977–2000: the EDEN survey. *J Invest Dermatol* (2003) **120**: 738–41.

16. Van de Kerkhof PCM, De Hoop D, De Korte J, Cobelens SA, Kuipers MV. Patient compliance and disease management in the treatment of psoriasis in the Netherlands. *Dermatology* (2000) **200**: 292–8.

17. Day S. Commentary: Treatment allocation by the method of minimisation. *Br Med J* (1999) **319**: 947–8.

18. Boateng F, Sampson A, Schwab B. Statistical analysis of possible bias of clinical judgements due to observing an on-therapy marker variable. *Stat Med* (1996) **15**: 1747–55.

19. Christiansen JV, Holm P, Moller R, Reymann F, Schmidt H. Etretinate (Tigason) and betamethasone valerate (Celeston valerate) in the treatment of psoriasis. A double-blind, randomized, multicenter trial. *Dermatologica* (1982) **165**: 204–7.

20. Weinstein GD. Safety, efficacy and duration of therapeutic effect of tazarotene in the treatment of plaque psoriasis. *Br J Dermatol* (1996) **135** (Suppl): 32–6.

21. Petersen LJ, Kristensen JK. Selection of patients for psoriasis clinical trials: a survey of the recent dermatological literature. *J Dermatol Treat* (1992) **3**: 171–6.

22. Ashcroft DM, Li Wan Po A, Williams HC, Griffiths CEM. Clinical measures of severity and outcome in psoriasis: a critical appraisal of their quality. *Br J Dermatol* (1999) **141**: 185–91.

23. Marks R, Barton SP, Shuttleworth D, Finlay AY. Assessment of disease progress in psoriasis. *Arch Dermatol* (1989) **125**: 235–40.

24. Feldman SR, Fleischer AB Jr, Reboussin DM, Rapp SR, Exum ML, Clark DR, Nune L. The self-administered psoriasis area and severity index is valid and reliable. *J Invest Dermatol* (1996) **106**: 183–6.

25. Krueger GG, Feldman SR, Camisa C, Duvic M, Elder JT, Gottlieb AB, *et al.* Two considerations for patients with psoriasis and their clinicians: what defines mild, moderate and severe psoriasis? What constitutes a clinically significant improvement when treating psoriasis? *J Am Acad Dermatol* (2000) **43**: 281–3.

26. Husted JA, Cook RJ, Farewell VT, Gladman DD. Methods for assessing responsiveness: a critical review and recommendations. *J Clin Epidemiol* (2000) **53**: 459–68.

27. Norman GR. Issues in the use of change scores in randomized trials. *J Clin Epidemiol* (1989) **42**: 1097–105.

28. Matthews JNS, Altman DG, Campbell MJ, Royston P. Analysis of serial measurements in medical research. *Br Med J* (1990) **300**: 230–5.

29. Temple R. Current definitions of phases of investigation and the role of the FDA in the conduct of clinical trials. *Am Heart J* (2000) **139**: S133–5.

30. Krueger GG. Psoriasis therapy–observational or rational? *New Engl J Med* (1993) **328**: 1845–6.

31. Gottlieb AB. Product development for psoriasis: Clinical challenges and opportunities. In: Roenigk HH, Maibach HI, eds, *Psoriasis*, 3rd edn. New York: Marcel Dekker (1998) 421–33.

32. Naldi L, Carrel CF, Parazzini F, Cavalieri d'Oro L, Cainelli T. Development of anthralin short-contact therapy in psoriasis: survey of published clinical trials. *Int J Dermatol* (1992) **31**: 126–30.

33. Louis TA, Lavori PW, Bailar JC, Polansky M. Crossover and self-controlled designs in clinical research. *New Engl J Med* (1984) **310**: 24–31.

34. Lambert MF, Wood J. Incorporating patient preferences into randomized trials. *J Clin Epidemiol* (2000) **53**: 163–6.

35. Kessels AG, Cardynaals RL, Borger RL, Go MJ, Lambers JC, Knottnerus JA, Knipschild PG. The effectiveness of the hair-restorer 'Dabao' in males with alopecia androgenetica. A clinical experiment. *J Clin Epidemiol* (1991) **44**: 439–47.

36. Peyri J. Ebastine in chronic urticaria: a double-blind placebo-controlled study. *J Dermatol Treat* (1991) **2**: 51–3.

37. Gupta MA, Johnson AM, Gupta AK. The development of an Acne Quality of Life scale: reliability, validity, and relation to subjective acne severity in mild to moderate acne vulgaris. *Acta Dermato-Venereol* (1998) **78**: 451–6.

38. Finlay AY. Quality of life measurement in dermatology: a practical guide. *Br J Dermatol* (1997) **136**: 305–14.

39. Charman C, Williams H. Outcome measures of disease severity in atopic eczema. *Arch Dermatol* (2000) **136**: 763–9.

40. Emerson RM, Charman CR, Williams HC. The Nottingham Eczema Severity Score: preliminary refinement of the Rajka and Langeland grading. *Br J Dermatol* (2000) **142**: 288–97.

41. Ashcroft DM, Li Wan Po A, Williams HC, Griffiths CEM. Quality of life measures in psoriasis: a critical appraisal of their quality. *J Clin Pharm Ther* (1998) **23**: 391–8.

42. Kantor J, Margolis DJ. Efficacy and prognostic value of simple wound measurements. *Arch Dermatol* (1998) **134**: 1571–4.

43. Lindholm C, Bjellerup M, Christensen OB, Zederfeldt B. Quality of life in chronic leg ulcer patients. An assessment according to the Nottingham Health Profile. *Acta Dermato-Venereol* (1993) **73**: 440–3.

44. Faust HB, Gonin R, Chuang TY, Lewis CW, Melfi CA, Farmer ER. Reliability testing of the dermatology index of disease severity (DIDS). An index for staging the severity of cutaneous inflammatory disease. *Arch Dermatol* (1997) **133**: 1443–8.

45. Chren MM, Lasek RJ, Quinn LM, Mostow EN, Zyzanski SJ. Skindex, a quality of life measure for patients with skin disease: reliability, validity, and responsiveness. *J Invest Dermatol* (1996) **107**: 707–13.

46. Kragballe K, Gjertsen BT, De Hoop D, Karlsmark T, van de Kerkhof PC, Larko O, Nieboer C, Roed-Petersen J, Strand A, Tikjob G. Double-blind, right/left comparison of calcipotriol and betamethasone valerate in treatment of psoriasis vulgaris. *Lancet* (1991) **337**: 193–6.

PSYCHIATRY

15

Overview

B.S. EVERITT

Biostatistics and Computing Department, Institute of Psychiatry, King's College, London, UK

The mentally ill have always been with us–to be feared, marvelled at, laughed at, pitied or tortured, but all too seldom cured.

Alexander and Selesnick, *The History of Psychiatry*, 1967. (Allen & Unwin, Sydney, Australia)

INTRODUCTION

In his dictionary of psychology, the late Professor Stuart Sutherland defines psychiatry as 'the medical speciality that deals with mental disorders'. An almost equally brief definition appears in Campbell's Psychiatric Dictionary, namely, 'the medical speciality concerned with the study, diagnosis, treatment and prevention of behaviour disorders'. In terms of either definition it would appear that psychiatry has a long history; Pythagoreans, for example, employed a form of music therapy with emotionally ill patients,[1] and Aretaeus (AD 50–130) observed mentally ill patients and did careful follow-up studies on them. As a result, he established that manic and depressive states often occur in the same individual and that lucid intervals generally exist between manic and depressive periods.

But a thousand years on such a seemingly enlightened approach to the mentally ill had been largely abandoned in favour of viewing the insane as wild beasts who should be kept constantly in fetters. Indeed according to Foucalt,[2] 'madness borrowed its face from the mask of the beast'. In early medieval times beating, incarceration and restraint were the 'treatments' endured by the majority of the mentally ill. Insanity was almost universally regarded as a spiritual trial which one had to undergo as a punishment for vice, a test of faith, or a method of purging sin–a form of Purgatory on Earth–which could be dealt with only by spiritual remedies such as exorcism or being locked up in a church overnight. Gradually other approaches to treatment were introduced although most were equally harsh, bleeding, vomiting and purging for mentally ill patients were common, as were more whimsical forms of treatment such as whirling or spinning a madman round on a pivot. These treatments were in addition to the continued use of manacles and chains for restraint. Apart from their harshness, what these treatments also had in common was that they were mostly ineffective.

It was not until the seventeenth century that the tide of opinion seems to have turned against rough treatment. For example, on 18 July 1646 the Court of Governors of Bethlem Hospital

Textbook of Clinical Trials. Edited by D. Machin, S. Day and S. Green
© 2004 John Wiley & Sons, Ltd   ISBN: 0-471-98787-5

ordered 'that no officer or servant shall give any blows or ill language to any of the mad folks on pain of loosing his place' and at the same hospital in 1677 the Governors propounded a rule that 'No Officer or Servant shall beat or abuse any Lunatik, nor offer any force to them, but upon absolute, Necessity, for the better governing of them'. As a substitute for coercion, some institutes housing the insane began to offer kindness, attention to health, cleanliness and comfort. Reformers such as John Monro pioneered the introduction of 'moral treatment' which stressed the value of occupation to combat the dangers of idleness, and the need for patients to be dealt with tenderly and with affection. Such an approach was now considered to be more likely to restore reason than harshness or severity.

But although there was an increasing desire for caring to replace constraint in dealing with the mentally disturbed, drugs such as corium, digitalis, antimony and chloral were still used to quieten patients, replacing physical fetters with pharmacological ones. And despite the best efforts of the advocates of the moral treatment approach, asylums housing the insane often remained depressing and degrading places until well into the twentieth century, as is illustrated by the following account of a visit by a newly appointed psychiatrist in 1953 to the chronic ward of a mental hospital in Cambridge in the United Kingdom:

> I was taken in by someone who had a key to unlock the door and lock it behind you. The crashing of keys in the lock was an essential part of asylum life then just as it is today in jail. This led into a big bare room, overcrowded with people, with scrubbed floors, bare wooden tables, benches screwed to the floor, people milling around in shapeless clothing. There was a smell in the air of urine, paraldehyde, floor polish, boiled cabbage and carbolic soap – the asylum smell. Some wards were full of tousled, apathetic people just sitting in a row because for twenty years the nurses had been saying 'sit down, shut up'. Others were noisy. At the back of the ward were the padded cells, in which would be one or two patients, smeared with faeces, shouting

obscenities at anybody who came near. A scene of human degradation.

And, as we shall see in the next section, several new twentieth century treatments were equally as harsh as those used 200 years earlier, and in the main, almost equally ineffective in producing a cure. One positive change from earlier times, however, was that now some clinicians began to take the first small steps to evaluating treatments scientifically by making qualitative and quantitative observations and measurements. Empiricism was, at last, about to play a role in psychiatric practice.

PSYCHIATRIC TREATMENT AND ITS EVALUATION: THE EARLY TWENTIETH CENTURY

In the 1920s Dr Henry A. Cotton[3] proposed a theory relating focal infection to mental disorders, in particular the functional psychoses. According to Dr Cotton:

> The so called functional psychoses we believe today to be due to a combination of many factors, but the most constant one is the intracerebral, bio-chemical cellular disturbance arising from circulating toxins originating in chronic foci of infection, situated anywhere in the body, associated probably with secondary disturbance of the endocrin system. Instead of considering the psychosis as a disease entity, it should be considered as a symptom, and often a terminal symptom of a long continued masked infection, the toxaemia of which acts directly on the brain.

Dr Cotton identified infection of the teeth and tonsils as the most important foci to be considered, but the stomach and in female patients, the cervix could also be sources of infection responsible, according to Dr Cotton's theory, for the mental condition of the patient. The logical treatment for the mentally ill resulting from Dr Cotton's theory was surgical elimination of the chronically infected tissue, all infected teeth and tonsils certainly and for many patients, colectomies. Additionally female patients might require enucleation of the cervix, or in some cases complete removal of fallopian tubes and ovaries. Such treatment was, according to Dr Cotton, enormously successful with, out of 1400 patients treated, only 42 needing to remain in hospital.

The focal infection theory of functional psychoses was not universally accepted, neither were the striking results said to have been obtained by the removal of these infections. So in 1922 Drs Kopeloff and Cheney[4] of the New York State Psychiatric Institute undertook a study to investigate Dr Cotton's proposed treatment in the spirit of, in their own words: 'an approach free from prejudice and without preconceived ideas as to the possible results'. To achieve this laudable if somewhat pious aim, Kopeloff and Cheney planned their study in the form of an experiment. All the patients were divided into two groups as nearly identical as possible. All members of one group received operative treatment for foci of infection in teeth and tonsils, while members of the other group received no such treatment and consequently could be regarded as controls. No doubt Kopeloff and Cheney's study would have been hard pressed to have gained ethical approval today, but despite its ethical and probable scientific limitations it did produce results (summarised here in Table 15.1) that cast grave doubts over removal of focal infections as a treatment for some types of mental illness, and indirectly at least, drove a nail into the coffin of Dr Cotton's theory as to the cause of these conditions.

Dr Cotton's suggested treatment for patients with functional psychoses was severe, but not more so than other 'physical therapies' which became popular in the 1930s and 1940s. Insulin coma, for example, required patients to be given large doses of insulin which, by lowering the blood sugar, induced a comatose state from which they would be rescued by a large dose of glucose (if they were amongst the lucky ones–some patients died). According to Sargant and Slater,[5] (reproduced with permission of Elsevier Science) 'reliable statistics are mostly in favour of the treatment', although this claim needs to be considered alongside their recommendation as to how to select patients for treatment:

> It is rarely indeed that facilities will exist for the treatment by a full course of insulin of all schizophrenics coming under observation, and it is therefore important not to waste the treatment on patients not very likely to respond while denying it to the favourable cases.

Perhaps the most severe of the physical therapies was a lobotomy, where the brain was cut with a knife. The operation was pioneered by Egas Moniz, a Lisbon neurologist, and later taken up enthusiastically by psychiatrists such as William Sargant of St. Thomas's Hospital in the United Kingdom. Evaluation of the effectiveness of the therapy was largely anecdotal, and even an enthusiast such as Sargant knew that the operation was often performed at a price:

> It is probable that the highest powers of the intellect are affected detrimentally, and if the patient shows little sign of this in his day-to-day behaviour it may be because the daily routine of existence makes little call on his best powers. We recognise too that temperamental qualities also are not unaffected, that

Table 15.1. Results from Kopeloff and Cheney's study[4]

	Demential praecox		Manic depressive	
	Controls	Operated	Controls	Operated
Number of cases	15	17	15	9
Recovered	–	–	5	4
Improved	5	5	8	1
Total benefited	5	5	13	5
Unimproved	10	12	2	4
Left hospital	3	5	6	3

the reduction in self-criticism may lead to tactless and inconsiderate behaviour, and that the more immediate translation of thought and feeling into action can show itself in errors of judgement. The damage, once done, is irreparable...

Sargant and Slater[5]

Both insulin therapy and lobotomies were slowly phased out as treatments for the mentally ill, but another of the physical therapies introduced in the mid-twentieth century, electric shock (ECT), remains in use to this day largely because it has been found to be effective in a number of studies (see next section). This treatment, introduced by Cerletti and Bini, consists of producing convulsions in a patient by means of passing an electric current through two electrodes placed on the forehead. The idea that such convulsions might help the mentally ill patient was not new; as long ago as 1798, for example, Weickhardt had recommended the giving of camphor to the point of producing vertigo and epileptic fits.

ECT was (and is) used primarily in the treatment of patients with severe depression. Early claims for its effectiveness bordered on the miraculous. Batt,[6] for example, reported a recovery rate of 87%. Fitzgerald[7] was only slightly less optimistic, suggesting the figure was 78%. In neither report however was there any attempt to gather data on recovery rates in concurrent controls. Despite this, other psychiatrists accepted the quoted recovery rates as an indication of the effectiveness of ECT. Typical is the following quotation from Napier:[8]

It is a remarkable advance that a type of case in which the outlook was formerly so problematical can now be offered with some confidence the prospect of restoration in a matter of weeks.

(Reproduced with permission of the British Journal of Psychiatry)

Some researchers attempted to evaluate ECT by comparing their results with those from historical controls or from concurrent patients who for one reason or another had not been offered the treatment of choice (ECT). But such studies largely only illustrated the weaknesses of such

an approach. That by Karagulla,[9] for example, compared results for six groups of patients. Two groups, men and women, had been treated at the Royal Edinburgh Hospital for Mental and Nervous Disorders in the years 1900–39 (before the advent of ECT). The other four groups had been treated in the years 1940–48, two (men and women) by ECT and two others (men and women) not using ECT. It requires little imagination to suppose that the historical controls seen during the period 1900–39 are of little use in evaluating ECT; any difference between the recovery rates for the periods 1900–39 and 1940–48 in favour of the latter could be explained by many other factors than treatment with ECT. The differences between the ECT groups and the concurrent controls are also virtually impossible to assess since the decision to use ECT on a patient was a subjective one by the clinicians involved. There is no way of knowing whether the treated and untreated groups are comparable.

But the evaluation of treatments in medicine in general and psychiatry in particular was about to be placed on a scientifically far firmer footing, by the introduction and then the increasing use and acceptance of the controlled clinical trial.

PSYCHIATRIC TREATMENTS AND THEIR EVALUATION: THE 1950s ONWARDS

Kopeloff and Cheney's study of removal of focal infections as a treatment for particular forms of mental illness has many aspects of a modern clinical trial, although it is missing that most essential component, random allocation. Kopeloff and Cheney decided themselves in regard to each patient whether they should be operated on or whether they should be a control.

It was Fisher who recognised the need for randomisation to treatment groups in medical, biological and agricultural experiments, and the eventual adoption of the principle into the evaluation of treatments has led to what Sir David Cox has called 'the most important contribution of 20th Century statistics', the randomised controlled clinical trial. In such trials patients are assigned to treatment groups according to chance. Prior to Fisher's randomisation principle being adopted, most of the early studies to compare competing treatment for the same condition involved arbitrary, non-systematic schemes for deciding which treatment a patient would receive. The first trial with a properly randomised control group was that for streptomycin in the treatment of pulmonary tuberculosis, carried out by Bradford Hill in 1947. The first psychiatrist to advocate the use of Fisher's experimental approach in the evaluation of psychiatric treatments, particularly the physical treatments, appears to have been Lewis.[10] (Reproduced with permission from Oxford University Press) In his paper he criticises past studies and of a controlled trial he concludes:

> An organised experiment would demand much that has not hitherto been practicable, including voluntary acceptance by independent hospitals and clinics of an agreed procedure for the selection, management, evaluation of mental state, and follow-up investigation of treated, as well as of control cases. Such an experiment, as R.A. Fisher (1942) has demonstrated, requires much forethought and self-discipline on the part of those who carry it out.

For many psychiatrists practising at the time this was not altogether welcome news. The physical therapies, such as insulin coma and psychosurgery remained in use, with advocates of these treatments retaining their enthusiasm, apparently untroubled by the usual requirements of rational scientific scepticism. Demands that clinical trial methodology be adopted to evaluate treatments whose effectiveness most psychiatrists already took for granted, fell largely on deaf ears.

But slowly matters did improve. In the early 1950s Miller and his colleagues randomly allocated ten schizophrenic patients to each of three alternative treatments, ECT, Pentothal and Pentothal plus non-convulsive stimulation, and assessed them before treatment began, after the cessation of treatment, and then again two weeks later.[11] Although the sample size was totally inadequate to demonstrate any significant treatment

differences, the use of randomisation represented a great improvement over earlier studies.

Other small trials of ECT were reported in the 1950s but it was not until 1965 that the MRC published the results of the first large-scale trial of the treatment. This was a multicentre trial involving 55 clinicians and 269 patients. As well as demonstrating the effectiveness of ECT in the treatment of depression, the MRC trial also showed that a large multicentre trial in psychiatry was feasible. The trial did, however, have some critics. In a letter to the *British Medical Journal*, Sargant[12] wrote:

> There is no psychiatric illness in which bedside knowledge and long clinical experience pays better dividends; and we are never going to learn how to treat depressions properly from double-blind sampling in an MRC statistician's office.
>
> (Sargant W Antidepressant drugs. Br Med J. (196) **1**; 1495. Reproduced with permission from the BMJ Publishing Group)

At the end of the 1940s and the beginning of the 1950s, the physical treatments introduced into psychiatry 30 years earlier still formed the core of most psychiatrists' treatment armoury. But matters were about to change; in the 1950s several entirely new types of drugs were to be introduced in psychiatric practice. In the main the discovery of these drugs was not based on a scientific knowledge of brain chemicals, rather their discovery was for the most part serendipity, resulting from acute observations made by clinicians such as Henri Laborit (the effects of the antihistamine promethazine, from which developed chlorpromazine), and John Cade who first described the value of lithium in manic depression by observing its effect on a number of patients. The tricyclic antidepressants and the Selective Serotonin Reuptake Inhibitors (SSRIs), which had fewer side effects in treating depression, were also discovered in the 1950s. Finally, almost by accident, Leo Sternback in 1957 identified the benzodiazepines for treating mild anxiety.

The need to establish whether or not these newly discovered compounds were effective in treating mentally disturbed patients greatly increased most psychiatrists' appreciation of the need to use clinical trials for evaluating treatments. And after 1960 the increasing need to satisfy regulatory authorities (prior to 1960 only the USA had such a body overseeing the introduction of new drugs into general use, but the thalidomide tragedy changed the situation dramatically) meant that the randomised controlled clinical trial has now become established as the 'gold standard' for evaluating competing therapies, although even as late as 1963 some psychiatrists were unwilling to accept that such an approach was necessary; this is from the preface of a 1963 edition of Sargant and Slater[5] commenting on controlled clinical trials:

> If they fail to demonstrate any differences between a placebo and a drug which everybody knows to be effective, this means only that the work has not been done well enough.

Fortunately it is difficult to imagine such a view being expressed in a major psychiatric text nowadays. Over the last 40 years the use of clinical trials in psychiatry, particularly for evaluating new drugs, has become widespread. A quotation from one of the psychiatric champions of this approach, Michael Shepherd,[13] remains almost the perfect model for the modern scientific view that psychiatrists should have in the evaluation of psychotropic drug therapies in particular, and in the evaluation of psychiatric treatments in general:

> The clinician is compelled to hold the balance between the scales of laboratory data on the one hand and stochastic theory on the other. Though his experience and judgement are essential it will be necessary for him to adopt a more experimental role in the future if he is to co-operate fully with the pharmacologist and the statistician whose techniques he should understand if full weight is to be given to observations made in the clinical setting.
>
> (Shepherd, 1959, reproduced with permission)

SUMMARY

Treatment of the mentally ill has made giant strides in the last 50 years. Drug treatment of schizophrenia, depression and anxiety disorders have, in randomised clinical trials, been found to be effective and have done much to alleviate the misery of these conditions. Drug treatment of mental illness works by altering in some way the chemistry of the body. Chlorpromazine, for example, has been shown to interfere with the action of the neurotransmitter dopamine. But the modern view of mental illness, that it has both psychological and physical dimensions, implies that effective treatment must aim to ease the suffering of the mind as well as correcting possible abnormalities of chemistry. And so, in the 1970s, behavioural psychotherapy began to be used to treat particular disorders. More recently cognitive therapy has been introduced. This provides a simple, straightforward treatment regimen which lasts weeks rather than years, and above all permits the patients to make sense of, and thus hopefully control, their psychological problems.

Clinical trials in psychiatry initially involved the evaluation of drug treatments. More recently, however, psychological therapies have been subjected to the rigours of the randomised clinical trial, and there has been a growing awareness that the theoretical and logistical problems of such trials differ from those of the average drug trial. Consequently three of the chapters in this section concentrate on clinical trials of psychological treatments as now used in psychiatry. In Chapter 17 Katherine Shear and Philip Lavori discuss the many problems associated with assessing treatments for anxiety, in particular how interventions work in the community settings where they will eventually be used. In Chapter 18 Nicholas Tarrier and Til Wykes give a masterly overview of how clinical trials have been used to evaluate the effectiveness of cognitive behavioural treatments of psychosis. Finally in Chapter 19 Graham Dunn considers the many issues that arise in applying clinical trial methodology to the use of psychotherapy for treating depression. The difficulties of undertaking clinical trials in this area are clearly identified in all the papers, but these difficulties should be seen as a challenge to psychiatrist and statistician alike, in what must been seen as the long term goal of alleviating the misery that is mental illness.

REFERENCES

1. Gordon BL. *Medicine Throughout Antiquity*. Philadelphia: Davies (1949).
2. Foucalt M. *Madness and Civilization: A History of Insanity in the Age of Reason*. London: Tavistock (1967) (transl. from the French by Richard Howard; originally published as *Histoire de la Folie*).
3. Cotton HA. The etiology and treatment of the so-called functional psychoses. Summary of results based upon the experience of four years. *Am J Psychiat* (1922) **2**: 156–91.
4. Kopeloff N, Cheney CO. Studies in focal infection: its presence and elimination in the functional psychoses. *Am J Psychiat* (1922) **2**: 139–56.
5. Sargant W, Slater E. *An Introduction to Physical Methods of Treatment in Psychiatry*. Edinburgh: Livingstone (1944).
6. Batt JC. One hundred depressive psychoses treated with electrically induced convulsions. *J Mental Sci* (1943) **89**: 289–96.
7. Fitzgerald OWS. Experiences in the treatment of depressive states by electrically induced convulsions. *J Mental Sci* (1943) **89**: 73–80.
8. Napier FJ. Death from electrical convulsion therapy. *J Mental Sci* (1944) **90**: 875–8.
9. Karagulla S. Evaluation of electrical convulsion therapy as compared with conservative methods of treatments of depressive states. *J Mental Sci* (1950) **96**: 1060–91.
10. Lewis AJ. On the place of physical treatment in psychiatry. *Br Med Bull* (1946) **3**: 22–34.
11. Miller DH, Chang J, Cumming E. A comparison between unidirectional current non-convulsive electrical stimulation given with Reiter's machine, standard alternating current electron shock (Cerletti method) and pentothal in chronic schizophrenia. *Am J Psychiat* (1953) **189**: 226–40.
12. Sargant W. Antidepressant drugs. *Br Med J* (1965) **1**: 1495.
13. Shepherd M. Evaluation of drugs in the treatment of depression. *Can Psychiat Assoc J* (1959) **4**: 120–8.

16

Alzheimer's Disease*

LEON J. THAL AND RONALD G. THOMAS

Department of Neurosciences, University of California San Diego, San Diego, CA 92037, USA

BACKGROUND

HISTORY

Descriptions of patients with dementia appear in the Bible, Roman and Greek writings, and Shakespeare. However, it was not until the early portion of the 20th century that Alzheimer's disease (AD) was identified as a specific disease entity. The index case, Frau Auguste D, a 50-year-old woman, was admitted to the Frankfurt Insane Asylum in 1901 (see Table 16.1, time-line). She was found to be suffering from a pre-senile dementia with memory loss, generalised cognitive impairment, delusions and hallucinations. Upon her death in 1906, brain examination revealed generalised cerebral atrophy and two microscopic lesions called plaques and tangles.[1] The disease was subsequently named 'Alzheimer's disease' by Kraepelin.[2] However, Kraepelin, the dominant figure of the day, defined AD as a presenile dementia occurring between the ages of 40 and 60 so that individuals who had similar clinical presentations in their later

years were considered to not have AD. Thus, AD was considered to be a rare disorder causing only presenile dementia.

Over the succeeding decades, advances were made largely based on pathological studies of AD. Amyloid-like staining was noted by Dirvy.[3] Terry[4] and Kidd[5] described the ultrastructure of the neurofibrillary tangle as a paired helical filament. In 1968, Blessed et al.[6] carried out autopsies in an elderly cohort and found cerebral atrophy as well as plaques and tangles. These authors concluded that these elderly subjects had AD and that there was no difference between early-onset and late-onset AD.

At that time, the prevailing opinion in the United States was that dementia after age 65 was primarily due to cerebral atherosclerosis. It was not until the mid-1970s that physicians and scientists in the US recognised that most elderly individuals with dementia suffered from AD. Katzman[7] noted the high prevalence of dementia and pointed out that AD was the fourth most common cause of death in the US. At the same time, modern neurochemical techniques were applied to the study of AD brain tissue. Three laboratories independently described the loss of cholinergic markers in AD.[8-10] At the same time,

* Supported by Alzheimer's Disease Cooperative Study Grant #AGO 10483.

Textbook of Clinical Trials. Edited by D. Machin, S. Day and S. Green
© 2004 John Wiley & Sons, Ltd ISBN: 0-471-98787-5

Table 16.1. AD timeline

1907	Index case, Frau Auguste D described by Alzheimer
1910	Kraepelin calls AD a rare presenile dementia
1927	Dirvy identified amyloid in the plaque
1963	Terry and Kidd describe the ultrastructure of the neurofibrillary tangle
1975	NIA established–AD is its primary focus
1976/77	Selective loss of cholinergic markers reported in AD
1976	Katzman reports that AD is the fourth leading cause of death in the US
1980	Alzheimer's Association formed
1984	Glenner sequences amyloid and postulates that it causes AD
1984	NIA initiated Alzheimer Centers programmes
1987	First gene for AD on chromosome 21
1991	Alzheimer's Disease Cooperative Study funded by NIA
1992	Presenilin 1 mutation on chromosome 14 for early-onset AD
1993	Tetrahydroaminoacridine (Cognex), first cholinesterase inhibitor is marketed
1993	Apo E_4 allele identified as a risk factor for late-onset AD
1995	Presenilin 2 mutation on chromosome 1 for early-onset AD
1996	Donepezil (Aricept), second AChE inhibitor, marketed
1997	Vitamin E and selegiline delay time to endpoints in AD including progression of disease
2000	Rivastigmine (Exelon), third AChE inhibitor, marketed

the National Institute on Aging (NIA) was formed in 1975 and its first director, Dr Robert Butler, identified AD as the most important disease of aging. In 1980, the Alzheimer's Association was formed to represent public interest in this disorder. It has subsequently grown to more than 250 national chapters.

Initially, the NIA focused on the funding of individual investigator grants and some programme project grants. Developments occurred rapidly, and in 1984, Dr George Glenner isolated amyloid from the blood vessel wall of Alzheimer tissue and postulated that amyloid was the causative agent of AD.[11] By 1987, the first gene for early-onset familial AD, which later was found to be the β-amyloid precursor protein gene, was linked to chromosome 21.[12] In 1993, an association was reported between the presence of the E_4 allelic variant of apolipoprotein E and the development of AD.[13] This was the first genetic risk factor described for late-onset AD. In the same year, the first acetylcholinesterase (AChE) inhibitor, tetrahydroaminoacridine (Cognex) was approved and marketed. This drug was developed based on the empirical observation of a decrease in cholinergic functioning originally made in 1976. During

this same time, two additional genes coding for presenilin 1, located on chromosome 14, and presenilin 2, located on chromosome 1, were found to be responsible for additional families with early-onset AD.[14,15] Additional cholinesterase inhibitors were approved in 1996 and 2000. In 1997, the first trial demonstrating a delay in time to endpoints was published using the antioxidant, vitamin E, and the monoamine oxidase inhibitor, selegiline.[16]

By 1984, the NIA recognised the need for the study of well-characterised brain tissue for patients with AD. It initiated the Alzheimer's disease centres programme by funding five centres in 1984 with gradual growth of the centres' programme to 30 by 2000. In 1991, the NIA also funded the Alzheimer's Disease Cooperative Study (ADCS) with a mandate to both develop new instrumentation for the testing of patients with AD and to carry out clinical trials for promising agents that would not be tested by the pharmaceutical industry, such as compounds lacking patent protection, compounds in the public domain for the treatment of other disorders, and molecules derived from individual investigator laboratories or small biotechnology companies.

Over the past four decades, interest in AD has markedly increased. Funding has increased to approximately $400 million per year by the Federal government. Citations in Index Medicus have increased from fewer than 100 in 1970 to more than 3000 per year by 2000.

EPIDEMIOLOGY

Epidemiological studies of AD have been extremely useful in defining prevalence, incidence and risk factors. Numerous prevalence studies have been carried out in the US, Europe and China. Overall, these studies indicate that the prevalence of AD is under 1% below the age of 65. After age 65, the prevalence rises rapidly, doubling with every five-year epoch. The prevalence exceeds 30% by age 90 (see Kawas and Katzman[17] for a review).

Epidemiological studies have also been useful in defining both risk and protective factors for the development of AD (Table 16.2). The most important risk factor is age. A second important risk factor is family history. This was recognised by Heston et al.[18] who noted that the cumulative risk for AD was significantly higher for parents and siblings of patients than for the general population as a whole. This finding has been subsequently confirmed by many other individuals.[19,20] The discovery of early-onset AD families further strengthened the importance of genetics as a risk factor. Finally, the association of the apo E, E$_4$ allele and AD represents a genetic risk for late-onset AD. In addition, a number of more minor risk factors have been identified including female sex, head injury and low education.

Table 16.2. Risk factors for AD

Major risk factors	Protective factors
Age	Higher education
Positive family history	NSAIDs
AD genes	Oestrogens
Minor risk factors	**Non-risk factors**
Low education	Aluminium
Head trauma	Vascular disease
Female sex	

Epidemiological studies have also identified the use of non-steroidal anti-inflammatory drugs (NSAIDs) and oestrogens as potential protective factors (see Kawas and Katzman[17] for a review). These epidemiologic observations plus studies on the basic biological mechanisms of NSAIDs and oestrogens led to the development of several clinical drug trials designed to determine whether or not NSAIDs or oestrogens can either slow the rate of decline in patients with established AD or prevent AD in normal elderly.

Epidemiological studies have also been useful in determining that exposure to aluminium and cerebrovascular disease are not associated with the development of AD.

GENETICS

Genetic inheritance of AD and familial clustering was first reported in the 1950s[21] and 1960s,[22] then confirmed in a pathological series in the 1970s.[23] Inheritance was complex but appeared to be autosomal dominant in a small proportion of cases, inherited as a complex trait in up to 50% of the population and sporadic in the remainder. Since these initial studies were carried out, inheritance for early-onset AD has been confirmed in patients carrying mutations for APP, presenilin 1 and presenilin 2. In addition, late-onset AD has been linked to the apo E, E$_4$ allele as a risk factor gene. Thus, at present, approximately one-half of known AD cases may have some underlying genetic component.

PATHOLOGY

The macroscopic pathology of AD consists primarily of cerebral atrophy and dilatation of the ventricles. The hallmarks of the disease are two microscopic lesions. The first, neurofibrillary tangles, are intraneuronal paired helical filaments consisting predominantly of hyperphosphorylated tau protein. The second is the senile plaque, a pathological inclusion in the neuropil consisting of damaged neuritic endings, compact and diffuse amyloid, and other proteins. The number of both plaques and tangles correlates moderately well with the degree of dementia. There is also a significant neuronal loss and loss of synapses. The loss of synapses correlates best with the severity of dementia (see Terry *et al.*[24] for a review).

PATHOGENESIS AND AETIOLOGY

At the present time, the cause of AD remains unknown. However, the best hypothesis at present is that misprocessing of amyloid and its deposition in the brain results in nerve cell damage followed by loss of neurons and the dementia syndrome. Data supporting this hypothesis is derived from studies of early-onset familial AD families. Individuals carrying obligate genes for AD on chromosomes 1, 14 and 21 all develop AD at an early age. In addition, fibroblasts transfected with DNA from these individuals either produce excess amounts of both a-beta 1-40 and 1-42 or undergo a shift in the ratio of a-beta production favouring the production of more a-beta 1-42. This shift is important since a-beta 1-42 is highly insoluble and represents the predominant form of a-beta present in the senile plaque. Individuals carrying one or two apo E_4 alleles also appear to deposit more a-beta in their brains than individuals lacking an E_4 allele. Finally, individuals with Down's syndrome carry an extra copy of chromosome 21, have three genes for amyloid, and overproduce this protein. All develop the pathological features of AD if they live long enough. Thus, the deposition of amyloid appears to be the central feature in the pathogenesis of AD. However, this hypothesis awaits formal testing (see Selkoe[25] for a review).

HISTORY OF CLINICAL AD TRIALS PRIOR TO 1976

Prior to the discovery of a cholinergic deficiency in the brains of patients with AD, drugs chosen for clinical testing in AD were chosen based on the premise that cerebrovascular insufficiency caused AD. Thus, numerous therapeutic modalities were tried including: vasodilators, anticoagulants, hyperbaric oxygen and cerebral metabolic-enhancing agents known as nootropics. None of these agents were proven to be efficacious for the treatment of AD, although the use of ergoloid alkaloids, a class of agents with both cerebral metabolic-enhancing and vasodilating activity, did produce a minor degree of improvement on subjective rating scales. With the demonstration of a cholinergic deficiency in AD, development of these compounds in the US largely ceased.

GENERAL ISSUES IN AD CLINICAL TRIALS

DIFFICULTY OF DIAGNOSIS

There are many problems associated with the development of drugs and the conduct of clinical trials in AD. At present, there is no biological marker for the disease during life. Thus, clinicians are never 100% certain of the diagnosis. However, recent clinicopathological series reveal that the diagnostic accuracy for AD now generally exceeds 80% and approaches 90%, especially for cases selected for clinical drug trials.[26-29] More recently, approximately 15–20% of AD patients have also been found to have extrapyramidal features. Examination of their brains reveals the presence of neocortical and subcortical Lewy bodies as well as abundant plaques but few tangles indicating the presence of dementia associated with Lewy bodies.[30-32] Thus, in any contemporary trial, approximately 10% of individuals will turn out to have another disease at autopsy and approximately 20% will have Lewy bodies accompanying the neuropathological changes of AD.

PATIENTS

Patients with AD always have memory impairment as the core feature. However, many other features may be present such as difficulties with language, praxis, visuospatial relations and behaviour. There is substantial heterogeneity in the clinical presentation of the patient population. In addition, patients decline at varying rates over time which leads to increased variability in response measures. These differences in patient population characteristics and change over time are largely responsible for the need to include reasonably large samples in AD clinical trials.

ENDPOINTS

The endpoints studied in AD clinical trials depend primarily on the question being asked in the trial. Early trials of cholinesterase inhibitors were designed to detect treatment–placebo differences in cognition over relatively short periods of time. For these trials, the primary endpoints consisted of a cognitive measure to determine the specificity of the agent on important cognitive endpoints and a clinical global impression to make certain that the overall effect was sufficiently robust to be clinically significant. Trials examining agents designed to alter the rate of decline have generally used a difference in slope or a difference at endpoint in cognitive and global measures. One recent trial used the time to development of functional endpoints such as institutionalisation, death, loss of activities of daily living (ADL) or progression to a more severe stage of dementia as a composite endpoint.[16] Finally, in primary and secondary prevention trials where enrolled patients are either normal or mildly cognitively impaired upon enrollment, the time from enrollment to diagnosis of AD is often used as the endpoint.

SURVIVAL ANALYSIS IN AD

While the use of endpoint differences and changes in the rate of decline are currently the most frequent approach being used in many AD studies, the use of survival analysis is becoming increasingly frequent. There are a number of inherent advantages to survival analysis in AD. First, endpoints can be real-life events rather than artificial constructs such as the amount of change on a psychometric test. Events such as death and institutionalisation require little interpretation and clearly possess face validity. Second, survival analysis naturally allows the combination of multiple endpoints; also, any patient who reaches one

of several prespecified endpoints or who terminates from the study provides useful data. Dropouts for advancing disease in a longitudinal study are less of a statistical problem because information concerning whether or not that individual reached an endpoint may be available. Third, the use of survival analysis allows patients who reach an endpoint (usually the diagnosis of AD) to exit the study and seek alternative treatments without impacting the statistical analysis. This feature may potentially enhance recruitment for long-term, placebo-controlled survival trials. Fourth, survival analysis allows for comparison of the entire group despite varying lengths of follow-up, i.e., no imputation. Fifth, it is usually more informative unless the incidence is low. The potential disadvantage of survival analysis in AD trials is that the time to reach certain endpoints (such as institutionalisation) is likely to be more variable and affected by social support systems than the rate of change on a cognitive measure. Also, if large numbers of patients drop out of the study without reaching the defined study endpoint, the validity of the study may be open to question. Some examples of useful endpoints or milestones in AD patients include death, institutionalisation, loss of basic ADLs, loss of instrumental ADLs and decline in the disease stage.

PHASE 1 TRIALS

Phase 1 trials for AD are carried out to determine the general tolerability of the agent and maximum tolerated dose. These trials commonly utilise fewer than 100 subjects exposed to drug. Early phase 1 trials are generally single dose exposure carried out in normal elderly subjects to determine the maximum tolerated dose. Subsequently, the tolerability of multiple daily doses is evaluated in brief trials lasting for one to two weeks. More recently, trials involving multiple daily dosing have been carried out in early AD patients rather than normal controls in so-called 'bridging studies'. The advantage of this approach is that if the metabolism of the drug differs between AD patients and healthy normal controls, the doses tolerated by AD patients will be found early in the drug development process. Early phase 1 studies focus on tolerability, side effects and pharmacokinetics. Subsequent phase 1 studies are often carried out to look for food interactions and interactions with other commonly used pharmaceutical products.

PHASE 2 TRIALS

Phase 2 trials are classically designed to explore the dose range of an agent and to establish an initial determination of efficacy. They generally utilise 100–500 subjects. Due to the time and cost involved in the drug development process, many sponsors are currently carrying out combined phase 2/3 studies. Most phase 2 studies are carried out as multi-arm, parallel, placebo-controlled trials. The maximum dose used in such a trial is approximately one-half to two-thirds of the maximum tolerated dose determined during phase 1 testing. Two, three or four doses are generally employed and compared to placebo. In some trial designs, an arm of an already-approved agent may be added as a positive control. Most phase 2 trials designed for symptomatic treatment are approximately six months in duration in order to meet both European and US regulatory guidelines. Endpoints in these trials are generally treatment–placebo differences on a cognitive scale, most commonly the Alzheimer's Disease Assessment Scale–Cognitive Component (ADAS-Cog), and a Clinician's Global Impression (CGI).

The number of subjects needed to demonstrate efficacy in clinical trials with continuous response measures depends on the relationship between the effect size sought, the standard deviation of the outcome measure, and other parameters such as type 1 error, type 2 error, drop-out rate, drop-in rate, and base rate for the control group. For example, for a treatment trial seeking to detect a four-point difference on the ADAS-Cog at six months assuming a standard deviation of nine, 100 subjects per group would be required in a two-arm trial with a power of 90% and an alpha (type 1 error) of 5%.

Few phase 2 trials are designed to examine the ability of the agent to slow decline in AD. Such efficacy-oriented studies are infrequently carried out because of the need for a large sample size and long duration. In general, studies designed to slow decline are carried out in phase 3 clinical trials. A few phase 2/3 trials have been carried out in an attempt to look for both cognitive and global improvement and for alteration in the rate of decline over the course of one year. For one-year trials designed to slow decline in AD, using a typical outcome measure in which the standard deviation of the rate of change is equal to the one-year decline, a typical study using 80% power and two-sided testing with an alpha (type 1 error) of 5% would require 63 subjects per group (assuming no drop-outs) comparing drug to placebo for significance to detect a 50% decrease in rate of decline (Table 16.3). Most studies are powered to detect 25–40% decreases in rate of decline and therefore require larger sample sizes.

PHASE 3 TRIALS

Many AD trials are currently carried out as combined phase 2/3 studies. Depending on the number of arms, these trials generally utilise 300–600 subjects per trial. A complete phase 3 programme (for an FDA new drug application) will include at least two pivotal trials and will utilise 1000–3000 subjects to both test efficacy and to determine the side-effect profile of the agent. In recent years, several different trial designs have been utilised. For short-term trials designed to improve cognition, three trial designs have been used: crossover designs, randomised control parallel designs (RCPD) and enrichment designs

Table 16.3. Same size calculations for AD slope trial

Reduction in rate of decline (%)	Subjects per group (N)	Total sample size (N)
25	251	502
50	63	126
75	28	56

(a notable variant of RCPD). The use of the crossover design presents a number of problems for the study of AD patients. This design assumes that there are no carry-over or period effects of the drug and that the treatment response is the same in both periods. This is rarely the case. The major advantage of this design is in the economy of subjects because each subject acts as its own control. However, because AD is not a static disorder but the change is over time, carry-over and period effects are often present and this design is now rarely used. Randomised, controlled, parallel design studies have two major advantages: the control population is concurrent (thus any period effects are balanced) and uncontaminated by drug exposure and there are no period effects. The disadvantage of this design is that more subjects are required to answer the central question. An enrichment design combines features of both crossover and parallel designs. It was used in several cholinesterase inhibitor trials including one of the US multicentre tacrine trials.[33] Patients demonstrating improvement after initial tacrine treatment were withdrawn from drug, washed out, and subsequently randomised to drug or placebo and analysed for response in a double-blind parallel phase. Non-responders were dropped from the trial prior to the double-blind phase, thereby resulting in enrollment of an enriched population in the double-blind phase. While this design has many advantages including individual dose titration for each patient, its major disadvantage is that all subjects are exposed to drug at some point during the study allowing for possible carry-over effects. Also, there is no placebo-treated population throughout the study on which to base an estimate of adverse events in the control population. Thus, parallel, placebo-controlled designs currently predominate in phase 3 symptomatic studies. These studies are similar to the description of phase 2/3 symptomatic studies described above.

Slowing decline in AD remains an important goal since if slowing can actually be accomplished, the treatment effect size will continue to increase with the duration of treatment. Natural history studies indicate that for most commonly used neuropsychological instruments, the annual rate of change is approximately equal to the one-year standard deviation of change. Thus, for the ADAS-Cog, the rate of change is approximately $7.0 +/- 7.8$ points per year.[34] Examination of rate of change studies indicates that the rate of decline on common instruments is reasonably constant during the middle stages of dementia but is slower in early and more severe dementia.[35] The rate of change is predictable for groups but quite variable for individual patients. Rate of decline is likely to be influenced by the distribution of disease subtypes such as the presence of the Lewy body variant of AD.[36] The gene dosage of apo E_4 does not appear to significantly alter the rate of decline over one year.[37] Knowledge of the rate of decline allows for the accurate computation of sample sizes for studies designed to slow cognitive decline in AD. Most contemporary phase 3 studies examining rate of decline in AD are designed to detect group differences of approximately 25–35% since most clinical investigators and AD advocacy groups believe that finding smaller effect sizes would not result in clinically useful drugs.

In addition to trials designed to slow decline in AD, one trial of vitamin E and selegiline[16] utilised survival analysis in a 2×2 factorial design to examine the time to important endpoints in patients with AD. One advantage of the 2×2 factorial design is that two agents can be tested simultaneously. In addition, interactions between the two agents can be examined. A third advantage of this design is that 75% of subjects are randomised to treatment thereby enhancing enrollment. The disadvantage of the 2×2 factorial design is that negative interactions (sub-additivity) can occur thereby reducing the 2×2 factorial design to a four-arm study which results in a significant loss of power in the analysis. In the 2×2 factorial design study of selegiline and vitamin E, the primary endpoint was the time to reach any of the following: death, institutionalisation, loss of basic ADLs and progression from moderate to severe dementia. Although this study was useful in determining that treatment could cause a delay in the time to these endpoints, this trial design could not resolve the issue as to whether or not the delay in the time to endpoints resulted as a consequence of drug treatment alone or a change in brain structure as a consequence of the potential neuroprotective effect of these two agents.

In an attempt to intervene earlier in the course of the disease, individuals with mild cognitive impairment (MCI) are currently being studied. Patients with MCI generally present with a memory complaint. When evaluated, they demonstrate the poor recall and rapid forgetting but are otherwise generally normal with respect to cognitive functioning and ADLs. However, patients identified with MCI convert to AD at a rate of 12–15% per year. In contrast, unselected normal subjects over the age of 65 develop AD at a rate of only 1% per year.[38] This high rate of conversion has allowed for the development of clinical trials of a reasonable size using the MCI patient population. The endpoint of such clinical trials is the time to development of clinically diagnosable AD analysed with survival analysis. Several such trials have been initiated recently examining the effects of vitamin E, cholinesterase inhibitors and NSAIDs to delay the time to the development of AD in patients with MCI.

PRIMARY PREVENTION TRIALS

Numerous studies have indicated that AD is uncommon before the age of 65. However, after the age of 65, the prevalence doubles approximately every five years reaching an average prevalence of over 30% by 90 years of age.[39,40] Given that the prevalence doubles every five years, delaying the onset of appearance of the disease by five years would result in a 50% reduction of prevalence in one generation. Delaying onset by 10 years would halve the prevalence again for a total reduction of 75%. Thus, primary prevention would yield the greatest cost benefit.

The earliest pathological changes of AD may occur 20–30 years before the clinical expression of disease.[41] Age-specific incidence of AD increases with aging (Table 16.4).

Table 16.4. Age-specific incidence of AD

Age	Incidence (%)	Cases/1000/yr
65–69	0.6	6
70–74	1.0	10
75–79	2.0	20
80–84	3.3	33
85–89	4.0	40

Thus, several strategies can be considered for primary prevention trials. In the first strategy, healthy individuals would be treated in an attempt to delay the onset of disease. The main advantage of this design is that the results would be generalisable to other healthy individuals. Because of the large sample size and high costs associated with this strategy, enrichment strategies should also be considered. These include enrolling: older subjects, subjects with a positive family history of AD, and subjects at risk because of the presence of an apo E_4 allele. Several primary prevention trials for AD are currently preparing to get underway utilising some of these strategies. A second strategy would be to find subjects who are already randomised to compounds of interest in trials for other indications to which cognitive endpoints could be added. This has already been successfully accomplished within the framework of the Women's Health Initiative (WHI) where approximately 8000 non-demented women over the age of 65 have been enrolled and randomised to hormone replacement therapy (HRT) to determine the effects of these agents on coronary artery disease and osteoporotic fractures. Cognitive endpoints have now been added to this trial to determine the effect of HRT on incidence of dementia. A third approach would be to randomise to drug treatment a non-demented population being studied for another purpose such as an epidemiological study of cardiovascular disease.

If individuals are entered into a study entirely on the basis of age, a large sample size will be required using population-based, non-enriched entry criteria. For example, for individuals at a mean age of 75 who have normal cognition on initial evaluation, dementia will appear at a rate of approximately 1.5% per annum. Over five years, the cumulative incidence of dementia would be 7.5%. For a two-arm study with alpha = 0.05 and power = 80%, 2000 subjects per group would be required to detect a 30% effect size, not accounting for losses secondary to death. With such low incidence, even these large samples will yield only 150 cases of dementia in the untreated group. If a drug reduced the incidence of AD by 50%, 75 cases would exist in the treated group. To allow for losses to follow-up and death, approximately 2500 subjects would be needed per group for a total sample size of 5000. These sample sizes would only allow for an 80% probability of detecting a 30% increase in disease incidence.

Several primary prevention trials to prevent dementia or AD have been initiated with most utilising an enrichment strategy.

1. Women's Health Initiation Memory Study (WHIMS)–8000 normal women >65 years of age randomised to HRT or placebo.
2. Preventing postmenopausal memory loss and Alzheimer's disease with Replacement Estrogens (PREPARE) study–900 normal elderly women with a family history of AD randomised to HRT or placebo.
3. Gingko study–3000 normal elderly subjects (age >75) treated with Ginkgo or placebo.
4. AD Anti-Inflammatory Prevention Trial (AD-APT)–2600 normal elderly subjects with a positive family history of AD randomised to one of two anti-inflammatory drugs or placebo.

MISCELLANEOUS ISSUES

PRIMARY, SECONDARY AND TERTIARY TREATMENTS

Treatment of existing symptoms represents tertiary treatment and is representative of all of the currently approved drugs for AD. Secondary treatment refers to treatment when minimal but not full-blown disease is present. This is best exemplified by the treatment of patients with MCI who have minimal symptomatology. Finally, primary prevention refers to intervention before any

clinical symptoms of disease appear. This will be the ultimate goal in treating AD.

SYMPTOMATIC VS STRUCTURAL CHANGE

Treatments that slow progression in AD may produce underlying structural change within the brain. One could logically reason that if treatment caused slowing of the rate of decline, it may have a permanent underlying effect on the brain. Unfortunately, a change in slope in a measure of cognition is insufficient evidence to prove that an underlying brain structural effect has occurred. Additional trial design manoeuvres must be utilised. The most widely utilised manoeuvre is that of withdrawal. If the effect induced by the drug is purely symptomatic, even though individuals are better at the end of the trial, they should decay back to the curve of untreated subjects when the drug is withdrawn (Figure 16.1). This was clearly demonstrated in the 26-week Aricept trial in which patients were removed from Aricept and cognitive scores dropped to placebo levels after a six-week wash-out.[42] An alternative clinical manoeuvre to demonstrate the same effect would be a randomised start design. In this experiment, half the group is started on drug and half started on placebo. If the drug has a purely symptomatic effect, individuals begun on placebo then crossed over to active drug will 'catch up' to those started on drug at the beginning of the trial. If the drug has a structural effect on the brain, individuals started on drug later in the course of the treatment period will fail to 'catch up'.

In addition to various trial manoeuvres, the demonstration of a structural change within the brain could be used to support a structural effect for a therapeutic agent. For example, in a rate of decline trial, the maintenance of hippocampal volume or the maintenance of a synaptic number, as demonstrated on an imaging study, would serve as a direct demonstration that a pharmacological agent produced a difference in brain structure. Finally, a biochemical marker could be utilised. For example, in Parkinson's disease if a 'dopaminergic sparing' agent were developed,

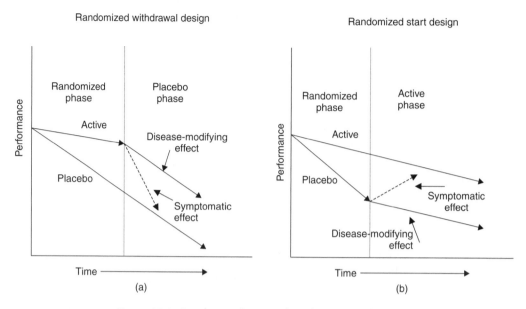

Figure 16.1. Randomised start and randomised withdrawal

it might be reflected in higher homovanillic acid levels in the cerebrospinal fluid after drug withdrawal at the end of the treatment period. For AD, a clear-cut biochemical marker does not yet exist.

N-OF-ONE DESIGN

This manoeuvre is not particularly useful for drug development but is often used in the clinical setting to determine continued response to drug. An example of an N-of-one design in an idealised setting would be to answer the question of whether or not a patient on a cognitive-enhancing agent, such as a cholinesterase inhibitor, is still responding to drug. This question is an important one since AD patients continue to decline while on treatment. After one or two years on treatment, the clinician is faced with the decision as to whether or not to continue treatment. In an idealised version, a patient could be blindly crossed over to placebo to examine for a withdrawal effect. If the patient was on a symptomatic treatment and continuing to respond, a decline in cognition should be observed following drug withdrawal. This manoeuvre could then be followed by blindly restarting the patient on

drug and looking for improvement. In reality, this manoeuvre is often carried out in the clinic with simple withdrawal of the agent, retesting, reintroduction and retesting but without the use of placebo. While still useful, the lack of a blinded crossover to placebo limits the interpretation of the results of this manoeuvre.

ETHICAL ISSUES

At present, available drugs to treat AD are symptomatic. Several agents are currently approved and before enrolling patients in any clinical trial, disclosure and discussion of these agents with the patient and their caregiver is necessary. In addition, vitamin E and selegiline have been reported to delay the time to endpoints in moderately advanced AD patients. The results of the vitamin E study also need to be discussed with patients before enrolling them in clinical trials since the use of both cholinesterase inhibitors and vitamin E is currently the standard of care in the US.

A vigorous debate has emerged in the US regarding the ethics of placebo-controlled trials. Some have argued that placebo-controlled trials are unethical since they deny patients the use of approved agents while enrolled in the trial. Individuals espousing this viewpoint claim that drug development can continue using add-on studies or by demonstrating equivalence of a new agent to an existing agent. Others argue that placebo-controlled trials are ethical since currently available agents are entirely symptomatic and do not alter the underlying course of the disease. In addition, patients are free to not enter placebo-controlled trials if they wish to receive currently approved medications. There is concern that comparator studies may result in the development and licensing of many marginal or ineffective agents since currently approved agents are of marginal efficacy and may produce negative results in some clinical trials. It is possible that if a new agent were compared to an approved agent and the true effect size in the approved agent was minimal, the newly tested drug would be approved even though the effect size may not have been sufficient to warrant approval in a placebo-controlled trial. A major drawback of using active control groups is the requirement of larger sample sizes. At present, most new agents being tested in the US are compared to placebo. If and when agents are developed that can clearly alter the course of the disease, long-term, placebo-controlled trials will become both unethical and socially unacceptable.

REFERENCES

1. Alzheimer A. Uber eine eigenartige Erkrankung der Hirnrinde. *Allgem Z Psychiatr-Gerich Med* (1907) **64**: 146–8.
2. Kraepelin E. *Psychiatrie: ein Lehrbuch fur Studierende und Artze.* Leipzig: Verlag v. Johann Ambrosius Barth (1910).
3. Dirvy P. Etude histochemique des plaques seniles. *J Belge Neurol Psychiat* (1927) **27**: 643–57.
4. Terry RD. Neurofibrillary tangles in Alzheimer's disease. *J Neuropathol Exp Neurol* (1963) **22**: 629–42.
5. Kidd M. Paired helical filaments in electron microscopy of Alzheimer's disease. *Nature* (1963) **197**: 192–3.
6. Blessed G, Tomlinson BE, Roth M. The association between quantitative measures of dementia and of senile change in the cerebral grey matter of elderly subjects. *Br J Psychiat* (1968) **114**: 797–811.
7. Katzman R. The prevalence of malignancy of Alzheimer's disease. *Arch Neurol* (1976) **33**: 217–18.
8. Davies P, Maloney AJF. Selective loss of central cholinergic neurons in Alzheimer's disease. *Lancet* (1976) **2**: 1403.
9. Bowen DM, Smith CB, White P, Davison AN. Neurotransmitter-related enzymes and indices of hypoxia in senile dementia and other abiotrophies. *Brain* (1976) **99**: 459–96.
10. Perry EK, Perry RH, Blessed G, Tomlinson BE. Necropsy evidence of central cholinergic deficits in senile dementia. *Lancet* (1977) **1**: 189.
11. Glenner GG, Wong CW. Alzheimer's disease: initial report of the purification and characterization of a novel cerebrovascular amyloid protein. *Biochem Biophys Res Commun* (1984) **120**: 885–90.
12. St. George-Hyslop PH, Tanzi RE, Polinsky PJ, *et al.* The genetic defect causing familial Alzheimer's disease maps on chromosome 21. *Science* (1987) **235**: 885–90.
13. Corder EH, Saunders AM, Strittmatter W, *et al.* Gene dose of apolipoprotein E type 4 allele and the risk of Alzheimer's disease in late onset families. *Science* (1993) **261**: 921–3.
14. Schellenberg GD, Bird TD, Wijsman EM, *et al.* Genetic linkage evidence for a familial Alzheimer's disease locus on chromosome 14. *Science* (1992) **258**: 668–71.
15. Levy-Lahad E, Wijsman EM, Nemens E, *et al.* A familial Alzheimer's disease locus on chromosome 1. *Science* (1995) **269**: 970–3.
16. Sano M, Ernesto C, Thomas RG, *et al.* A controlled trial of selegiline, α-tocopherol, or both as treatment for Alzheimer's disease. *New Engl J Med* (1997) **336**: 1216–22.
17. Kawas CH, Katzman R. Epidemiology of dementia and Alzheimer's disease. In: Terry RD, Katzman R, Bick KL, Sisodia SS, eds, *Alzheimer Disease.* Philadelphia: Lippincott Williams & Wilkins (1999) 95–114.
18. Heston LL, Mastri AR, Anderson VE, White J. Dementia of the Alzheimer type. Clinical genetics, natural history, and associated conditions. *Arch Gen Psychiat* (1982) **38**: 1085–90.
19. Heyman A, Wilkinson WE, Stafford JA, Helms MJ, Sigmon AH, Weinberg T. Alzheimer's disease: a study of epidemiological aspects. *Ann Neurol* (1984) **15**: 335–41.
20. Amaducci LA, Fratiglioni L, Rocca WA, *et al.* Risk factors for clinically diagnosed Alzheimer's disease: a case–control study of an Italian population. *Neurology* (1986) **36**: 922–31.

21. Sjogren T, Sjogren H, Lindgren GH. Morbus Alzheimer and morbus Pic: a genetic, clinical, and patho-anatomical study. *Acta Psychiat Neurol Scand* (1952) **8**: 9–152.

22. Larsson T, Sjogren T, Jacobsen G. Senile dementia: a clinical, sociomedical and genetic study. *Acta Psychiat Scand* (1963) **39**(Suppl 167): 1–259.

23. Heston LL. The genetics of Alzheimer's disease. *Arch Gen Psychiat* (1977) **34**: 976–81.

24. Terry RD, Masliah E, Hansen LA. The neuropathology of Alzheimer's disease and the structural basis of its cognitive alterations. In: Terry RD, Katzman R, Bick KL, Sisodia SS, eds, *Alzheimer Disease*. Philadelphia: Lippincott Williams & Wilkins (1999) 188–203.

25. Selkoe DJ. Molecular pathology of Alzheimer's disease: the role of amyloid. In: Growdon JH, Rossor MN, eds, *The Dementias* Boston: Butterworth Heinemann (1998) 257–84.

26. Wade JPH, Mirsen TR, Hachinski VC, Fishman M, Lau C, Merskey H. The clinical diagnosis of Alzheimer's disease. *Arch Neurol* (1987) **44**: 24–9.

27. Morris J, McKeel D, Fulling K, Torack R, Berg L. Validation of clinical diagnostic criteria for Alzheimer's disease. *Ann Neurol* (1988) **24**: 17–22.

28. Burns A, Luthert P, Levy R, Jacoby R, Lantos P. Accuracy of clinical diagnosis of Alzheimer's disease. *Br Med J* (1990) **301**: 1026.

29. Galasko D, Hansen L, Katzman R, Wiederholt W, Masliah E, Terry R, Hill LR, Lessin P, Thal LJ. Clinical–neuropathological correlations in Alzheimer's disease and related dementias. *Arch Neurol* (1994) **51**: 888–95.

30. Dickson D, Davies P, Mayeux R, *et al*. Diffuse Lewy body disease. *Acta Neuropathol* (1987) **75**: 8–15.

31. Hansen L, Salmon D, Galasko D, *et al*. The Lewy body variant of Alzheimer's disease: a clinical and pathological entity. *Neurology* (1990) **40**: 1–8.

32. Perry R, Irving D, Blessed G, Fairbairn A, Perry E. Senile dementia of Lewy body type. *J Neurol Sci* (1990) **95**: 119–39.

33. Davis K, Thal L, Gamzu E, *et al*. A double-blind, placebo-controlled multicenter study of tacrine for Alzheimer's disease. *New Engl J Med* (1992) **327**: 1253–9.

34. Thal LJ, Carta A, Clarke WR, *et al*. A one-year multicenter placebo-controlled study of acetyl-l-carnitine in patients with Alzheimer's disease. *Neurology* (1996) **47**: 705–11.

35. Stern RG, Mohs RC, Davidson M, *et al*. A longitudinal study of Alzheimer's disease: measurement, rate, and predictors of cognitive deterioration. *Am J Psychiat* (1994) **151**: 390–6.

36. Klauber MR, Hofstetter CR, Hill LR, Thal LJ. Patterns of decline in the Lewy body variant of Alzheimer's disease. *Arch Psychiat Shanghai News* (1992) **4**(Suppl): 50–3.

37. Growdon JH, Locascio JJ, Corkin S, Gomez-Isla T, Hyman BT. Apolipoprotein E genotype does not influence rates of cognitive decline in Alzheimer's disease. *Neurology* (1996) **47**: 444–8.

38. Petersen RC, Smith GE, Waring SC, Ivnik RJ, Tangalos EC, Kokmen E. Mild cognitive impairment: clinical characterization and outcome. *Arch Neurol* (1999) **56**: 303–8.

39. Rocca WA, Hofman A, Brayne C, *et al*. Frequency and distribution of Alzheimer's disease in Europe. A collaborative study of 1960–1990 prevalence findings. *Ann Neurol* (1991) **30**: 381–90.

40. Evans DA, Funkenstein HH, Albert MS, *et al*. Prevalence of Alzheimer's disease in a community population of older persons. *Am Med Assoc J* (1989) **262**: 2551–6.

41. Braak H, Braak E. Diagnosis of Alzheimer's disease: development of cytoskeletal changes and staging of Alzheimer related intraneuronal pathology. *Neurobiol Aging* (1994) **15**: S141.

42. Rogers SL, Farlow MR, Doody RS, Mohs R, Friedhoff LT. A 24-week, double-blind, placebo-controlled trial of donepezil in patients with Alzheimer's disease. Donepezil Study Group. *Neurology* (1996) **50**: 136–45.

17

Anxiety Disorders

M. KATHERINE SHEAR[1] AND PHILIP W. LAVORI[2]

[1]Western Psychiatric Institute and Clinic, Pittsburgh, PA 15213, USA
[2]VA Medical Center, Menlo Park, CA 94025 2539, USA

INTRODUCTION

Anxiety disorders are the most prevalent psychiatric conditions in the community with a lifetime community prevalence of 20–30%.[1] These disorders can be seriously impairing, reducing quality of life and causing disability. Recent studies suggest some forms of anxiety are associated with early mortality. Many who suffer from anxiety disorders have other serious medical problems, such as depression, pulmonary disease, cardiovascular illness and neurological conditions. Prevalent and debilitating, anxiety disorders are serious, persistent illnesses that warrant treatment. Clinical trials are needed to establish efficacy of promising interventions and to determine the best ways to deliver efficacious treatments in different contexts.

Methods for conducting efficacy trials in anxiety disorders have evolved over the past few decades. Reliable diagnostic instruments and symptom severity scales have been developed and tested. Strategies for medication administration have been identified and manuals written to standardise these procedures. Cognitive behavioural treatment methods have been specified and explained in manualised format. Treatment training and adherence measures are available. These methodological advances mean that studies of the efficacy of new interventions can be conducted efficiently and with confidence.

Given the availability of efficacious treatments, researchers are now turning their attention to studies that test these interventions in the community settings where they will be used, and in clinical contexts (such as maintenance of response) that go beyond the phase of acute illness that is the focus of most efficacy studies. With this shift in focus, new methodological problems appear. Generic problems that need to be addressed in designing such studies, often known as effectiveness studies, have been described in the literature.[2] In this chapter we discuss methodological issues pertaining to effectiveness studies of anxiety disorders. We identify some key features of these disorders and consider the problems they create for study questions and study design. Solutions to methodological problems in clinical trials often require trade-offs, and the problems we discuss are posed in this way. We provide our view of the best way to manage these

Textbook of Clinical Trials. Edited by D. Machin, S. Day and S. Green
© 2004 John Wiley & Sons, Ltd ISBN: 0-471-98787-5

problems, and in some cases, make suggestions for methodological innovations.

Clinical researchers regularly make methodological choices regarding subject recruitment, selection and characterisation of subjects, procedures for enrollment, assignment to experimental group, experimental manipulation, outcome assessment and follow-up process. Methods chosen will place specific limits upon what can be learned from a study. Thus, it is fundamental that study methodology be driven by the question the researcher seeks to answer. However, unlike efficacy studies, in effectiveness studies, the question is not always clear. Defining the study question is the first problem for the effectiveness researcher. Most experienced clinical researchers are expert in conducting efficacy studies to answer the question 'Does a new treatment produce better results than a control condition for a well-defined condition, under tightly controlled circumstances of use?' Both psychosocial and pharmacological treatment researchers have successfully undertaken such studies, and thus are poised to test efficacy hypotheses for new interventions.

The field of effectiveness research is far less developed. Investigators move forward in unmarked terrain as they decide upon the most important next questions. For example, a study of Long Term Strategies in the Treatment of Panic Disorder (MH045963-6) currently in progress under the direction of the authors is designed to answer the question 'Should non-responders to an initial trial of CBT receive medication or an additional dose of CBT?' This important question is not addressed by efficacy studies of either medication or psychotherapy. Having articulated such a question, decisions must be made about what methodological approach should be used, and what problems to anticipate. For example, Principal Investigators of the Long Term Strategies Panic study had to confront the issue of what the right duration of the initial CBT trial might be, and what level of non-response to initial trial should be chosen to define intake into the randomised maintenance trial. Decisions such as these are not trivial, since neither the most important questions, nor the best way to approach a given question, is obvious. Given this ambiguity, we suggest anxiety disorder researchers might be guided by some of the key features of these disorders (Table 17.1). We discuss the methodologic relevance of five such features: (1) anxiety disorders are characterised by high community prevalence; (2) diagnostic boundaries are ambiguous, both between pathological and normal anxiety and among the different anxiety disorders; (3) phobic fear and avoidance is prevalent in these disorders; (4) anxiety disorders are treatable using either medication or cognitive–behavioural interventions; and (5) anxiety disorders frequently co-occur with other disorders. Each of these features will affect decisions about the research question and the choice of methods.

FEATURES OF ANXIETY DISORDERS THAT IMPACT STUDY METHODOLOGY

HIGH COMMUNITY PREVALENCE

Anxiety disorders are highly prevalent in the community. The high prevalence means there are many patients in need of treatment. Epidemiological studies document that most of these patients do not present for care in a specialty mental setting.[3] Instead, they can be found in a range of community service settings. Even among those who do seek specialty mental health treatment, only a subset will be enticed to an academic medical clinic, regardless of the incentives provided. For those who seek treatment at a community mental health setting, usual practice diagnostic procedures cannot be relied upon to identify anxiety disorders.[4] It is clear that we need to know how to recognise and treat the people with anxiety disorders who most researchers never see. Put another way, we need to study those who do not participate in studies. This obvious paradox underscores the principle that effectiveness studies will not be straightforward.

The job is not simply a matter of running an efficacy study in one or more community settings. Doing so would be important only if there are serious questions about whether patients in such settings respond to proven treatments.

If this is the case, it is important to frame the specific questions the study should answer, based on the reasons for predicting response differences. For example, if researchers suspect severity is an important treatment moderator, it might be important to conduct a standard randomised efficacy trial in settings with patients of varying severity. Likewise, some patients have co-occurring symptoms or syndromes, such as serious medical illness, along with an anxiety disorder such as panic disorder. It might make sense to recruit patients from medical clinics into an efficacy trial in order to study the influence of the medical illness on the treatment of the target condition. Other examples of parameters that might be predicted to render uncertain outcome with a proven efficacious treatment include organisational features of the setting or socio-economic status of the patient. Specific considerations like these ought to drive the important design decisions such as where the research will be conducted and in how many different kinds of settings.

A different kind of research question might be driven by the subject paradox (how to study patients who do not participate in studies), for example 'What is the most successful way of recruiting and engaging individuals who do not seek treatment in a research clinic?' The investigator might compare a public education programme to a professional educational intervention. Or, the research aim might focus on evaluating alternative screening strategies in different settings. Another example might be 'How much diversity of setting should be incorporated into a study?' In addressing this question the researcher might investigate the variation of clinical presentation, treatment acceptance, or outcome across different ethnic or socio-economic groups. Alternatively, the investigators might examine the effect of different organisational structures or the impact of the organisational

Table 17.1. Implications of features of anxiety disorders for research design

Feature	Research issues
1. High community prevalence	Settings: which and how many Recruitment: reaching the unstudied patient Assessment: measuring outside the research clinic Awareness: bridging the patient's knowledge gap Human subjects protection: make or buy Technology: the right machine for the setting Comorbidity: adjusting to increased variability
2. Poorly defined nosologic boundaries	Normal vs disordered: a question of excess Differential diagnosis: core symptoms overlap Pluripotency: treatments with broad efficacy Double counting: symptoms Endpoints: ranking outcomes Aiming low: focus on preventing relapse Stability: the time frame for outcome
3. Phobic fear and avoidance	Evasion: measuring the avoidant subject Fear: recruiting the anxious subject Identification: personal choice vs avoidance
4. Discordant models of the disorders	Acknowledgement: both models have treatment successes Control: paying attention to the other intervention Comparing: accommodating preference for modality Targets: agreeing on the goals Dissemination: thinking ahead about the audience

climate[5] on outcomes or study the implementation of organisational interventions to optimise the likelihood of dissemination of a treatment.[6]

Whatever studies are done, it is clear that for anxiety disorders, researchers need to extend their reach if they seek to make an impact on the great majority of individuals who suffer from these conditions. Methods need to be devised to study patients in primary care and specialty medical settings, dental offices, churches, schools, community centres, and a range of other community service or support settings (e.g. domestic violence or homeless shelters, or even highly utilised commercial operations such as supermarkets[7] or department stores). The use of such settings to deliver care may be particularly relevant for patients with anxiety disorders who have phobic restrictions, and are unable to travel outside a restricted area.

Designing a new clinical trial for an anxiety disorder outside of an established research centre raises other problems. Investigators make deliberate decisions about where to recruit, assess and treat patients, as well as whether to carry out any of these activities in more than one kind of setting. Existing clinical research methods for recognising and recruiting affected individuals may be too cumbersome to work in a setting where research activities are not customary. For example, a busy primary care practice or even a mental health facility may not be oriented towards identifying and tracking individuals who meet criteria for anxiety disorders. Frequently staff in such places are very busy, very dedicated and sometimes opinionated about what is best for their patients. The researcher who comes to study usual practice may be seen as challenging the skills, competence or even integrity of the staff. Still, recent studies in primary care[8] have succeeded in overcoming these barriers and have done much to provide information to inform processes to optimise care.

Protocol-driven treatments face additional barriers to acceptance in settings other than the research clinic. Assessment of outcomes is hard enough in a research clinic; assuring good follow-up and reliability of measurement in

non-traditional research settings will tax the ingenuity of the next generation of effectiveness researchers. Recent work using adaptive testing methods holds promise as a technique. Given these challenges, it is tempting to suggest that researchers concentrate on one research setting, and hope or assume that results will generalise. But the decision to limit the setting has uncertain implications for interpreting and generalising results. There is a trade-off between generalisability and the cost of dealing with heterogeneity of setting. These costs must be borne, and the methodological challenges met, in order to produce research-grade answers to the question of effectiveness.

In working in almost any non-mental health community setting, the investigator must address stigma and self-criticism that can be associated with the idea of having a mental disorder. Researchers need to take steps to minimise the difficulties that may be caused by identifying a person as ill, especially when the person in question has not already identified their symptoms as problematic. In such a situation, the news may come as an unwelcome surprise, or may be perceived as insulting or embarrassing. The newly diagnosed individual may feel suddenly stigmatised and this may lead to a rejection of the diagnosis and/or the researcher bearing the news. There may be anger or discouragement towards the community setting in which the person sought help. The researcher needs to be sensitive to these possibilities and proactive in dealing with untoward reactions associated with identification of an anxiety disorder. For example, if there is a decision to recruit subjects in a non-psychiatric setting such as a church or supermarket, the researcher would need to include an introductory phase of the work that addresses fears and stigma associated with a diagnosis. This can be done in a variety of ways. A community educational phase might be undertaken prior to initiation of recruitment. Individual or group consciousness raising might be offered. Focus groups are a very useful strategy being increasingly used by researchers. In this situation, small groups of individuals with different types of anxiety might be invited to participate in a focus group. Participants are paid and the group leader might guide the group in discussion of topics such as the meaning of having an anxiety disorder, the perceived response of others, including family, friends and/or the community at large. A focus group might also be asked to discuss how researchers might best approach undiagnosed people in the community who suffer from these disorders, or the group might be asked how to best present treatment options, or how to explain and encourage participation in research. Thus armed, the researcher will be more successful in recruiting and retaining subjects for a clinical trial. An example of a very innovative approach to the problem of community recruitment[9] utilised an intensive telephone engagement strategy in which mothers of inner city minority children were invited to identify and problem-solve an important difficulty they were experiencing. Only after the intake recruiter had successfully helped with this practical problem did they explain the availability of services for other kinds of problems. This approach was shown to significantly increase attendance at the first clinic appointment. Whatever the approach, it is clear that the prospective patient research volunteer must be given opportunities to understand their anxiety symptomatology as a treatable condition underlying what may be just an awareness of limitation or fear. These individuals further need to decide for themselves which treatment programme they wish to access. The researcher needs to present a clinical trial in this context.

Sometimes stigma can be best addressed at the level of the service provider—such as a primary care physician, or administrators and service providers in different kinds of agencies. In order to access patients in a given facility it may be very important to first understand the headaches of the facility administrators. A researcher who takes the time to both identify and respond to the problems faced by those attempting to deliver care will be rewarded with a much higher level of enthusiasm and support for the research project. Researchers in the field of services research have understood and successfully accomplished this

kind of work.[10] Partnering with administrators in different service agencies to find ways to improve their efforts is likely to provide easier access to subjects and better support for implementation of study procedures. Careful attention to such issues can determine the feasibility of the study.

Assessment Strategies in Community Settings

The standard research diagnostic interview and follow-up batteries were designed to achieve careful, reliable descriptions of different well-specified phenotypes of psychiatric illness. While highly successful in meeting this goal, such instruments have not been designed to maximise efficiency and minimise patient and staff burden. These extensive and time-consuming inventories will not survive transplantation into a primary care setting, a hospital emergency room or a dental office, let alone a church or school. Instead, radically simplified tools must be developed that utilise innovative statistical and psychometric methods (e.g. adaptive testing) and/or study sample sizes must be increased to compensate for extra variance.

The assessment strategy used in a community setting may need to be altered in other ways as well. No matter how prevalent an anxiety disorder may be in the community, it will be lower in the community setting, compared to the prevalence in the enriched intake stream of a specialty anxiety clinic. The odds on a disease may easily vary fivefold or more from clinic to community. Given that the specificity and sensitivity of the diagnostic instruments will be no better in the community setting, and may well be worse, the 'Bayes factor' of the test (sensitivity divided by $1 -$ specificity) will be smaller in the community setting. For example, if the sensitivity and specificity both decline from 90% to 80% then the Bayes factor declines from $0.9/(1 - 0.9) = 9$ to $0.8/(1 - 0.8) = 4$. If both the prior odds of disease and the Bayes factor are lower, the positive predictive value will also be lower (the odds of disease given a positive test are just the prior odds of disease times the Bayes factor). In the numerical example above, given only a fivefold difference in prior odds, the posterior odds on disease given a positive test may vary by an order of magnitude from clinic to community, making interpretation of intake diagnosis problematic. Multi-step diagnostic procedures may be necessary to avoid over-diagnosis.[11]

Research Recruitment

Study subjects volunteer to participate in research. In a clinical trial, the manner of presentation of treatment options may make or break a study. The highly selected population of patients who present to an academic centre often come preconditioned to the value of research protocols, and may have specifically sought out the clinic because of its reputation as a research centre. The potential research volunteer in a community setting has not voted for research 'with his feet', and may need a gradual, informative and upbeat approach, to accept the idea of protocol-driven treatment and randomisation. Institutional review boards may well regard placebo control as especially unattractive in such a context, and may also be concerned about 'overselling' the potential benefits of research to patients. Yet, there is reason to believe that the patient in the community context may be the one with the most to gain from participation in research, because of the likelihood that her illness would otherwise go unrecognised, or the equally disadvantageous likelihood of inadequate treatment.

Context-Relevant Treatment Protocols

To optimise study results, strategies must be developed for providing protocol treatments in a context-relevant manner. This may include adjusting to the absence of third-party payers, or making use of setting-specific para-professional personnel for some of the interventions. Or, it may mean incorporating 'escalation' strategies into the treatment protocol, so that subjects identified with substantial needs are transferred to a more traditional setting.

Practical and Administrative Issues

Human subjects review may need to be coordinated among several kinds of organisations. Some may be willing to enter into agreements to accept the investigator's home institutional review, others may need to develop their own review processes and obtain Federal-Wide Accreditation. Template agreements that have been shown to work would be a valuable resource.

The investigator must choose methods of data capture and processes for the data edit cycle that work in diverse settings at sites that are distant from the coordinating institution. Data monitoring, correction of errors and tracking of follow-up are all affected. Technological limitations need to be respected. For example, fax-based methods may be more easily deployed than internet-based methods, especially in settings where a fax machine is already in use. On the other hand, as personal digital assistants become ubiquitous, patient follow-up may be individualised, remote and remotely cued. We can imagine technology that rings a telephone number or sends an instant message, asking for self-report follow-up, and that can schedule and connect the subject with a live interviewer, all implemented on the same small wireless device, that might be cheap enough to give away as a free incentive to participation.

Despite the difficulties associated with exporting clinical trials to the community, it is clear that the next generation of clinical research in anxiety disorders needs to be rolled out into the settings where individuals with these disorders live and work. In addition to the many issues related to the setting of a study in the community, there are many design considerations related to which patients should be included in a given study. Patients in different community settings are likely to be heterogeneous in different ways, and to differ from patients who seek treatment at traditional research clinics. Existing studies document a high rate of comorbidity among anxiety disorders, between anxiety disorders and depression, and between anxiety disorders and medical illnesses. There is also comorbidity of anxiety disorders with for example psychotic disorders[12] and substance abuse.[13,14] Such comorbidity may increase the likelihood that a patient seeks treatment at research clinics, and therefore it is possible that studies in the community will have to deal with less comorbidity than studies in the research clinic. Nevertheless, an effectiveness researcher must decide how to manage comorbidity. There are many consequences of decisions to include or exclude comorbidities from study eligibility criteria. There are a variety of assessment considerations that are different in comorbid versus non-comorbid subjects. Symptoms of co-occurring depression or substance abuse may be difficult to disentangle from anxiety symptoms. Many medical disorders produce symptoms of autonomic nervous system activation, as do anxiety disorders. Such medical comorbidity may be especially likely in primary care or medical clinic settings. The trade-off between heterogeneity and its attendant increase in measurement variance, and homogeneity and its attendant restrictions on generalisability, must be carefully considered. In addition, rigid exclusion criteria may be less acceptable in community settings than in the specialty research clinic; patients who are surprised by a diagnosis may be disappointed if they are ruled out from studies by being 'too complicated'. An alternative for the researcher is to simply accept comorbidity and heterogeneity of the population and evaluate a treatment that targets a specific symptom, behavioural pattern or symptom cluster, without regard to the context in which it occurs. To make this decision the researcher accepts the 'noise' this will cause in the system and powers the trial accordingly.

Other considerations related to patient heterogeneity include the fact that illness severity and typical background treatment history may vary across settings. Patients in some settings may have already received multiple treatments, while in other settings they may be treatment naïve. Given the findings from multiple studies that have documented that affective and anxiety disorders are under-recognised and under-treated in the community, it is likely that patients recruited from non-mental health settings will

have had little exposure to proven efficacious treatment. Often such patients have sought help from clergy or other informal sources. In the case of anxiety disorders, the awareness of the 'irrationality' of symptoms often means these individuals suffer in silence, embarrassed to reveal their self-perceived defects. Such patients are often enormously relieved when they learn that their disorder is understood. Even when treatment has apparently been offered, it may be less vigorous than the versions that have been proven efficacious in clinical trials. Inadequate doses and durations of pharmacotherapy may be the rule, and specific psychotherapies may be offered in name only. It may be particularly important not to assume (for example) that a patient has demonstrated a lack of response to treatment, and therefore be ruled out as ineligible.

If patients are identified in settings other than the specialty clinic, they may not view their anxiety disorder (which may be news to them) as the main problem they should be concerned with (along with their hypertension, macular degeneration, current spousal abuse or arthritis). They may be unwilling to make accommodations in schedules and may have needs for unusual availability of research staff in time and space. Some patients may not understand the usual standard procedures for treatment in a mental health clinic. They may need to be approached in an accommodating way.

POORLY DEFINED NOSOLOGIC BOUNDARIES

A second feature of anxiety disorders is that the boundaries between normal and pathological anxiety and among the pathological disorders are ill defined. Unlike most psychiatric disorders, the symptoms that comprise the diagnostic criteria for anxiety disorders are recognisable in normal people every day. The pathological state is defined by excess. However, the definition of excess is not precise. Because anxiety is a normal emotion, it is not always clear where the boundary between normal and pathological lies. This is particularly true in the context of stressful life events and ongoing difficulties. The boundary with normal may arise in defining a clinical population in need of treatment. Boundary issues are also relevant to treatment targets and definition of remission. In general, there is no consensus on what comprises remission of an anxiety disorder. We discuss this problem and suggest some ways it might be addressed. The problem of the boundary between normal and pathological is not a question raised only in the area of anxiety disorders, but rather is a continued question in the ongoing discussion related to definitions of psychopathology. A recent paper[15] provides a good summary of current issues. As these authors point out, it is also relevant to consider the relationship between mental and physical disorders. These considerations are important for clinical researchers to keep in mind but a detailed discussion of the various issues is beyond the scope of this chapter.

However, as noted above, anxiety is a normal emotion, and so its pathological state must be distinct from normal variation. It is best to experience anxiety in moderation. While anxiety can be disabling in excess, a deficiency of anxiety can also be impairing. The question of how much anxiety is optimal is not a philosophical one. Rather, it is one of the conundrums that currently face the clinical trials investigator. Namely, the investigator must decide how much symptom relief is optimal and how much is sufficient to declare a meaningful response to treatment. Given that anxiety is normal, is there some expected floor for the intensity of anxiety symptoms, or is symptomatic anxiety qualitatively different?

Another design question relates to the level of anxiety that results in optimal long-term outcome. Still another relates to the definition of remission of a given disorder. The field has not reached consensus on how to define remission for any of the anxiety disorders. This is a critical methodological problem that needs to be addressed. Investigators need to consider whether there is a way to overshoot the mark or is less always more? This is a serious question, as researchers are not agreed upon whether it

is useful to have some anxiety symptoms in order to keep coping functions operative and/or provide 'toughening up' experiences. Perhaps some continued symptomatology is a good idea to encourage continued exposure. The continued presence of low-level symptoms may increase the chances that the patient does not become complacent[16] and/or provide opportunities to confirm the absence of more severe symptoms.

On the other hand, since anxiety disorders are clearly debilitating, perhaps it is best to eliminate symptoms as fully as possible. Perhaps if we leave residual symptoms, this indicates that we have not eliminated the underlying vulnerability and relapse will be more likely. Ideally, we would like to eliminate pathological anxiety while leaving 'normal' anxiety intact. Yet this distinction may be difficult to define. If we have a pharmaceutical compound that reduces anxiety, might we overshoot the mark? If so, would that be as problematic as undertreatment? Common sense, and the results of a famous study,[17] suggest that a moderate level of anxiety is associated with optimal performance in situations like test-taking. Laurence Olivier is known to have suffered, as many actors do, from tremendous stage fright. His view of this was that this fear was an essential motivator that ensured his performance would be undertaken with the highest possible focus and concentration. Every researcher knows that the approach of the deadline for grant submission generates substantial anxiety which again motivates the highest possible level of energy and productivity.

Threshold issues relate to the decision to begin as well as the decision to end treatment. At what point do we declare anxiety to be at a clinically significant level that warrants intervention? If Laurence Olivier experienced intense anxiety at each performance, should he be treated? The goal of treatment of an unhappy but successful person should be first and foremost to prevent failure (inability to perform, because of paralysing fear or shoddy performance, because of cavalier attitude) while, if possible, reducing the discomfort of unhappiness. In this context we echo a famous quote of Freud, concerning the goals of psychoanalysis vis-à-vis unhappiness. Anxiety clearly exists on a continuum yet a treatment decision is a binary one. We do not attempt to administer a partial treatment. The decision of who to treat, of the minimal level of symptomatology an eligible subject may have will have implications for interpreting and acting on study results. It is likely that there is a distance from the boundary with normality associated with optimal effect of treatment. The closer to the boundary, the more likely the study will show non-specific or placebo effects. The farther from the boundary (i.e. the more severe and complicated the symptoms are) the less likely that the treatment will be fully effective. One consideration in deciding who to treat in a research study of anxiety disorders is the life context and the personal context in which the anxiety disorder symptoms arise.

Considerations Related to Life Context and Individual Psychology

Because of the salience of environmental stimuli as a trigger for normal anxiety, and the importance of coping mechanisms and social supports as responses to anxiety, it might be argued that these context measures are of particular importance in anxiety studies. Little is known about the relationship between onset, course and treatment of anxiety disorders and these external factors. There is a need to examine what the nature of these relationships may be. For example, it is not known whether faulty coping mechanisms play a role in the vulnerability to one or another of the anxiety disorders. If so, perhaps this should be a target of a treatment intervention. If not, perhaps coping skills are variable across individuals and/or across stressors and may act as a moderator of treatment response. In this case, improving coping may be a strategy for treatment of non-responders.

Strong social support is well known to be an important contributor to a sense of safety. Anxiety disorder patients experience the world as more dangerous. Safety is not necessarily the opposite of danger, but a sense of safety can mitigate the perception of likelihood of danger and/or the perception of consequences of the danger. Anecdotally, some anxiety disorder patients are thought to have unusually good interpersonal skills. Turning to others may be one way a patient with panic disorder copes with a world perceived as persistently and unpredictably frightening. For other individuals with anxiety disorders, anxiety may be exacerbated by relationships with others. A patient with social phobia fears scrutiny by others and this may motivate them to avoid relationships or to concentrate on developing a small group of 'safe' people. Someone with OCD may fear contamination from others, or an OCD patient may fear harming other people. Either may lead them to have reduced social contacts and less overall sense of safety. It is also possible that deficits in internal representations of other people can lead to problems in regulation of emotions. This can contribute to anxiety symptoms and perhaps even to the onset of anxiety symptomatology. There is some indication that relationships with others help regulate neuroendocrine and autonomic nervous system functioning. Whether to include measures of social support and attachment into clinical trials in anxiety disorders is a decision researchers must begin to consider. Such information is an additional patient burden. However, it may be difficult to determine optimal interventions for patients in the community if researchers do not begin to address some of these issues.

Also ill defined are boundaries between different diagnostic categories with similar symptomatology, and frequent comorbidity. Given the fact that fears, worries, somatic symptoms and behavioural manifestations are shared across disorders, distinctions can sometimes be blurred. There have been changes in diagnostic criteria sets since DSM III, especially for panic disorder and generalised anxiety disorder (see below). There has also been a change in the relationship between panic and agoraphobia, and between these disorders and other DSM IV anxiety disorders. These changes reflect growing recognition of the occurrence of panic and phobic symptoms across disorders. In addition, the core generalised anxiety disorder (GAD) symptom, worry, is also frequently found in other anxiety disorders and in depression. The content of worry apparently differs in depression and GAD.[18] However, this is a nuance for an assessment strategy, and again, time is required to tease this apart.

The diagnostic groups that comprise the anxiety disorders share cognitive manifestations of fear or worry, behavioural manifestations of efforts to cope with the anxious thoughts (phobia or compulsions), and somatic symptoms that often accompany the anxiety. Yet each disorder has a different 'flavour' of symptoms, and each may reflect different aetiological underpinnings. The similarities have implications for clinicians and researchers alike and will have a bearing on the design of new treatments and dissemination of efficacious interventions. As study intake moves into the community, we can expect the diagnostic overlap to increase, if only because mild versions of disorders are harder to separate than severe ones. Efficacy studies have focused on specific diagnostic groups, rather than on anxiety as a loose complex of symptoms. This means that the ostensible usefulness of study results depends on clear, reliable identification of the specific disorders in patients, at best a dubious proposition in the community setting. However, it should be recognised that while the efficacy studies have been carried out in carefully constructed 'pure cultures', the results of those studies show a startling uniformity of options for treatment across the spectrum of anxiety disorders. It may be that the careful and expensive nosologic dissection characteristic of the first generation of clinical trials is added to the precision and power of those studies, but may be relaxed in the next generation of effectiveness studies, making a virtue of necessity.

We now know how to reliably identify anxiety disorders and we know how to provide efficacious acute interventions, but these demonstrations have occurred only in the research clinic. The traditional decision point for clinical intervention, i.e. clinical (DSM IV) diagnosis, is fairly clear, though there are remaining controversies about psychiatric diagnosis. For the most part, these are beyond the scope of this paper. Researchers have developed tools to use for screening, diagnosis and severity ratings of anxiety symptoms. Ensuring that clinicians are aware of these and that the instruments are user-friendly is a focus of current work. There are many existing publications related to different assessment instruments, so we will not provide this information here. Instead, we suggest that even with a good instrument, there are some difficulties in establishing clearly a single target condition, and that the attempt may be a useless diversion of effort if discriminatory precision is less important than inclusiveness of intake.

The high rate of co-occurrence of anxiety disorders is an area of confusion that concerns the diagnostic nomenclature. For this and other more theoretical reasons, there is controversy in the field with regard to whether different DSM IV diagnoses describe truly distinct illness categories. Moreover, even if they are different, their co-occurrence creates measurement problems. For example, if a patient in treatment for a panic disorder has a co-occurring specific phobia of heights, should avoidance of bridges be rated a symptom of panic disorder, of height phobia or both?

As noted above, it may be possible to aim current established treatments on the generic symptoms that occur across the disorders: fear or worry, somatic symptoms and behavioural changes such as avoidance or compulsive ritualising. The broad spectrum effects of serotonin-active medications lend themselves to such an approach, as do the psychosocial treatments which may reduce generic cognitive, somatic and behavioural symptoms across disorders. An investigator planning a community study needs to decide whether to test treatments in the classical disorder-specific trial or in a more broadly-based group of patients defined by the common symptoms and behaviours of the anxiety disorders. We think that the latter choice deserves serious consideration.

Defining Outcomes and Measuring Results

Katschnig and Amering[19] point to the considerable complexity of symptoms in panic disorder, suggesting that spontaneous and situational panic attacks, anticipatory anxiety, phobic avoidance, disabilities, comorbid depression and substance abuse must be considered. One might add to this the presence of other anxiety disorders, personality disorders and physical illnesses. These authors list methodological difficulties that emerge from this complexity. They raise questions such as which of the phenomena are most important in assessing course and outcome, what are the relevant time intervals for symptom assessment, at what point should the clinician consider that the illness has transitioned to a remitted state? Such considerations are relevant for each anxiety disorder. All are comprised of multiple domains of symptoms, including panic, anticipatory anxiety, worry, phobia, obsessions or compulsions. Since the diagnostic criteria do not require the presence of each of these, it is possible to meet criteria for one or another anxiety disorder with prominent symptoms in one domain and none in another. Over time this may change. In some situations different domains within a disorder may be negatively correlated. For example, an individual may experience a reduction in panic attacks while becoming increasingly phobic. Is this improvement or worsening of the overall condition? A patient with OCD may experience a decrease in obsessions as the compulsive behaviours grow and become instantiated. Should this be considered a change in severity? A person with a phobia may experience lower overall impairment and/or fear as their phobic behaviour become more fixed, and they begin to accommodate the phobia in their lives. Does this mean the phobia is in partial remission? What if the intensity of symptoms is actually worse than when the disorder was first diagnosed, and yet there is less impairment? Similarly, if an individual with OCD has prominent obsessions and intermittent compulsions are they better off, worse off, or the same as if the opposite is true? What is the role of impairment and/or quality of life in determining outcome? What criteria should we use for illness severity? What about treatment response or remission? It is clear that response entails a clinically significant, noticeable change in symptom levels while remission entails a return to functioning with symptoms at a level that they cause no noticeable distress. Studies are underway to identify precise markers of these important clinical transitions.

The fact that the symptoms of a single disorder do not necessarily travel together creates difficulties in defining the endpoint for a treatment. Such a 'carousel course' (Figure 17.1) of symptoms leads to assessment quandaries that can be daunting. Again, taking the case of panic disorder with agoraphobia, if a patient starts treatment with several full panic attacks per week, and then has a marked reduction in panic attacks, but continues to have frequent limited symptom episodes, and remains moderately agoraphobic, how much improved is the patient compared to baseline? How should life context be factored into assessment of illness severity? If a social phobic gets a new job which requires less public performance than previously, but the job is below his or her level of competence, social anxiety symptoms may diminish noticeably but is the patient really better?

Several authors have drawn attention to these problems and the general recommendations have been to use composite measures of severity over an extended period of time. Such composite measures are available for most of the disorders, and most are quite user-friendly: The Yale–Brown Obsessive Compulsive Scale has been widely used and is available in a self-report format. The same is true for the more recently developed Panic Disorder Severity Scale. The Social Phobia Inventory (SPIN) is also brief and comprehensive. There is little agreement in the field about the one or two best measures for each disorder. The same measures can sometimes be used for screening diagnosis and outcome though it makes sense to pick the instrument most relevant to the goal of the assessment. The use of a composite measure presupposes that it is possible in principle to rank order the outcomes of the patients, although there may be many outcomes that are distinct but not ordered. From a statistical point of view, the ability to reliably order patient outcomes into as few as four or five categories

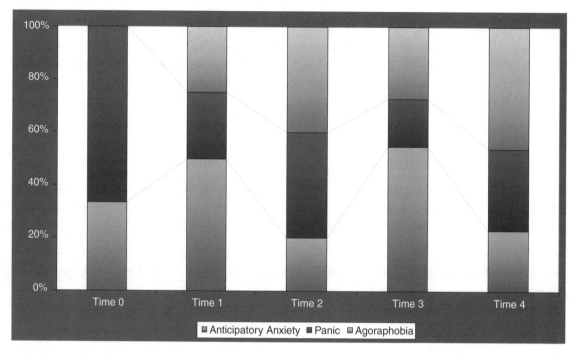

Figure 17.1. Panic disorder as an example of a 'carousal' symptom pattern

provides considerable increase in the power to detect treatment differences, compared to a simple dichotomy of response/no response. There are diminishing returns even to perfectly reliable orderings with more than five levels. Given even modest unreliability, it may not pay to push composite measures beyond a few levels of discrimination. The challenge posed by the 'carousel course', and the pleiotropic outcomes, of anxiety disorder is fundamental: the ability to rank patient outcomes is the most basic feature of scientific measurement and study.

As studies extend into the community, they will explore the less severe forms of the disorder, and may be even more vulnerable to the problem discussed above. This raises the possibility that the target of measurement should not be improvement (alone) but prevention of significant worsening. The advantage of this approach is that it may move the measurement into a more reliable regime, in which there is less controversy about the meaning of the outcome. The disadvantage is that it may also require large sample

sizes, in order to detect modest effects on low probability outcomes.

Choosing a Time Frame for Outcome Assessment

The specifics of time frame are also controversial. While a group of senior panic disorder researchers achieved consensus on a recommendation of an optimal period of four weeks for assessment of symptoms, and a minimum of two weeks, these recommendations are not always followed. In fact, frequently symptom status is reported without specification of the time frame of the assessment. The issues around time course are further complicated by variability between domains and within a domain, depending on life circumstances. Some domains of symptoms, such as phobic symptoms, are very stable, and a change in them, even over a fairly brief period, e.g. a few weeks, can be an indicator of change in illness severity or course. (A caveat here is the change in life context.) However, other symptoms are very unstable. For example, it is typical for panic attacks to occur in clusters and then to subside. The problem is further compounded by difficulties inherent in rating panic frequency. Anticipatory anxiety can be far worse if there is a specific environmental demand to confront an anxiety-provoking situation. For example, if a social phobic must go to a wedding. This raises the question of the time frame over which different types of symptoms should be assessed, and the situations in which the symptoms should be evaluated. Again, a focus on long-term prevention of serious worsening may help.

We do not have definitive answers to these myriad questions, but suggest that we should be paying attention to these assessment challenges. It may be possible to undertake secondary data analyses that target these questions. In the meantime, we suggest that outcome assessment must take into consideration multiple domains to make a meaningful judgment of response or remission. Further, it makes sense to establish and publish conventions for raters so that others can understand clearly results of studies. Reports of study results rarely describe conventions for rating phobia, including changes in life context and/or situational demands. Many published panic disorder studies use panic attack frequency as the only outcome. Reporting conventions should be broadened to address these issues.

Phobic Fear and Avoidance

A third issue specific to anxiety disorders is the occurrence of phobic symptomatology. One of the trickiest problems in anxiety disorders treatment is the assessment and management of avoidance. Avoidance is a natural reaction to fear and is usually successful in reducing anxiety in the short run. However, the longer-term effect is virtually always to increase anxiety. Avoidance also causes substantial functional impairment. Avoidance may lead a social phobic to seriously curtail his or her education, or resist career development because of fear of speaking in a group. The net result can be highly significant to income and productivity. Thus, avoidance is both a coping mechanism and a symptom. By its nature, it can be difficult to measure, since many anxiety disorder patients try to avoid thinking about anxiety-provoking situations, in addition to avoiding confronting these situations. This means that asking a person if there is anything they are avoiding often results in under-reporting. It is necessary to inquire about avoidance by asking specific questions, and this can be time-consuming. Some behaviour therapists argue that phobias can only be assessed using a behavioural challenge protocol. However they are measured, it is clear that phobic symptoms are important as they are among the strongest and most consistent predictors of long-term outcome.

Avoidance can also play a role in silencing anxiety symptoms and reducing the impetus to seek help. This may be one way that phobic symptoms act to worsen the course of illness. Silencing of symptoms is also reminiscent of the hypertension analogy where serious consequences result from lack of awareness of symptoms and difficulty adhering to treatment regimens. In fact, phobic avoidance has now been found, like hypertension, to be a predictor of cardiovascular mortality, at least for men. A further issue related to the silencing of distress is that it can be difficult to distinguish pathological from normal avoidance behaviours. Phobic symptomatology may become so integrated into the patient's life that it seems normal. Avoidance of some situations may be treated as though they are simply life choices. The patient may say that he or she simply does not enjoy shopping in a mall when the fact is that they are afraid to go to a mall because they may have a panic attack. The problem of distinguishing normal from pathological anxiety is broader than the issues related to phobia.

This realm of symptoms causes methodological problems that involve both assessment and treatment. Phobic symptoms entail avoidance of cues that evoke fear, anxiety or other dysphoric affects. An individual with phobic avoidance will make every effort to evade exposure to the feared situation. Evasion often extends to thinking or talking about the situation. This means that the phobic individual cannot be counted on to talk about their symptoms spontaneously. In fact, to obtain a clear picture of the extent of behavioural avoidance often requires a detailed inquiry. Such an assessment takes time and is not desirable in many community settings. An investigator must decide whether this time is worth the trade-off of information. The answer to this question will be influenced by the type of study and the population being studied. However, it is important for researchers to be aware that more co-occurring phobia has been consistently associated with poorer response to treatment and greater likelihood of relapse.[20,21] The clinical significance of phobic symptoms underscores the need to attend to this component of anxiety symptomatology.

THE TWO CULTURES: DISCORDANT MODELS OF THE ANXIETY DISORDERS

A fourth characteristic of anxiety disorders is based upon the fact that there are two powerful models of these disorders that are not yet fully integrated. Specifically, neurobiological (generally biomedical) and learning theory (generally academic psychological) researchers use different paradigms to explain symptom onset and to guide treatment. When studying treatment in community settings, it is important that neither group ignore the other. In anxiety disorders, perhaps more than any other conditions, there is a need to build on information obtained from both of these academic disciplines, given that each field can claim clinical results.

Incorporating Information from Biomedicine and Academic Psychology in Study Designs

Anxiety disorders are unusual in that they have been the focus of intensive and more or less independent study by both biomedical/psychiatric and behavioural/psychological researchers. Efficacious treatments have been devised by each group. Yet, most treatment studies test interventions in one, but not both areas. The existence of two very different types of efficacious intervention for each of the anxiety disorders

presents some especially challenging methodological issues for which there is no simple solution. The practice of ignoring the findings of the other modality when conducting studies is increasingly problematic. If not specifically instructed, pharmacotherapists may vary widely in their knowledge and use of efficacious behavioural interventions. This variation can be highly problematic for a treatment study. On the other hand, much effort must go into controlling the interaction of the pharmacotherapists with the patient. Researchers must decide how much behavioural intervention the medication therapist should administer. Complicated and time-consuming procedures are often required to ensure that such interventions are provided uniformly.

On the other hand, patients in the community often receive medication that can be efficacious for treating anxiety disorders, even before presenting to the cognitive behavioural therapist for treatment. Investigators must decide how to manage this situation. Should such patients be eliminated from a CBT trial? Should they be eligible and left on medication that is not fully effective? Or should all medication be discontinued? Each of these decisions is problematic since a partially effective medication can affect outcome whether it is continued or discontinued. Omission of this increasingly large group of patients, on the other hand, can also be an important threat to generalisability of the study.

Another problem for researchers is how to decide whether to compare medication and psychosocial treatments, and if so, to decide how best to do so. There is clearly a need in the field to address this problem, but the solution to the problem is not trivial. Among the problems are that patients often have treatment preferences. Many will simply refuse to participate in a study in which they must agree to be assigned to a treatment modality at random. Others will agree and drop out when they receive an unwanted treatment assignment. There are a number of possible designs for a comparison treatment study. These include a full factorial design (Figure 17.2) in which each active treatment is compared to an

	Active medication	Placebo medication	No pill
Active psychotherapy	X	X	X
'Placebo' psychotherapy	X	X	X
No psychotherapy	X	X	X

Figure 17.2. Full factorial design

inactive (placebo) control treatment and no treatment, and the two treatments are combined in all possible combinations. While this is the most complete design it is often impractical because of the treatment combinations (or lack of treatment) or because of the number required. It is difficult to undertake such a study at a single site and then there are problems with multiple sites in equivalence of providing all treatments and in minimising patient heterogeneity. An alternative class of designs has been described recently[22] that allows patients and investigators to describe preferences in advance of randomisation and then be randomised within their preference set ('equipoise stratum').

Other design issues are related to the different putative underpinnings of symptoms as conceptualised from different points of view. These different viewpoints sometimes translate to different treatment targets. For example a CBT approach to panic disorder focuses on underlying fear of bodily sensations, while the pharmacotherapist targets bursts of autonomic arousal. Pharmacotherapists and psychosocial researchers typically use different assessment strategies, and may or may not accept those of the other camp. In recent years, a series of multisite studies undertaken as a collaboration between neurobiologic and cognitive behavioural scientists has produced a more comfortable meeting ground for both groups. Still, there are disagreements.

In addition to the scientific differences, there are social and political differences between the two groups of researchers that can complicate methodological decisions in treatment trials. The investigators need to be clear about who the audience for their results will be. Design decisions may influence who will listen to their results. Ideally, a study can be designed so that it will be convincing to any treatment researcher. However, there are turf issues that may influence the mutual acceptance. Clinicians and researchers from one camp may feel the other is poaching on their turf. This is more likely to occur if there is insufficient attention to the issues of efficacy of the alternative treatments.

Guild issues are prominent in this field, and few pharmacotherapists understand the principles and techniques of administering cognitive behavioural treatment. Similarly many psychosocial researchers are not well informed about pharmacotherapy. Investigators from each group tend to have strong allegiance to the unique validity of their own methods. At times, there has been rancour and contentiousness between them, though this has improved in recent years. In the few instances that there has been a head-to-head comparison of medication and cognitive behavioural treatment, they have been similar in efficacy. It is not yet clear when or how combination treatments might be best administered. There is a need to take into consideration both biomedical and behavioural–psychological perspectives in designing treatment studies.

CONCLUSIONS

Although proven efficacious treatments have been identified for each of the anxiety disorders, the work of clinical trials remains unfinished. There are many unanswered questions, and much left to study in order to inform clinicians about how to optimise treatment decisions for patients with these debilitating conditions. In spite of achievements in documenting treatment efficacy over the past decades, treatment research has just scratched the surface. Innovations are needed in treatment development and in dissemination of proven interventions. To accomplish this there is a need for innovations in methodology. Efficacy studies, designed to meet US FDA regulatory needs,[23] will continue to have a role in the clinical research pipeline. But, there is a need for new clinical methods to support studies before and after efficacy. It is not our purpose to provide a comprehensive review of such methods. Rather, we have focused on a few key issues in anxiety disorders that require special consideration.

Existing clinical trials in anxiety disorders, like those in other areas of psychiatry, have provided information telling us which treatments are active in reducing target symptoms. Unanswered are a myriad of critical questions that relate to daily life decisions in the clinic. For example, do impairments as well as symptoms respond to efficacious treatments? If so, what is the time course of response? What is the optimum dose and duration of treatment to achieve maximal results? How often can we produce remission with existing treatments? What is the best way to define remission? Is maintenance treatment needed after remission is achieved? If so, how long? What if a patient does not achieve symptom remission? How should such a patient be managed over the

long run? Do patients with complex comorbid conditions respond to treatment in a way that is similar or different than those with less comorbidity? Can a clinician be confident that proven efficacious treatments are appropriately utilised in a patient whose symptoms meet criteria for the target disorder, but who differs in demographic characteristics, social supports, or other ways from those seen in efficacy studies? How closely must procedures in the community follow those used in research studies in order to achieve the same results?

These and other questions like them are often broadly grouped under the rubric of 'effectiveness' studies. We focus especially on characteristics of anxiety disorders that make these decisions complicated and that comprise methodological challenges for researchers. We confess that we may raise more questions than we can answer. However, where possible, we will at least provide suggestions about possible ways to address the problems.

Decisions about primary, secondary and tertiary prevention interventions are not so well specified. There is accumulating evidence for psychological and neurobiological precursor states for anxiety disorders and for psychosocial risk factors. This information raises hopes for the possibility of primary prevention. Clearly it would be advantageous to be able to intervene early, before the development of the disorder and, ideally, even before the onset of a precursor state. Once established, anxiety disorders are chronic relapsing conditions. With or without treatment, patients are likely to experience symptoms that wax and wane, to meander in and out of full-fledged symptom states in different configurations, to experience temporary, partial or incomplete states of remission. We need more information about how to manage anxiety disorders, once established, in order to best prevent complications and recurrence of full symptomatic episodes.

REFERENCES

1. Kessler RC, McGonagle KA, Zhao S, Nelson CB, *et al.* Lifetime and 12-month prevalence of DSM-III-R psychiatric disorders in the United States:

Results from the National Comorbidity Survey. *Arch Gen Psychiat* (1994) **51**(1): 8–19.

2. Hohmann A, Shear MK. Community based intervention research: coping with the noise of real life in study design. *Am J Psychiatr* (2002) **159**: 201–7.

3. Kessler RC, Soukup J, Davis RB, Foster DF, Wilkey SA, Van Rompay MI, Eisenberg DM. The use of complementary and alternative therapies to treat anxiety and depression in the United States. *Am J Psychiat* (2001) **158**(2): 289–94.

4. Shear MK, Greeno C, Kang J, Ludewig D, Frank E, Swartz HA, Hanekamp M. Diagnosis of non-psychotic patients in community settings. *Am J Psychiat* (2000) **157**(4): 581–7.

5. Glisson C, Hemmelgarn A. The effects of organizational climate and interorganizational coordination on the quality and outcomes of children's service systems. *Child Abuse Neglect* (1998) **22**(5): 401–21.

6. Rosenheck R. Stages in the implementation of innovative clinical programs in complex organizations. *J Nerv Ment Dis* (2001) **189**(12): 812–21.

7. Swartz H, Shear MK, Frank E. *Supermarket Psychotherapy*. Psych Services (in press).

8. Roy-Byrne PP, Katon W, Cowley DS, Russo JE, Cohen E, Michelson E, Parrot T. Panic disorder in primary care biopsychosocial differences between recognized and unrecognized patients. *Gen Hosp Psychiat* (2000) **22**(6): 405–11.

9. McKay M, McCadam K, Gonzales J. Addressing the barriers to mental health services for inner city children and their caretakers. *Commun Mental Health J* (1996) **32**(4): 353–61.

10. Essock S, Goldman H. Outcomes and evaluation: system, program and clinician level measures. In: Minkoff K, Pollack D, eds, *Managed Mental Health Care in the Public Sector: A Survival Manual. Chronic Mental Illness*, Vol. 4. Amsterdam: Harwood Academic (1997) 295–307.

11. Dohrenwend BP, Shrout PE. Toward the development of a two-stage procedure for case identification and classification in psychiatric epidemiology. *Res Commun Mental Health* (1981) **2**: 295–323.

12. Dixon L, Green-Paden L, Delahanty J, Lucksted A, Postrado L, Hall Jo. Variables associated with disparities in treatment of patients with schizophrenia and comorbid mood and anxiety disorders. *Psychiat Serv* (2001) **52**(9): 1216–22.

13. Kandel DB, Huang F-Y, Davies M. Comorbidity between patterns of substance use dependence and psychiatric syndromes. *Drug Alcohol Depend* (2001) **64**(2): 233–41.

14. Brady KT. Comorbid posttraumatic stress disorder and substance use disorders. *Psychiat Ann* (2001) **31**(5): 313–19.

15. Widiger TA, Sankis LM. Adult psychopathology: issues and controversies. *Ann Rev Psychol* (2000) **51**: 377–404.

16. Fava GA, Rafanelli C, Ottolini F, Ruini C, Cazzaro M, Grandi S. Psychological well-being and residual symptoms in remitted patients with panic disorder and agoraphobia. *J Affect Disord* (2001) **65**(2): 185–190.

17. Yerkes RM, Dodson JD. The relation of strength of stimulus to rapidity of habit formation. *J Comp Neurol Psychol* (1908) **18**: 459–82.

18. Diefenbach GJ, McCarthy-Larzelere A, Williamson DA, Mathews A, Manguno-Mire GM, Bentz BG. Anxiety, depression, and the content of worries. *Depress Anxiety* (2001) **14**: 247–50.

19. Katschnig H, Amering M. The long-term course of panic disorder and its predictors. *J Clin Psychopharm* (1998) **18**(6, Suppl 2) 6S–11S.

20. Scheibe G, Albus M. Predictors and outcome in panic disorder: a 2-year prospective follow-up study. *Psychopathology* (1997) **30**: 177–84.

21. Cowley DS, Flick SN, Roy-Byrne PP. Long-term course and outcome in panic disorder: a naturalistic follow-up study. *Anxiety* (1996) **2**: 13–21.

22. Lavori PW, Rush AJ, Wisniewski SR, Alpert J, Fava M, Kupfer DJ, Nierenberg A, Quitkin FM, Sackeim HA, Thase ME, Trivedi M. Strengthening clinical effectiveness trials: equipoise-stratified randomization. *Biol Psychiat* (2001) **50**(10): 792–801.

23. Rubinow DR. Practical and ethical aspects of pharmacotherapeutic evaluation. In: Ginsburg BE, Carter BF, eds, *Premenstrual Syndrome: Ethical and Legal Implications in a Biomedical Perspective*. New York: Plenum Press (1987) 47–55.

18

Cognitive Behaviour Therapy

NICHOLAS TARRIER[1] AND TIL WYKES[2]

[1]School of Psychiatry and Behavioural Sciences, University of Manchester, Manchester M23 9LT, UK
[2]Institute of Psychiatry, De Crespigny Park, London SE5 8AF, UK

BACKGROUND

We have chosen in this chapter to provide an overview of the difficulties for the investigation of psychological therapies using the methodology of randomised control trials. In order to do so we have selected studies of a new treatment for psychosis, cognitive behaviour therapy (CBT). This is a new therapy that, following a period of development, has now resulted in four large randomised control trials.

Cognitive behaviour therapy is a therapy that targets the symptoms of one disorder, schizophrenia. The lifetime risk is 1%. This disorder is characterised by a cluster of specific symptoms that are typically divided into two categories, positive and negative. Positive symptoms include auditory hallucinations and delusions, both of which produce much distress. Negative symptoms include lack of drive, emotional apathy as well as poverty of speech and social withdrawal.

In many, if not most, cases the disorder follows a relapsing course.[1] A significant proportion, but not all, people suffering from the disorder have poor outcomes, i.e. with high levels of dependence on continuing psychiatric care, low

levels of financial independence and little social fulfillment. There is some underlying variation in the disorder,[2] which is probably affected by interactions with other clinical, social and environmental demands and supports such as life events (death of parent), absence of a supportive family (or presence of a critical one) and economic conditions (high unemployment).

Several different sorts of psychological therapies have been developed to address the following outcomes:

- Total number of symptoms
- Distress caused by symptoms
- Relapse
- Social functioning
- Family engagement
- Quality of life
- Skills/thinking style, e.g. problem solving, coping skills.

The currently accepted treatment for the positive symptoms of schizophrenia is medication. This has been shown to reduce them significantly and does reduce relapse. However, it also has costs as well as benefits in that there is the risk

Textbook of Clinical Trials. Edited by D. Machin, S. Day and S. Green
© 2004 John Wiley & Sons, Ltd   ISBN: 0-471-98787-5

ng side effects such as tremor, rest-
d uncontrollable mouth movements.
ffects disappear on stopping the med-
there is the chance that the mouth
movements will develop into a condition known
as tardive dyskinesia that is irreversible. Some
patients, about one-third, also continue to experience positive symptoms despite adequate doses
of medication. It is these symptoms that were the
targets for change in this further development of
a psychological therapy, CBT.

Because of the potential risks of long-term
medication and the unpleasant side effects also
experienced on short-term treatment, consumers
of mental health services have been extremely
positive about the development of psychological
treatment. This has led to further pressure on
funders of health service research to provide
more data on acceptable alternatives or adjuncts
to medication treatment. Hence the recent trials
of CBT in the UK sponsored by either the
UK Department of Health directly, government
research agencies or large UK research charities.

WHAT IS COGNITIVE BEHAVIOUR THERAPY?

The main developmental roots for CBT have been
in depression and anxiety. This began over 20
years ago but more recently the approach has
been applied to people with schizophrenia. This
later development produced changes in the way
the intervention is presented, although the underlying model of change may be similar to that
adopted for the other disorders. The main aim of
the intervention is to reduce distress, disability
and emotional disturbance as well as the relapse
of the acute symptoms.[3] Cognitive behaviour
therapies are active and structured therapeutic
methods and should be distinguished from psychoeducation which tends to be simple, didactic
and educational. Brief educational packages have
been shown to be ineffective either with families[4]
or with individual patients.[5]

Although there are specific components of
CBT that would be accepted by all its proponents,
these ingredients may be given in different
proportions by different groups of professionals
and for different individuals within a single
service. Below is a list of the ones that we have
identified as being used by most groups:

- Engagement with the client.
- Problem identification.
- Agreeing on a collaborative formulation of the problems to be assessed.
- Use of alternative explanations to challenge delusional and dysfunctional thoughts.
- Establishing the link between thoughts and emotions.
- Encouraging the patient to examine alternative views of events.
- Encouraging the patient to examine the link between thoughts and behaviour.
- Use of behavioural experiments to reality test.
- The setting of behavioural goals and targets.
- Developing coping strategies to reduce psy-chotic symptoms.
- Development and acquisition of relapse pre-vention strategies.

Some groups have also included:

- Improvement in self-esteem.
- Increasing social support and social networks.
- Schema focused therapy.

TREATMENT DEVELOPMENT

New treatments usually evolve through a number
of stages. Initially the problem is identified and
suggestions, involving theoretical and pragmatic
elements in varying degrees, are advanced for its
solution. Innovative case studies are carried out.
Replications and developments in other case studies and case series follow. The next stage consists
of uncontrolled and small exploratory controlled
trials. These are often innovative but methodologically weak. Finally the 'gold standard' of evaluation, the large randomised controlled trial (RCT),
is carried out if the new treatment is showing sufficient promise. RCTs are increasingly large and
methodologically rigorous and therefore more
expensive, often now involving numerous sites
and large numbers of patients. A further theme

is that of identifying what is responsible for the improved outcome following the treatment; that is, the trial includes an explanatory element. Trials that identify the key components responsible for the changes are essential to the further devel- opment of treatment and ... ation of the tr... alth
... he-
... ent
... nt
... th
... e
... n

... f
si
th
wo
a
pat
mo
sion
1970
et al. ... recent decad ... controlled trials were carried ou ... small trials with methodological weaknesses were initially published. For example, Tarrier *et al.*[10] compared coping training with problem solving but assessments were not blind and drop-outs were not included in the analysis. Garety *et al.*[11] compared cognitive behaviour therapy to treatment-as-usual but again assessments were not blind and group allocation was not random. Drury *et al.*[12,13] evaluated cognitive therapy with acutely ill patients, but the treatment included individual and group treatment of patients and families while assessments were neither independent nor blind. However, three medium size methodologically robust trials of CBT variants have been carried out with chronic schizophrenic patients,[14–16] and one large multi-site trial with recent onset acute patients (the SoCRATES Trial[17]). It is therefore appropriate to review not only these trials but also the changes in clinical trial methods in this field in order to begin to define the most optimal strategy for the future evaluation of this and other psychological therapies.

WHY CARRY OUT CLINICAL TRIALS OF PSYCHOLOGICAL TREATMENTS?

PURPOSES AND OUTCOMES

There are a number of different beneficiaries from clinical trials. From the health services perspective there is an increase in knowledge about what treatments are likely to provide the most benefits (see section on Evidence-Based Practice below). In addition, for clinical academics there may be elements of the design of ... trial that will allow certain models of aetiology ... treatment efficacy to be tested which can ... form theories of the disorder as well as leading ... improvements in treatment. For therapists ... trial may produce clinical improvements ... mean that the participants can make health ... s and for the patients the treatments may ... de them with changes that are valued, such ... creased social inclusion. So it cannot be assumed that there is a single purpose for carrying out a clinical trial. These different purposes change the type of trial performed, particularly in relation to how outcomes are defined. We have set out a number of different outcomes below which may be variously valued by different groups (in the list respectively health service, clinical academic, therapist and participant) and which could be targets in CBT trials. It cannot be assumed that all groups will value all outcomes to the same extent, or that the same outcome would be measured in the same way from the different viewpoints. For instance, symptoms can be measured as a simple change over treatment, by a threshold amount or by the effects on the emotional life of the patient, for example the distress caused by the symptom.

Possible outcomes of treatment:

- The occurrence or frequency of a particular event: e.g. number of relapses, time to relapse (survival functions).
- The use of services or other resources: e.g. days spent in hospital, use of community mental health care.
- Improvement in symptoms at a level assumed to be of clinical significance: e.g. at least 20% or 50% improvement, return to within normal range.
- Change in a single symptom or other continuous outcome that is considered central or primary to the disorder: e.g. severity of delusions or hallucinations.
- Change in psychopathology that is general or secondary to the disorder: e.g. scores on a standard measure of psychopathology, severity of distress or anxiety.
- Changes to other important aspects of the person's life: e.g. social functioning, number of friends, quality of life.

Trials are also expensive and so the chances of funding are dependent on the types of trials wanted by the funding agencies. The main beneficiary (and funding) of clinical trials is the health service who would prefer pragmatic rather than model testing trials. But in the UK there has also been a new trend that may also affect the type of trial – the inclusion of mental health service users (consumers) and, where appropriate, carers on the trial management committees. There are examples of this; users and carers were represented in this way on a trial of CBT in dual diagnosis patients[18] and of effectiveness of family interventions,[19] and also on the research steering group which generates the research designs for the Centre for Recovery in Severe Psychosis

at the Institute of Psychiatry in London. The involvement of service users in clinical trials in the UK is now defined in guidelines provided by the Consumers in Research Unit within the Department of Health. This new undertaking does not seem to be prevalent in other countries.

The difficulty for research into psychological treatments is that studies are usually funded from public resources even at the early stages. This is in contrast to trials of medications where particular companies are not only required to carry out specific research for licensing but are also likely to benefit financially from the results of trials. Unlike drugs, psychological treatments do not have a specific product champion and therefore have to compete with other health care trials for scarce resources.

THERAPEUTIC RELEVANCE

In addition to the list of possible outcomes above there are other measures that may be essential in the assessment of outcome in a trial. For instance, if one of the hypotheses is that the therapy works through a specific mechanism then a sole outcome measure without recourse to either qualitative and/or process measures would not provide a test of this hypothesis. This is an extension of the sorts of questions stipulated by a clinical academic but is also essential to the health services. It may be that the treatment provides its effects through a simple mechanism which could be provided in a less sophisticated way, that is not requiring high levels of training and supervision.

It has been suggested that psychological therapies may all work through a common pathway: that the non-specific effects of psychotherapy may account for much of the effect of treatment outcome.[20,21] This is hardly surprising as psychological therapies have much in common with each other – they involve, for example, an interaction, negotiation of goals, an agenda for each session. The improvement could be produced by these commonalities and not through the specific model of therapy adopted. For example, treatments that were designed as non-specific placebo controls (e.g. befriending in Sensky et al.[16] and supportive counselling in Tarrier *et al.*[15]) performed much better than expected, although never better than CBT. Therefore, the choice of a comparison group is extremely important. If psychological therapy is compared to treatment-as-usual (TAU), which includes less individual attention than the psychological therapy, its effectiveness may be due to shared common themes of psychological therapy not to ingredients of a particular therapy. Tarrier *et al.*[10] investigated the effects of expectation of therapeutic benefit by the use of a demand and counter-demand manipulation. Half of the participants were told that they should expect therapeutic benefit to accrue with their progress through treatment (demand condition) and the other half were told that they should expect benefit but that it would not be apparent until after the end of treatment and post-treatment assessment (counter-demand condition). This manipulation of expectancies had no effect on clinical measures, suggesting that at least the anticipation of treatment benefit was not influential in this patient group.

Alternatively, as psychological therapies include specific attributes in common it may be wrong to conclude, in a comparison of two types of psychological therapy, that CBT is not the best form of therapy when the two treatments do not differ significantly from each other. There is always the danger that the study will be underpowered to demonstrate an advantage of CBT when the non-specific control group does better than expected. However, CBT may be significantly better than TAU, whereas the alternative may not give such an advantage. When the health services have to decide which of several forms of psychological therapy to choose to add to their therapeutic armantarium, selecting CBT would be their best choice.

ACUTE CARE, MAINTENANCE THERAPY AND DURABLE EFFECTS

Schizophrenia is most often a chronic relapsing condition. If we take the metaphors from treatments with medication then psychological therapy could be provided in a number of different ways.

- Acute antibiotic treatment which kills off the bacteria causing the disease (intensive psychological treatment which changes a key factor in the psychological make-up of the individual, e.g. cognitive behaviour therapy for panic disorder[22]).
- Acute treatment of symptom exacerbations and maintenance treatment, e.g. asthma treatment with steroids followed by maintenance with Salbutamol and/or sodium chromoglycate (CBT for chronic depression[23]).
- Prophylactic treatment for malaria (e.g. debriefing treatments for possible post-traumatic stress disorder[24]).

Psychological therapy often sets itself the same target as treatment using antibiotics, with an acute phase followed by a follow-up during which there is no active treatment. This protocol mainly resulted from the lack of specialist input in the health services, making it imperative to ration services. It also follows a set of expectations that come from the behavioural tradition in the treatment of psychological problems and recent CBT interventions for anxiety disorders where interventions are brief and the effects durable. For example, Figure 18.1 shows the effects of imipramine and CBT for panic disorder from a trial by Clark *et al.*[22] In their trial the drug and the psychological treatment had similar effects at the end of treatment, but psychological treatment had a more permanent effect and the differences between the two treatments were significant at follow-up. The improvement was predicted by the change in cognitions following treatment. In other words, the psychological treatment changed a maintenance factor for the disorder.

This expectation of intensive treatment producing durable gains may not be appropriate for schizophrenia as it is a relapsing condition that, in some cases, may have a deteriorating course. Furthermore, residual symptoms may be present between episodes of exacerbation. Residual positive symptoms at discharge are a risk factor for relapse.[5] Many maintenance and causal factors have been proposed and are in multiple domains, such as social, biological as well as

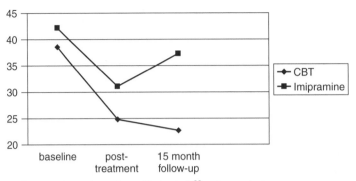

Source: Reproduced from Clark et al.,[22] with permission.

Figure 18.1. Psychological treatment for panic disorder

psychological. It is possible that CBT could have a successful effect on one of these factors but fail later when other factors become crucial in the progress of the disorder. This would be shown as a successful outcome at post-treatment but a lack of durability of gains at follow-up. However, the usual interpretation of this pattern of results is that the effect on the disorder was only temporary. If gains were 'only temporary' in a group of patients who were chosen because their symptoms were 'residual' then even this 'temporary' gain would be welcome. This set of results, rather than dismissing the treatment effect, actually generates a further question–how do we maintain the gains made during treatment when treatment is withdrawn?

The therapeutic protocol adopted for schizophrenia with medication is to provide medication intensively at the acute stage that is followed by maintenance treatment at lower dose of similar drugs. It may be that psychological treatment needs to be provided in an equivalent way.

An alternative mechanism and pattern of results for CBT could be improvement in one factor, such as self-esteem, which then allows further improvements in other factors to occur, such as increased social support through the extension of a support network by increased social contact. This would produce an improvement at post-treatment and even greater gains at follow-up. However, it would appear that CBT was not only durable but conferred greater benefits

as time passes, although it would not be clear to the research team how this latter improvement came about. This poses the question of how do we explain increases in effect size post-therapy which cannot be explained merely by the loss to follow-up of those people for whom the therapy conferred hardly any benefit at all.

Trials of acute CBT have shown significant effects of therapy mostly at the cessation of treatment but always after a follow-up period. Figure 18.2 provides data from Gould et al.[25] of the effect sizes of seven trials calculated from the following equation:

$$\text{Effect size} = (M_t - M_c)/\text{SD}_c$$

where M_t is the mean of the treatment group, M_c is the mean of the control group and this is divided by the standard deviation of the control group of participants.

The mean effect size for the trials studied by Gould et al. is 0.65 (95% CI 0.56–0.71). This average is called a medium to large effect size according to Cohen[26] (p. 40). Patients continued to improve over the follow-up period with the combined effect size cited by Gould et al.[25] of 0.93 for the four studies reporting a follow-up period. These results are encouraging given that schizophrenia is a relapsing condition where life events and other stressors may trigger new episodes of illness. However, the interpretation of the results of individual trials has since changed, mainly because the accepted standards for trials have changed. Several trials that make up this figure are methodologically weak with difficulties in random assignment, blindness of ratings, adequate outcome assessment and problematic or unsophisticated analyses (see below).

FAIRNESS AND CHANGING STANDARDS IN TRIAL DESIGN AND REPORTING

Standards have changed and what was reported in papers a number of years ago would have been adequate and satisfactory for the times. However, there are now clear guidelines on how trials should be reported, formalised in the CONSORT Statement.[27,28] CONSORT is a checklist and flow diagram that were designed to improve the quality of reports of randomised controlled trials. The checklist gives detailed instruction on describing the study's method and design, assignment and randomisation, masking (blinding), participant flow and follow-up, and analysis. The flow diagram provides readers with a clear picture of the progress of all participants in the trial, from the time they are referred to the trial until the end of their involvement. It

should include the number assessed for eligibility for the trial, reasons for exclusion, who was randomised and what happened to them prior to final assessment and analysis of the trial results.

These standards on reporting, by implication, provide strong recommendations to researchers about what they need to consider and action when designing and managing a trial. Table 18.1 contains a list of those points of the design or analysis that can seriously bias the interpretation of the results.

The majority of the current CBT trials do not conform to the reporting guidelines as set out in here. For some trials the significant discrepancies between Table 18.1 and the trial may lead to a biased interpretation of the results. For example, in Drury et al.[12,13] it is not clear what specific therapy is provided as a variety of different components were being tested at the same time. In Garety et al.[11] the participants were not randomly allocated to treatment groups. Kuipers et al.[14] had no blind assessment of treatment outcomes. Sensky et al.[16] recruited by repeatedly canvassing local services for referrals. However, the current meta-analyses do show that despite these methodological difficulties there seem to be significant changes in overall symptoms following treatment with CBT.

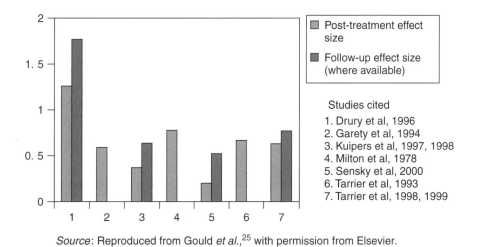

Source: Reproduced from Gould *et al.*,[25] with permission from Elsevier.

Figure 18.2. Effect sizes of CBT trails

Table 18.1. Items that should be included in reports of randomised trials

Heading	Subheading	Descriptor
Title		Identify the study as a randomised trial
Abstract		Use a structured format
Introduction		State prospectively defined hypothesis, clinical objectives, and planned subgroup or covariate analyses
Methods	**Protocol**	**Describe**
		Planned study population with inclusion or exclusion criteria
		Planned interventions: their nature, content and timing
		Primary and secondary outcome measure(s) and the minimum important difference(s), and indicate how the target sample size was estimated
		Reasons for statistical analyses chosen, and whether these were completed on an intention-to-treat basis
		Mechanisms for maintaining intervention quality, adherence to protocol and assessment of fidelity
		Prospectively defined stopping rules (if warranted)
	Assignment	**Describe**
		Randomisation (e.g. individual, cluster, geographic)
		Allocation schedule method
		Method of allocation concealment
	Masking (blinding)	**Describe**
		Mechanism for maintaining blind and allocation schedule control
		Evidence for successful blinding
Results	**Participant flow and follow-up**	Provide a trial profile summarising participant flow, numbers and timing of randomisation assignment, interventions, and measurements for each randomised group
	Analysis	State estimated effect of intervention on primary and secondary outcome measures, including a point estimate and measure of precision (confidence interval)
		State results in absolute numbers when feasible (for example, 10/20, not 50%)
		Present summary data and appropriate descriptive and interferential statistics in sufficient detail to permit alternative analyses and replication
		Describe prognostic variables by treatment group and any attempt to adjust
		Describe protocol deviations
	Discussion	State specific interpretations of study findings, including sources of bias and imprecision (internal validity) and discussion of external validity, including appropriate quantitative measures when possible
		State general interpretation of the data in light of the available evidence

Source: Modified from Begg *et al.*[27] and Moher *et al.*[28]

EVIDENCED-BASED PRACTICE

There is considerable current enthusiasm for evidence-based health care in general and mental health care, but there is a current debate on how evidence-based practice can be consistently implemented in routine settings both in the UK[29] and abroad.[30,31]

Evidence-based practice is the delivery of interventions for which there is strong scientific evidence that they improve relevant patient outcomes. Although the type of scientific evidence does vary, the gold standard for treatment outcome is the RCT. Where several trials exist they can be considered together through meta-analysis. Knowledge concerning evidence-based practice accrues through the accumulating results of efficacy and effectiveness studies.

Thus the purpose of evidence-based practice is (a) to ensure that the wealth of research evidence informs clinical practice so that those who are in receipt of treatment will receive the treatment that is the best available and represents the current knowledge base, and (b) to ensure that planning and policy is determined by empirical evidence, for those purchasing services to be able to make informed choices and for those receiving services to be empowered by such knowledge. Furthermore, the establishment of an evidence-based practice knowledge base of what works allows the practice of mental health services and individual clinicians to be compared to the evidence base. This increases accountability and establishes guidelines for good practice and improves the quality of mental health services. Limitations in evidence also set the research agenda for the future.

There are, however, critics of the collation of data for evidence-based practice. This mainly focuses around the use of specific meta-analytic techniques that have very limited entry criteria. The Cochrane database, for example, provides valuable searches and evaluations of randomised control trials with strict criteria for entry. Although the evidence may be strong for a particular practice it may be based on a very small number of studies. The main criteria for exclusion are the lack of randomisation of the participants within the trial and the lack of data on all those participants who entered the trial. Although clearly the results of such trials should be less weighted in the final evaluation, such information may be valuable when few other data are available.

TRIALS METHODOLOGY AND AIMS

Efficacy trials are devised to test whether the therapy has an effect overall on the outcomes of interest. They are carried out in relatively controlled environments, usually by sophisticated university based research teams, and often involve highly expert therapists. For CBT trials the outcomes of interest are a reduction in overall psychotic symptoms, reductions in relapse or reduced rates on admission to hospital, reduced psychopathology and improvements in functioning. These trials may also include various control groups and process measures to help understand why the treatments work. An effectiveness trial attempts to more closely resemble the real world of routine services, inclusion criteria are wider so the sample treated is more heterogeneous and includes the atypical patients, and the therapists are recruited from the routine services. The measured outcomes are reduced to the minimum and tend to be gross measures that are clinically significant such as relapse or hospital admission; health economic measures to assess cost are also desirable. In special cases an equivalence trial may be designed, in which a new treatment is expected to match the clinical efficacy of an established treatment but may have other benefits, for example in terms of acceptability or cost. These trials have special methodological features that distinguish them from simple comparative trials.[32]

PARTICIPANT SAMPLES

Recruitment Bias

Figure 18.3 shows how the patient flow in a study should be described. The box of particular interest is the one at the very top that describes those who have been assessed for eligibility. In order to prevent bias in recruitment the best method for ascertaining samples of patients for a trial is to recruit them from a cohort of patients in contact with a service that covers a geographic area (as in Tarrier et al.[15] and Lewis et al.[17]). This ensures that the people who are in the trial do represent those who have the disorder. In the UK it is largely assumed that those patients with schizophrenia in contact with the services will represent those with the disorder requiring clinical intervention. For example, Tarrier et al.[15]

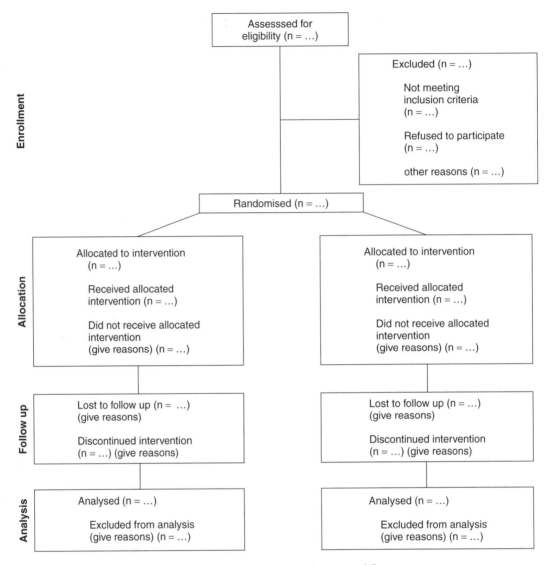

Figure 18.3. Participant recruitment and flow

screened all patients who might have a diagnosis of schizophrenia in a number of NHS trusts,
selected those who achieved predetermined criteria and examined their notes further. All putative
candidates following this procedure were inter-
viewed to ascertain whether they satisfied the
entry criteria. This method has been used as a
gold standard and other trials of CBT have used
the data from Tarrier et al.[15] to compare with
their study sample in order to conclude that their

sample was representative (see Sensky et al.[16]).
What a comparison of samples allows is just
that–if the samples are similar then the results
of the trials can be usefully compared, but this
information cannot be used as evidence of sample
representativeness.

Convenience samples which recruit from clinic
attenders or, even more problematically, patients
referred to the project by their clinicians are at
risk of selection bias. The referrer may only select

those possible participants who they view as good candidates for the treatment or conversely patients who are difficult or treatment refractory. Recruitment of referred patients is unfortunately the norm.[14,16] Even though it may be possible to compare the recruited sample to the whole population of patients who may be eligible in terms of socio-demographic and clinical service contact, this will not be enough data to rule out a systematic bias. In the treatment of panic disorder, Klein[33,34] has argued vigorously that in comparisons of psychotherapy verses drug, a pill placebo–drug comparison is necessary to ensure that the sample is not atypical since the efficacy of the drug (in this case imipramine) is well established. This is largely an argument about how representative or typical any sample is, given a reliance on convenience samples.

Selection

There are a number of different factors that need to be considered as part of the recruitment process such as service delivery system, academic support, socio-economic status of the area and geography (urban, suburban and rural area). It is unlikely that these will have a specific interaction with the outcome from therapy, but as these factors will affect the generalisation of the trial results it is probably important for the sample to represent a variety.

But ethnicity and cultural mix may potentially affect therapy outcomes. As we know very little about how to target psychological therapy to different cultural groups, it seems reasonable to start investigating a new treatment with a culturally homogeneous group and in later trials modify to accommodate cultural diversity, if such modification would be a requirement of effectiveness in cultural subgroups.

Diagnosis

In psychological therapies, especially in the field of psychosis, there has been a dilemma about whether to adopt medical diagnosis as entry criteria to studies. Some clinical psychologists (e.g.

Bentall et al.[35]) would prefer the adoption of symptomatic entry criteria as schizophrenia is a term covering a group of people with a wide variety of abnormal experiences. So some trials have as their entry criteria a specific symptom experienced as distressing rather than membership of a single diagnostic category.[11,36] However, even in these studies some patients were excluded on the basis of diagnosis because of not fulfilling other criteria (see below), and it was certainly the view of one of the authors (TW) that in feasibility studies of group CBT some patients with diagnoses other than schizophrenia, e.g. personality disorder or bipolar affective disorder, did not respond in similar ways to the patients with diagnoses of schizophrenia or schizoaffective disorder. Current CBT studies have generally included patients from the schizophrenia spectrum and it is certainly the view of some CBT therapists that the type of therapy offered to people with bipolar affective disorder is different from that designed for schizophrenia.[37]

Even when diagnosis is used there are too many different systems to choose from (e.g. clinical case note diagnosis, research diagnoses (RDC), DSMIV, ICD10, etc.). The choice of a different system will change the characteristics of the sample. For instance, if people are drawn on RDC criteria they will not necessarily be as chronic as those fulfilling the DSMIV criteria.

Exclusion Criteria

As well as criteria for inclusion into trials most studies also exclude people on the basis of specific issues. In trials of psychological therapy for psychosis one usual criterion is that the people who enter the trial are those whose symptoms have remained despite adequate doses of medication. The group chosen on this basis is extremely chronic and refractory and provides an extremely stringent test of the efficacy of psychological treatment.

A further thorny issue is that of co-morbid substance abuse. Most studies will exclude individuals when the abuse is severe, but the criteria for severity are rarely set out clearly so that it is impossible to compare between trials. Patients who are recruited from inner city areas are unlikely to be free of recreational drug use. A small consumption of cannabis may not affect the therapy efficacy, but it is not clear whether any use of class A drugs affects the therapeutic effect of psychological treatment. A more recent trial has been designed to test the efficacy of CBT and family intervention to treat dual diagnosis patients (those diagnosed as suffering from schizophrenia and substance abuse) in which the substance abuse is thought to increase the risk of poor outcomes in the primary disorder.[18] In this case severe substance abuse was an entry criterion.

Again some people may have a co-morbid organic condition such as epilepsy that may warrant exclusion, although most trials again would evaluate whether the organic condition is primarily responsible for the symptoms of the disorder which they are trying to alleviate. Deteriorating brain disorders such as Alzheimer's disease may be a reasonable exclusion criterion as CBT relies on the carry-over of changes in one session to subsequent sessions. Similarly, people who have learning disabilities may also have some difficulties with CBT as it is currently devised, although therapists have extended treatment for depression to the learning disabilities field. Current trials also do not support the idea that lower IQ prevents therapeutic changes.[38] But all current trials do have a lower cut-off for IQ, usually around 65.

Drop-out or Lost to Follow-up

Two main issues affect the inferences about the trial results. The first is the effect of those people who drop out of the therapy and the second is those people who are lost to contact at any stage of the trial. Different systems of dealing with drop-outs can be adopted. Some systems assume that the person would not have changed at all since leaving the trial (LOCF), but this approach has its problems.[39] But assuming that the group who drop out would have performed in the same way as those who remained also produces difficulties. Drop-outs may be those people who

might never have achieved any change following therapy. Clearly if a treatment produces high levels of drop-outs this might imply something about the acceptability of treatment. A precise description of drop-outs is required but, from the trials submitted so far this is missing in all but a few cases.

More research on drop-outs is clearly required. But in the area of mental health in particular, the research is difficult, if not impossible, to carry out. The new guidelines on research governance[40] do not allow for the harassing of people who have dropped out of trials for their reasons for dropping out or for data on their current health status. However, it is not only of interest academically, as it provides some information on the veracity of the theory underlying the disorder, but also essential to inform the health services. For example, Tarrier et al.[41] reported that patients who dropped out of treatment tended to be male, unemployed and unskilled, single, with a low level of educational attainment and a low premorbid IQ. They had a lengthy duration of illness although at the time of discontinuation they were not severely ill and functioned at a reasonable level. They were likely to be paranoid but not suspicious of the therapist. They were unlikely to be grandiose. They did not understand the rationale for therapy or the potential for benefit but feared it could make them worse.

It is not clear whether it is appropriate or ethical to collect personal information that is kept for routine monitoring purposes for a person who has dropped out of a trial. This information may consist of health service contacts kept on health care databases such as case notes as well as information from third parties. For trials involving people with severe disorders, third-party information from key workers is nearly always included as part of the measurement of outcome. The lack of data on drop-out may affect the relevance and benefit of the trial results to the wider community. It may therefore be unethical not to collect as much of it as possible. The interpretation of new legal rights such as the new UK Human Rights Act should make the position of researchers clearer, but it is also possible that the idiosyncratic interpretations made by local

Research Ethics committees will lead to further confusion in this already complicated area.

PLATFORM AND ORDNANCE

A naval military analogy between the vehicle of delivery, the platform (e.g. battleship, frigate, etc.) and what is delivered, the ordnance (e.g. shell, missile, etc.) is helpful in understanding the difference between service organisation and therapy.[42] In terms of this analogy the platform would be aspects of the mental health service, such as assertive outreach, case management and so on; whereas ordnance would consist of different types of therapeutic intervention, such as CBT and family interventions. This distinction is useful in clarifying what is being tested. For example a trial of different service organisations (platforms) would be the UK 700 trial,[43] in which 708 psychotic patients in four centres were randomly assigned to standard or intensive case management. In this trial the only specific difference between the two trial limbs was the number of patients the case managers had in their case loads. No investigation was made about the therapeutic input that the case managers implemented. The results indicated that there was no advantage in clinical or social outcomes of intensive case management. In contrast there are examples of therapy trials in which a comparison was made between CBT plus routine care, supportive counselling plus routine care, and routine care alone for chronic patients[15] and acute patients.[17] In these trials patients are recruited across a number of sites so that variations in routine care and service delivery are accommodated. It may be questioned whether trials of services are of much value if they do not include effective therapies. A battleship is unlikely to perform well in a naval engagement firing a bow and arrow!

BACKGROUND SERVICES

The background mental health services and their accessibility may affect trials in a number of ways. Recruitment may be affected by what services are already available and who has access to them. For example, recruitment is likely to be different if there is free universally available health care provided by a service committed to research and development. A large proportion of the population will use this service and potentially be available for recruitment and eligible for the trial. This is essentially what happens in the UK National Health Service. This case is very different when health care is provided, funded by reimbursements in a fragmented manner to certain groups of the population by private services who are unlikely to be committed to research. In this case the proportion of the population available for recruitment will be much reduced and biased towards certain subgroups who may, for whatever reasons, have no access to private care. Here recruitment is likely to be highly selective and potentially biased. The provision of different services to different income groups or other population subgroups mitigates against representativeness of trial populations in the USA, Australia and some European countries[44,45] and compromises the value of such trials.

RANDOMISATION

Purpose

To give an equivalent chance of a recruit being in any of the groups in the trial design. Some researchers think that one of the purposes is to balance the groups on every factor that may be relevant to the treatment response, but purely random allocation will not provide such matching. If there is strong evidence that a particular factor may affect the outcome then this should be included as a factor in the analysis. In the past researchers have said they have provided evidence of the equivalence of their samples in analyses of pre-treatment group comparisons and on the basis of finding no statistically significant differences on factors pertinent to the treatment response have then not included these factors in their analyses of therapeutic outcome. The current advice is not to carry out such pre-treatment comparisons but to include pertinent factors in the outcome assessment. However, there is a need for a clear description of the people who dropped out of treatment in relation to those who remained as this may bias the interpretation of the results.

For studies of psychological treatments in psychosis the most relevant factors are listed below.

- The *chronicity of the illness*, measured in months or years since first diagnosis, is likely to affect treatment outcome because it is well known in the field of psychiatry that those with longer illnesses may be less likely to change. Tarrier *et al.*[15] found that this modestly predicted treatment outcome in an intensive CBT trial.
- The *duration of untreated psychosis* (DUP) is the time spent experiencing symptoms prior to the diagnosis and treatment of the disorder. Several studies suggest that DUP affects the success of other treatments, particularly medication, and it may be that this is also a factor in the efficacy of psychological disorders.
- The *severity of the symptoms* has been shown to affect treatment outcome.[15,38] In the London–East Anglia trial the best outcomes following CBT were found for those people who said they were not absolutely certain that their delusions were true. The effect of this same factor was also alluded to several years ago in a small trial by Watt *et al.*[46] But, although the outcome at post-treatment was affected by this factor there was no measurable influence at follow-up nine months after the end of therapy.[47]
- *Gender* was investigated by Gould *et al.*[25] in their meta-analysis of CBT trials. They found no relationship between effect size and the proportion of men in the trial but as they themselves point out no data were available for the specific outcomes for men and women that precludes a definitive evaluation. However, young men are usually thought to have a poorer outcome and are more likely to drop out.[41]
- *Intellectual status* has been suggested by critics of psychological therapy to be a bar

to significant treatment effects. Although one recent study has not found this to be true,[38] trialists should consider this factor in their analysis if only to counter such criticisms.

- *Interactions with other treatments* need to be considered where these are variables within the group of patients entered into the trial. The most pertinent for CBT studies is the issue of the use of medication. Medication is now often divided into two main types, typical antipsychotics which have been available for a number of years and atypical antipsychotic medications which have become available recently. Most published CBT studies were carried out before the wide availability of these newer medications. However, medication was not a predictor of outcome in Garety *et al.*[38] or Tarrier *et al.*[15] Kuipers *et al.*[47] comment that in their CBT group, because symptomatic improvement would be achieved, these patients would be less likely to be prescribed clozapine (an atypical antipsychotic) and would generally be prescribed lower doses of medication. These predictions, although only a trend towards significant, were shown in their data. Pinto *et al.*[48] chose their sample on the basis of a failure of at least two medications to reduce positive symptoms. In their study, which was not methodologically strong, the effect size was extremely large with the combined effect of CBT and the new medication (clozapine) producing an effect size of 2.18.[49] This suggests that medication should be taken into account in randomisation or at least in subgroup analyses.

Entry to the study may be stratified if the variable has a known interaction with treatment or the variable can be used as a covariate in the analyses. Being clear about which variables may interact with psychological treatment is essential at the outset of the trial because the trial must be defined and have a sufficiently large sample to be adequately powered to test for these effects.

Details

Details of the process of randomisation must be supplied in the paper. For instance in Kuipers *et al.*[14] a randomised permuted blocks allocation was adopted in each centre which contributed participants to the trial. Other studies with multiple centres (e.g. Sensky *et al.*[16]) randomised participants at each centre, this they then argued allows them to control for within-centre effects and allows them to test between-centre effects of treatment efficacy.

Blindness

In clinical trials blindness usually refers to two aspects of the trial. The first relates to the allocation of participants to the different treatment limbs so that the allocation process is independent and concealed from those involved in the assessment or treatment. This prevents people from choosing who to put into the trial on the basis of the patient's own preference, resulting in more enthusiastic people being in the treatment arm, or the research worker's preference which may result in those with more favourable prognoses being allocated to the experimental treatment.

The second use of the word blindness relates to the concealment of which treatment the participant received from those involved with assessment, especially of outcome. This is an extremely important issue and one that is difficult to ensure. The aim is to prevent any bias, conscious or otherwise, entering the assessment process through knowledge of which treatment the participant received. For example, knowledge that the hypothesis to be tested was that CBT would be better that treatment-as-usual because previous studies had demonstrated this may bias an assessor to rating the patient as more improved if they knew the patient had received CBT.

The importance of adequate concealment was demonstrated in a study by Moher *et al.*[50] who examined the quality of concealment in treatment trials in circulatory and digestive disease, mental health, obstetrics and childbirth. The examined trials had already passed a number of quality assessments and been included in a number of meta-analyses. They found that trials with poorer quality blinding were associated with an increased estimate of benefit of 34%. This replicated a similar earlier finding of Schulz *et al.*[51] who also reported exaggerated treatment efficacy of 30–40% in trials with inadequate concealment. There is good evidence that the poorer the trial methodology the better, and more inflated, the treatment results obtained.

The assessment and treatment procedures must be separate and independent, in other words the person who carries out the assessment should be different from the person who delivers the treatment. This is not always the case in published trials, for example Brooker *et al.*[52,53] trained mental health nurses in family intervention and assessed the effectiveness of the intervention by having the nurses perform the assessments. It could be argued that any problem of bias could be avoided in cases such as these by performing the assessments through patient self-report. However, this does not address the problem of social approval that may introduce bias where patients give results they think their therapist would want to receive.

Independent assessors and therapists will not ensure that assessors remain naive to treatment allocation. Accidental knowledge of allocation can be minimised by using separate administrative procedures and geographically separating therapists from assessors in terms of office location and administrative procedure. This should prevent assessors bumping into patients about to receive therapy and such similar accidents. Patient allocation should be multiply coded so that learning of one patient's allocation does not break the whole trial code. Patients should be instructed not to reveal any detail of their treatment or who has treated them to the assessors at the start of the trial and before each assessment. It is unlikely that this will be fool-proof but it will minimise revelations. See Tarrier *et al.*[15] for further details of efforts to maintain blindness in a clinical trial of CBT.

Opinions differ as to whether verification of maintenance of blindness is desirable. It is possible to ask assessors to guess the allocation of trial participants. This can be used as evidence of successful blindness.[15,54] Assessors should not be informed that they will be asked to guess as this would prime them to the task. Guessing is less likely to be successful when there are more than two treatment groups. With two groups, or even more than two, an assessor could adopt a strategy that patients who improved should be in the experimental treatment group because this would be in line with the study hypothesis. If the trial had been successful this strategy would have been correct and the assessor would most likely have guessed right in many cases although for the wrong reasons. This would not be an indication that the assessor knew of the treatment allocation and was hence biased in their assessment but that they knew who improved which aided them in guessing group allocation. The problem for the trial investigators here would be that their assessors appear not to have been blind. If the assessors were not able to guess correctly using this strategy it would probably mean that the experimental treatment had not been effective and the trial was a failure anyway. Having assessors guess allocation holds the investigators hostage to fortune, although with multiple treatment groups it can be effective in demonstrating blindness.

Even if assessors do maintain blindness to treatment allocation they will still be aware of the timing of the assessment, pre-, post-treatment or follow-up. Thus the only way to ensure blindness of both treatment allocation and assessment time is to separate the gathering of information from its rating. Thus all assessment interviews should be audio-taped independently of their rating and rating should be carried out by a different assessor who is unaware of the allocation or assessment. This would also allow the audio-tapes to be edited of any accidental revelation

of identifiers. To be successful interviews need to follow a protocol as to the procedure of the interview so that adequate and sufficient information is available to make ratings. In most studies of CBT in general and for psychosis in particular, the process for blind allocation is rarely described, for example Kuipers et al.[14] In contrast, Sensky et al.[16] and Tarrier et al.[15] both describe the method for ensuring blindness and the maintenance of allocation of subjects to groups.

PROTOCOL

Design Protocol

There are various ways of testing whether a particular treatment is efficacious but the accepted method is to compare the treatment with a placebo control that allows for a comparison of client expectations of improvement during therapy with the active ingredient itself. We have discussed above the importance of these non-specific factors in psychological treatments. Social contact, social support and the modelling of interpersonal behaviour are all an integral part of psychological therapy. Tests of the effectiveness of individual CBT have used a variety of designs. Table 18.2 below gives the outline of the main recent trials.

There are a variety of designs that will allow the examination of both the effectiveness and specificity of the effect of CBT above the effects found for psychological interventions in general in this group. The results show that there are significant effects over treatment-as-usual. There is also one study[16] that shows a

Table 18.2. Designs for randomised control trials of CBT for psychosis

Comparison with treatment-as-usual	Comparison with alternative 'placebo' therapy	Comparison with 'placebo' therapy and treatment-as-usual
Garety et al.[11]	Sensky et al.[16]	Tarrier et al.[10]
Kuipers et al.[14,47]	Drury et al.[12,13]	Tarrier et al.[15,73]
Barrowclough et al.[18]		SOCRATES[17]

difference between CBT and a 'placebo' therapy (befriending), but only at follow-up. However, Tarrier et al.[15] found a significant difference between CBT and TAU but no overall difference between the two therapies at any stage of the study.[55] Analysis of specific symptoms found that there was a significant advantage of CBT over supportive counselling in the treatment of hallucinations.[56]

Treatment Protocol

It is essential to have a clear and unambiguous treatment protocol for psychological treatments. However, even when a manual is available it is much harder to evaluate exactly whether the protocol has been adhered to. In treatments with medication this process is relatively easy as the dose and timing of the treatment can be verified using simple procedures. For psychological treatment the verification process relies on taped interviews of treatment sessions that are then rated later for fidelity with the treatment protocol. However, there are several problems that may interfere with this process. Firstly the patient must agree to the recording of the session and in some studies, e.g. Chadwick et al.,[57] the patients refused to have any sessions taped. Once taped sessions have been collected the independent rating must answer a number of questions:

- Does the session represent the treatment to be provided? In other words is it possible to differentiate the experimental treatment from the placebo treatment. Sensky et al.[16] and Tarrier et al.[15] were able to show that their independent assessors was able to assign 100% and 97% of the tapes rated to the appropriate treatment arm.
- Is the experimental treatment manual being adhered to? This requires that the researchers have a specific rating scale that will allow the rating of key areas of their treatment. Haddock et al.[58] has developed a rating scale (the Cognitive Therapy Scale for Psychosis–CTS-Psy) to assess quality of therapy. This allows assessment of general (e.g. interpersonal effectiveness) and specific (e.g. guided discovery)

aspects of therapy to be assessed. However, the scale allocates equal weighting to all items. There is, as yet, no empirical evidence to support such equal weightings, and it may well be, for example, that 'agenda setting' is less important than the 'choice of intervention'.

- Does the progression of therapy cover all the key topics of the manual? This requires that several sessions of therapy are recorded at different times and that the content of these is scored for the timing of the interventions in the treatment programme. This is probably the most important part of rating CBT trials because although it can be clear how many sessions are provided to a patient it is not clear whether the content given is the same. CBT researchers (personal communications, including one of the authors, NT) observe that some patients are able to travel through the whole manual whereas others cover much less. So although the therapy duration may be equivalent, exposure to the complete protocol can be different. This dosage of treatment may be an important factor in defining treatment outcome as some patients are clearly getting more treatment than others. However, the number of treatment sessions is not related to effect size as presented in Gould et al.[25]

Progression through therapy may be affected by a number of factors such as the level of disturbance or cognitive impairment of the patient. Therapists will also differ in their ability to progress therapy and their skills in different aspects–determined by skills, training, profession, trial provided training (see Tarrier et al.[59]). So far in CBT trials these factors have not been investigated in any detail.

INDIVIDUALISED TREATMENTS

Turkington and Siddle[60] claim that a case formulation is essential to treating psychotic patients successfully. We do not disagree that a case formulation is desirable but with psychotic patients it is not always possible and a purely symptomatic approach has to be adopted on occasions.[61] In spite of our support for case formulation the evidence from general adult mental health that a case formulation is necessary is poor and the results equivocal. Schulte *et al.*[62] treated a mixed group of 120 phobic patients with a standardised treatment and individualised behaviour therapy based on functional behaviour analysis. They also included a yoked control group in which treatment was based not on the individual's assessment but that of the yoked patient. The standardised treatment group showed the most improvement and patients who acted as yoked controls improved as well as the other patients. Similarly Emmelkamp *et al.*[63] allocated 22 obsessive–compulsive patients to either tailor-made cognitive behavioural therapy or standardised exposure *in vivo* therapy. There were no significant differences between groups but the group sizes were small ($n = 11$ in each group). Jacobson *et al.*[64] treated 30 distressed marital couples with either a manual-based version of marital therapy or a clinically flexible version of the same treatment in which treatment plans were individually based and the number of treatment sessions were not specified. Both treatments resulted in significant improvements at post-treatment but at six-month follow-up the couples treated with the structured format were more likely to have deteriorated and flexibly treated couples were more likely to have maintained their treatment gains. There appears little advantage of case formulation-based treatment over a standard package. This result is not surprising given the sample sizes of these studies. Standard treatment programmes are effective for a wide range of psychological disorders and even if an individualised treatment was superior the difference in effect sizes will most probably be small and the sample size to significantly demonstrate such a difference would necessarily be large. Therefore, the studies that have been done are massively underpowered. To substantiate this Tarrier and Calam[65] have estimated the sample sizes required to show significant differences with 80% power and 0.05 significance level based on the data provided in the published report of Emmelkamp *et al.*[63] On the basis of their data

the numbers in each group required to show a significant difference for the five outcome measures would be between 25 and in excess of 15 000, with a median of 800 patients in each treatment group. The issue of case formulation-based treatment versus protocol-based treatment is unlikely to be resolved by a direct head-to-head comparison, which would be too large and costly.

TREATMENT COMPONENTS

CBT treatments also differ in other ways from each other. Although they have a basic set of ingredients the emphasis may be placed differently. For example, the different emphases on behavioural activation and cognitive schema in the changes in thinking thought to be the cause of the treatment effect. Changing behaviour can have an effect on thinking as studies of CBT for panic disorder have discovered.[22] Patients in the Clark study were treated with behavioural activation programmes that are embedded in CBT. They showed that the prediction of outcome was dependent on one main factor, cognitions about their bodily sensations. The behavioural experiments seemed to have an effect on cognition. But, other groups in the field of psychosis emphasise more distal stimuli such as the developmental path of the delusion. The particular component of CBT that accounts for most of the variance in outcome has not yet been differentiated and these more subtle differences are not used in meta-analyses of the treatment studies. Figure 18.4 shows the effect sizes taken from Gould *et al.*[25] on a scale devised by ourselves on the amount of behavioural activation that the treatment emphasises. As can be seen from the graph the effect size is increased when more behavioural activation is included. It may be that a simple change in behaviour via a behavioural experiment may provide enough evidence to reduce delusional conviction. For instance Birchwood and Chadwick[66] suggest that the perceived powerfulness of an auditory hallucination directly predicts the distress experienced. Adopting one successful coping strategy may provide enough evidence to reduce the perceived power of an auditory hallucination and increase the amount of perceived

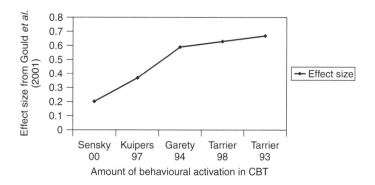

Figure 18.4. How much 'B' in CBT for psychosis

control the patient has over their symptoms. Wykes *et al.*[67] provides some evidence of this relationship in a waiting list control trial of group CBT for auditory hallucinations. If this is true then successful behavioural experiments should always be included and should predict successful treatment outcome. As yet no study has attempted to measure this process.

Turkington and Siddle[60] maintain that cognitive therapy with psychotic populations will result in long-term improvement because it involves schema change whereas cognitive behaviour therapy (as carried out by Tarrier *et al.*[15]) will result in short-term change only. They go on to say that 'schema change seems vital in terms of the durability of any achieved benefits' (p. 302). However, there is little evidence that schema are causative in psychosis or that change is important for treatment effects (see Figure 18.4). The direct transport of Beck's model of depression to psychosis in the absence of evidence for its explanatory value in this population has been criticised.[68] The evidence for the effect of schema work on outcome is anyway sparse even in the area of depression for which it was designed. Jacobson randomised 150 people to three treatment arms: (i) behavioural activation, (ii) behavioural activation and work on dysfunctional thoughts, and (iii) total CBT with work on cognitive schema. The results of this trial showed no differences in outcome either at post-treatment or follow-up between the three groups. The effect of the other components of CBT was no different to

the effects of behavioural activation alone (see Figure 18.5).

OUTCOMES

Current thinking from methodologists on trials in psychiatry is that designs should be simplified and that outcome measures should be kept to a minimum. In particular the use of rating scales should be restricted to 'one or two which are best understood' (Johnson,[69] p. 229). Follow-up should be carried out on 'few occasions rather than many' and entry criteria should be as broad as possible.[69] This advice is rather in conflict with that given previously which suggests that, in the treatment of psychosis, multiple outcomes which reflect the complex nature of the disorder and its effects should be used[70] and that data on the process of therapy are essential. The multiple effects of therapy may, but not necessarily, have a common outcome in relapse prevention or total symptoms. For instance cognitive therapy should affect cognition, CBT should affect cognitions and behaviour, and family interventions should affect families' interactions. All these effects could in some way change the outcome of the disorder but via multiple pathways. Because of these multiple effects, multiple outcomes may be recommended in order to differentiate the route to effectiveness in explanatory trials.

All current trials measure overall symptoms. However, they all do so in different ways and even when the measure appears to be a standard

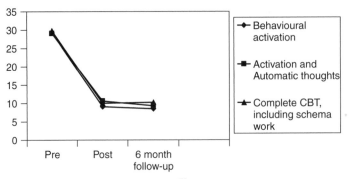

Source: Data from Jacobsen *et al.*[75]

Figure 18.5. Evidence of the effect of schema work in depression

measure (e.g. BPRS[71]) it is often adapted. For instance Kuipers *et al.*[14] added items to the BPRS making it difficult to compare their results with others adopting the conventional version of the same instrument. The use of non-standard instruments to measure awareness of stigma, coping skills, etc. prevents comparisons being made and does need replication with standardised rating scales with no known psychometric properties.

In all medical trials a statistically significant difference in outcome may provide little benefit to the patients. What needs to be defined for trials of CBT for psychosis is the clinical significance of outcomes. This was alluded to earlier in this chapter. Clinically significant outcomes may be reductions in the distress associated with the disorder. Currently clinical significance is defined as the sorts of improvements that are achieved in drug trials–20% change in symptoms. This may be a low threshold for what could be achieved through psychological therapy. Many trials of psychological therapy adopt only a statistically significant test of effectiveness, but Tarrier *et al.*[15] and Sensky *et al.*[16] adopt a 50% change criterion for their measures, although Kuipers *et al.*[14] use the lower threshold of 20%. Where trials use such a threshold of achieving clinical significance or not, comparisons can be made by comparing the Numbers Needed to Treat (NNT), which represents the number of patients that need to be treated to achieve one clinically significant outcome.[72]

CONCLUSIONS

Because psychological therapy has no product champion as found in the drug industry, pragmatic trials are needed initially to convince people that therapy is worthwhile. However, these need to be followed by explanatory trials that can establish the specificity of the treatment. Currently the trials in the field of psychosis have mainly been pragmatic and these have shown that the therapy is worthwhile with improvements in positive and negative symptoms at post-treatment and follow-up in some studies. However, the trials that have been designed to test the specificity of treatment have not been so successful. Very few differences emerge between CBT for psychosis and alternative therapies are shown at post-treatment. Of the two studies with long follow-ups one showed an advantage for CBT over the alternative therapy[16] but the other showed equivalent benefits of both therapies (CBT and supportive counselling) over routine care.[55,73] One resolution of this conflict may be the nature of the therapy chosen. In the Sensky *et al.*[16] study the comparison condition was befriending which is described as a therapy with equivalent amounts of therapist contact but where the content was a discussion focusing on neutral topics such as hobbies, sports and current affairs where the therapist is instructed to be empathic but non-directive. Even this therapy was associated with reductions in symptoms at the end of therapy that may be a testament to the paucity of the social contact and lack of warm relationships of people with continuing active psychosis. However, the effects of this therapy were not sustained to a follow-up where the patients in the comparison therapy condition actually got worse. In the Tarrier et al.[15] study the comparison therapy chosen was supportive counselling in which the therapist tried to achieve a supportive relationship which fostered rapport and provided emotional support. This therapy proved to be successful in reducing symptoms over the course of the therapy and follow-up. This result suggests that some of the essential ingredients of CBT encompassed within the counselling framework may be either shared with supportive counselling or are as effective as these other ingredients. It is of course possible that within the model of schizophrenia which encompasses a vulnerability stress model that the two forms of therapy may work via different pathways. Supportive counselling may work by emphasising self-esteem through rapport within the therapeutic relationship. Unlike befriending this support produces more stable changes that are durable to follow-up. However, it should be noted that supportive counselling did significantly worse at treating hallucinations when compared to CBT on this symptom alone.[56]

Currently there is no evidence that cognitive behaviour therapy works via a cognitive system, although training in coping skills has been shown to improve coping.[74] None of the studies have yet produced analyses showing that the cognitive change established during therapy is the key to later improvement. In fact few have even provided analyses which test this possibility. Because of the complex nature of the aetiology of psychosis with its multiple causal processes it may be impossible to identify a single route to change. There may be many idiosyncratic routes that will only be established in large trials with several hundred patients included. One such trial is taking place in Manchester, the Socrates trial.[17] In this trial hundreds of acute patients who are at the beginning of their illness have been provided with therapy and followed up over a long period. It is only through these sorts of studies that it

will be possible to establish routes to change that can then inform the development of therapy. It is only by these later developments that it will be possible to develop training and therefore provide larger numbers of people with psychosis with effective psychological therapy.

REFERENCES

1. Wiersma D, Nienhuis FJ, Sloof CJ, Geil R. Natural course of schizophrenic disorders: a 15 year follow-up of a Dutch incidence cohort. *Schizophr Bull* (1998) **24**: 75–85.
2. British Psychological Society. *Recent Advances in Understanding Mental Illness and Psychotic Experiences*. Leicester: British Psychological Society (2000).
3. Fowler D, Garety P, Kuipers E. Cognitive therapy for psychosis: formulation, treatment, effects and service implications. *J Mental Health* (1998) **7**: 123–33.
4. Tarrier N, Barrowclough C, Vaughn C, Bamrah JS, Porceddu K, Watts S, Freeman HL. The community management of schizophrenia: a controlled trial of a behavioural intervention with families. *Br J Psychiat* (1988) **153**: 532–42.
5. Cunningham-Owens DG, Carroll A, Fattah S, Clyde Z, Coffey I, Johnstone EC. A randomised, controlled trial of a brief educational package for schizophrenic outpatients. *Acta Psychiat Scand* (2001) **103**: 362–9.
6. Beck AT. Successful outpatient psychotherapy with a schizophrenic with delusion based on borrowed guilt. *Psychiatry* (1952) **15**: 305–12.
7. Tarrier N. Psychological treatment of schizophrenic symptoms. In: Kavanagh D, ed., *Schizophrenia: An Overview and Practical Handbook*. London: Chapman & Hall (1992).
8. Tarrier N. Modification and management of residual psychotic symptoms. In: Birchwood M, Tarrier N, eds, *Psychological Approaches to Schizophrenia: Innovations in Assessment, Treatment and Services*. Chichester: John Wiley & Sons (1992).
9. Haddock G, Tarrier N, Spaulding W, Yusupoff L, Kinney C, McCarthy E. Individual cognitive-behaviour therapy in the treatment of schizophrenia: a review. *Clin Psychol Rev* (1998) **18**: 821–38.
10. Tarrier N, Beckett R, Harwood S, Baker A, Yusupoff L, Ugarteburu I. A trial of two cognitive behavioural methods of treating drug-resistant residual psychotic symptoms in schizophrenic patients. I: Outcome. *Br J Psychiat* (1993) **162**: 524–32.

11. Garety P, Kuipers E, Fowler D, Chamberlain F, Dunn G. Cognitive-behaviour therapy for drug resistant psychosis. *Br J Med Psychol* (1994) **67**: 259–71.

12. Drury V, Birchwood M, Cochrane R, Macmillan F. Cognitive therapy and recovery from acute psychosis. I. Impact on psychotic symptoms. *Br J Psychiat* (1996) **169**: 593–601.

13. Drury V, Birchwood M, Cochrane R, Macmillan F. Cognitive therapy and recovery from acute psychosis. II. Impact on recovery time. *Br J Psychiat* (1996) **169**: 602–7.

14. Kuipers E, Garety P, Fowler D, Dunn G, Bebbington P, Freeman D, Hadley C. London–East Anglia randomised controlled trial of cognitive-behavioural therapy for psychosis: 1. Effects of the treatment phase. *Br J Psychiat* (1997) **171**: 319–27.

15. Tarrier N, Yusupoff L, Kinney C, McCarthy E, Gledhill A, Haddock G, Morris J. A randomised controlled trial of intensive cognitive behaviour therapy for patients with chronic schizophrenia. *Br Med J* (1998) **317**: 303–7.

16. Sensky T, Turkington D, Kingdon D, Scott JL, Scott J, Siddle R, O'Carroll M, Barnes TRE. A randomised controlled trial of cognitive-behavioral therapy for persistent symptoms in schizophrenia resistant to medication. *Arch Gen Psychiat* (2000) **57**: 165–72.

17. Lewis SW, Tarrier N, Haddock G, Bentall R, Kinderman P, Kingdon D, Siddle R, Drake R, Everitt J, Leadley K, Benn A, Glazebrook K, Haley C, Akhtar S, Davies L, Palmer S, Faragher B, Dunn G. Randomised controlled trial of cognitive-behaviour therapy in early schizophrenia: acute phase outcomes. *Br J Psychiat* (2002) **181**(Suppl 43): 91–7.

18. Barrowclough C, Haddock G, Tarrier N, Lewis S, Moring J, O'Brian R, Schofield N, McGovern J. Randomised controlled trial of motivational interviewing and cognitive behavioural intervention for schizophrenia patients with associated drug or alcohol misuse. *Am J Psychiat* (2001) **158**: 1706–13.

19. Barrowclough C, Tarrier N, Sellwood W, Quinn J, Mainwaring J, Lewis S. A randomised controlled effectiveness trial of a needs based psychosocial intervention service for carers of schizophrenic patients. *Br J Psychiat* (1999) **174**: 506–11.

20. Horvath A, Symonds D. Relationship between working alliance and outcomes in psychotherapy: a meta-analysis. *J Counsel Psychol* (1991) **38**: 139–49.

21. Wampold BE, Mondin GW, Moody M, Stich F, Benson K, Ahn H. A meta-analysis of outcome studies comparing bona fide psychotherapies: empirically, "all must have prizes". *Psychol Bull* (1997) **122**: 203–15.

22. Clark DM, Salkovskis PM, Hackmann A, Middleton H, Anastasiades P, Gelder M. A comparison of cognitive therapy, applied relaxation and imipramine in the treatment of panic disorder. *Br J Psychiat* (1994) **164**: 759–69.

23. Paykel ES, Scott J, Teasdale JD, Johnson AL, Garland A, Moore R, Jenaway A, Cornwall PL, Hayhurst H, Abbott R, Pope M. Prevention of relapse in residual depression by cognitive therapy. *Arch Gen Psychiat* (1999) **56**: 829–35.

24. Yammey G. Psychologists question debriefing for traumatised employees. *Br Med J* (2000) **320**: 140.

25. Gould RA, Mueser KT, Bolton E, Mays V, Goff D. Cognitive therapy for psychosis in schizophrenia: an effect size analysis. *Schizophr Res* (2001) **48**: 335–42.

26. Cohen J. *Statistical Power Analysis for the Behavioral Sciences*. Hillsdale, NJ: Lawrence Erlbaum (1988).

27. Begg C, Cho M, Eastwood S, Horton R, Moher D, Olkin I, Pitkin R, Rennie D, Schulz KF, Simelk D, Stroup DF. Improving the quality of reporting of randomized controlled trials: The CONSORT Statement. *J Am Med Assoc* (1996) **276**: 637–9.

28. Moher D, Schulz K, Altman D. The CONSORT Statement: revised recommendations for improving the quality of reports of parallel group randomisation. *J Am Med Assoc* (2001) **285**: 1987–91.

29. Geddes J, Reynolds S, Streiner D, Szatmari P, Haynes B. Evidence-based practice in mental health. *Evidence-Based Mental Health* (1998) **1**: 4–5.

30. Barlow DH. Health care policy, psychotherapy research and the future of psychotherapy. *Am Psychol* (1996) **51**: 1050–8.

31. Drake RE, Goldman HH, Leff HS, Lehman AF, Dixon L, Mueser KT, Torrey WC. Implementing evidence-based practices in routine mental service settings. *Psychiat Serv* (2001) **52**: 179–82.

32. Jones B, Jarvis P, Lewis JA, Ebbutt AF. Trials to assess equivalence: the importance of rigorous methods. *Br Med J* (1996) **313**: 36–9.

33. Klein DF. Preventing hung juries about therapy studies. *J Consult Clin Psychol* (1996) **64**: 81–7.

34. Klein DF. Discussion of 'methodological controversies in the treatment of panic disorders'. *Behav Res Ther* (1996) **34**: 849–53.

35. Bentall RP, Jackson HF, Pilgrim D. Abandoning the concept of schizophrenia: some implications of validity arguments for psychological research into psychotic phenomena. *Br J Clin Psychol* (1989) **27**: 303–24.

36. Wykes T, Parr A-M, Landau S. Group treatment for auditory hallucinations – a waiting list controlled study. *Br J Psychiat* (1999) **175**: 180–5.

37. Lam D, Bright J, Jones S, Hayward P, Schuck N, Chisholm D, Sham P. Cognitive therapy for bipolar illness – a pilot study of relapse prevention. *Cognit Ther Res* (2000) **24**: 503–20.

38. Garety P, Fowler D, Kuipers E, Freeman D, Dunn G, Bebbington P, Hadley C, Jones S. London–East Anglia randomised controlled trial of cognitive-behavioural therapy for psychosis. II Predictors of outcome. *Br J Psychiat* (1997) **171**: 319–27.

39. Everitt BS. The analysis of longitudinal data: beyond MANOVA. *Br J Psychiat* (1998) **172**: 7–10.

40. Department of Health. *Research Governance Framework for Health and Social Care.* Department of Health, UK (2001).

41. Tarrier N, Yusupoff L, McCarthy E, Kinney C, Wittkowski A. Some reason why patients suffering from chronic schizophrenia fail to continue in psychological treatment. *Behav Cognit Psychother* (1998) **26**: 177–81.

42. Marshall M. A systematic review of the effectiveness of acute day hospitals versus admission. Paper presented at The Making Mental Health Services Effective: Now and Tomorrow Conference, 7–8 September 2000, Manchester, UK (2000).

43. Burns T, Creed F, Fahy T, Thompson S, Tyrer P, White I, & the UK 700 Group. Intensive versus standard case management for severe psychotic illness: a randomised trial. *Lancet* (1999) **353**: 2185–9.

44. Wykes T, Tarrier N, Lewis S. *Outcome and Innovation in the Psychological Treatment of Schizophrenia.* Chichester: John Wiley & Sons (1998).

45. Tarrier N. What can be learned from clinical trials? Reply to Devilly and Foa (2001). *J Consult Clin Psychol* (2001) **69**: 117–18.

46. Watt F, Powell G, Austin S. Modification of delusional beliefs. *Br J Med Psychol* (1983) **46**: 359–63.

47. Kuipers E, Fowler D, Garety P, Chisholm D, Freeman D, Dunn G, Bebbington P, Hadley C. London–East Anglia randomised controlled trial of cognitive-behavioural therapy for psychosis. III Follow-up and economic evaluation at 18 months. *Br J Psychiat* (1998) **171**: 319–27.

48. Pinto A, La Pia S, Mennella R, Giorgio D, DeSimone L. Cognitive-behavioral therapy and clozapine for clients with treatment-refractory schizophrenia. *Psychiat Serv* (1999) **50**: 901–4.

49. Rector NA, Beck AT. Cognitive-behavioral therapy for schizophrenia: an empirical review. *J Nerv Ment Dis* (2001) **189**: 278–87.

50. Moher D, Pham B, Jones A, Cook DJ, Jadad AR, Moher M, Tugwell P, Klassen TP. Does quality of reports of randomised trials affect estimates of intervention efficacy reported in meta-analyses? *Lancet* (1998) **352**: 609–13.

51. Schulz KF, Chalmers I, Hayes RJ, Altman DG. Empirical evidence of bias: dimensions of methodological quality associated with estimates of treatment effect in controlled trials. *J Am Med Assoc* (1995) **280**: 178–80.

52. Brooker C, Tarrier N, Barrowclough C, Butterworth A, Goldberg D. Training community psychiatric nurses for psychosocial intervention: report of a pilot study. *Br J Psychiat* (1992) **160**: 836–44.

53. Brooker C, Falloon I, Butterworth A, Goldberg D, Graham-Hole V, Hillier V. The outcome of training community psychiatric nurses to deliver psychosocial intervention. *Br J Psychiat* (1994) **165**: 222–30.

54. Basoglu M, Marks I, Livanou M, Swinson R. Double-blindness procedure, rater blindness, and ratings of outcome. *Arch Gen Psychiat* (1997) **54**: 744–8.

55. Tarrier N, Kinney C, McCarthy E, Humphreys L, Wittkowski A, Morris J. Two year follow-up of cognitive-behaviour therapy and supportive counselling in the treatment of persistent positive symptoms in chronic schizophrenia. *J Consult Clin Psychol* (2000) **68**: 917–22.

56. Tarrier N, Kinney C, McCarthy E, Wittkowski A, Yusupoff L, Gledhill A, Morris J. Are some types of psychotic symptoms more responsive to CBT? *Behav Cognit Psychother* (2001) **29**: 45–55.

57. Chadwick P, Sambrooke S, Rasch S, Davies E. Challenging the omnipotence of voices: group cognitive behavior therapy for voices. *Behav Res Ther* (2000) **38**: 993–1003.

58. Haddock G, Devane S, Bradshaw T, McGovern J, Tarrier N, Kinderman P, Baguley I, Lancashire S, Harris N. An investigation into the psychometric properties of the Cognitive Therapy scale for psychosis (CTS-Psy). *Behav Cognit Psychother* (2001) **29**: 93–106.

59. Tarrier N, Barrowclough C, Haddock G, McGovern J. The dissemination of innovative cognitive-behavioural treatments for schizophrenia. *J Mental Health* (1999) **8**: 569–82.

60. Turkington D, Siddle R. Improving understanding and coping in people with schizophrenia by changing attitudes. *Psychiat Rehab Skills* (2000) **4**: 300–20.

61. Tarrier N, Haddock G. Cognitive-behaviour therapy for the treatment of schizophrenia: a case formulation approach. In: Hofman SG, Thompson MC, eds, *Handbook of Psychological Treatments*

for Severe Mental Disorders. New York: Guilford Press (2001).

62. Schulte D, Kunzel R, Pepping G, Schulte-Bahrenberg T. Tailor-made versus standardised therapy of phobic patients. *Adv Behav Res Ther* (1992) **14**: 67–92.

63. Emmelkamp PMG, Bouman TK, Blaauw E. Individualised versus standardised therapy: a comparative evaluation with obsessive–compulsive patients. *Clin Psychol Psychother* (1994) **1**: 95–100.

64. Jacobson NS, Schmaling KB, Holtzworth-Munroe A, Katt JL, Wood LF, Follette VM. Research-structured vs clinically flexible versions of social learning-based marital therapy. *Behav Res Ther* (1989) **27**: 173–80.

65. Tarrier N, Calam R. New developments in cognitive-behavioural case formulation. Epidemiological, systemic and social context: an integrative approach. *Cognit Behav Psychother* (2002) **30**: 311–28.

66. Birchwood M, Chadwick P. The omnipotence of voices: testing the validity of cognitive model. *Psychol Med* (1997) **21**: 1345–53.

67. Wykes T, Reeder C, Corner J, Williams C, Everitt B. The effects of neurocognitive remediation on executive processing in patients with schizophrenia. *Schizophr Bull* (1999) **25**: 291–308.

68. Patience DA. Cognitive-behaviour therapy for schizophrenia. *Br J Psychiat* (1994) **165**: 266–7.

69. Johnson T. Clinical trials in psychiatry: background and statistical perspective. *Stat Meth Med Res* (1998) **7**: 209–34.

70. Barrowclough C, Tarrier N. Psychosocial interventions with families and their effects on the course of schizophrenia: a review. *Psychol Med* (1984) **14**: 629–42.

71. Ventura J, Green M, Shaner A, Liberman R. Training and quality assurance with the Brief Psychiatric Rating Scale: the drift busters. *Int J Meth Psychiat Res* (1993) **3**: 221–44.

72. Sackett DL, Richardson WS, Rosenberg W, Haynes RB. *Evidence-Based Medicine*. London: Churchill Livingstone (1998).

73. Tarrier N, Wittkowski A, Kinney C, McCarthy E, Morris J, Humphreys L. The durability of the effects of cognitive behaviour therapy in the treatment of chronic schizophrenia: twelve months follow-up. *Br J Psychiat* (1999) **174**: 500–4.

74. Tarrier N, Sharpe L, Beckett R, Harwood S, Baker A, Yusupoff L. A trial of two cognitive behavioural methods of treating drug-resistant residual psychotic symptoms in schizophrenic patients. II: Treatment-specific changes in coping and problem-solving skills. *Social Psychiat Psychiat Epidemiol* (1993) **28**: 5–10.

75. Jacobson NS, Dobson KS, Truax PA, Addis ME, Koerner K, Gollan JK, Gortner E, Prince SE. *J Consult Clin Psychol* (1996) **64**: 295–304.

19

Depression

GRAHAM DUNN

Biostatistics Group, School of Epidemiology & Health Sciences, University of Manchester, Manchester, UK

INTRODUCTION

The purpose of the present chapter is to explore the pitfalls in and challenges to the valid estimation of the effects of psychotherapies. Although 'depression' appears in the title, the discussion will be relevant to psychological treatments for any mental illness (including psychotic disorders such as bipolar depression and schizophrenia). Most of the illustrative examples, however, will refer to the treatment of depression. Right from the start, despite pointing out all of its potential problems, I will assume that by far the best way of trying to estimate treatment effects is via the use of a *randomised controlled trial* (RCT). I have little sympathy with the increasingly popular view that we can learn much of real value about treatment effects from systematically collected outcome data in routine clinical practice (see Dunn[1] for a critique of this view). Nor do I have any sympathy for the often-heard view that RCTs and the use of statistical methods are inappropriate vehicles for the evaluation of something as complex as psychotherapy. As we have written elsewhere: 'Clinicians who claim that statistical methods are inappropriate for the evaluation of psychotherapies because they are limited to analysing means, or do not account for individual differences, are simply revealing their ignorance of statistics and of recent developments in statistical methodology'.[2]

A belief in the fundamental role of randomisation, however, does *not* imply that the naïve implementation of RCTs in outcome research cannot lead to some invalid or unsafe conclusions. The design of the trial and statistical analysis of the results have to be appropriate to the setting. Psychotherapy involves complex interactions between patient and therapist and sometimes (as in group therapy) involves the interaction of a group of patients with each other as well as with their therapist. It is not as simple as taking a tablet! A psychotherapy trial is likely to be far more complex, both in its implementation and in the analysis and interpretation of the subsequent results, than most drug trials. There are also far more opportunities for invalid inferences concerning treatment effects.

First, and often primarily, we are concerned with *internal validity*: the valid estimation of a causal effect of treatment from the data actually collected (given set of patients, therapists, treatment centres and psychotherapy actually delivered). Are the group differences we see the causal effects of treatment? Or can they be explained by other factors? Later we may be concerned with *external validity*: generalisation of the inferred causal effects to other patients, therapists, treatment centres and, perhaps, other forms of psychotherapy. To help clarify the discussion I have made much use of Rubin's counterfactual model of causality and its use in the estimation of treatment effects.[3,4] The kernel of the present discussion, applied to the problems of patient choice and non-adherence to treatment, can be found in Dunn.[5]

THE CAUSAL EFFECT OF TREATMENT

Mr Smith has suffered from severe depression, on and off, for several years. Six months ago his family doctor advised him to undergo a course of psychotherapy. He accepted this advice, has had several what he thinks were very helpful sessions with the psychotherapist, and now is feeling considerably better. Let's assume, for the sake of argument, that he has a total score of 10 points on the Beck Depression Inventory (BDI),[6] having started with a score of 20 six months ago. What is the effect of psychotherapy? How do we measure this effect? Putting it another way, what proportion, if any, of the drop from 20 to 10 points might be attributed to the receipt of therapy? Or perhaps I should have written: 'What proportion might *validly* be attributed to the receipt of therapy?' But, before we attempt to answer this question, let us consider another patient, Mrs Jones, who also suffers from chronic depression. Like Mr Smith, she was advised to have psychotherapy by her family doctor six months ago but, for various reasons, she never managed to keep any of her appointments and has not received any help from the therapist. A third patient, Mr Adams, refused outright to have anything to do with the therapist. Mrs Jones' present BDI score is 12 and that for Mr Adams is 15. For Mrs Jones and Mr Adams one might ask what would have been the effect of therapy offered if they had actually received it? What might their BDI scores have been?

In the above paragraph we are trying to find a way to estimate what may be called the *causal effect* of a treatment. The essence of the solution to the problem is a comparison. For each of the three patients, Mr Smith, Mrs Jones and Mr Adams, there are two possible outcomes of the referral to see a psychotherapist. The first is to receive therapy and have the severity of depression measured after a given interval after the onset of the course of treatment. The second is to fail to get the offered help, but again have the severity of depression measured after the allotted time. Let the variable T represent treatment received. It has two possible values, $T = t$ (therapy) and $T = c$ (no therapy). I use 'c' for no therapy to indicate that it can be regarded as a control condition. Let i indicate the identity of the patient ($i = 1$ for Mr Smith, 2 for Mrs Jones and 3 for Mr Adams). Finally, let $Y_T(i)$ indicate the final BDI score for patient i after receiving treatment option T. There are two *potential* outcomes for each of the three patients, as indicated in the following table:

Patient	BDI with therapy	BDI without therapy
Mr Smith	$Y_t(1)$	$Y_c(1)$
Mrs Jones	$Y_t(2)$	$Y_c(2)$
Mr Adams	$Y_t(3)$	$Y_c(3)$

We define the causal effect of the receipt of therapy as the difference between the BDI score for the ith patient after therapy and the corresponding BDI score after receiving no therapy. That is, by the difference $Y_t(i) - Y_c(i)$. It is a random variable that varies from one patient to another. Unfortunately, it can never be observed. The obvious problem is that each patient receives one of the treatment conditions, or the other, but not both. Either the patient receives psychotherapy or he/she does not. That is, the ith patient provides a value for either $Y_t(i)$ or $Y_c(i)$, but not both. Mr Smith provides $Y_t(1)$ but not $Y_c(1)$, Mrs Jones provides $Y_c(2)$ but not $Y_t(2)$, and so on. We provide a statistical solution to this problem in the following section, but we will re-emphasise the point that the causal effect of psychotherapy is the comparison of the outcome actually observed with that which would have been observed if, *contrary to fact*, the other treatment option had been taken.

Similar arguments apply to the comparison of the effects of different types of psychotherapy, or to the comparison of a specific type of psychotherapy with, for example, a psychopharmacological intervention such as a tricyclic antidepressant. The essence is always to try to get an estimate of the difference between the patient's observed response with that which would have been observed if the patient had received the alternative treatment.

COMPARISON OF GROUP AVERAGES AND THE ROLE OF RANDOMISATION

Now let's assume that we have access to a large population of eligible patients – the target population about which we wish to draw causal inferences about the value of psychotherapy or counselling. And let us concentrate on the *average causal effect* (ACE)[3,4] of the therapy for this target population. The average for the population is called an expected value in statistics and the ACE can therefore be written as:

$$ACE = E[Y_t(i) - Y_c(i)] \qquad (1)$$

where the expectation $E[\cdot]$ is over all values of i. From the mathematical properties of expectations (averages) it follows that:

$$ACE = E[Y_t(i)] - E[Y_c(i)] \qquad (2)$$

This simple formula shows us that information on *different* patients can be used to estimate $E[Y_t(i)]$ and $E[Y_c(i)]$ separately and the difference between these two expectations (averages) can be used to estimate the average of the differences (i.e. the ACE). We *can* observe the $Y_t(i)$'s in patients receiving therapy and we can also observe the $Y_c(i)$'s for those in the control condition. All that we need is to be sure that the observed averages for the treated (therapy) and untreated (control) patients are unbiased

estimates of $E[Y_t(i)]$ and $E[Y_c(i)]$, respectively. In general, however, the average of the $Y_t(i)$'s for the *whole* of the population (i.e. all possible i's) is *not* the same as the average of the $Y_t(i)$'s for those patients who have happened to receive the treatment (psychotherapy). Expressed mathematically:

$$E[Y_t(i)] \neq E[Y_t(i)|T = t] \neq E[Y_t(i)|T = c] \qquad (3)$$

and

$$E[Y_c(i)] \neq E[Y_c(i)|T = t] \neq E[Y_c(i)|T = c] \qquad (4)$$

where '|' means 'given that'. To summarise, the ACE is defined by the difference between $E[Y_t(i)]$ and $E[Y_c(i)]$ but what we actually observe are the estimators of $E[Y_t(i)|T = t]$ and $E[Y_c(i)|T = c]$. How do we ensure that our observed averages are also valid estimators of $E[Y_t(i)]$ and $E[Y_c(i)]$? If we are able to do this then we have replaced an impossible-to-observe causal effect on an individual patient with a possible-to-estimate average of the causal effects for our target population.[4]

If both $E[Y_t(i)] = E[Y_t(i)|T = t]$ and $E[Y_c(i)] = E[Y_c(i)|T = c]$ then the potential outcomes (both the $Y_t(i)$'s and the $Y_c(i)$'s) are statistically independent of the mechanism of assigning (or choosing) treatment options. Otherwise, they are not. If either the patient's family doctor, or the patient himself, or both, were to decide which treatment option to choose then it is almost certain that this choice will not be statistically independent of the *potential* outcome. This is the familiar problem of *confounding*. The difference in *observed* outcomes may arise from the fact that the patients with the best (or worst) prognosis, on average, might be the ones that opt for therapy. The observed outcomes in this situation might tell us something about the selection mechanism (treatment choice) but are not very informative about the causal effect of therapy. Knowing the values of all of the prognostic variables, together with a little knowledge of experimental design, might lead us to match or stratify the patients prior to estimation of the treatment effects. But we cannot guarantee that we are aware of all possible confounders. There is always the possibility that we have not thought of, or forgotten, something that is vitally important. Although we may be able to convince ourselves that we have not missed an important confounder, the only way we can ensure that we can convince a sceptical reviewer is to allocate treatment options *randomly*. Random allocation ensures that both $E[Y_t(i)] = E[Y_t(i)|T = t]$ and $E[Y_c(i)] = E[Y_c(i)|T = c]$ providing that t and c are the *allocated* treatments (not, necessarily, those actually received). Randomisation is the only sure way of coping with all confounders, and it copes with them irrespective of whether we are aware of them or not. Randomisation does not guarantee that treatment groups will be exactly comparable in any given comparison, but it does ensure that on average there will be comparability. Our conclusion is that if we wish to be sure that we are estimating the desired ACE we need an RCT.

An essential corollary of randomisation is that we obtain outcome data on all of the randomised patients and that we calculate our group averages from the patients as they were randomised and *not* according to whether they actually received or adhered to the treatment option that they were allocated to. This is the *intention-to-treat* (ITT) principle (see, for example, Sheiner and Rubin[7]). If we do not use ITT then the fundamental assumptions concerning our estimates of the causal effect of treatment (ACE) no longer hold. Loss to follow-up (i.e. a failure of the patient to provide outcome data) is a major threat to all RCTs but, in this part of the discussion we will simplify matters by assuming that outcome has, indeed, been obtained for all patients entering the trial. But what if some of the patients choose a treatment option other than the one they were randomly assigned to? Or perhaps some patients adhere to the allocated treatment much less than others – they turn up to the occasional session of therapy, for example, but not all of those which had been planned. This will clearly dilute (attenuate) the effect we wish to estimate. In fact, our ACE estimator (the difference between the observed mean outcomes for the two

randomly allocated groups) provides us with an estimate of the causal effect of *offering* treatment (i.e. randomisation) rather than the effect of actually receiving it. It is a valid estimator of a causal effect but many investigators (particularly psychotherapists!) might claim that it is an estimator of the wrong effect. As an estimator of the causal effect of receiving therapy the ITT estimate is likely to be biased. However, many other investigators might be convinced that this is the estimator of real interest – it measures the effect of a decision to treat in a given way and is therefore vitally important for people involved in making these decisions (or, at the very least, those paying for them!). It is the standard approach to the analysis of drug trials and that usually expected by the regulatory authorities such as the US Food and Drug Administration (FDA) and the UK National Institute for Clinical Excellence (NICE).

CHOICE OF, AND ADHERENCE TO, AN APPROPRIATE FORM OF PSYCHOTHERAPY

What constitutes the active treatment for our required comparison? There are several common forms of psychotherapy that are regularly used for patients with depression, including behaviour therapy, cognitive behaviour therapy (CBT),[8] interpersonal psychotherapy (IPT),[9] brief dynamic psychotherapy.[10] Usually the therapy involves the treatment of individual patients, but there is also the possibility of working with groups of patients with similar problems, or with the patient and his or her family. For a general review, see for example, Scott[11] or Roth and Fonaghy.[12] If our aim is to evaluate the efficacy of one of these forms or models of treatment, or to compare its efficacy with another model of psychotherapy or even pharmacotherapy, then it must be self-evident that we need to be able to describe explicitly and precisely what treatment using any of the specified models actually involves; i.e. they must be standardised. Crits-Christoph and Gladis[13] give two main reasons for standardisation. First, from a clinical viewpoint, there is a need to be able to describe what actually seems to work (or does not) so that clear treatment recommendations can be made to other potential therapists. Second, from a research viewpoint, therapies need to be replicable. Standardisation of psychotherapies, however, is not easy, and it is a topic beyond both the scope of the present chapter and the competence of the present writer. Briefly, it involves the creation of a detailed treatment manual, the selection and subsequent training of appropriate therapists in the use of the manual, certification of therapists based on adherence to the treatment model, and continued assessment of therapist adherence and competence during a clinical trial.[13] Clearly, when critically appraising the results of a particular RCT, we need to be able to convince ourselves that the therapy has been undertaken as intended, and that the therapy as given was exactly what it is said to be. For this we need a published treatment manual and a well-validated method of measuring adherence to the therapy as described in the manual.

CHOICE OF AN APPROPRIATE CONTROL GROUP

Standardisation of psychotherapy might be thought to be a difficult problem but it is often far more difficult to come up with a valid and convincing control condition. Crits-Christoph and Gladis[13] consider this as perhaps the single most vexing problem for research into the outcome of psychotherapy. Too often, we see that researchers have used 'no treatment' or 'waiting-list' controls. Too often we see the phrase 'routine care' used for the control condition when, in many circumstances it implies routine neglect. It is important that when patients are invited to take part in an RCT they are convinced that they will receive adequate levels of advice, support and care if they are allocated to the nominal control condition. Otherwise, why should they consent to randomisation? Otherwise, why should an ethics committee grant its approval for the trial? It is also important that the test psychotherapy is being compared to a care package that might be regarded as potentially as

good as the therapy on offer. The test therapy, for example, might involve supportive counselling in addition to the specific elements implied by the psychotherapeutic model, and the natural control condition would be the receipt of the same level of support in the absence of the psychotherapeutic elements under test. If, however, we wish to evaluate supportive counselling itself, then we still have a problem. Trialists often refer to 'equipoise' in justification of randomisation in an RCT. To maintain equipoise we need to be convinced that the control group patients are at least provided with the best-available routine care and that they are not allocated to a condition that might cause harm.

I will illustrate the choice of control groups by referring to a particularly well-known and influential psychotherapy trial. The National Institute of Mental Health (NIMH) Treatment of Depression Collaborative Research Program (TDCRP)[14] involved the use of four treatment arms. Groups 1 and 2 received CBT and IPT, respectively. Group 3 received pharmacotherapy with imipramine (administered double blind) together with a care package called 'clinical management (CM)'. Finally, Group 4 received a pill placebo (again administered double blind) and CM. Elkin et al.[14] state that 'The CM component of both pharmacotherapy conditions was introduced into the study to ensure standard clinical care, to maximize compliance, and to address ethical concerns regarding the use of a placebo on depressed patients. The CM component provided guidelines, not only for the management of medication and side effects and review of the patient's clinical status, but also for providing the patient with support and encouragement and direct advice if necessary. Although specific psychotherapeutic interventions were proscribed (especially those that might overlap with the two psychotherapies), the CM component approximated a "minimal supportive therapy" condition.'

The essence of the imipramine–CM and placebo–CM conditions was to provide a fully standardised package of clinical care, either of which could be used as a control group for the evaluation of the efficacy of the psychotherapies. So, the two major questions addressed by the

CRP study were '(1) Is there evidence ... fectiveness of each of the psychothera- ... compared both with the standard refer- ... eatment of imipramine–CM and with the placebo plus CM (PLA–CM) control condition? (2) Are there any differences in the effectiveness of the two psychotherapies?' These questions emphasise the comparative nature of this and any other well-designed RCT. When one asks questions about the effectiveness of psychotherapy one should always add the rider 'relative to what?' A valid and well-standardised control condition is as vital to the comparison as is the standardised package of therapy. Crits-Christoph and Gladis,[13] referring to the TDCRP trial, comment that whilst the placebo–CM is perhaps not the ideal control condition for psychotherapy, it serves a practical function. That is, if a specific psychotherapy can do no better than the placebo–CM control should the psychotherapy be pursued as a treatment option? Beware of authors who make claims about the improvement of patients in a particular treatment group without reference to that in other comparison groups. Roth and Fonaghy's[12] (p. 64) comment that the small differences between the four TDCRP trial groups, in terms of their outcome, is due to the unexpectedly good outcome under placebo–CM (explained by the fact that it contains non-specific elements of psychotherapy) seems to be missing the point.

CHOICE OF ASSESSMENT METHOD AND OUTCOME MEASURES

It is very difficult to see how one could possibly design a so-called double blind RCT in the field of psychotherapy evaluation. The patients are likely to know what is going on, unless they have been deceived by their therapists, and it would be rather bizarre if the therapists were unaware of what treatment was being offered! Blind assessment by a third party (a clinician or research worker not involved in the provision of therapy or clinical support) is often the preferred option, but even here it is frequently difficult to maintain blindness. The therapists themselves should not undertake the assessment of outcome. One should always bear in mind, however, that irrespective of who carries out the assessment, there is always the possibility of subjective biases in the assessments. The Hamilton Rating Scale for Depression, HRSD[15] and the Beck Depression Inventory, BDI[6] are the two most commonly used measures of depressive symptoms in RCTs for the treatment of depression. In fact, they are frequently both used within the same RCT to assess different aspects of symptomology. The HRDS is a clinician-rated measure, based on an interview with the patient, which gives more weight to the 'biological' or somatic symptoms of depression, whilst the BDI is a patient-completed questionnaire which concentrates more on the cognitive aspects. There have been suggestions that different forms of therapy (drugs as opposed to psychological treatments, for example) might have a differential effect on these outcome measures (drugs doing better according to the HRDS and the BDI favouring CBT, for example). The expected treatment group by outcome measure interaction needs to be specified (and preferably published) as part of the trial protocol and, if it is regarded as being important, the trial needs to be powered accordingly. In reality, it is hard to imagine a convincing justification for a trial of the size and expense needed for such a test.

What about missing outcome assessments? Drop-outs and other sources of missing data lead to real problems for the valid estimation of the effects of treatment. A detailed discussion of this topic is beyond the scope of the present chapter, but it must be stressed that the only effective way of dealing with missing data is to ensure that there are none. Investigators should make every effort to ensure that outcome data (however brief) are collected on *all* of the patients randomised, irrespective of their subsequent treatment history. In particular, data collection should not be abandoned simply because the patient has not taken up the offer of therapy or has not adhered to the prescribed course of treatment.[16,17] There is no logical reason why patients should refuse to be assessed even though they have decided that therapy is not for them, although, in practice, the two types of protocol violation are likely to go together.

But what if you have drop-outs and haphazardly missing data? What is the best way of dealing with them in the statistical analysis? If we use a naïve complete-case analysis (that is, base the inferences concerning causal effects on those patients with complete data) then we are likely to have two problems: lack of statistical efficiency (low statistical power) and bias. Bias may be caused, for example, by the drop-outs not occurring completely at random. Ideally, analyses should be available on all available data (and should include where possible all patients randomised to the competing treatment arms) and should compensate for the observed patterns of drop-out. Possibilities for dealing with the missing values include imputation (ranging from rather crude and unsatisfactory methods – at least from the point of view of estimation – such as last-observation-carried-forward to the much more realistic stochastic imputation methods including hot-decking and multiple imputation), the use of inverse probability weighting and, finally, a full likelihood analysis based on statistical models for both the missing data process and for the outcome given that it has been assessed. For further details, readers are referred to a series of reviews in *Statistical Methods in Medical Research*, **8**(1), particularly the primer on multiple imputation by Schafer.[18] The use of inverse probability weights is widespread in survey statistics but has only occasionally been used to allow for drop-outs in RCTs. The use of this technique in longitudinal clinical trials is explained and illustrated in Everitt and Pickles.[19] Its use is also illustrated in a recent depression trial by Dowrick *et al.*[20] Finally, a discussion of the analysis of longitudinal data with drop-outs, paying particular attention to the NIMH TDCRP trial, is provided by Gibbons *et al.*[21]

CENTRE, GROUP AND THERAPIST EFFECTS

It is clear that the outcome of psychotherapy is dependent upon characteristics of the therapist.

These include training and experience of the therapist, degree of adherence to the therapeutic model (use of a manual, for example) and the capacity to develop a therapeutic alliance with the patient (see, for example, Crits-Christoph *et al.*[22] and Roth and Fonaghy[12]). In a multi-centre RCT there are also likely to be differences in the effectiveness of the collaborating clinical centres. Therapists in some centres may have considerably more experience in the use of a given treatment approach than in others, reflected, for example, in their degree of adherence to a given therapeutic model. In addition, if patients are treated as groups rather than individually there are also likely to be differences between groups arising not only from the characteristics of the patients and of the therapist but also from interactions between the patients.[23] If they get on well together the group might thrive. If, on the other hand, there is a particularly disruptive or difficult patient within a particular group then the group as a whole may not do as well as it might otherwise have done.

Consider a hypothetical single-centre RCT with two treatment arms. In Group A all the patients receive CBT individually from an internationally respected pioneer of CBT, Dr Garner. In Group B all the patients, again individually, receive supportive counselling (SC) from a recently-trained community psychiatric nurse, Mr Martin. Let's assume that Dr Garner's patients do considerably better than those of Mr Martin. What can we infer about the causal effect of CBT from such a trial? What are the threats to the validity of the trial? Dr Garner is likely to be a very experienced, highly-skilled and highly-motivated 'brand champion'. Mr Martin, on the other hand, lacks experience. Is the observed difference due to the difference in abilities and experience of the two therapists, or is it an effect of CBT? We cannot tell. The two effects are completely confounded in this simple design. This is a severe threat to the internal validity of the trial. If, however, we believe that the observed differences are an effect of CBT, then what? We still cannot be sure that there is not some attribute of Dr Garner that enables him to be particularly successful in delivering this particular variant of CBT. Could other clinicians use the same model and achieve the same or, at least, comparable results? We do not know. This is a threat to the external validity or generalisability of the trial's findings.

In practice, many RCTs, which otherwise have admirable design characteristics and quality control procedures, involve the use of only two or three highly-skilled and experienced therapists. They are often the academic clinicians who have been involved in the development or modification of the therapy under evaluation. Does this invalidate the findings of these trials? No, but it does limit their generalisability. They should, perhaps, be regarded as the equivalent of the pharmacotherapist's 'Phase II' drug trials, being a necessary preliminary to the design and conduct of a full 'Phase III' evaluation using a large and representative sample of therapists. It would be inappropriate and certainly difficult to justify a large multi-centre trial involving large numbers of therapists without first being able to establish that the 'experts' or 'brand champions' are able to achieve promising results. If the latter cannot demonstrate worthwhile effects then it would be pointless to move on to the larger trial. If they can, however, we then (but only then) need to ask how well the therapy might work in routine clinical practice.

In a large multi-centre trial we need to involve as many therapists as possible. Each therapist is likely to be based in only one of the centres and to be delivering treatment in only one arm of the trial (i.e. therapists are *nested* within both centres and treatments), but it is possible for a therapist to deliver more than one of the forms of therapy in a comparative trial (i.e. therapists, like centres, are *crossed* with treatments). These designs have implications for the statistical analysis and for the validity of statistical inferences based on these analyses.[24–26] Both centre and therapist effects should be incorporated into an appropriate statistical model. Using the notation of Roberts,[26] such a model, for a quantitative outcome measure, for example, will have the form:

$$y_{ijk} = \alpha + \lambda_j + \sum_p \beta_p x_{ijkp} + u_{jk} + \varepsilon_{ijk} \qquad (5)$$

Here y_{ijk} is the outcome of the ith patient of the kth therapist within the jth treatment arm of the trial. Assuming that λ_j is zero in the control arm, λ_j is the effect of the treatment effect for the jth arm of the trial. Each x_{ijkp} is the baseline measurement of the pth patient characteristic (such as a demographic or other prognostic variable, including treatment centre) and β_p is the corresponding regression coefficient. The term u_{jk} is the average effect of the kth therapist within the jth treatment arm of the trial. It is a random variable (i.e. randomly varying from one therapist to another) with an assumed mean of zero and variance of σ_j^2. This variance may vary from one arm of the trial to another (there is no *a priori* reason why the variation between therapists within different arms of the trial should be the same) and, in particular, if the control arm does not involve the use of therapists at all, then, for the controls $\sigma_j^2 = 0$ (i.e. in this situation there are no therapist effects in the control group). In the case of the possibility of one or more arms of the trial involving group therapies, the statistical model would be even more complex.

Models such as that described in equation (5) are called *random effects, random regression* or *multilevel* models.[27] Technical details of their use are beyond the scope of this chapter and interested readers are referred to Roberts[26] for an illustration of their use in the context of RCTs involving therapist effects. What readers should note, however, is that failure to allow for appropriate therapist effects in the statistical analysis (assuming that they are present in the data) is likely to lead to spurious statistical significance (i.e. the stated p-values will be too low) and estimated confidence intervals or standard errors for treatment effects that are too optimistic (i.e. smaller than they should be). A corollary of this is that, even when the analysis is correct, a trial whose sample size has not been determined after allowance for the possibility of therapist effects is very likely to be underpowered (too small!). This is the same problem as those faced by the designers of cluster randomised trials (see, for example, Donner[28]). Again, Roberts[26] provides details of the required adjustments to sample size calculations, on the assumption that therapist variation is the same for each of the arms of the trial.

But there is more to the problem of therapist effects than can be solved by the technical device of allowing for them in an appropriate statistical model. Nor is the main problem one of generalising from the impact of therapists in a given trial to the wider community of therapists. We started the discussion in the present section by comparing the outcome of CBT as delivered by Dr Garner with that of SC as delivered by Mr Martin. We pointed out that the required treatment effect is fully confounded with the difference between the two therapists. Now let us move on to a larger trial in which each of the patients in Group A receives CBT from a randomly selected therapist from a team of, say 50, experienced and highly competent cognitive therapists. Each of the patients in Group B, on the other hand, receives SC from a randomly selected therapist from a team of experienced and highly competent interpersonal therapists. We still have a problem. Again, the required treatment effect (the difference between outcomes for CBT and SC) cannot be disentangled from the difference between the average effects of the two groups of therapists. In general, the λ_j in equation (5) can either be interpreted as the average of the within-Group j therapist effects or as an effect of therapy j – that is, the two interpretations are equivalent. 'At the present time, researchers and consumers of psychotherapy research findings are left with a basic dilemma when interpreting the findings of studies focusing on the efficacy of specific treatments: how to disentangle the effects due to the therapeutic approach from those due to the particular therapists who have carried out the approach. It is particularly pressing when different therapists carry out each of the treatments in a comparative outcome study.'[29]

The cognitive therapists and counsellors in the above hypothetical trial (or even in a real one such as the NIMH TDPRC study) might differ in lots of ways and these therapist differences may be the causal effects of the treatment difference,

not the difference in psychotherapeutic approach. Consider therapeutic competence, for example. The CBT therapists might, for example, be either more or less competent than their SC counterparts. But how could we assess this? How could we possibly compare the competence of Dr Garner as a cognitive therapist, for example, with that of Mr Martin as a counsellor. It is akin to asking whether I am more competent as a statistician than my scientific colleague is as a laboratory worker. And moving to a crossed design (both types of therapy being offered by every therapist) does not solve our problem. If Dr Garner, for example, were to be experienced and highly competent as both a cognitive therapist and an interpersonal therapist we still would not be able to compare the competencies in the two approaches. Elkin[29] (Reproduced with permission of Oxford University Press) concluded that 'We may never be able to truly "disentangle" the effects due to the therapist from those due to the therapy, because they may often be inherently intertwined and also very interactive with particular patient attributes.'

'The treatment conditions being compared … are, in actuality, "packages" of particular therapeutic approaches and the therapists who chose and are chosen to administer them.'[30] The interpretation of the results of RCTs should explicitly acknowledge this fact. As well as very carefully defining both the treatment and the control conditions, authors should provide critical information about the therapists carrying out the treatments, and the information should be included in the dissemination concerning supposedly empirically validated results.[29] The latter is particularly important when we come to systematic review and/or meta-analysis of the results from a disparate collection of individual trials, and in the formulation of any subsequent clinical guidelines based upon the results of these trials.

WHAT WORKS FOR WHOM?

The question implies a belief that there is no constant treatment effect. That is, it implies that a given form of treatment has a greater effect on some patients than it does on others; that the receipt of psychotherapy A will be more beneficial for Mr Smith than the receipt of psychotherapy B, for example, but that B might be better than A for Mrs Jones. Mr Smith has a particular attribute (presenting symptoms, clinical or family history, for example) that indicates therapy A. Mrs Jones, on the other hand, has characteristics that indicate therapy B. In the epidemiological literature this is called 'effect modification' – a particularly useful term as it should remind us that 'causal effect' implies comparison of observed outcome with that which would have been observed under different circumstances. In terms of statistical modelling (analysis of variance, or covariance, for example) it will provide an example of a treatment group by patient attribute interaction, where the attribute could be one of a potentially vast range of measures made on the patients at or prior to randomisation. Supposed examples of such interactions are rarely convincing. Even if based on a valid statistical analysis (i.e. a test of an appropriate two-way interaction) they are usually 'discovered' as part of a *post hoc* 'fishing trip'. More frequently their existence has been based on an invalid analysis. All too often the investigators are looking for a so-called 'predictor of outcome' by searching in the relevant treatment group for patient attributes associated with good outcome. This tells us nothing about effect modification – the same attributes might lead to the better outcomes within the control group(s). One should *always* remember that valid inferences from an RCT involve *comparison* of the randomised groups. Here we are concerned with the question 'Does the treatment effect (e.g. comparison of outcomes in Groups A and B) depend on, say, patient attribute C?' The identity of attribute C should be clearly specified in the trial protocol, together with a prior estimate of the size of the proposed interaction. The sample size for the trial should then be determined such that there is sufficient power to detect this interaction through the use of an appropriate statistical significance test. One good candidate for attribute C might be patient preference,[31] but there is little, if any,

methodologically sound work in this area. Crits-Christoph and Gladis[13] comment that two of the largest randomised clinical trials ever undertaken to evaluate psychotherapies (although not specifically for depression) failed to provide much support for specified patient – treatment interactions.[22,32]

ESTIMATION OF CAUSAL EFFECTS IN AN RCT WITH PATIENT CHOICE

Consider a hypothetical RCT in which 200 eligible depressed patients have been randomly allocated to receive either counselling plus routine care ($T = t$) or routine care alone ($T = c$). For simplicity, assume that all of the 100 patients allocated to routine care receive exactly that (they do not have access to counselling unless they have been allocated to that treatment arm of the trial). Of the 100 patients offered counselling, however, only 70 accept the offer. A fixed time interval after randomisation (six months, say) the patients' clinical status (improved versus not improved) is assessed and used as the primary outcome of the trial. The effects of either treatment allocation or treatment actually received are to be estimated from the differences between average outcomes as before, the only difference being that we are averaging binary outcomes (1 = improved; 0 = not improved, say) to obtain observed proportions. The results of this hypothetical trial are summarised in Table 19.1 (note that we have simplified the issue by assuming there are no drop-outs).

The estimate of the ITT effect is both simple and familiar. The proportion of those receiving counselling who improve is 0.70 (i.e. 70/100) and the corresponding proportion for the control

Table 19.1. Results of a hypothetical trial of counselling

	$T = t$		$T = c$	
	Improved	Total	Improved	Total
Comply	60	70		
Do not comply	10	30		
Overall	70	100	50	100

group is 0.50 (i.e. 50/100). The difference (the ACE for being offered counselling) is 0.20. For readers who prefer NTT (the reciprocal of the difference between the two proportions), this is 5 (i.e. 1/0.20). But what about estimating the causal effect of receiving treatment? There are two commonly used, but invalid, methods of analysis—analysis *per protocol* or analysis *as treated*. There is also the correct (correctness, of course, being vitally dependent on the validity of a few key assumptions) but much less familiar estimator – the *complier average causal effect* (CACE).[33–35] The per protocol analysis compares the outcome in those people in the counselling group who actually receive counselling with that in the control group (i.e. it excludes patients who have violated the treatment protocol from the analysis). Here the difference is $60/70 - 50/100 (= 0.36)$. The as treated analysis compares outcome in those patients who receive counselling with that in those who do not receive it (all patients are included in this analysis). Here it is $60/70 - 60/130 (= 0.40)$. The problem with both of these estimators is that it is impossible to interpret them as a causal effect in the sense of comparing potential outcomes *on the same patient*. The patient groups are not comparable. The estimated effects are merely associations, subject to confounding. And association, as you all know, does not imply causality!

What about the CACE? This is an estimate of the difference between the outcome in the compliers (i.e. those who accepted and received the offered counselling) with that which would have been expected *in the same patients* if they had not been offered counselling. This is where we need two key assumptions.[36,37] The first one is easy to defend for a randomised trial. The second needs a bit more careful thought.

Assumption 1: the proportion of patients who are *potential* compliers is the same in the two randomly allocated groups. This follows directly from the random allocation mechanism.

Assumption 2: the proportion of potential non-compliers who improve is independent of treatment allocation. In other words, it makes no difference to the outcome of a patient who would

refuse the offer of counselling whether or not they are in the group actually offered counselling. The offer, in itself, is not beneficial.

Assumption 1 allows us to estimate the proportion of potential compliers in the control group. In our example it is 70/100. The estimated number of non-compliers in the control group is 30 and the number of compliers is 70.

Assumption 2 allows us to estimate the proportion (number) of patients who improve amongst the non-compliers in the control group. In our example the number of patients who improve in this group is estimated to be 10 (the proportion is 10/30). Now, there were a total of 50 patients who were observed to improve in the control group and therefore the estimated number of potential compliers who improve in the control group must be 40 (that is $50 - 10$). Otherwise the numbers do not add up! So, the proportion of patients improving in the counselling group amongst those who actually receive counselling is 60/70. The proportion in the corresponding control group (i.e. those who would have accepted the offer) is estimated to be 40/70. The CACE estimator is the difference between these two proportions, $60/70 - 40/70 (= 0.29)$. The corresponding NNT is 3.5.

Note that in the above example the potential compliers did better than the non-compliers, irrespective of which treatment arm they were allocated to. This is not unexpected and not too difficult to rationalise. But now consider a second, more 'difficult' example. The results of a second hypothetical trial are shown in Table 19.2. The ITT effect (ACE) is estimated by $50/100 - 30/100 (= 0.20)$. The corresponding NTT is 5. The CACE estimate is $35/70 - 15/70 (= 0.29)$.

Table 19.2. Results of a second hypothetical trial of counselling

	$T = t$		$T = c$	
	Improved	Total	Improved	Total
Comply	35	70		
Do not comply	15	30		
Overall	50	100	30	100

The corresponding NNT is again 3.5. But note that this time the potential compliers in the control group are doing a lot worse than the non-compliers (15/70 vs 15/30). Again, this is reasonably straightforward to rationalise. The patients who accept the offer of counselling are those with the worst prognosis or, equivalently, those that turn it down (or would turn it down if offered it) are those who are getting better anyway. The latter do not need treatment. But what this should do is prompt the data analyst to ask whether Assumption 2 is really justified. Might the offer of help on its own be of benefit? And if so, of how much benefit? Or perhaps those patients in the control group who would have accepted the offer feel let down (resentful demoralisation) and do worse than they would otherwise have done if they had known nothing about the possible offer of help.

In practice, we do not have to work right through the estimation from first principles in the above way. It can be shown that the required estimates can be obtained from the following simple formula:[33,38,39]

$$CACE = \frac{\text{ITT estimate for outcome}}{\text{ITT estimate for receipt of treatment}}$$
(6)

This formula applies in situations where both of the measures of outcome and treatment received are binary (i.e. both the ITT effects are differences between proportions) or where both are quantitative (i.e. both the ITT effects are differences between means), or one is binary and the other quantitative. So, for the first example above, $CACE = (70/100 - 50/100)/(70/100 - 0) = 0.29$, as before.

RANDOMISED CONSENT AND PATIENT PREFERENCE DESIGNS

A serious issue in the design of RCTs concerns the amount of information given to the patient about the aims of the trial. So-called informed consent is a prerequisite for most trials but it is not always obvious what 'informed consent'

actually means or whether, strictly speaking, it is ever possible. In the context of our example illustrating the effect of patient compliance to a treatment offer, is it ever ethically justified to randomise and then only seek consent to treat in the group allocated to receive therapy? This is an example of Zelen's[40] original form of the randomised consent design. All patients in the trial are asked to provide outcome data, of course, but those in the control group may never know that they had taken part in a trial. Is this really a serious ethical problem? This design would circumvent the potential problem of resentful demoralisation amongst the controls. I will not attempt to answer the question raised.

In an attempt to solve some of the serious problems surrounding the issue of patient preference, Brewin and Bradley[41] (see also Bradley[42] and Silverman and Altman[43]) have proposed what they describe as the *patient preference design*. In this design, eligible patients are told about the reasons for the trial and the treatments on offer. Patients who do not have a strong preference (that is, they are prepared to be randomised) are entered into a conventional RCT. Those patients with a strong preference are offered the treatment of their choice. So, for the comparison of two treatments, A and B, for example, the patient preference trial finishes up with four groups: those who prefer A; those without preference who are randomly allocated to A; those who prefer B; those without preference who are randomly allocated to B. In the context of the present discussion, the comparison of the randomly allocated groups can lead to an ACE or CACE estimate as described above. But what can the two patient preference groups provide? Merely an estimate of association. Like per protocol or as treated estimators, they do not appear to be able to provide estimates of causal effects. And for this reason they cannot be used to check the (external) validity of the estimates of causal effects provided by the randomised groups. Whether the difference between the two preference groups is the same as or completely different from that provided within the core RCT, so what? What does it tell us? That there are selection effects? The treatment effect may, indeed, be different in those patients without a strong preference (i.e. those prepared to be randomised) when compared to the rest, but the rest cannot provide the valid information from which we can test whether it is true. But perhaps readers should see the results of such a trial and decide for themselves. An example of the use of a patient preference design is provided by a recently published trial of counselling for depression.[44,45]

Another design possibility which, in my view, has much more promise is to simply ask the participants of a conventional RCT what their preferences are prior to randomisation. The aim here is not to allow patient preference to influence treatment received (but in the presence of non-compliance this will be inevitable) but to incorporate patient preferences into the analysis of the resulting data. This has been tried by Torgerson et al.[31] Although the latter authors do not pursue all of the possibilities in terms of estimating treatment effects, the design offers ways, at least partially, of testing the validity of the assumptions necessary for the above CACE estimator, or, equivalently, looking for a poor prognosis/demoralising effect in the potential compliers of the control group. Getting preference information prior to randomisation would also improve the precision of the estimates of the CACE, but this is well beyond the scope of the present chapter – for further information, see Fisher-Lapp and Goetghebeur.[39] The latter article will also provide a suitable entry to the literature on adjustment for partial compliance (i.e. regression models for the response in terms of levels of compliance).

CONCLUSIONS

The design and analysis of a convincing RCT for the estimation of the effects of psychotherapy are difficult. It is not safe to simply assume that the theoretical and logistical problems are similar to those of the average drug trial. Life here is much more complex. Psychotherapy (at least in its individual form) involves the interaction of two people (the patient and the therapist) and it is the involvement of these two people that is the essence of the complexity. Added to this are the problems of the choice of adequate control groups (in particular, the absence of a convincing placebo) and the impossibility of conducting a trial that is double blind. In the critical appraisal of such trials we should not, perhaps, be searching for methodological perfection but, instead, be aware of the pitfalls to valid inferences concerning treatment effects and temper our judgements accordingly (and this applies just as much to the trials that we have been involved in as it does to the trials of other investigators).

This chapter has not considered systematic review and meta-analysis of trials of psychotherapies but the authors (and appraisers) of such studies should be fully aware of all the methodological pitfalls of the individual trials. A meta-analysis of a series of trials that have naïvely ignored random therapist effects, for example, or ignored the structure of a group therapy trial, simply summarises the faulty analyses of the originals. Unfortunately, the consumers of meta-analyses (particularly if they are produced under the auspices of such august bodies as the Cochrane Collaboration) seem to place far too much faith in their findings. Consumers need to be aware that the authors of systematic reviews are capable of missing subtle (or not so subtle) methodological flaws in the original trials. Consumers should resist taking the conclusions of the authors of these meta-analyses, and the clinical guidelines that result from them, on trust. In order to critically appraise a published systematic view one needs to know about not only the mechanism (and quality) of the review itself, but also have a detailed knowledge of what the reviewers should have been looking for in the way of methodological problems in the original trials. Reporting guidelines such as CONSORT[46,47] are having a substantial impact on the quality of clinical trials, and on the appraisal methodologies of systematic reviewers. In the case of psychotherapy trials, however, the CONSORT recommendations only cover a small part of the key components of the trial. Sticking to CONSORT guidelines is necessary for a good trial report, *but is not sufficient*. I hope the present chapter succeeds in stimulating readers to think of other aspects of such trials that need to be equally well reported.

REFERENCES

1. Dunn G. Statistical methods for measuring outcomes. In: Tansella M, Thornicroft G, eds, *Mental Health Outcome Measures*. London: Gaskell (2001) 5–18.
2. Garety P, Dunn G, Fowler D, Kuipers E. The evaluation of cognitive behaviour therapy for psychosis. In: Wykes T, Tarrier N, Lewis S, eds, *Outcome and Innovation in Psychological Treatment of Schizophrenia*. Chichester: John Wiley & Sons (1998) 101–18.
3. Rubin DB. Estimating causal effects of treatments in randomized and nonrandomized studies. *J Educ Psychol* (1974) **66**: 688–701.
4. Holland PW. Statistics and causal inference (with discussion). *J Am Stat Assoc* (1986) **81**: 945–70.
5. Dunn G. The challenge of patient choice and non-adherence to treatment in randomised controlled trials of counselling or psychotherapy. *Understand Stat* (2002) **1**: 19–29.
6. Beck AT, Ward CH, Mendelson M, *et al*. An inventory for measuring depression. *Arch Gen Psychiat* (1961) **4**: 561–71.
7. Sheiner LB, Rubin DB. Intention-to-treat and the goals of clinical trials. *Clin Pharmacol Ther* (1995) **57**: 6–15.
8. Fennell MJV. Cognitive-behaviour therapy for depressive disorders. In: *New Oxford Textbook of Psychiatry*. Oxford: Oxford University Press (2000) 1394–405.
9. Markovitz JC, Weissman MM. Interpersonal psychotherapy for depression and other disorders. In: *New Oxford Textbook of Psychiatry*. Oxford: Oxford University Press (2000) 1411–20.
10. Ursano RJ, Ursano AM. Brief individual psychodynamic psychotherapy. In: *New Oxford Textbook of Psychiatry*. Oxford: Oxford University Press (2000) 1421–32.
11. Scott J. Psychological treatments for depression: an update. *Br J Psychiat* (1995) **167**: 289–92.
12. Roth A, Fonaghy P. *What Works for Whom? A Critical Review of Psychotherapy Research*. New York: The Guilford Press (1996).
13. Crits-Christoph P, Gladis M. The evaluation of psychological treatment. In: *New Oxford Textbook of Psychiatry*. Oxford: Oxford University Press (2000) 1259–69.
14. Elkin I, Shea T, Watkins JT, *et al*. National Institute of Mental Health Treatment of Depression Collaborative Research Program (1989). *Arch Gen Psychiat* (1989) **46**: 971–81.
15. Hamilton M. A rating scale for depression. *J. Neurology Neurosurgery & Psychiatry* (1960) **23**: 56–61.
16. Lavori PW. Clinical trials in psychiatry: should protocol deviation censor patient data? *Neuropsychopharmacology* (1992) **6**: 39–48.
17. Siqueland L, Chittams J, Frank A, *et al*. The protocol deviation patient: characterization and implications for clinical trials research. *Psychother Res* (1998) **8**: 287–306.
18. Schafer D. Multiple imputation: a primer. *Stat Meth Med Res* (1999) **8**: 3–15.
19. Everitt BS, Pickles A. *Statistical Aspects of the Design and Analysis of Clinical Trials*. London: Imperial College Press (1999).
20. Dowrick C, Dunn G, Ayuso-Mateos J-L, *et al*. Problem solving treatment and group psychoeducation for depression: a multicentre randomised controlled trial. *Br Med J* (2000) **321**: 1450–5.
21. Gibbons RD, Hedecker D, Elkin I, *et al*. Some conceptual and statistical issues in analysis of longitudinal psychiatric data. *Arch Gen Psychiat* (1993) **50**: 739–50.
22. Crits-Christoph P, Siqueland L, Blaine J, *et al*. Psychological treatments for cocaine dependence: National Institute for Drug Abuse Collaborative Cocaine Treatment Study. *Arch Gen Psychiat* (1999) **56**: 493–502.
23. Burlinghame G, Kircher J, Taylor S. Methodological considerations in group psychotherapy research: past, present and future practices. In: Fuhriman A, Burlinghame G, eds, *Handbook of Group Psychotherapy and Counseling*. New York: John Wiley & Sons. (1994) 41–80.
24. Martindale C. The therapist-as-fixed-effect fallacy in psychotherapy research. *J Consult Clin Psychol* (1978) **46**: 1526–30.
25. Crits-Christoph P, Mintz J. Implications of therapist effects for the design and analysis of comparative studies of psychotherapies. *J Consult Clin Psychol* (1991) **59**: 20–6.
26. Roberts C. The implications of variation in outcome between health professionals for the design and analysis of randomized clinical trials. *Stat Med* (1999) **18**: 2605–15.
27. Goldstein H. *Multilevel Statistical Models*, 2nd edn. London: Arnold (1995).
28. Donner A. *Design and Analysis of Cluster Randomization Trials in Health Research*. London: Arnold (2000).
29. Elkin I. A major dilemma in psychotherapy outcome research: disentangling therapists from therapies. *Clin Psychol: Sci Pract* (1999) **6**: 10–32.

30. Elkin I, Parloff MB, Hadlet SW, Autry JH. National Institute of Mental Health Treatment of Depression Collaborative Research Program: background and research plan. *Arch Gen Psychiat* (1985) **42**: 305–16.

31. Torgerson DJ, Klaber-Moffett J, Russell IT. Patient preferences in randomised trials: threat or opportunity? *J Health Serv Res Policy* (1996) **1**: 194–7.

32. Project MATCH Research Group. Matching alcoholism treatments to client heterogeneity: Project MATCH posttreatment drinking outcomes. *J Studies Alcohol* (1997) **58**: 7–29.

33. Angrist JD, Imbens GW, Rubin DB. Identification of causal effects using instrumental variables (with discussion). *J Am Stat Assoc* (1996) **91**: 444–55.

34. Little R, Yau LHY. Statistical techniques for analyzing data from prevention trials: treatment of no-shows using Rubin's causal model. *Psychol Meth* (1998) **3**: 147–59.

35. Little R, Rubin DB. Causal effects in clinical and epidemiological studies via potential outcomes: concepts and analytical approaches. *Ann Rev Public Health* (2000) **21**: 121–45.

36. Bloom HS. Accounting for no-shows in experimental evaluation designs. *Eval Rev* (1984) **8**: 225–46.

37. Sommer A, Zeger SL. On estimating efficacy from clinical trials. *Stat Med* (1991) **10**: 45–52.

38. Cuzick J, Edwards R, Segnan N. Adjusting for non-compliance and contamination in randomized clinical trials. *Stat Med* (1997) **16**: 1017–29.

39. Fisher-Lapp K, Goetghebeur E. Practical properties of some structural mean analyses of the effect of compliance in randomized trials. *Contr Clin Trials* (1999) **20**: 531–46.

40. Zelen M. A new design for randomized clinical trials. *New Engl J Med* (1979) **300**: 1242–5.

41. Brewin C, Bradley C. Patient preferences and randomised clinical trials. *Br Med J* (1989) **299**: 313–15.

42. Bradley C. Designing medical and educational intervention studies. *Diabet Care* (1993) **16**: 509–18.

43. Silverman WA, Altman DG. Patient's preferences and randomised trials. *Lancet* (1996) **347**: 171–4.

44. Ward E, King M, Lloyde M, *et al*. Randomized controlled trial of non-directive counselling, cognitive-behaviour therapy, and usual general practitioner care for patients with depression. I: Clinical effectiveness. *Br Med J* (2000) **321**: 1383–8.

45. Bower P, Byford S, Sibbald B, *et al*. Randomized controlled trial of non-directive counselling, cognitive-behaviour therapy, and usual general practitioner care for patients with depression. II: Cost effectiveness. *Br Med J* (2000) **321**: 1389–92.

46. Moher D, Schultz KF, Altman DG. The CONSORT statement: revised recommendations for improving the quality of reports of parallel-group randomized trials. *Ann Int Med* (2001) **134**: 657–62.

47. Altman DG, Schultz KF, Moher D, *et al*. The revised CONSORT statement for reporting randomized trials: explanation and elaboration. *Ann Int Med* (2001) **134**: 663–94.

REPRODUCTIVE HEALTH

20

Contraception

GILDA PIAGGIO*

Department of Reproductive Health and Research, World Health Organisation, Geneva, Switzerland *The views
expressed in this paper are solely those of the author and do not necessarily reflect the views of the World
Health Organization.

INTRODUCTION

Contraception deals with the prevention of pregnancy. The basic pillar of family planning is
a wide spectrum of contraceptive methods that
enables men and women to make informed
choices about timing and size of family. Effective and safe methods should be available such
that they fit the needs of women and men in
very diverse social and cultural settings worldwide. There should be reversible methods that protect against sexually transmitted infections, can be
controlled by women, can be used by adolescents
and by breast-feeding women. The choice of a
contraceptive method involves personal decisions
and depends on the stage of life, family situation
or civil status, age, preferences and health profile
of individuals and couples. Contraceptive research
and development has resulted in a variety of available methods and continues to address important
issues to fill gaps in the available portfolio and in
knowledge about method safety and effectiveness.

Contraceptives are generally used by healthy
individuals to prevent pregnancy and some also
serve prophylactic purposes. They need to be

very safe so that it does not offset the benefits
obtained from their use, and this emphasizes the
importance of addressing the safety concerns.
Both contraceptive efficacy and risks should be
well defined to enable the user and the prescriber
to make the best choice of a contraceptive
method.[1]

The development of effective and safe methods
of contraception poses special challenges. First,
to achieve an understanding of the complex physiology of reproduction. Second, the effectiveness
of many methods depends on a successful interaction between men and women. Some methods
have to be used by the man or the couple but
failure (pregnancy) is always observed in the
woman. Third, for some methods, behavioural
and social factors are critical, determining compliance, which is very difficult to assess.

Contraceptive methods can in general be classified into hormonal and non-hormonal methods. Hormonal methods used by women include
oral contraceptive pills (OCs), injectable preparations, implants, hormone-releasing devices (vaginal rings and progestogen-releasing IUDs) and
post-coital oral pills (visiting pills and emergency

Textbook of Clinical Trials. Edited by D. Machin, S. Day and S. Green
© 2004 John Wiley & Sons, Ltd ISBN: 0-471-98787-5

contraceptive (EC) pills). Non-hormonal methods used by women include intrauterine devices (IUDs), barrier methods (diaphragm and female condom), spermicides, natural methods (calendar and lactational amenorrhoea) and sterilisation, as well as immunocontraceptives, that are being developed. Hormonal male methods consist of injectable preparations and implants, still under development. Non-hormonal ones comprise condoms, withdrawal and sterilisation (vasectomy and vas occlusion), while immunocontraceptives or vaccines are under development.

These broad classes of contraceptive methods differ in the length of the acting period, in the mechanism of action, in the interval and way of administration or insertion, in the possibility of control by the woman, in their effectiveness and in their possible effects on health and indications for their use. They also differ in the way they meet the interests of men and women in different social and cultural settings.

CONTRACEPTION METHODS: AN OVERVIEW

Table 20.1 presents a list of currently used contraceptive methods with the interval of action required, the pregnancy rates under typical and perfect use and the main safety concerns. Extensive and detailed descriptions of old and new contraceptive methods are available.[2,3] A comprehensive review of the literature on contraceptive efficacy was done by Trussell and Kost.[4]

HORMONAL CONTRACEPTIVES FOR WOMEN

Hormonal methods prevent conception by inhibiting ovulation or preventing implantation or changing the quality of cervical mucus and thus preventing sperm access to the cervix. Oral methods exert their action if administered within a cycle, while injectable preparations, implants and hormone-releasing devices are long-acting.

Oral Contraceptives

OCs comprise combined oral contraceptives (COCs) and progesterone-only pills (POPs).

Modern low-dose COCs contain a combination of oestrogen and a progestin (20 to 35 mcg of oestrogen and 150 mcg or less of levonorgestrel, or 200 to 300 mcg of norgestrel or 400 to 1000 mcg of norethindrone or the equivalent of another progestin). There are monophasic formulations, with constant daily doses of oestrogen and progestin, biphasic ones, in which the dose of progestin changes in each of two periods and triphasic ones, in which the dosages change in each of the three seven-day periods of pill intake during the 21 days of pill cycle.

COCs prevent conception through the suppression of ovulation via hypothalamic and pituitary effects and progestin-mediated alterations in the consistency and properties of cervical mucus. It is still unconfirmed if the mechanism of action also includes alterations in the endometrial lining and of tubal transport mechanisms.

POPs have a lower dose of progestin than do COCs (75 mcg of norgestrel or 350 mcg of norethindrone). They prevent conception through a combination of mechanisms including suppression of ovulation, alteration of cervical mucus, of the endometrium and of the fallopian tubes.

Synthetic oestrogens were first developed in the early 1930s and the more potent ethinyl oestradiol in 1938, while synthetic orally active progestins were first produced in the early 1950s. In this decade the first generation progestins, like ethynodiol and lynesterol were developed. OCs became available in the United States in 1959. A major breakthrough in the development of OCs was the finding that the oestrogen and progestin acted synergistically to inhibit the pituitary. This allowed the transition from high-dose to low-dose, of both the oestrogen and the progestin. Low-dose oestrogen COCs have less frequent complaints about breast tenderness, nausea and leg cramps.[5] Information on efficacy and common side-effects was obtained from randomised clinical trials (RCTs),[6,7] one of them comparing COCs and POPs.[7] The progestins that have been most widely studied are norethindrone (or norethisterone) and levonorgestrel (second-generation). Around the 1990s, three new progestins have

Table 20.1. Contraceptive methods available, their characteristics, typical failure and discontinuation rates and safety concerns

Type	Method	Duration of action	Typical one year pregnancy rate per 100 woman-years	Perfect one year pregnancy rate per 100 woman-years	Safety concerns
Hormonal for women					
OCs	COCs	Daily	6–8	0.1	Cardiovascular diseases, depression, hepatic adenomas
	POPs	Daily	1 (breastfeeding)	0.5	Unknown
Injectables	DMPA	3-month	0.3	0.3	None
	NET-EN	2-month	0.3	0.3	None
	Combined	once-a-month	0.3	0.3	Same as for COCs for severe pathologies
Implants	Norplant	5-year	0.1	0.1	Infection at implant site
	Jadelle	5-year			Infection at implant site
	Implanon	3-year			Infection at implant site
Vaginal rings	Combined	3–12 months	<3	<3	Vaginal irritation (at insertion) Lesions
	Low-dose Lng	3–12 months	4.5	3.2	Vaginal irritation (at insertion) Lesions
Non-hormonal for women					
IUD	Copper	8–10 yrs	0.8	0.6	Increased menstrual bleeding, anaemia Uterine perforation PID 20–30 days post-insertion
	Lng-releasing	5–7 yrs	Not available	Not available	STD risk
Barrier	Female condom	Coitus-related	21	5	None
	Diaphragmw/ spermicide	Coitus-related	20	6	Toxic shock syndrome Urinary tract infections
	Cervical cap	Coitus-related	20 (nulliparous) 40 (parous)	9 (nulliparous) 26 (parous)	Toxic shock syndrome
Spermicides	Spermicides	Coitus-related	26	6	Vaginal infection and irritation
Natural	Periodic abstinence	Daily	20	1–9	None
	Lactational amenorrhoea	Duration of breastfeeding	2	0.5	None
Sterilisation	Female	Permanent	0.5	0.5	Infection, anesthesia complications
Non-hormonal for men					
Barrier	Male condom	Coitus-related	14	3	
Natural	Withdrawal	Coitus-related	19	4	
Sterilisation	Male (vasectomy)	Permanent	0.2	0.1	Cancer of prostate and testes

been introduced (third-generation): norgestimate, desogestrel and gestodene.

OCs are likely to affect lipid and carbohydrate metabolism and the coagulation system, which seem to be predictive of cardiovascular problems. The effect of low-dose OCs on these physiological functions has been shown to be non-existent or small.[8–11] Another safety concern regards cancer. Some studies have reported that the use of hormonal contraceptives is protective of cancer

of the ovary and the endometrium.[12] However, a possible link between the use of OCs for a long period and breast cancer risk among young women and cancer of the cervix is still a concern. Side-effects of COCs are nausea, headaches, dizziness, spotting, weight gain, breast tenderness and chloasma. For POPs, the main side-effect is menstrual irregularities.

The association between OCs and cardiovascular diseases, namely venous thrombosis (VTE), ischaemic heart disease and cerebrovascular disease, has been the object of a controversy. There seems to be a small increase in the risk of VTE, larger for the OCs containing third-generation progestins compared to those containing second-generation progestins. However, 'modern, low oestrogen dose OCs are extremely safe if used appropriately in young women'.[13] The most recent evidence suggests that myocardial infarction and stroke are rare and limited to women who smoke cigarettes or have hypertension or other cardiovascular risk factors.

OCs constitute the most common form of steroidal hormonal contraception and it is also the most common method of reversible contraception in countries other than China. It is estimated that 60 to 80 million women are OC users worldwide.[14] COCs are a safe method of contraception, only not to be recommended for women with cardiovascular diseases, diabetes mellitus, cancer or smoking.[15] POPs can be taken by lactating women, but are not recommended in cases of thromboembolism or vein thrombosis.

OCs require daily attention by the woman and they have a high discontinuation rate: in programmes, it has been reported that less than 50% of the women who start use continue treatment after one year.[16,17] Both COCs and POPs are very effective under perfect use,[15] and under typical use they are still effective (Table 20.1).

Injectable Preparations

The most common injectable contraceptive is the progestin-only preparation depot-medroxyprogesterone acetate (DMPA), that provides contraceptive protection for three months. Norethisterone enantate (NET-EN) is also a progestin-only preparation that provides protection for two months. Combined oestrogen–progestin once-a-month injectable contraceptives are Cyclofem, which combines DMPA with an oestrogen, and Mesigyna, which combines NET-EN with an oestrogen. Injectable preparations are long-acting and require the intervention of health care professionals to administer the injection.

The mechanism of action of DMPA is suppression of ovulation and changes in the cervical mucus and the endometrium. Combined injectable preparations seem to have a mechanism of action similar to COCs.

DMPA was first used as a contraceptive in the 1960s. Subsequently other alternative injectable contraceptives were developed among which NET-EN gained widespread use. Once-a-month injectables were developed with the purpose of overcoming the inconvenience of the disruption of the menstrual bleeding pattern of progesterone-only preparations. WHO undertook the evaluation and optimisation of the dose and oestrogen/progesterone ratio of Cyclofem and Mesigyna.[18] Also, the Chinese Injectable No. 1, with a complicated administration schedule, was developed in China. A multicentre trial was important to decide between the 100 mg or 150 mg dose for DMPA.[19] A number of clinical trials showed that NET-EN was highly effective.[20] Other trials determined that NET-EN needs to be administered every two months and also compared DMPA and NET-EN.[21]

Regarding safety concerns, a large multicentre study provided reassurance that the use of DMPA was not associated with cancer[22] and thus DMPA was registered in the United States as a long-acting contraceptive.[23] Headache is a common complaint, side-effects are weight gain and delay in the return of fertility. Menstrual irregularities are frequent, including prolonged and heavy bleeding, mostly during the first months of use, and long periods of amenorrhoea.

About 16 million women worldwide are users of injectable contraceptives: 13 million DMPA users in 90 different countries, 1 million NET-EN users and 2 million once-a-month injectables users in Latin America and China, and introductory studies are being conducted in several other countries.[24]

Progesterone-only contraceptives can be taken by breastfeeding women when they do not have access to other methods. It is not recommended for women with multiple risk factors for arterial cardiovascular disease or with unexplained vaginal bleeding. A theoretical concern is the effect on the neonate for breastfeeding women <6 weeks postpartum.

Injectable contraceptives are very effective: 0.3 pregnancies per 100 woman-years in the first year of use for DMPA, NET-EN and combined injectables[15] (Table 20.1).

Implants

Implants used for contraception in women consist of a silicone rubber tube or capsule inserted subdermally in the arm, containing a steroid or progestin released through it at a constant rate for several years. Implants are thus long-acting and require the intervention of health care professionals for insertion and removal. Norplant is the most widely used implant, consisting of six levonorgestrel-releasing rods with contraceptive action during five years. Jadelle is a two-rod levonorgestrel implant with a five-year duration. Implanon is a single implant releasing 3-keto-desogestrel during three years. Another single implant releases ST 1435, a progestin rapidly metabolised, making the implant suitable for lactating women.

The mechanism of action, similarly to that of POPs, includes a combination of effects, there being indications that ovulation suppression is not the only one,[25] since only about 50% of women show suppression of progesterone levels.[26]

Norplant became available in the United States in 1991, after regulatory approval based on large clinical trials, which provided information on discontinuation rates and side-effects.[27] Norplant II is a two-rod levonorgestrel implant easier to insert and remove and less conspicuous than Norplant, with a modified manufacturing design, but its development was stopped after trials comparing it with Norplant showed lower efficacy. The pregnancy rates were found to depend on the type of tubing used to manufacture the implant, the soft tubing being an improvement over the hard tubing.

The main safety concern of implants is infection at the implant site, otherwise they are considered safe. The main side-effect observed among Norplant users is disturbances in the menstrual bleeding pattern, with episodes of prolonged and heavy bleeding, mostly during the first months of use. Common complaints are headache, weight gain, mood change and depression. The safety of Norplant has been confirmed.[28]

It is estimated that one million women are Norplant users. Patterns of use are similar to other progestogen-only contraceptives. It is very effective, with 0.1 pregnancies per 100 woman-years in the first year of use.[15]

Vaginal Rings

Vaginal rings are devices releasing either a combination of a progestin and an oestrogen or only a progestin, of which the most common are levonorgestrel and progesterone.

The mechanism of action of levonorgestrel-releasing rings is similar to that of POPs, but with an increased effect on cervical mucus.

The first ring was progesterone-only, then the progesterone dose was reduced and combined rings were developed. Several designs were studied before an active core ring surrounded by an active silastic membrane was developed, leading to multi-compartment rings. A low-dose levonorgestrel contraceptive ring (20 mcg/day) was studied in WHO multicentre trials.[29,30]

Safety concerns related to the levonorgestrel ring are menstrual disturbances, vaginal symptoms, lesions and repeated expulsion.

Vaginal rings are attractive because they can be discontinued easily by the woman herself and are thus under her control, they do not require daily attention like the OCs, and they are not coitus-related like the condoms. The one year pregnancy rates of combined rings were less than 3 pregnancies per 100 woman-years in a multicentre trial[31] (Table 20.1).

Emergency Contraception

Emergency contraception (EC) based on pills is a post-coital method that is recommended up to three to five days after an act of unprotected intercourse. The standard EC method was the Yuzpe regimen of COCs (ethinylestradiol 100 mcg and levonorgestrel 0.5 mg or *dl*-norgestrel 1.0 mg repeated 12 hours later). A superior regimen consists of two 0.75 mg doses of levonorgestrel 12 hours apart[32] or a single 1.5 mg dose.[33] Single doses of the anti-progestin mifepristone, ranging from 10 mg to 600 mg is another method. EC is a back-up method and cannot be used regularly.

Regarding the mechanism of action, if unprotected intercourse occurs within a few days of ovulation, the only time when fertilisation can occur, ECs will exert their effect prior to implantation being completed (day 6–7 after fertilisation) and thus an established pregnancy would not be disrupted.[34,35] If EC is administered when a woman is already pregnant there is evidence from a study with pregnant women that 'ethinyl oestradiol is not a reliable abortifacient ... and that its efficiency as a postcoital contraceptive may be limited to a relatively short period following ovulation prior to implantation'.[36]

Although EC started in the 1980s in Europe with the Yuzpe regimen, it was only in 1997 that the FDA in the United States declared the regimen safe and effective.[37] The standard EC method until the late 1990s was the Yuzpe regimen, when levonorgestrel was shown in a trial to be more effective and have a better side-effect profile.[32] It has been registered in 1999 in the United States and is available now in at least 80 countries around the world. Mifepristone started to be used as an EC method at the dose of 600 mg. RCTs have shown that 10 mg can be used instead of higher doses, with a reduced effect of delay of menses observed with higher doses.[38]

EC pills are relatively benign and they pose no serious safety concerns. Nausea and vomiting are common with high-oestrogen regimens. Levonorgestrel and mifepristone regimens have a better side-effect profile than the Yuzpe regimen.[32,38] A concern with mifepristone is the delay of menses, mainly with high doses.[38]

In women receiving EC up to 72 hours after unprotected intercourse, 1.1% pregnancy rates have been observed after levonorgestrel with typical use and 3.2% after Yuzpe.[32] With the coitus-to-treatment interval extended to 120 hours, pregnancy rates were 1.1% to 1.3% after mifepristone

doses ranging from 10 mg to 600 mg.[38] With perfect use, the corresponding figures in the cited trials were 0.8% after levonorgestrel, 1.9% after Yuzpe and 0.3% to 1% after mifepristone.

NON-HORMONAL CONTRACEPTIVES FOR WOMEN

IUDs

Intrauterine devices (IUDs) are inert intrauterine rings or plastic devices with or without drug loading (copper or levonorgestrel). They are long-acting and require the intervention of health care professionals for insertion and removal. IUDs inserted after an unprotected coitus are also effective as EC.

The mechanism of action of IUDs is to inhibit sperm and ovum transport and fertilisation.

IUDs were first introduced for contraceptive purposes at the beginning of the 1900s. The first IUD consisted of a loop of silk thread. Then a metal copper-releasing ring was developed. In the 1960s plastic coils became popular, like the Lippes Loop. The IUD used in the 1970s, the plastic Dalkon Shield, was associated with high pregnancy rates and high infection rates. Safety problems with old devices included the risk of contracting pelvic inflammatory disease, and that of septic abortion and infertility, with consequent high discontinuation rates. Randomised clinical trials (RCTs) published in 1975 compared the Dalkon Shield with the Lippes Loop D and the new Copper-7 and Copper-T 200. The superiority of collared Copper-T was thus established.[39–41] In the early 1980s trials were conducted including NOVA T, MLCu250, Copper-T 220C and MLCu 375.[42] In other trials the Copper-T 380 showed superiority over the MLCu 375.[43–44] Many IUD trials were conducted in China to try to design copper IUDs adapted to Chinese women. A major development was that of steroid-releasing IUDs. Devices releasing 20 mcg/day of levonorgestrel have been shown to be very effective.[47]

High efficacy and low risk have been observed for copper IUDs and the levonorgestrel-releasing IUD in large trials[47–50] and there has been a progressive increase in effectiveness with continued research.[26]

IUDs are the most commonly used contraceptive methods after sterilisation, and the most commonly used reversible method in China. It is estimated that about 120 million women are IUD users worldwide.[51] The method is not recommended for pregnant women and those with current sexually transmitted infections or at risk of acquiring them.

Compliance is not a problem with IUDs, but there could instead be discontinuation for several reasons. New copper devices and the new hormone-releasing IUD combine low pregnancy rates with low discontinuation rates. One-year pregnancy rates for the most efficient IUDs are <1 per 100 woman-years for the copper IUDs, 0.1–0.2 for the levonorgestrel-releasing IUD and 0.6–0.8 for the TCu-380A IUD.[15]

Barrier Methods

Barrier methods used by women are the diaphragm, the female condom and spermicides. The importance of developing effective dual protection barrier methods that provide protection against sexually transmitted diseases (STDs) has increased in the last years with the spread of the HIV/AIDs epidemic. Condoms are barrier methods providing this feature of dual protection.

Barrier methods prevent conception by avoiding contact between sperm and the ovum. They act as a mechanical barrier (condom, diaphragm) or by inactivating the sperm (spermicides) or both (diaphragm with spermicide and cervical cap).

The female condom has become an important alternative because it is under the woman's control and can provide women with the ability of protecting themselves against STDs in situations where men refuse to use condoms. It is coitus-related and thus pregnancy can be the result of either method failure or inconsistency of use. Effectiveness: 5 pregnancies per 100 woman-years in the first year of use under perfect use (effective), 21 under typical use (only somewhat effective).[15]

The diaphragm is an elastic membrane with cavity rim, which may be attractive to potential users but it lacks the advantage of protection against STDs. A new microbicide-releasing diaphragm is being developed to address this concern. Safety concerns for the diaphragm are a history of toxic shock syndrome and allergy to latex.[15] It is effective under perfect use (Table 20.1).

Spermicides are in the form of creams, jellies, foams in pressurised containers, foaming tablets or suppositories. They are not very effective when used by themselves, but can be used in combination with other methods. Effectiveness: 6 pregnancies per 100 woman-years in the first year of use if used correctly and consistently (effective), 26 under typical use (only somewhat effective).[15] Self-administered topical preparations with spermicidal and microbicidal activities are being studied, that provide both contraceptive and anti-infection protection and are under the control of the woman. The cellulose sulphate gel is one such preparation.

The cervical cap or sponge is a mushroom cap-shaped device releasing a spermicide and whose concave side is applied over the cervix. Its maximal insertion time is 24 hours. It is effective under perfect use (Table 20.1).

Natural Methods

Periodic abstinence restricts intercourse to the infertile phase of the woman's cycle, which depends on the ability of the woman to identify the fertile period.[52] It acts through prevention of fertilisation. It is effective under perfect use (Table 20.1).

The lactational amenorrhoea method is an accepted method of contraception when the interest of the woman is birth-spacing, since it has been observed that breastfeeding women within six months of delivery who are amenorrhoeic have <2% risk of becoming pregnant.[53] Effectiveness: 0.5 pregnancies per 100 woman-years in the first year of perfect use (very effective), 2 under typical use (effective).[15]

Sterilisation

Sterilisation in women is an effective surgical procedure involving the blockage of the fallopian tubes, which transport mature ova from the ovaries to the uterus. The most widely practised techniques are minilaparotomy and laparoscopy. Sterilisation is the only permanent contraceptive method and the most prevalent, 180 million couples have been reported to be sterilised (male or female). Research is in progress to develop a non-surgical procedure. Effectiveness: 0.5 pregnancies per 100 woman-years in the first year of use (always very effective).[15]

ImmunoContraceptives

Research is in progress for the development of a female vaccine based on the human chorionic gonadotrophin molecule (hCG), for action after fertilisation and before implantation.

HORMONAL CONTRACEPTIVES FOR MEN

Hormonal injectable methods for men that reduce the production of spermatozoa are based on weekly injections of testosterone. Research is in progress for the development of a longer-acting injectable preparation, namely at four-week intervals. Preparations based on DMPA and testosterone and on NET-EN and testosterone are under study.

Implants for men are also under investigation. A depot androgen/progestin combination has recently demonstrated high contraceptive efficacy with satisfactory short-term safety and recovery of spermatogenesis.[54] In this trial, a hormonal implant was given every four months to replace testosterone and the progestin DMPA was injected every three months.

NON-HORMONAL CONTRACEPTIVES FOR MEN

Barrier Methods

Condoms used by men are tubes closed spherically on one side, normally made of a latex membrane 0.06 to 0.07 mm thick.[55] Most are lubricated, and some contain spermicides. The feature of dual protection and the mechanism of action are the same as those described for the female condom.

Research on the male condom has dealt with efficacy and acceptability issues. Old condoms were made of hard material, acceptability was low and they were not very resistant to adverse storage conditions. Improvement has been made with the latex condoms. A new polyurethane condom was compared with latex condoms in RCTs.[56]

Male condom is the most widely used of barrier methods but its use is not more widespread because it is often not accepted, mainly by the male partner. Condoms have practically no risk of side-effects. The only concern has been allergy to latex in latex condoms.

Effectiveness: 3 pregnancies per 100 woman-years in the first year of use if used correctly and consistently (effective), 14 under typical use (only somewhat effective).[15]

Natural Methods

Withdrawal, or *coitus interruptus*, is a low effectiveness method (Table 20.1) which depends on the man successfully withdrawing the penis from the vagina before ejaculation starts, and thus preventing fertilisation.

Sterilisation

Vasectomy in the male is a simple surgical procedure, but it is questionable in some cultural settings due to the incision and non-reversibility. Research is in progress for the development of a reversible procedure.

A possible association between vasectomy and prostate cancer was a safety concern, but observational studies have shown that if there is such an association, the increased risk in vasectomised men compared to non-vasectomised men is small.[57]

Sterilisation is the only permanent contraceptive method for men. Effectiveness: 0.1–0.2

pregnancies per 100 woman-years in the first year of use (always very effective).[15]

ImmunoContraceptives

Research on vaccines for men is in progress based on antibodies that neutralise the biological effect of the gonadotrophin hormone-releasing hormone (GnRH) and follicle-stimulating hormone (FSH), with a resulting oligospermia or azoospermia.

CLINICAL TRIAL METHODS IN CONTRACEPTION

Observational studies constitute the source of information for comparisons of efficacy, discontinuation rates or safety across broad classes of contraceptive methods, for example implants and IUDs. Women cannot usually be randomised to different broad classes of methods because the woman's choice of contraceptive is determined by social, cultural and personal reasons. An exception to this was one large RCT which allocated women at random to OCs or to vaginal methods (consisting of diaphragms, jellies, creams or foams).[58] However, results were difficult to interpret because there were many women switching methods and lost to follow-up.[59,60]

RCTs, on the other hand, have been an important tool to find new safe and efficient regimens or devices within each broad class and improve existing ones by answering questions about the best compound, the best dose, the best interval or route of administration (compounds) or the best physical properties (devices).

Sometimes partially randomised trials are used to compare two types of hormonal contraceptives within the same broad class with a non-hormonal one, used as a placebo control group. For example, in a WHO trial (data not published) on the effect of two injectable contraceptives (DMPA and NET-EN) on lipid and lipoprotein metabolism, women requesting an injectable contraceptive were allocated at random to the two preparations, and a group of non-hormone-releasing IUD users was the control. In another

WHO trial under preparation, two types of implants will be compared with regard to efficacy in preventing pregnancies, allocating at random the type of implant to women choosing implants. To assess the effect of hormones on the bleeding pattern, IUD users or sterilised women will constitute a control group.

Clinical trials generally include an insufficient number of women to provide conclusive information on rare events, like cancer and cardiovascular diseases.[26] However, a careful documentation of serious adverse events and predisposing risk factors in the conduct of clinical trials should always be provided.[1]

General principles applying to the conduct of clinical trials and post-registration assessment of steroidal contraceptive drugs have been established.[1,61] The development of a new contraceptive method involves a long process until it is registered and reaches the market. The methodology used depends on the stage of development and will be treated separately for Phase I/II and Phase III trials.

PHASE I/II TRIALS

Objectives

Phase I trials deal with drug safety and aim to determine an acceptable drug dosage, and also study drug metabolism and bioavailability. In contraceptive research, Phase I trials are conducted to investigate the pharmacology of steroidal contraceptive or other contraceptive drugs in healthy volunteers.[61] Phase I trials must be preceded by initial toxicity studies in rodents and pharmacokinetic studies in primates, which give an indication for the dose used in the first clinical study.[61]

When a contraceptive has been assessed to be safe in Phase I trials, its research progresses to Phase II trials, using the optimal dose and administration schedule. Contraceptive Phase II trials are small-scale investigations into the effectiveness and safety of a contraceptive method, carried out on closely monitored patients. They have the goal to establish its mechanisms of action, metabolic effects and provide preliminary estimates of the frequency of common side-effects, its effectiveness and its acceptability. It is recommended to previously conduct repeated-dose toxicity and reproduction studies in animals. Phase II studies are conventionally subdivided into Phase IIA, studies on the pharmacology of the drug in patients and Phase IIB, definitive dose-finding studies.[61]

Since steroidal contraceptives are used by healthy people, it is desirable to assess the minimum effective dose at the initial stages of clinical testing.[61] This can be done already in Phase I trials instead of in later stages. The direct assessment of efficacy in small trials is not possible because with reasonably effective contraceptives pregnancy is a rare event. There exist surrogate variables for efficacy of a steroid drug for pregnancy prevention. Phase I trials on contraceptives, therefore, are often also used to look at these surrogates of efficacy in addition to safety issues, so that Phase I and Phase II trials are combined to evaluate both safety and endocrinological endpoints. Examples of surrogates of efficacy are hormone levels as indicators of inhibition of ovulation in contraceptives for women, sperm concentration in long-acting androgen–progestogen formulations for men as an indicator of inhibition of spermatogenesis, and amount of serum hCG antibodies in immunocontraceptive trials for women. Serological and clinical diagnoses of pregnancies are also conducted.

In the case of hormonal contraceptives for women, the following clinical pharmacological parameters should be studied to assess the inhibition of ovulation:[1]

1. Hormonal activity: the nature and hormonal activity of a steroid contained in the contraceptive and its principal metabolites should be described.
2. Pharmacological action on ovarian function: the mechanism by which the contraceptive effect is attained should be described. This involves, in the first place, a description of the ovarian function in women with normal ovulatory function, measuring plasma concentration of ovarian steroids and gonadotrophins

and conducting ultrasound of ovaries. Thus, information is obtained on the extent to which ovarian function is suppressed. Time to onset of action and to return to normal ovarian function after discontinuation should be studied.

3. Other pharmacological effects on the reproductive system: effects on the endometrium and on the cervical mucus.
4. Effects on other endocrine systems: pituitary, adrenal, thyroid.
5. Metabolic effects: effects on hemostatic variables, plasma lipids and carbohydrate metabolism. For products not containing an oestrogen and suppressing oestrogen secretion, effect on bone mineral density and bone metabolism.

Design

For contraception in women, recruitment into Phase I trials is conducted among volunteers of reproductive age, not pregnant or lactating, regularly menstruating, identified in family planning clinics or selected community groups, who are IUD users or sterilised, and therefore, not at risk of becoming pregnant. Users of other hormonal contraceptives than the one being studied are not acceptable because the method might interfere with the assessment of clinical and laboratory parameters. Other selection criteria depend on the contraceptive being studied. For example, for contraceptive vaccines, acute hypersensitivity to the carrier should be excluded, and if reversibility cannot be assured, participants should be no younger than 25 years and have had children previously.

A series of sequential studies using different dose levels are conducted to assess the minimum effective dose. These studies involve doses that are two or three times the initial dose. For each dose level, a study is conducted in 10–20 healthy volunteers.[61]

Selection criteria for Phase II trials on women, different to those mentioned for Phase I trials, are being currently exposed to the risk of pregnancy and have proven fertility. At this stage, if volunteers participating in Phase I studies are IUD users and they are willing to continue, then the IUD should be removed to assess efficacy.

Phase IIB trials require about 50–100 subjects to assess efficacy and side-effects of the dosage determined in early trials (Phase I–IIA).

Examples

Examples of Phase I and Phase II clinical trials are the ones conducted with injectable preparations to evaluate well-known potent synthetic progestins in combination. A Phase I trial tested the use of progesterone as an alternative.[62]

Several examples for injectable contraceptives are summarised in a review by Newton et al.[24] An early pharmacological trial on Cyclofem with 11 women involved one pre-treatment cycle, a 3-month treatment phase with an injection of Cyclofem every 28 days and then a 3-month recovery phase. It confirmed that ovulation was inhibited and that inhibition of luteal activity persists after the last injection for several cycles.[63]

A comparative non-randomised study of Cyclofem and Mesigyna with 15 women, 8 receiving Cyclofem and 7 Mesigyna, involved one pre-treatment cycle, three treatment cycles of 28 days and a 90-day follow-up period. The results showed that the suppressive effect of Cyclofem was greater than Mesigyna.[64]

A four-arm trial of reduced dose of medroxyprogesterone acetate and oestradiol cypionate in Cyclofem recruited 88 women into the following groups: Cyclofem full dose, Cyclofem half dose, DMPA full dose, DMPA half dose. All four preparations were found to be effective in inhibiting ovulation for at least one month after the injection, and the combined preparations showed more regular bleeding patterns.[65]

Metabolic Studies

Specific Phase II studies on biochemical variables are conducted when required. These variables include lipid and lipoprotein metabolism, coagulation, fibrinolysis and platelet function as well as other physiological events such as vaginal blood loss.[61] The parallel group designs have been the most common design in this type of study, but factorial designs have also been used. Newton et al.[24] describe examples of these studies for injectable once-a-month preparations. The crossover design has been used in a metabolic study to compare three different progestogens (norgestrel, norethisterone and medroxyprogesterone) in treatment periods of 3-week duration immediately preceded by 3 weeks of 'wash out'.[64]

Ethical Considerations

When conducting Phase I/II trials, the fact that contraceptive methods are used by healthy individuals implies a different risk/benefit assessment compared with therapeutic drugs for life-threatening diseases. This justifies the assessment of the minimum effective dose at early stages of development.

When volunteers are advised on the risks and benefits of the study in order to seek their informed consent, the specific risks of receiving a steroidal contraceptive should be explained.

PHASE III TRIALS

Objectives

After a contraceptive is shown to be reasonably effective in Phase II trials, it is essential to compare it with the current standard contraceptive(s) within the same broad class in a large trial involving a substantial number of patients, with the goal of establishing its efficacy.[26] Phase III trials permit more refined estimates of safety, effectiveness and acceptability in comparison with a standard. In contraceptive research, this information provides the basis for introducing a hormonal contraceptive into family planning practice in field trials in various settings, as a prerequisite for registration with drug regulatory authorities (see introductory trials in the other Issues section later).

Design and Trial Size

The most common design to compare methods within each broad class of contraceptives has been the parallel group design, with simple randomisation in single-centre trials, and stratified by centre in multicentre trials. This was the case for the development of OCs,[5–7] injectables,[18,19,22,32,33,38,55,67] implants,[27] IUDs,[40–46] condoms[68] and EC regimens.[32,38,56]

The control used in RCTs to compare efficacy of methods is typically an active control, since a placebo control would not be ethical. Examples of comparisons of new versus standard, respectively, are the following: NET-EN versus DMPA (injectables), Norplant II versus Norplant (implants), steroid-releasing versus copper IUDs, polyurethane condom versus latex condom, Yuzpe versus levonorgestrel regimens (EC). Placebo controls have been used to assess efficacy of a treatment to improve the bleeding pattern disrupted by the use of progestin-only contraceptives.

In contraceptive trials, the main end-point for efficacy is based on pregnancies, a rare event. The number of subjects required per group to detect as significant a difference between groups corresponding to a doubling of the rate, in a two-sided 5% level test, with 80% power, is usually large (1140 for a control rate of 2%, 4700 for a control rate of 0.5%).

When the effect of two factors is of interest and if an interaction is likely to be present, the sample size needed is approximately double in a four-arm 2×2 trial than in a two-arm trial comparing the two doses of only one component. This might be a reason for which factorial designs have not been commonly used in contraceptive efficacy trials. In the study of bleeding patterns among users of progestogen-only contraceptives, an example of a factorial design is provided by a trial comparing the effect of low-dose aspirin and vitamin E alone or in combination on Norplant-induced prolonged bleeding.[69]

For registration of a steroidal contraceptive, some regulatory agencies require clinical trials with 200 (FDA) or 400 subjects completing two years of observation, while some others require even less.[26] It is clear that this number does not provide sufficient power to detect a difference in rare events with the control. Nor does it provide sufficient precision for a confidence interval estimation of a rare event: 5 events observed in 200 subjects gives a rate of 2.5% with 95% CI of 1% to 10%. On the other hand, the Committee for Proprietary Medicinal Products (CPMP) recommends that 20 000 cycles be observed, which at 13 28-day cycles per year is equivalent to 1540 women-years or 770 women followed completely for two years. This calculation is based on the criterion that the difference between the upper 95% confidence limit for the Pearl index (number of pregnancies per 100 women-years) and the point estimate does not exceed 1.[1]

Recruitment

Participants in Phase III contraceptive trials are usually recruited in family planning clinics. A majority of attendants requesting contraception in family planning clinics (other than STD clinics) are healthy. On arrival, subjects (women or men) or couples requesting or using the method under study are screened for eligibility. An eligibility criterion common to contraceptive efficacy trials is good general health, but others are specific to the contraceptive method, depending on the corresponding safety concerns and eligibility criteria.[15]

Trial participants are not therefore a random sample from women in reproductive age, and their particular characteristics affect external validity, making difficult the generalisation of results to wider populations.[4,70] First, women choosing a particular broad class of contraceptive are likely to be self-selected. For example, implants are often selected by older women. Second, clinicians are likely to select different types of women for different contraceptives. Third, women who are long-term users of a method and are happy with it do not come to the clinic and are less likely to be enrolled.

According to current ethical principles, all eligible subjects have to provide informed consent before being enrolled into the trial. In contraceptive trials, obtaining this consent from adolescents is problematic because some countries require a minimum legal age to provide consent. Consent from relatives is not always possible due to the need to maintain confidentiality in sensitive issues like contraception.

Randomisation, Allocation Concealment and Blinding

Randomisation in contraceptive RCTs is achieved in a similar way to RCTs in other areas, by the use of a computer-generated randomisation sequence. In multicentre trials the randomisation is usually stratified by centre, done in blocks, and prepared centrally. Treatments are allocated by assigning the next consecutive subject number in the randomisation sequence to the next enrolled subject.

Allocation concealment strategies include sealed opaque envelopes (unblinded trials) and packing of drugs by a central company (blinded trials). Many multicentre multinational RCTs have included settings with poor telecommunication systems, in which central telephone randomisation as a strategy for allocation concealment was not a feasible option.

Most clinical trials comparing implants, IUDs and other devices cannot be blinded because insertion or placement of the device usually implies that both the administrator and the user will see it, touch it or smell it. The situation is similar in sterilisation trials in which surgical procedures are compared. Some trials comparing IUDs or sterilisation techniques can be blinded to the woman but not to the device or procedure administrator. Depending on the treatments being compared, many clinical trials comparing injectable preparations, drugs for EC and possibly spermicides can be blinded to users, treatment administrators and outcome evaluators ('double blind').

Blinding in contraceptive trials can avert bias after treatment allocation by preventing the following causes of bias. First, it is possible that the health care provider or the user will tend to discontinue one treatment more than the other. Second, ascertainment bias could be introduced in the evaluation of subjective outcomes, like lesions in contraceptive rings trials. The delay in the recognition of pregnancy, the imprecision in the estimate of the date of conception and the occurrence of chemical pregnancies noted above are sources of uncertainty which also pave the way for the introduction of ascertainment bias. Bias could still be present even in blinded trials due to unblinding caused by ancillary information, like differential side-effects from the treatments being compared. For example, in EC trials, higher doses of a compound might cause nausea more frequently than lower doses.

Effectiveness and Efficacy of Contraceptive Methods: Theoretical Model

Effectiveness of a method can be defined as 'the proportionate reduction in fecundability caused by the use of a method'.[4] As such, it is not measurable because one would have to compare the rate of conception under use of the method with that in the same population not practising contraception nor lactating. The common use of effectiveness is to denote how well a method works. Sometimes efficacy is used with this meaning.

Steiner et al.[71] proposed a theoretical model (see also Refs. 4 and 51) in which the couple's ability to conceive and the timing and frequency of intercourse determine the unobservable pregnancy rate in the absence of contraception. In the presence of (perfect or imperfect) contraceptive protection this pregnancy rate is reduced, determining the 'typical' pregnancy rate. This typical rate is composed of the perfect use pregnancy rate and the imperfect use pregnancy rate, weighted by the proportion of each type of user.

A measure of efficacy that implies a comparison with the same treated population under placebo is the proportion of pregnancies prevented out of the expected pregnancies, or preventable fraction, given by 1− observed pregnancy rate/expected pregnancy rate.

The contraceptive method efficacy is the preventable fraction under conditions of perfect use, and the effectiveness is the preventable fraction under conditions of typical use. The difference between these two rates depends on both the pregnancy rates under each condition and the proportions of the two types of users.[52]

Estimation of Pregnancy Rates and Efficacy in Non-coitus Related Methods

Sterilisation, which acts continuously and is permanent, and methods which act continuously but are reversible, like IUDs and long-acting hormonal methods, are non-coitus related methods in the sense they do not require any particular action by the user to be effective.

If there is no daily monitoring of follicular growth or urinary metabolites, the estimates of efficacy by the preventable fraction are constructed with external estimates of probabilities of conception[72] and with data on pattern and timing of intercourse. The latter is difficult to obtain in large trials comparing regular use contraceptives, therefore the common measure of how well a contraceptive method works in preventing pregnancy is failure, or the occurrence of pregnancy in the period of time during which the contraceptive is used.[4] Thus, efficacy in this loose sense is evaluated in the woman and (inversely) measured in number of pregnancies per woman-time of observation (typically per 100 woman-years).

For reversible methods (for example IUDs and long-acting hormonal methods), the assessment of the pregnancy status might be difficult due to the following sources of uncertainty:[52,70] (1) when the decision to stop using a method is made, the pregnancy might be recognised after the method is stopped; (2) imprecision in the estimate of the date of conception when the estimate is based on the date of start of the last menstrual period; (3) occurrence of early 'chemical' pregnancies, of which a considerable percentage is lost before reaching the stage of clinical pregnancy and (4) early foetal losses, which might be unnoticed by the woman.

In clinical trials comparing regular contraceptives, women are usually required to return to the clinic at specified intervals during a follow-up period. The timing of reporting pregnancies varies among women. It is important that the method of counting pregnancies does not depend on this timing. The 'active follow-up' prevents this problem by defining a cut-off date and contacting women three months later to learn their pregnancy status at the cut-off date.[70]

One of the main problems affecting data quality is the loss to follow-up in trials comparing regular use contraceptives, that require long periods of follow-up. Bardin and Sivin[26] discuss the bias introduced in comparative trials by the failure to observe all subjects through the completion of the study. The magnitude of the bias depends on the proportion of subjects lost to follow-up and the outcome mean or proportion in this group.

The estimation of the pregnancy rate using the Pearl index has been shown to be not appropriate due to the decline in fertility of the cohort being followed with duration of the contraceptive use. This decline in fertility has been illustrated by Sivin and Schmidt[42] from long-term studies, where a progressive increase in the effectiveness of each device with age was observed, as well as a wider difference in failure rates among devices and a progressive increase in effectiveness with continued research.

Life table techniques have been the recommended analysis technique for years, using the single decrement method, in which women who exit for other reasons than pregnancy are censored at the time of exit.[52,70,73] The estimation of the pregnancy rate is given by the cumulative life table rate (net rate). The daily life table method, using the Kaplan–Meier product-limit estimate of the cumulative pregnancy rate (net rate) gives similar results and leads naturally to the logrank test to compare groups.[73]

A difficulty in the estimation of pregnancy rates is the presence of other reasons of discontinuation. For IUDs, the commonly analysed discontinuation reasons are expulsion, medical removal (due to pain, bleeding or pelvic inflammatory disease), non-medical removal (wish to become pregnant, no further need of contraception) and loss to follow-up. The use of net rates from life table techniques deals with competing causes by censoring. This approach has been criticised by Tai et al.[74] because it assumes independence of the different reasons for discontinuation. They argue that the estimates obtained by this approach are overestimates of the rate for each of the reasons, as can be seen by the fact that the sum of the probabilities of discontinuation due to all the reasons is greater than one. They are hypothetical rates that would occur if discontinuations for other reasons could not take place. Tai et al. recommend the use of cumulative incidence rates, that estimate the pregnancy rate in the presence of competing causes. They also argue in favour of the competing risk methodology to compare cumulative incidences between two methods (two IUDs). Farley discussed these recommendations, concluding that 'Kaplan–Meier estimates are more appropriate when estimating the effectiveness of a contraceptive method, ... (and the) cumulative incidence estimates are more appropriate when making programmatic decisions regarding contraceptive methods'.[75]

Behavioural Patterns and the Estimation of Efficacy of Contraceptive Methods

Methods that are used around the time of intercourse, like barrier methods and spermicides, are coitus-related and require a high degree of user compliance with the correct way of using the method in order to prevent pregnancy reliably.[52] For these methods, a pregnancy can be the result of either a method failure or lack of use or incorrect use. OCs are not coitus-related but have to be taken daily by women, posing similar types of problems. Similarly, periodic abstinence relies for its effectiveness on rules of when to abstain from sexual intercourse in order to avoid pregnancy, and users may depart from these rules.

In order to separate a method failure from a lack of use or an incorrect use of a method which is coitus-related, investigators denoted pregnancies in which the method had not been used or had been incorrectly used as 'user failures'. Pregnancies in which the method had been correctly used were denoted as 'method failures'. Trussell[70] illustrated the inadequacy of computing pregnancy rates corresponding to these two sources using the same denominator that includes all exposure from both 'perfect' and 'imperfect' use. He proposed to collect information on 'imperfect' use for all months of exposure, or alternatively obtain information on correct and consistent use at the end of the trial, and calculate separate rates for 'perfect' users and for 'imperfect' users.

For comparative trials, this issue is addressed by conducting a stratified analysis by imperfect and perfect use. The comparison of the effectiveness between treatments for all cycles (whether perfect or imperfect use took place) provides the treatment effect under conditions of typical use. The comparison of the efficacy between treatments is given by a subgroup analysis with cycles of perfect use.

Estimation of Pregnancy Rates, Effectiveness and Efficacy of Emergency Contraceptives

In trials comparing EC methods, it is feasible to know the pattern and timing of intercourse: protocols usually require a single unprotected act of intercourse, and its date is reported by the woman, as well as the date of start of the last menstrual period. A crude estimate of efficacy is the proportion of observed pregnancies (number of pregnancies divided by the number of women treated), but this measure is affected by the distribution of timing of intercourse with respect to the woman's cycle. The number of pregnancies occurring in the same population under no use of method is unobservable. It is estimated by the expected number of pregnancies, calculated by multiplying the number of women having unprotected intercourse on each day of the menstrual cycle by the probability of conception on that day, using external probabilities of conception.[72] The proportion of pregnancies prevented, or preventable fraction, is given by (1 − [observed pregnancies/expected pregnancies]). A technique for the construction of confidence intervals for the preventable fraction is available, using variance–covariance matrices from the external estimates of conception probabilities.[72] The day of ovulation, and thereof the day of the cycle in which intercourse took place, is usually estimated from the date of the last menstrual period as reported by the women, and thus subject to imprecision.

The success of EC depends on not having further unprotected acts of intercourse during the same cycle, since the EC treatment does not prevent pregnancies resulting from these acts.[32,38] Therefore user compliance can affect the effectiveness of the method. If the EC treatment includes two doses, its success also depends on the treatment compliance, i.e., on the woman taking the second dose (at home) at the correct interval. The estimation of typical and perfect use is therefore relevant in EC trials. When comparing groups, this has been achieved by two analyses, one including all subjects and a subgroup analysis with perfect users.

Caveats in Comparing Efficacy and Effectiveness Between Groups: Intention-to-Treat and Subgroup Analysis

In RCTs, the comparison of estimates of effectiveness obtained with two treatments corresponds to an intention-to-treat (ITT) analysis (in the absence of lost to follow-up), while that of efficacy corresponds to a subgroup analysis of perfect users. In large RCTs, the proportions of perfect and imperfect users are likely to be similar in the treatments being compared, so that differences in effectiveness between two treatments will depend mainly on differences between the pregnancy rates under the two treatments. Thus, the comparisons of effectiveness between treatments within the RCT are not biased (internal validity).

On the other hand, the comparison of efficacy between treatments has the limitations of a subgroup analysis. In the first place, the advantages of randomisation are lost, since imperfect users are excluded from the analysis. When the subgroup analysis is based on subject characteristics that are not affected by treatment, like baseline variables, each smaller subgroup is like a smaller randomised trial.[76] But when the subgroup is defined by a variable observed after randomisation and potentially affected by the treatment, then the treatment effect may influence classification into the subgroup. The treatment effect observed in the subgroup would then be biased. This caveat is illustrated by an RCT to compare mifepristone and levonorgestrel for EC. The main variable to define perfect use is adhering to the protocol requirement of not having further acts of unprotected intercourse before the start of next menses. Mifepristone is known to delay ovulation and thus is associated with a delay in the start of menses, while levonorgestrel is not.[33,38] This provides women under both regimens with a differential opportunity to violate the requirement, and then the effects of treatment under perfect

use and under typical use are likely to be of different magnitude. In the second place, unless the trial was designed to have sufficient power at the subgroup level, a relevant treatment effect in the subgroup will not be detected, or the confidence interval estimate of the effect will be imprecise. Stratification into perfect and imperfect users is another way of reporting results.[32,38]

Assessment of Side-effects and Acceptability of Contraceptive Methods

In women using contraceptives regularly, information on side-effects and complaints such as nausea, vomiting, diarrhoea, fatigue, dizziness, headache, lower abdominal pain and breast tenderness, as well as adverse events, can be collected in follow-up visits. Differences between groups in events which have a rate of 5 or more per 100 can be detected with small trials. Rates of 1 to 5 per 100 require larger trials. Detection of differences for lower rates would require even larger trials.[26]

Side-effects of EC are complaints (or signs and symptoms) of nausea, vomiting, diarrhoea, fatigue, dizziness, headache, lower abdominal pain and breast tenderness, and are treated as binomial proportions. Delay in the return of next menses, a time-to-event outcome, is undesirable because it gives the opportunity for more acts of unprotected intercourse and is a source of anxiety for the woman. It has been found to be a concern with mifepristone, mainly with high doses.

Acceptability of a contraceptive method depends not only on the characteristics of the method but on the service delivery setting and the socio-demographic and economic factors of a particular country.[24] It can be assessed by questions to the user regarding satisfaction, willingness to recommend the method to others and to pay to have access to the method. Many side-effects of regular use contraceptives are reflected in discontinuation. Some of these discontinuation reasons are related to the acceptability of the method by the user. For long-acting hormonal methods, for example, the main discontinuation reason is disturbances in the menstrual bleeding pattern, largely determined by cultural and social factors. An Egyptian study on the acceptability of once-a-month injectable contraceptives found differences between women discontinuing and those continuing in all measures of acceptability.[77] Factors important in determining acceptability were: age, contraceptive history, learning about injectables, the husband's attitude and knowing about another user's satisfaction.

OTHER ISSUES

Vaginal Bleeding Patterns

Hormonal contraception is often associated with disturbances in the vaginal bleeding pattern. These disorders are common with the use of progestogen-only hormonal methods and they do not imply a health risk *per se*, since it has been shown that the amount of blood loss is not a problem. They may be tolerated by the woman, and this depends on cultural and behavioural patterns. The measurement of bleeding patterns can be achieved by direct questions to women, by their completing menstrual diaries or by measuring blood loss.[26]

The most used method of analysis of menstrual diaries is the reference period method,[78] which was standardised by WHO using a 90-day reference period.[79] It consists in analysing bleeding/spotting records in women's menstrual diary cards by taking fixed-length segments of time (the reference period, for which a 90-day segment has been used as a convention) and deriving measures of bleeding pattern, or indices. The following 10 indices have been recommended:[80] number of bleeding/spotting days, number of spotting days, number of bleeding/spotting episodes, number of spotting-only episodes, mean, range and maximum value of lengths of bleeding/spotting episodes, mean, range and maximum value of lengths of bleeding-free intervals. These indices have been analysed using box–whisker plots and non-parametric analysis techniques. To summarise the information provided, Belsey and Carlson[81] conducted a principal component analysis with data from women using different contraceptives, and concluded that most of the essential information about a woman's bleeding

pattern was contained in four indices: number of bleeding/spotting episodes, mean length of episodes, mean length of bleeding-free intervals and the range of bleeding-free interval lengths. Based on the indices, the following clinically important patterns are derived:[80] no bleeding (amenorrhoea), prolonged, frequent, infrequent and irregular bleeding.

The 90-day reference period method was applied to diary data collected from women treated with Cyclofem, Mesigyna, a low-dose levonorgestrel-releasing ring and DMPA taking part in Phase III WHO clinical trials. Among women using once-a-month injectable and the levonorgestrel-releasing ring the incidence of acceptable patterns was higher than among DMPA users, although the patterns were different from those of normally menstruating women.[82]

Several placebo controlled RCTs have been conducted to investigate the therapeutic effectiveness of one or more treatments for bleeding irregularities. An example is given by a trial comparing the bleeding pattern of untreated DMPA users with groups treated with ethinyl oestradiol or oestrone sulphate.[83]

Equivalence Trials

In equivalence trials, the objective is to show that a new contraceptive or contraceptive device that has advantages with regard to side-effects, user preference or cost has equivalent efficacy to that of the standard one. Failure to detect a difference in a conventional significance test does not imply equivalence and a significant difference may correspond to equivalence within a margin of clinical relevance (or margin of equivalence, denoted by Δ). A confidence interval for the difference between the methods, on the absolute or relative scale, on the other hand, is meaningful because it contains all likely values for the effect. If these are all smaller than Δ, then the methods can be considered equivalent.

For trials in the reproductive field, it has been reported that the first difficulty encountered with the corresponding trials was that the 'equivalence' nature of the trial had not been recognised by the design teams. Therefore no statement of an equivalence hypothesis with the specification of the margin of equivalence had been formulated, nor had the sample size been calculated with the objective to demonstrate equivalence. This resulted in underpowered trials to demonstrate equivalence within a clinically relevant difference. In only a few cases was an equivalence hypothesis stated with a clear specification of the margin of equivalence.[84]

An example of an equivalence trial is given by the WHO Yuzpe-levonorgestrel trial.[32] The Yuzpe regimen using combined oral contraceptives had been used in EC as an effective method to prevent unwanted pregnancy. However, like other regimens containing oestrogen, it is associated with side-effects like nausea and vomiting. The progestogen regimen levonorgestrel was shown to be better tolerated and equally or more effective, and it was recommended as a better alternative to the Yuzpe regimen. Another example is a trial establishing the equivalence between a single dose and a split dose of 1.5 mg levonorgestrel for EC.[33]

Introductory Trials and Phase IV Trials

Introductory trials are field studies to assess acceptability, effectiveness, continuation of use, side-effects and service-related needs of a method in specific populations, in the context of family planning services.[61] They are expanded Phase III trials. Some countries may require to conduct these trials in a network of 5–10 centres, including an acceptability component. Such studies might involve 1000 to 5000 subjects.

Phase IV trials are those conducted after a drug has been approved for marketing, to further investigate adverse effects of the drug. Very rare events cannot be rigorously assessed before the contraceptive drug reaches the market because even Phase III trials do not have sufficient power. Strategies for post-registration surveillance of contraceptive drugs are reports of adverse reactions, large-scale experimental studies, formal epidemiological studies and indirect correlational studies.[61] The most commonly used consists of epidemiological studies. Post-registration RCTs are costly, lack sufficient power

to detect uncommon but important reactions, cannot last long enough to identify long-term effects and the experimental group cannot be compared to a placebo.[61,85] This last limitation implies that when comparing two active treatments through an RCT, the absence of effect does not mean that either has no risk compared to a placebo. Another limitation of RCTs as a strategy at this stage of development of the contraceptive is that RCTs are conducted on healthy women and the risk of adverse reactions might be relevant in women with risk conditions.[60]

Systematic Reviews

Systematic reviews on contraceptive methods are available in the Cochrane Library.[86] A search was done using the word 'contraception', obtaining 45 hits out of 1456 total. A systematic review was included in the list if it included comparisons of efficacy, side-effects or acceptability of these methods or effectiveness of treatments for bleeding irregularities induced by them. Trials including contraceptives as treatment for complications or diseases and those comparing treatments for complications due to contraceptive use other than bleeding irregularities were not included. Subfertility trials were not included. The title and if necessary the abstract were examined to assess whether the review was eligible. The 22 reviews satisfying these criteria are listed in Table 20.2.

As an example, the systematic review 'Interventions for emergency contraception' included 33 trials, most of which were conducted in China. The authors conducted 46 meta-analyses with different comparisons and various outcomes comprising efficacy (pregnancies) and side-effects, including delay of menses. For the mifepristone dose-comparisons they grouped the doses used in different trials in low, mid and high doses.[87]

ACKNOWLEDGEMENTS

The author is greatful to Dr TMM Farley for useful discussions regarding the structure of the chapter, and to Dr P D Griffin for proof-reading the section on Phase I/II trials.

The UNDP/UNFPA/WHO/World Bank Special Programme of Research, Development

Table 20.2. Systematic reviews in The Cochrane Database of Systematic Reviews addressing efficacy or side-effects of contraceptive methods

Method	Stage	Review
OCs	Complete review	Biphasic versus monophasic oral contraceptives for contraception
	Complete review	Biphasic versus triphasic oral contraceptives for contraception
	Protocol	Triphasic versus monophasic oral contraceptives for contraception
	Protocol	Skin patch and vaginal ring versus combined oral contraceptives for contraception
	Protocol	Comparison of acceptability of low-dose oral contraceptives containing norethisterone
Injectables	Protocol	Treatment of vaginal bleeding irregularities induced by progestin-only contraceptives
Implants	Protocol	Subdermal implantable contraceptives versus other forms of reversible contraceptives as effective methods of preventing pregnancy
EC	Complete review	Interventions for emergency contraception
IUDs	Complete review	Frameless versus classical intrauterine device for contraception
	Complete review	Hormonally impregnated intrauterine systems (IUSs) versus other forms of reversible contraceptives as effective methods of preventing pregnancy
Barrier	Complete review	Condom effectiveness in reducing heterosexual HIV transmission
	Complete review	Diaphragm versus diaphragm with spermicides for contraception
	Complete review	Sponge versus diaphragm for contraception
	Protocol	Cervical cap versus diaphragm for contraception
	Protocol	Female condom for preventing heterosexually transmitted HIV infection in women
	Protocol	Non-latex versus latex condoms for contraception
Lactational amenorrhoea	Protocol	Lactational amenorrhoea for family planning
Sterilisation	Complete review	Minilaparotomy and endoscopic techniques for tubal sterilisation

and Research Training in Human Reproduction, Department of Reproductive Health and Research, WHO, Geneva, Switzerland, supported the author during her work on this chapter.

REFERENCES

1. Committee for Proprietary Medicinal Products (CPMP). Clinical investigation of steroid contraceptives in women. The European Agency for the Evaluation of Medicinal Products (2000).
2. Van Look PFA, Pérez-Palacios G. *Contraceptive Research and Development 1984 to 1994*. Oxford: Oxford University Press (1994).
3. Rabe T, Runnebaum B. *Fertility Control – Update and Trends*. Berlin: Springer-Verlag (1999).
4. Trussell J, Kost K. Contraceptive failure in the United States: a critical review of the literature. *Stud Fam Plann* (1987) **18**(5): 237–83.
5. Dionne P, Vickerson F. A double-blind comparison of two oral contraceptives containing 50 mu g. and 30 mu g. ethinyl estradiol. *Curr Ther Res Clin Exp* (1974) **16**(4): 281–8.
6. WHO Task Force on Oral Contraceptives. A randomized, double-blind study of six combined oral contraceptives. *Contraception* (1982) **25**: 231–41.
7. WHO Task Force on Oral Contraceptives. A randomized, double-blind study of two combined and two progesterone-only oral contraceptives. *Contraception* (1982) **25**: 243–52.
8. Fotherby K. Update on lipid metabolism and oral contraception. *Br J Fam Plann* (1990) **15**: 23–6.
9. Gaspard UJ. Metabolic effects of oral contraceptives. *Am J Obstet Gynecol* (1987) **157**: 1029–41.
10. Runnebaum B, Rabe T. New progestogens in oral contraceptives. *Am J Obstet Gynecol* (1987) **157**: 1059–63.
11. Sabra A, Bonnar J. Hemostatic system changes induced by 50 mcg and 30 mcg estrogen/progestogen oral contraceptives. *J Reprod Med* (1983) **28**: 85–91.
12. WHO. Oral contraceptives and neoplasia. Report of a WHO Scientific Group, 817. WHO Technical Report Series (1992).

13. Farley TMM, Meirik O, Collins J. Cardiovascular disease and combined oral contraceptives: reviewing the evidence and balancing the risks. *Human Reprod Update* (1999) **5**(6): 721–35.

14. Rabe T, Runnebaum B. The future of oral hormonal contraception. In: Rabe T, Runnebaum B, eds. *Fertility Control – Update and Trends*. Berlin: Springer-Verlag (1999) 73–89.

15. RHR/WHO. Improving access to quality care in family planning: medical eligibility criteria, second edition. WHO/RHR/00.02 (2000).

16. Hagenfeldt K. Contraceptive research and development today: an overview. In: Van Look PFA, Pérez-Palacios G, eds. *Contraceptive Research and Development 1984 to 1994*. Oxford: Oxford University Press (1994) 3–22.

17. Rivera R. Oral contraceptives: the last decade. In: Van Look PFA, Pérez-Palacios G, eds. *Contraceptive Research and Development 1984 to 1994*. Oxford: Oxford University Press (1994).

18. WHO Task Force of Long-Acting Systemic Agents for Fertility Regulation. A multicentred phase III comparative study of two hormonal contraceptive preparations given once-a-month by intramuscular injection. II. The comparison of bleeding patterns. *Contraception* (1989) **40**(5): 531–51.

19. WHO Task Force of Long-Acting Systemic Agents for Fertility Regulation. A multicentred phase III comparative trial of 150 mg and 100 mg of depot-medroxyprogesterone acetate given every three months: Efficacy and side-effects. *Contraception* (1986) **34**: 223–35.

20. Hall P. Long-acting formulations. In: Diczfalusy E, Bygdeman M, eds. *Fertility Regulation Today and Tomorrow*. New York: Raven Press (1987) 119–41.

21. WHO Task Force of Long-Acting Systemic Agents for Fertility Regulation. A multinational comparative clinical trial of long-acting injectable contraceptives: norethisterone enantate given in two dosage regimens and depot-medroxyprogesterone acetate, final report. *Contraception* (1983) **28**: 1–20.

22. WHO Collaborative Study of Neoplasia and Steroid Contraceptives. Breast cancer and depot-medroxyprogesterone acetate: a multinational study. *Lancet* (1991) **338**: 833–8.

23. WHO Collaborative Study of Neoplasia and Steroid Contraceptives. Depot-medroxyprogesterone acetate (DMPA) and risk of epithelial ovarian cancer. *Int J Cancer* (1991) **49**: 191–5.

24. Newton JR, d'Arcangues C, Hall PE. Once-a-month combined injectable contraceptives. *J Obstet Gynaecol* (1994) **14**: S1–34.

25. Croxatto HB, Diaz S, Miranda P, Elamsson K, Johansson ED. Plasma levels of levonorgestrel in women during longterm use of Norplants. *Contraception* (1980) **22**(6): 583–96.

26. Bardin CW, Sivin I. Lessons learnt from clinical trials. In: Michal F, ed. *Safety Requirements for Contraceptive Steroids*. WHO (1989) 400–13.

27. Sivin I. International experience with Norplant and Norplant-2 contraceptives. *Stud Fam Plann* (1988) **19**: 81–94.

28. International Collaborative Post-Marketing Surveillance of Norplant. Post-marketing surveillance of Norplant((R)) contraceptive implants: II. Non-reproductive health(1). *Contraception* (2001) **63**(4): 187–209.

29. Koetsawang S, Ji G, Krishna U, Cuadros A, Dhall GI, Wyss R, *et al.* Microdose intravaginal levonorgestrel contraception: a multicentre clinical trial. I. Contraceptive efficacy and side effects. World Health Organization. Task Force on Long-Acting Systemic Agents for Fertility Regulation. *Contraception* (1990) **41**(2): 105–24.

30. Koetsawang S, Ji G, Krishna U, Cuadros A, Dhall GI, Wyss R, *et al.* Microdose intravaginal levonorgestrel contraception: a multicentre clinical trial. II. Expulsions and removals. World Health Organization. Task Force on Long-Acting Systemic Agents for Fertility Regulation. *Contraception* (1990) **41**(2): 125–41.

31. Sivin I, Mishell DR Jr, Victor A, Diaz S, Alvarez-Sanchez F, Nielsen NC, *et al.* A multicenter study of levonorgestrel–estradiol contraceptive vaginal rings. I-Use Effectiveness. An international comparative trial. *Contraception* (1981) **24**(4): 377–92.

32. WHO Task Force on Postovulatory Methods of Fertility Regulation. Randomised controlled trial of levonorgestrel versus the Yuzpe regimen of combined oral contraceptives for emergency contraception. Task Force on Postovulatory Methods of Fertility Regulation. *Lancet* (1998) **352**(9126): 428–33.

33. Von Hertzen H, Piaggio G, Ding J, Chen J, Sonj S, Bártfai G, *et al.* Low dose mifepristone and two regimens of levonorgestrel for emergency contraception: a WHO multicentre randomised trial. *Lancet* (2002) **360**: 1803–10.

34. Wilcox AJ, Weinberg CR, Baird DD. Timing of sexual intercourse in relation to ovulation: effects on the probability of conception, survival of the pregnancy, and sex of the baby. *N Engl J Med* (1995) **333**(23): 1517–21.

35. Wilcox AJ, Weinberg CR, Baird DD. Post-ovulatory ageing of the human oocyte and embryo failure. *Human Reprod* (1998) **13**(2): 394–7.

36. Bacic M, Wesselius dC, Diczfalusy E. Failure of large doses of ethinyl estradiol to interfere with early embryonic development in the human

species. *Am J Obstet Gynecol* (1970) **107**(4): 531–4.

37. Grimes DA. Emergency contraception – expanding opportunities for primary prevention. *N Engl J Med* (1997) **337**(15): 1078–9.

38. WHO Task Force on Postovulatory Methods of Fertility Regulation. Comparison of three single doses of mifepristone as emergency contraception: a randomised trial. Task Force on Postovulatory Methods of Fertility Regulation. *Lancet* (1999) **353**(9154): 697–702.

39. Tatum HJ. Comparative experience with newer models of the Copper T in the United States. In: Hefnawi F, Segal SJ, eds. *Analysis of Intrauterine Contraception*. New York: American Elsevier Publications (1975) 155–63.

40. Jain AK. Safety and effectiveness of intrauterine devices. *Contraception* (1975) **11**(3): 243–59.

41. Sivin I, Stern J. Long-acting, more effective copper T IUDs: a summary of U.S. experience, 1970–75. *Stud Fam Plann* (1979) **10**(10): 263–81.

42. Sivin I, Schmidt F. Effectiveness of IUDs: a review. *Contraception* (1987) **36**(1): 55–84.

43. Champion CB, Behlilovic B, Arosemena JM, Randic L, Cole LP, Wilkens LR. A three-year evaluation of TCu 380 Ag and multiload Cu 375 intrauterine devices. *Contraception* (1988) **38**(6): 631–9.

44. Cole LP, Potts DM, Aranda C, Behlilovic B, Etman ES, Moreno J, *et al.* An evaluation of the TCu 380Ag and the Multiload Cu375. *Fertil Steril* (1985) **43**(2): 214–7.

45. Rowe P. Clinical performance of copper IUDs. Proceedings of a meeting: a new look at IUDs. In: Bardin CW, Mishell DR, eds. *Proceedings from the Fourth International Conference on IUDs*, Newton, MD. Butterworth Heinemann (1994) 13–31.

46. Sastrawinata S, Farr G, Prihadi SM, Hutapea H, Anwar M, Wahyudi I, *et al.* A comparative clinical trial of the TCu 380A, Lippes Loop D and Multiload Cu 375 IUDs in Indonesia. *Contraception* (1991) **44**(2): 141–54.

47. Sivin I, Stern J, Coutinho E, Mattos CE, el Mahgoub S, Diaz S, *et al.* Prolonged intrauterine contraception: a seven-year randomized study of the levonorgestrel 20 mcg/day (LNg 20) and the Copper T380 Ag IUDS. *Contraception* (1991) **44**(5): 473–80.

48. Luukkainen T, Allonen H, Nielsen NC, Nygren KG, Pyorala T. Five years' experience of intrauterine contraception with the Nova-T and the Copper-T-200. *Am J Obstet Gynecol* (1983) **147**(8): 885–92.

49. WHO Task Force on the Safety and Efficacy of Fertility Regulation. The TCu 380A, the TCu 220C, Multiload 250 and Nova T IUDs at 3, 5 and 7 years of use. Results from three randomized trials. *Contraception* (1990) **42**: 141–58.

50. WHO. Long-term reversible contraception. Twelve years of experience with the TCu380A and TCu220C. *Contraception* (1997) **56**(6): 341–52.

51. Wagner H. Intrauterine contraception: past, present and future. In: Rabe T, Runnebaum B, eds. *Fertility Control – Update and Trends*. Berlin: Springer-Verlag (1999) 151–71.

52. Farley TM. Reproduction. In: Armitage P, Colton T, eds. *Encyclopedia of Biostatistics* (1998).

53. Labbok M, Jennings VH. Advances in fertility regulation through ovulation prediction during lactation (lactational amenorrhoea method) and during the menstrual cycle. In: Van Look PFA, Pérez-Palacios G, eds. *Contraceptive Research and Development 1984 to 1994*. Oxford: Oxford University Press (1994).

54. Turner L, Conway AJ, Jimenez M, Liu PY, Forbes E, McLachlan RI, Handelsman DJ. Contraceptive efficacy of a depot progestin and androgen combination in men. *J of Clinical Endocrinology and Metabolism* (2003) **88**(10): 4659–67.

55. Rabe T, Vladescu E, Runnebaum B. Contraception: historical development, current status and future aspects. In: Rabe T, Runnebaum B, eds. *Fertility Control – Update and Trends*. Berlin: Springer-Verlag (1999) 29–72.

56. Population Council Center for Biomedical Research. *Annual Report 1991*. New York: The Population Council (1991).

57. Farley TMM, Meirik O, Metha S, Waites GMH. The Safety of vasectomy: recent concerns: Bulletin of the World Health Organization (1993) **71**(3-4): 413–9.

58. Fuertes-de la Haba A, Bangdiwala IS, Pelegrina I. Success of randomization in a controlled contraceptive experiment. *J Reprod Med* (1973) **11**(4): 142–8.

59. Potts M, Feldblum PJ, Chi I, Liao W, Fuertes-de La HA. The Puerto Rico oral contraceptive study: an evaluation of the methodology and results of a feasibility study. *Br J Fam Plann* (1982).

60. Skegg DCG. The epidemiological assessment of safety of hormonal contraceptives: a methodological review. In: Michal F, ed. *Safety Requirements for Contraceptive Steroids*. WHO (1989) 21–37.

61. Special Programme of Research, Development and Research Training in Human Reproduction. Guidelines for the toxicological and clinical assessment and post-registration surveillance of steroidal contraceptive drugs. In: Michal F, ed. *Safety Requirements for Contraceptive Steroids*. WHO (1989) 415–54.

62. Garza-Flores J, Fatiikun T. Future directions in fertility regulation. In: Negro-Vilar A, Pérez-Palacios G, eds. *Reproduction, Growth and*

Development. New York: Raven Press (1991) 383–97.

63. Fotherby K, Benagiano G, Toppozada HK, *et al.* A preliminary pharmacological trial of the monthly injectable contraceptive Cycloprovera. *Contraception* (1982) **25**: 261–72.

64. Aedo AR, Landgren BM, Johannisson E, Diczfalusy E. Pharmacokinetic and pharmacodynamic investigations with monthly injectable contraceptive preparations. *Contraception* (1985) **31**: 453–69.

65. WHO Task Force of Long-Acting Systemic Agents for Fertility Regulation. A multicentred pharmacokinetic, pharmacodynamic study of once-a-month injectable contraceptives. I. Different doses of HRP112 and of DepoProvera. *Contraception* (1987) **36**(4): 441–57.

66. Silfverstolpe G, Gustafson A, Samsioe G, Svanborg A. Lipid metabolic studies in oophorectomized women: effects of three different progestogens. *Acta Obstet Gynecol Scand* (1979) Suppl 88: 89–95.

67. WHO Task Force of Long-Acting Systemic Agents for Fertility Regulation. A multicentred phase III comparative study of two hormonal contraceptive preparations given once-a-month by intramuscular injection: I. Contraceptive efficacy and side effects. World Health Organization. *Contraception* (1988) **37**(1): 1–20.

68. Family Health International. Contraceptive technology and family planning research. Family Health International (1992).

69. d'Arcangues C, Piaggio G, Brache V, Ben Haissa R, Hazelden C, Mossai R *et al.* Effectiveness of Vitamin E and low-dose aspirin, alone or in combination, on Norplant induced prolonged bleeding. *Contraception* (2004) (in press).

70. Trussell J. Methodological pitfalls in the analysis of contraceptive failure. *Stat Med* (1991) **10**(2): 201–20.

71. Steiner M, Dominik R, Trussell J, Hertz-Picciott I. Measuring contraceptive effectiveness: a conceptual framework. *Obstet Gynecol* (1996) **88**(3 Suppl): 24S–30S.

72. Trussell J, Rodriguez G, Ellertson C. Updated estimates of the effectiveness of the Yuzpe regimen of emergency contraception. *Contraception* (1999) **59**(3): 147–51.

73. Farley TM. Life-table methods for contraceptive research. *Stat Med* (1986) **5**(5): 475–89.

74. Tai BC, Peregoudov A, Machin D. A competing risk approach to the analysis of trials of alternative intra-uterine devices (IUDs) for fertility regulation. *Stat Med* (2001) **20**(23): 3589–600.

75. Farley TM, Ali MM, Slaymaker E. Competing approaches to analysis of failure times with competing risks. *Stat Med* (2001) **20**(23): 3601–10.

76. Yusuf S, Wittes J, Probstfield J, Tyroler HA. Analysis and interpretation of treatment effects in subgroups of patients in randomized clinical trials. *JAMA* (1991) **266**(1): 93–8.

77. Hassan EO, el Nahal N, el Hussein M. Acceptability of the once-a-month injectable contraceptives Cyclofem and Mesigyna in Egypt. *Contraception* (1994) **49**(5): 469–88.

78. Rodriguez G, Faundes-Latham A, Atkinson LE. An approach to the analysis of menstrual patterns in the critical evaluation of contraceptives. *Stud Fam Plann* (1976) **7**(2): 42–51.

79. Belsey EM, Farley TM. The analysis of menstrual bleeding patterns: a review. *Contraception* (1988) **38**(2): 129–56.

80. Belsey EM, Machin D, d'Arcangues C. The analysis of vaginal bleeding patterns induced by fertility regulating methods. World Health Organization Special Programme of Research, Development and Research Training in Human Reproduction. *Contraception* (1986) **34**(3): 253–60.

81. Belsey EM, Carlson N. The description of menstrual bleeding patterns: towards fewer measures. *Stat Med* (1991) **10**(2): 267–84.

82. Fraser IS. Vaginal bleeding patterns in women using once-a-month injectable contraceptives. *Contraception* (1994) **49**(4): 399–420.

83. Said S, Sadek W, Rocca M, Koetsawang S, Kirwat O, Piya-Anant M, *et al.* Clinical evaluation of the therapeutic effectiveness of ethinyl oestradiol and oestrone sulphate on prolonged bleeding in women using depot medroxyprogesterone acetate for contraception. World Health Organization, Special Programme of Research, Development and Research Training in Human Reproduction, Task Force on Long-acting Systemic Agents for Fertility Regulation. *Human Reprod* (1996) **11** Suppl 2: 1–13.

84. Piaggio G, Pinol AP. Use of the equivalence approach in reproductive health clinical trials. *Stat Med* (2001) **20**(23): 3571–7.

85. Petitti DB, Shapiro S. Strategies for post-registration surveillance of contraceptive steroids. In: Michal F, ed. *Safety Requirements for Contraceptive Steroids*. WHO (1989) 335–47.

86. The Cochrane Library (Issue 4). Oxford: Update Software (2002).

87. Cheng L, Gulmezoglu AM, Ezcurra E, Van Look PFA. Interventions for emergency contraception. The Cochrane Library. 2001. Oxford: Update Software (2001).

21

Gynaecology and Infertility

SILADITYA BHATTACHARYA[1] AND JILL MOLLISON[2]

[1]Department of Obstetrics and Gynaecology, University of Aberdeen, Aberdeen, UK
[2]Department of Public Health, University of Aberdeen, Aberdeen, UK

INTRODUCTION

The randomised clinical trial is widely accepted as the gold standard for scientific evaluation of treatments. In the current climate of clinical governance, data from clinical trials are considered to represent the highest level of evidence that can be used to inform effective treatment strategies. Yet, there are fewer trials in gynaecology in comparison with other disciplines. Those reported in the literature account for a minority of published papers in major journals.[1] Gynaecological trials incorporate a wide spectrum of clinical conditions and proposed interventions. Women can differ substantially in terms of age, physical and psychological disability; while treatments can range from drug therapy to surgical procedures, from information provision to physiotherapy and dietary advice. The aim of this chapter is to examine, test and explore the basic principles of clinical trials in gynaecology. An overview of different types of trials is provided and reference will be made to specific challenges, including identification of sample populations, choice of appropriate outcomes and tools, randomisation and arrangements for follow-up. Examples

are drawn from general gynaecology, infertility and fertility control. Trials in obstetrics, contraception and gynaecological oncology, which are discussed elsewhere, will be excluded from our discussion.

TAXONOMY OF CLINICAL TRIALS

Clinical trials may be classified in a number of ways (see Table 21.1). Some of these are discussed below.

PHASE I CLINICAL TRIALS

These preliminary studies generally address drug safety rather than efficacy, and may be performed on healthy volunteers. Examples include studies of drug metabolism and bio-availability of recombinant gonadotrophins in infertile women.[2] Most phase I trials are either directly or indirectly supported by the pharmaceutical industry and involve relatively small numbers of subjects. Women are required to adhere to a strict protocol and agree to fairly extensive evaluation often involving multiple investigations such as blood

Textbook of Clinical Trials. Edited by D. Machin, S. Day and S. Green
© 2004 John Wiley & Sons, Ltd ISBN: 0-471-98787-5

Table 21.1. Taxonomy of clinical trials

Phased trials	Phase I
	Phase II
	Phase III
	Phase IV
Conduct	Pragmatic
	Explanatory
Design	Parallel group
	Crossover
	Factorial
	Patient preference
	Cluster randomisation
Randomisation	True
	Quasi-randomisation

counts, biochemistry, endocrine profile and liver and kidney function tests. In this context, it may be useful to be aware of the fact that finding 'normal' subjects for such trials in reproductive medicine can sometimes be challenging as a large proportion of young, fit, healthy women may either be on oral contraception or actively trying for a pregnancy.

PHASE II CLINICAL TRIALS

These are also fairly small-scale investigations into the efficacy and safety of a drug and require close monitoring of each patient. Sometimes they can be employed as a screening process to screen drugs, which are either potentially inactive or toxic. They may also be used to determine the most appropriate dose and route of administration of a drug. Examples of these types of trials include those involving the use of misoprostol for medical termination of pregnancy.[3] Where patient acceptability of the route of administration, i.e. vaginal, oral or sublingual, is an important outcome, these trials may need to break out of the traditional mould of strictly controlled explanatory trials and assume the pragmatic approach associated with phase III trials.

PHASE III CLINICAL TRIALS

After a drug has been shown to be reasonably effective it is essential to compare it with the current standard management for the same condition in a large trial involving a substantial number of patients. This is also the design used for non-pharmacological interventions, which are increasing in number. The majority of the trials referred to in this chapter are phase III trials. This is the point of evaluation following which interventions are introduced into clinical practice.

PHASE IV CLINICAL TRIALS

Even after a treatment finds general acceptance, unanswered questions about its safety and long-term effectiveness continue to be addressed in the context of phase IV trials. The long-term implications of new methods of treatment of menorrhagia such as endometrial ablation are still under evaluation a decade after the results of the first phase III trials were reported. Medium-term data have been presented in a number of publications.[4,5]

PRAGMATIC AND EXPLANATORY TRIALS

In terms of design, clinical trials are often described as either explanatory or pragmatic. Explanatory trials measure efficacy – the benefit a treatment produces under ideal conditions. Pragmatic trials measure effectiveness – the benefit the treatment produces in routine clinical practice.[6] Examples of the former include evaluation of drugs used to treat menorrhagia or those used to undertake medical termination of pregnancy. The aim is to assess the outcome of a new drug under controlled conditions using a homogeneous group of patients. Eligibility criteria are strict, and protocol violations are not allowed. In an explanatory trial comparing recombinant follicle stimulating hormone with a urinary preparation, any woman who fails to receive the appropriate drug in the prescribed dose will be excluded from the study on grounds of protocol violation.

In contrast, a pragmatic trial aims to mirror the normal variations between patients that occur in real life. For example, a pragmatic trial of medical versus surgical treatment for menorrhagia will include all women with a subjective complaint of heavy menstrual loss. Women randomised to drug treatment, who find the intervention unacceptable and elect for surgery, do not face disqualification from the trial. This somewhat relaxed policy is justified on the grounds that women's decisions to reject their allocated treatment are likely to reflect real-life situations and can actually be interpreted as a measure of dissatisfaction. Furthermore, the treatment offered to patients in the surgery arm may not be identical, as operations may be performed by more than one surgeon, each with a slightly different technique. A similar attitude would apply to a pragmatic trial of physiotherapy for prolapse or counselling for premenstrual syndrome, where identical interventions cannot be guaranteed by different physiotherapists or counsellors.

There are other differences between the two types of trials. Blinding is more likely to be used in an explanatory trial such as one comparing oral metformin with placebo in women with polycystic ovarian syndrome. Pragmatic trials may also be blinded, but this is often not feasible (for example, in surgical versus medical trials), nor always desirable. There is also less of a compulsion to use placebos, as the objective is to compare the new intervention, not with a placebo, but with the 'gold standard' or best of the existing treatments. Clinician and patient biases caused by the absence of blinding may not necessarily be detrimental to the trial, but could actually be seen to be part of the response to treatment. The outcome in a pragmatic trial such as one comparing oral clomiphene citrate (a drug treatment) versus expectant management in unexplained infertility incorporates the total difference between the interventions that are being evaluated. This may include the effect of the treatment as well as the associated placebo effect as this best reflects the likely clinical response in practice.[6]

TRIAL DESIGN

SIMPLE PARALLEL GROUP

This is the simplest and commonest trial design involving a comparison between two groups, i.e. an experimental versus a control group. As this type of trial is most easily understood by researchers as well as patients, examples abound. Occasionally a trial may have three arms, e.g. intrauterine insemination (IUI) versus ovarian stimulation + intrauterine insemination versus in vitro fertilisation (IVF) for the treatment of unexplained infertility.[7] Sample sizes for such trials will be dictated by the minimum significant difference in outcome between any two arms. Due to the nature of the interventions, expected differences between the arms will vary. The number of women required to show a clinically significant difference in pregnancy rates between IUI and IVF is smaller than that necessary to show a difference between IUI and stimulated IUI, and will ultimately be the one chosen for this trial.

CROSSOVER

Crossover trials have the advantage of using women as their own controls, thus reducing the sample size required. Women are randomly exposed to either the control or the intervention arm first, followed by the other. Often a 'washout period' is introduced between the two arms to reduce the risk of contamination. Unfortunately this design is more suited for medical treatments of chronic conditions as opposed to surgical trials or infertility trials. In the first group the practicalities of the situation render such a design impossible. In the second, a definite outcome such as pregnancy has the natural effect of preventing women from completing later phases of the trial.[8] In such situations, exaggerated estimates of treatment effect can occur, leading to erroneous clinical decisions. From a practical point of view, only data from the first phase of the crossover trial may be valid. However, this design may well be suitable for exploring drug treatment of chronic conditions such as premenstrual syndrome or sexual function.

FACTORIAL

Factorial designs are often efficient as they can address two questions within the context of a

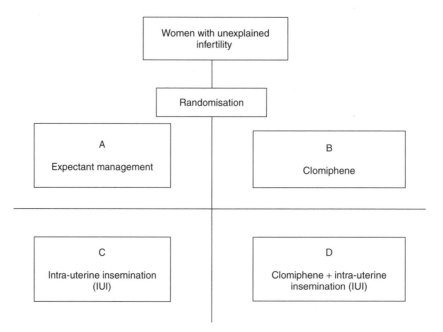

Figure 21.1

single trial. Women with unexplained infertility can be randomised to receive either expectant management (no treatment), insemination alone, clomiphene alone or clomiphene and insemination treatment as shown in Figure 21.1.

When the two treatments (factors) do not interact with one another, this design has the advantage of requiring half the number of patients that would be required if two parallel RCTs were to be conducted. The advantage is self-evident. In this case, the effect of IUI alone can be assessed by comparing groups C and D with A and B, while the effect of clomiphene can be evaluated by comparing B and D versus A and C. The advantage is self-evident. In this case, the effect of IUI alone can be assessed by comparing groups C and D with A and B, while the effect of clomiphene can be evaluated by comparing B and D versus A and C.

CLUSTER RANDOMISED TRIALS IN GYNAECOLOGY AND INFERTILITY

A potential problem that can occur with randomised controlled trials is where the intervention is not targeted at individual patients, but at groups of patients. This can happen where the intervention is an information package for the management of menorrhagia in primary care[9] or a clinical guideline for the management of infertility.[10] In these studies, randomising patients to receive management using the information package or clinical guidelines would have introduced contamination, since GPs would have been expected to manage both study (information leaflet, clinical guidelines) and control patients. Potentially this could underestimate the true effectiveness of the intervention. Therefore, clusters of patients (e.g. general practices) were randomly allocated to receive intervention (e.g. information leaflets, clinical guidelines) or control. Cluster randomisation should only be carried out when there is a strong justification for doing so.

The primary implication of cluster randomised trials is that the measurements on individuals are not statistically independent of one another; that is measurements from individuals within the same cluster will be correlated to one another. This has implications in the design (e.g. sample size), conduct (e.g. informed consent), analysis and reporting. Cluster randomised trials should adjust for this clustering when determining the number of patients required. The sample size that would be required if patients were to be randomised must be inflated by a factor which takes into account the extent of the clustering and the size of the cluster.[11] The extent of the correlation is measured by the intra-cluster correlation coefficient (ICC)[12] and researchers are required to have some indication of this, in order that the study can be adequately powered. Studies that fail to adequately inflate the sample size will suffer from a type II error.

Similarly, the correlated responses obtained from each cluster have an implication for the statistical analysis, since standard statistical tests (e.g. t-test) assume that observations are independent of one another. There are a number of approaches to analysing cluster randomised trials and these are detailed elsewhere.[13] Failure to account for the correlated responses in the analyses will result in an increased type I error.

Clustering of outcomes can also occur in infertility trials where alternative treatments are being compared. For example, in randomised controlled trials comparing IVF with ICSI the unit of allocation varies between patients,[14] oocytes[15] and cycles.[16] Often, outcomes such as implantation rate and fertilisation rate are considered. These are both expressed as percentages out of the total number of oocytes retrieved. Hence, in trials that randomise patients (couples) or cycles and report implantation or fertilisation rates, there will be clustering of the outcome since oocytes are clustered within patients or cycles.[14,16] Hence, in these studies adjustment should be made in the analysis to adjust for the correlated outcomes assessed (on each oocyte) within patients (or cycles). In trials that randomise by patients and report fertilisation of implantation rates, some adjustment is required. However, for outcomes such as live birth rate or pregnancy rate no adjustment is required since the percentages are expressed out of the total number of patients randomised. Bhattacharya et al.[16] randomised cycles and reported implantation rates per transferred

embryo. However, they noted that the difference in implantation rates was likely to be wider than that reported due to failure to adjust for the clustering of embryos/oocytes transferred to each woman. Studies where oocytes have been randomised have no clustering implications since oocytes retrieved from the same women are randomly allocated to receive ICSI or IVF.

When conducting randomised controlled trials in infertility, consideration should be given to the unit of randomisation and the outcome measures to be applied. When there is implicit clustering in the data, the statistical analysis should account for this using the methods described above.[13]

QUASI-RANDOMISED TRIALS

These are controlled experimental studies where treatment allocation is performed on the basis of patient unit numbers or days of the week when the patients are recruited. Although this design of treatment allocation affords an element of chance, it cannot be considered to be genuine randomisation. This type of design may still appeal to those involved in laboratory trials involving incubation or cryopreservation of human embryos. In these cases, it may be easier and cheaper to use a certain protocol for all embryos on alternate days or alternate weeks rather than change the protocol or a freezer setting for each embryo or each woman. The consequent loss of allocation concealment will lead to serious inclusion bias as some patients may be deliberately excluded. This, is turn, can exaggerate treatment effects.

PATIENT PREFERENCE TRIAL

A potential problem in some randomised trials arises when patients or their clinicians refuse to be randomised on grounds of strong treatment preferences. Exclusion of these patients may affect the generalisability of the results as participants may not be representative. Yet recruitment of these patients may introduce substantial bias especially when it is impossible to blind them. In addition, compliance and satisfaction may be higher with the preferred intervention.[17]

This is particularly so when the 'new' treatment is only available within the context of the trial or when, as in trials in unexplained infertility, one of the arms comprises a 'no treatment' or 'expectant management' group. Dissatisfaction with the allocation may lead to differential compliance and follow-up resulting in groups which cannot then be assumed to be similar. The outcome measures could also be affected by how satisfied patients are with their allocated treatment. The effect of patient preference on outcome would depend to a great extent on the specific outcomes being assessed. If the principal outcome is death or live birth, then the effect of patient preferences is likely to be small. If the principal outcome is satisfaction with care, then the effect of patient preference is large.[18] Under such circumstances the conventional randomised trial will underestimate the relationship between the intervention and the outcome, i.e. show the minimum effect size. Conversely a comparison between two groups of patients who have chosen their treatment and thus optimised their treatment choice will be considered to represent the maximum effect size. An intervention in question will have an effect size between the minimum and maximum as derived from the randomised and the preference part of a partially randomised patient preference trial.[18]

To deal with patient preferences within a trial, the use of a partially randomised patient preference (PRPP) trial has been suggested.[19] Patients with strong preferences are allowed their desired treatment. Those without such views are subjected to randomisation. For example in a trial of medical and surgical termination of pregnancy we end up with four groups–randomised to medical, randomised to surgical, prefer medical and prefer surgical.

Potential disadvantages with PRPP trials include effects of the trial size. The size of a total PRPP cohort will need to be much larger than for a conventional randomised controlled trial. As already mentioned, the size of the randomised cohort needs to be the same as in a conventional trial. In addition, the number of patients in the non-randomised preference arms needs to be of equivalent size. The numbers quickly add up to generate a total sample size double that for a conventional trial. This has the predictable effect of adding to the cost and duration of the trial. Entry of a disproportionate number of patients into either the randomised or the preference arms is also a problem, as the trial will not be completed unless the appropriate number have been recruited into the two components of the trial. The situation may be further complicated by patients favouring one treatment over another, making comparison of the two groups in the preference arm more difficult.

A further problem with this approach lies in the analysis. Any comparison using the non-randomised groups is unreliable because of unknown and uncontrolled confounders. Patient preference designs have been used in trials of termination of pregnancy[20,21] and menorrhagia.[22] The evidence to support the use of PRPP trials compared with conventional randomised trials is limited. A randomised comparison of the two strategies by Cooper et al.[22] suggested that the extra cost and complexity were not justified in the context of medical versus surgical treatment of menorrhagia.

A conventional randomised trial could address the effect that patient preference has on outcome by recording this information before allocation.[23] This would allow resources to be concentrated on recruiting as many patients as possible into the randomised comparison group but would allow stratification of the results by initial preference.

EQUIVALENT TRIALS

Often in reproductive health care the aim is to show that one treatment is as effective (equivalence), or no less effective (non-inferior), as another. The methodology for equivalence trials differs to that of superiority trials in design, analysis and interpretation. In designing equivalence trials, attention must be given to defining an equivalence margin. This is the difference in effect that would be deemed to be 'clinically insignificant'.[24] In comparison with superiority trials, larger sample sizes are needed to demonstrate equivalence. In the analysis of equivalence trials, conventional statistical testing has little relevance and interpretation of results should be conducted though use of confidence intervals in relation to the predefined equivalence margin.[25] Statistical significance is demonstrated if the upper and lower limits of the 95% confidence interval do not cross the equivalence margin.[25] In superiority trials, the most conservative analysis is by intention to treat (ITT). In an equivalence trial, however, a 'per protocol' (PP) analysis is usually considered statistically more conservative. This is because an ITT analysis may blur the comparison between groups and lead to an increased chance of declaring the two treatments as equivalent when they are not. The decision about which should be the primary form of analysis (ITT or PP) in an equivalence study is not straightforward.[26] It depends on the particular characteristics of the study, including the definitions adopted for the ITT and PP analyses and the risk of bias.[27]

PERFORMING AN RCT

SYSTEMATIC REVIEW

A systematic review of the literature is an essential component of the pre-trial work-up. It enables the researcher to define the clinical question in the light of work that has gone before and assess the need for a trial. It also provides vital information about the limitations of previous trials, outcome measures used and nature of follow-up. This is useful in planning the design of the proposed study. A recent systematic review[28] has identified typical problems associated with previous trials in unexplained infertility including small sample sizes, inappropriate outcome measures (pregnancy rates per cycle) and lack of cost data. Similar information relating to other topics in gynaecology can also be obtained from Cochrane reviews.

DEFINING THE STUDY POPULATION

Definition of the study sample is a vital part of any clinical trial. Unfortunately this aspect of trial design can be contentious. The diagnostic criteria of many gynaecological conditions continue to generate debate amongst clinicians. Disagreement about the definition of a particular condition can lead to dismissal of the conclusions of a trial as irrelevant. Certain terms continue to pose particular problems. For example, infertility which is defined as 'the lack of pregnancy after one year of regular unprotected coital exposure' refers to the lack of an exposure, i.e. pregnancy rather than a particular disorder. There may be contributory factors from both sexes, and definitions of subgroups such as unexplained infertility or polycystic ovarian syndrome vary widely. Variation in laboratory procedures (such as semen analyses) may affect the diagnosis of male infertility while the investigations used for tubal patency (laparoscopy versus hysterosalpingogram) may have an effect on the identification of endometriosis in infertile women.

With menorrhagia, the problem is different. The conventional textbook definition of menorrhagia (menstrual blood loss >80 mls) is impractical and the pragmatic approach is to include all women with a subjective complaint of heavy menstrual loss. This encourages a situation where critics can question the external validity of trials where women have been included either on the basis of objective measurement of menstrual blood loss or on pragmatic grounds with increased self-reported bleeding. Some purists will argue that efficacy of treatments for menorrhagia cannot be evaluated accurately without patients with 'genuine' pathology. However, the outcome of such trials may not necessarily be applicable to the vast majority of clinical situations where menstrual loss is not routinely measured. From a clinical point of view, it is probably more useful to use a pragmatic approach and recruit all women on the basis of a subjective complaint of menorrhagia.

Studies on urinary incontinence also require appropriate definition of the population group, as it is well known that women who attend urodynamic clinics constitute a small proportion of the total number of women in the community suffering from urinary incontinence. Although there is no way of completely avoiding selection bias, explicit description of the eligibility criteria allows the readers to draw their own conclusions regarding the applicability of the data to their own specific contexts. Those performing secondary research can also use these data to assess heterogeneity between trials.

A specific problem associated with infertility trials is the question of how to deal with the male partner. Conventionally it is the woman who undergoes treatment, and it is she who is considered to be the participant in trials and subjected to recruitment, randomisation and follow-up. However, in trials where satisfaction, acceptability and costs are outcomes, it is perhaps appropriate to seek the male partners' views as well.

An important aspect of the choice of the study population involves the effect of the participants on generalisability of the findings. Although study participants may meet eligibility criteria, participation is voluntary and volunteers may differ from the general population in terms of general health, co-interventions, educational level, motivation and ability to follow a protocol. Ethnic minorities may be missed on account of unfamiliarity with the language of the questionnaires used.

INTERVENTIONS

Due to its unique mix of medical and surgical workload, gynaecology offers a number of diverse interventions that need to be tested in the context of clinical trials. Some examples are shown in Table 21.2.

DEFINING OUTCOMES

For any trial, it is crucial to have an *a priori* hypothesis and a clinically relevant primary outcome on which the power calculation is based. This essential primary step prevents the sacrifice of quality for expediency and discourages opportunistic and inappropriate manipulation of collected data. Outcomes of choice include those that are purely clinical, as well as others which may be patient-centred or economic. The precise nature of the primary and secondary outcomes will depend on the type of trial and

Table 21.2. Types of interventions subjected to clinical trials in gynaecology

Intervention	Examples of trials
Packages of care	Information packages in use in general practice for appropriate treatment and referral in menorrhagia The value of guidelines in infertility for general practitioners
Surgical techniques	Hysterectomy versus endometrial ablation Different types of endometrial ablation, e.g. TCRE versus Laser
Drug trial	Placebo versus tranexamic acid for menorrhagia
Comparison of different treatment modalities	Medical versus surgical termination of pregnancy Mirena IUS versus endometrial ablation for menorrhagia Expectant treatment versus IVF for unexplained infertility
Laboratory techniques	*In vitro* fertilisation (IVF) versus intra-cytoplasmic sperm injection Alternative methods of cryopreservation of human embryos
Place of care	One-stop specialist clinic versus general clinic Out-patient versus in-patient endometrial ablation
Investigations	Effectiveness of methods of screening for chlamydia trachomatis Hysterosalpingography as a test of tubal patency The post-coital test in the diagnosis of infertility Hysteroscopy in the diagnosis of menorrhagia

its clinical context. This may involve different levels of observation and analysis, incorporating the individual, the family and the community.[29]

CLINICAL OUTCOMES

Clinical outcomes are essential components of any clinical trial. They should be meaningful to other clinicians and have a direct bearing on the women's appreciation of the burden of disease. Generally speaking, outcomes which are represented as discrete or categorical variables are often more meaningful than continuous outcomes. For example, the proportion of women requiring blood transfusion after hysterectomy is seen to be a more clinically relevant outcome than the volume of blood lost during the procedure. The proportion of women in whom the uterus is empty at 24 hours may be a more meaningful outcome than the mean number of hours required for medical termination. In reproductive medicine, many clinical trials have tended to choose surrogate markers such as number of oocytes retrieved or fertilised as primary outcome rather than live birth or pregnancy. The reason for such a choice is not difficult to guess. Fewer participants are required to achieve a 'significant' difference if the outcome is represented as a continuous variable (such as number of oocytes) instead of a dichotomous variable such as live birth. This in turn reduces the sample size and costs, allowing a single centre to perform a trial that would otherwise require far higher levels of funding and a multi-centre approach.

Explanatory trials usually rely on a single clinical outcome. For example, in a trial comparing drug treatments for menorrhagia, menstrual blood loss in millilitres may well be an appropriate primary outcome. Other physiological or biochemical outcomes such as haemoglobin level, volume urinary loss, extent of endometriosis visualised by laparoscopy, number of ovarian follicles seen on ultrasound scan and serum estradiol levels following ovarian stimulation may also be used in different situations. Unfortunately, they may not always correlate well with the clinically relevant outcomes–certainly from the patients' perspective. In certain cases, costs and a need to opt for a modest and realistic sample size dictate the need for surrogate outcomes in preference to more robust but less common substantive outcomes. Thus bone mineral density rather than the incidence of hip fracture may be chosen as a principal outcome in trials of hormone replacement therapy.[30]

Pragmatic trials usually require the evaluation of more than one outcome measure in order to come to a decision about the effectiveness, risks, costs and acceptability of an intervention. For example, in surgical trials of menorrhagia outcomes should include satisfaction with treatment, menstrual flow, pain, premenstrual syndrome and period of recovery. Sometimes when the impact of a disease spreads beyond the individual to a wider group such as the family, GPs or carers, outcomes may need to be expanded to include a wider group. This may be relevant in trials of urinary incontinence or HRT. It is however important to remember that it is the primary outcome on which the power calculation is usually based, and the one that the trial is best designed to address.

QUALITY OF LIFE

Quality of life (QOL) is now accepted by most clinicians as an important outcome in clinical trials.[31] However the term is sometimes used loosely and without a clear understanding of what it means.[32] Since QOL is considered to be a complex concept comprising physical, emotional and other dimensions, most questionnaires in common use not only assess the detailed aspects of QOL but also provide a summary score for overall health status.[33] Generic measures such as short form health survey (SF-36)[34] broadly assess physical, mental and social health and can be used to compare conditions and treatments. Although the number of such instruments in current use is rapidly increasing, there is a remarkable level of consistency between them.[33]

Other methods include tools focusing on a single aspect such as pain, anxiety as well as individualised measures in which patients themselves define and rate the most important aspects of their quality of life.[35] A number of condition-specific tools, which can be used either independently or to supplement generic measures, have been developed.[36] Examples include the King's College Questionnaire for Urinary Incontinence[37] and Menstrual Distress questionnaire.[38] The Endometriosis Health Profile-30[39] and The Menopause Rating Scale (MRS).[40]

A systematic review by Sanders *et al.*[41] showed that despite the plethora of instruments, the prevalence of reporting on quality of life remains low, increasing from 1% in 1980 to 4% in 1997. There is also a general unwillingness to ask patients to supplement questionnaire-based data with personal responses, and lack of appreciation about the critical importance of response rates.

Patients themselves can find it difficult to distinguish between quality of life and health status or to rate their health without a point of reference. At the same time, the effects of age and changing expectations need to be adjusted for when interpreting QOL scores. Overall, QOL offers a superior way of assessing treatment success in trials involving general gynaecology (such as menorrhagia, urinary incontinence, menopause, pre-menstrual tension) where interventions are targeted at women with benign but debilitating illnesses that compromise several key areas of day-to-day life. On the other hand, women seeking fertility treatment or abortion services are not necessarily unwell. The aim of treatment is to enhance their physical and mental well-being rather than correct a pre-existing deficit in health status. Existing instruments do not discriminate between these two broad groups and further refinements are needed with respect to assessing positive aspects of general and sexual health as opposed to the conventionally used negative aspects.[42] Meanwhile, simple global questions on self-reported health or QOL continue to be useful as prognostic measures for stratification of treatment allocation and as important outcome measures alongside purely clinical outcomes.

PATIENT SATISFACTION

There continues to be a general lack of agreement about the mechanisms which produce satisfaction, as well as the meaning of the word 'satisfaction' itself which has been defined as an 'evaluation based on the fulfillment of expectations'.[43] The conventional view is that satisfaction reflects the sum total of a number of patient-related factors, including expectations, characteristics and psychosocial determinants.[44] Over the past few years, patient satisfaction has become increasingly accepted as a measure of quality in health services and a valid outcome in randomised clinical trials.[45] This is particularly significant in the current climate of delivery of health care which aims to provide a patient-centred service with greater public involvement in planning.[46] The purpose of patient satisfaction measurement is to describe health care services from the patient's point of view, measure the 'process' of care and evaluate health care.[44] The particular strength of using satisfaction as an outcome is related to the unique circumstances of certain gynaecological trials such as those used for menorrhagia where not only the interventions but also the clinical outcomes may be dissimilar. In a trial of hysterectomy versus endometrial ablation, women would be expected to be amenorrhoeic following hysterectomy but not after ablation. Here, comparison of amenorrhoea rates is unlikely to be helpful in comparing the two groups, while satisfaction is not only a robust measure of treatment success, but also incorporates the sum total of a woman's experience of the alternative treatment arms including discomfort, recovery time and side-effects. A similar argument can be used to justify the use of the same outcome for trials comparing surgical and non-surgical treatment of urinary incontinence.

Despite their widespread use in clinical trials, assessment of patient satisfaction has been criticised on theoretical and methodological grounds and their practical use questioned.[47] Relatively few patients express open dissatisfaction with treatment.[48] Indeed satisfaction rates of 80% or more are reported by most hospital-based studies.[49] There is also little evidence to indicate that expressions of satisfaction result from the fulfillment of expectations; in some situations it is difficult to establish the fact that expectations exist at all. High satisfaction ratings do not necessarily mean that women have had good experiences in relation to the service as satisfaction may well make allowances for mitigating circumstances. If the aim is to provide women with a voice, it is important not to rely on satisfaction with treatment as a single outcome but to prioritise methods of accessing women's experience of interventions and the meaning and value they attach to them.[47] There are no off-the-shelf questionnaires that are completely satisfactory[50] and qualitative studies have demonstrated that high satisfaction rates cannot be taken as proof of positive experience. Many tools mentioned in the literature are not validated, while many expressions of satisfaction may not be evaluations at all.[51,52] Dissatisfaction may be more useful as a minimum level of negative experience and may be of potential use in benchmarking exercises. At the moment most clinical trials in gynaecology attempt to measure satisfaction using a number of direct and indirect questions. Some of these questions have been repeated at various points during follow-up to assess change in satisfaction rates over time. Despite the obvious shortcomings of the existing system, there has been an opportunity to refine and validate some of these questionnaires through repeated use in a series of related trials.[4] Acceptability has been measured by direct questions and by other tools such as the Semantic Differential technique in the context of menorrhagia and termination.[20-22]

In other areas such as infertility, satisfaction with treatment is more difficult to assess as the effect of the desired outcome (live birth) is predominant even where treatment is invasive or unpleasant. Conversely there is dissatisfaction with treatment where the outcome is failure to fall pregnant. Some attempts have been made in recent trials to specifically address separately satisfaction with 'treatment' as opposed to satisfaction with 'outcome'. This area is deserving of further study.

ECONOMIC EVALUATION

With the emergence of new methods of treatment comes an increasing awareness of the need to study not just the clinical effectiveness but also the cost-effectiveness of alternative treatments. Pragmatic clinical trials are the standard approach not only for evaluating interventions, but also comparing costs.[53] The costs of treatments are usually estimated using information about the quantities of the resources used. For example the resources used for hysterectomy include the staff time involved, the consumables used and the length of the subsequent in-patient stay. To estimate the cost of treatment, information about this resource use is combined with unit cost estimates, which provide a fixed monetary value to each cost-generating item.[54] The total cost is then the weighted sum of quantities of resources used where weights are unit costs. Carrying out an economic evaluation alongside a randomised trial allows detailed information to be collected about the quantities used by each patient in the study. Such information allows a cost for each patient, producing a patient-specific cost data. This is turn reduces the extent to which comparison between the groups is based on assumptions about resource use. However randomised trials are not necessarily the only way or necessarily the best way to address economic questions.[55] There is an important role for other methods, including modelling.

In the context of RCTs however there is an urgent need to revise the way in which health economic outcomes are addressed within a clinical trial. While cost outcomes are generally regarded as secondary outcomes, the rationale for a formal sample size calculation with adequate power for the planned analysis is still relevant given the large variability in costs between individuals.[56] This is even more relevant where subsets are used for cost data for practical reasons. A recent review has identified an urgent need to improve the statistical analysis and interpretation of cost data in RCTs.[54] This is particularly relevant to the provision of descriptive statistics relating to costs. As cost data are typically skewed, the median can be interpreted as the typical cost for individuals. However, it is the mean cost that is important for policy decisions as it is this value, multiplied by the number of patients, which gives an estimate of the total cost of an intervention.

Table 21.3 provides some examples of outcome measures used in different types of gynaecological

Table 21.3. Outcomes in gynaecological trials

Clinical area	Outcomes	Comments
Infertility	• Live birth rate per couple • Live birth rate per treatment • Clinical pregnancy rate per couple • Clinical pregnancy rate per treatment • Biochemical pregnancy rate • Fertilisation rate • Implantation rate • Multiple pregnancy • Morbidity (e.g. ovarian hyperstimulation) • Costs	Although live birth per couple is the most robust outcome, it demands large sample sizes and a longer duration of follow-up. Live birth/clinical pregnancy rate per treatment is still used in many trials. Multiple pregnancy and its effect on maternal and perinatal morbidity is increasingly being acknowledged as an important outcome of fertility trials.
Menorrhagia	• Satisfaction • Acceptability • Quality of life • Menstrual blood loss • Bleeding and pain scores • Morbidity • Repeat surgery • Haemoglobin level • Amenorrhoea rates • Costs	Satisfaction and QOL are clinically more useful than objective measurement of menstrual blood loss or amenorrhoea rates, especially when trials compare treatments such as hysterectomy which guarantees amenorrhoea versus the Mirena intrauterine system or endometrial ablation which do not. Satisfaction with treatment may not correspond to amenorrhoea rates. Long-term follow-up is important in the evaluation of all new technologies.
Urogynaecology	• Satisfaction • Acceptability • Quality of life • Symptom relief • Objective measurement of urinary loss • Surgical morbidity, repeat surgery • Length of hospital stay • Urodynamic assessment • Costs	Symptom relief and objective assessment of bladder function may not necessarily correspond with quality of life or satisfaction. Long-term follow-up is necessary for effective evaluation of treatments.
Hormone replacement therapy	• Hip fracture • Cardiovascular disease • Menopausal symptoms • Quality of life • Satisfaction • Acceptability • Bone mineral density • Serum lipid profile • Side-effects and morbidity	Historically, surrogate outcomes like lipid profile and bone density have been more popular than rates of cardiovascular disease or fracture.
Termination of pregnancy	• Efficacy: evacuation of the uterus • Acceptability • Morbidity • Quality of life • Costs	Quality of life is difficult to assess in the context of termination. Long-term follow-up difficult.

trials. A crude list such as this is useful, if only to illustrate the specific demands of different clinical areas. Overall, due to the limitations of using 'pure' clinical outcomes in benign gynaecology, 'satisfaction' and 'quality of life' (however defined) have found widespread acceptance as appropriate outcomes. In other areas such as infertility, 'satisfaction' is meaningless without the promise of live birth while even the most invasive and uncomfortable treatment may be perceived to be entirely acceptable if it leads to pregnancy. In general, even when relevant, purely clinical outcomes may lead to potential conflicts between the clinicians' and patients' points of view. A number of health state measures incorporating validated and reliable scales have been developed to address this very issue.[57] These may be generic or disease-specific. Most pragmatic trials will use a number of outcomes from the above categories. At the same time, it is best, in very large trials, to concentrate on a few simple outcomes – for reasons of convenience and efficiency.[58] There is also a statistical drawback to the use of multiple outcomes. The greater the number of outcomes, the higher is the possibility of one of them reaching statistical significance on the basis of chance alone. It is important to consider relevance of outcome measures to the stakeholders. It is thus important to predefine primary and secondary outcomes. The extent to which a trial changes practice will depend on the outcomes chosen.

SAMPLE AND SAMPLE SIZE

The sample size refers to the number of women needed to provide adequate power (usually 80% to 90%) in order to show that the findings of the trial are not merely due to chance. The sample size for each trial is usually calculated with the primary outcome in mind. Although secondary outcomes are often investigated and subgroup analyses performed, the power of an RCT to provide conclusive answers to these may be limited. The statistical approach to determining sample size is the power calculation, which determines how likely the study is to produce a statistically significant result for a difference

between groups of a certain magnitude. It is important to ensure that the study is designed to detect significant differences if they exist. Conversely if the statistical power is low, the results of the trial will be questionable as the numbers may have been too small to detect genuine differences. In general, a clinically significant difference in the primary outcome should be identified as the point of reference for a sample size calculation. Intimate knowledge of the clinical area is crucial for this. For example a 20% difference in satisfaction rate between two forms of treatment for incontinence may be considered to be clinically important. Conversely, against a background of low live birth rates, a difference of 5% to 10% may be enough to change clinical practice in an infertility trial.

In determining the sample size adequate attention should also be paid to the possibility of sample attrition and the need for any future subgroup analysis. For example, in abortion trials, a high non-response to follow-up should be anticipated and the sample size inflated accordingly.[21] In infertility trials, where it may be clinically important to assess the effect of the intervention in different clinical groups, a similar exercise will ensure meaningful subgroup analysis. At the same time, aiming for unrealistically large sample sizes is counterproductive and should be avoided. With a large sample size it is almost always possible to reject any null hypothesis (type I error). Conversely samples which are too small have a high risk of failing to demonstrate a real difference (type II error). The latter is more frequent in gynaecological trials. In small trials, a subgroup analysis based on tiny numbers of patients should be perceived as a hypothesis generating exercise.

RANDOMISATION

Randomisation involves allocating women to groups such that individual characteristics do not influence the nature of the intervention. For example in a trial of treatments for menorrhagia, the aim is to avoid bias by distributing factors that may influence outcome, such as age, parity, dysmenorrhea, premenstrual syndrome and uterine fibroids, randomly between treatment groups. It is anticipated that any difference in outcome is purely due to the treatment and not influenced by one or more of these other characteristics. Random allocation does not guarantee that the groups will be *identical* but it does ensure that any differences between them are due to chance alone.

Randomisation also facilitates the concealment of the type of treatment from the researchers and subjects to further reduce bias in treatment comparison. Thus it ensures that women with a higher BMI (body mass index) are not preferentially allocated to endometrial ablation rather than hysterectomy. In addition, it leads to treatment groups which are random samples of the population sampled and thus makes valid the use of standard statistical tests based on probability theory.

While the simplest method of randomisation is tossing a coin, in practice, this is not an accepted method of treatment allocation. The main reason for this is the lack of an audit trail that makes it difficult to confirm that the random allocation was done correctly. For these reasons the random allocation should be determined in advance, preferably by using pseudorandom numbers generated by a mathematical process. After the randomisation list has been prepared (by someone who will not be involved in recruitment), it must be made available to researchers. Although the process of randomisation can occur at the recruitment point this is preferably done at long range, by telephone or even the internet. If envelopes are used, these must be opaque, as researchers could theoretically hold envelopes to a lamp in order to read what is written inside. For the same reason these envelopes should be sequentially numbered so that the recruiter has to take the next envelope. Differences in outcome between treatment groups are considerably larger in trials where allocation concealment is not strictly enforced as this produces a clear bias. Telephone randomisation, either by means of an operator or a computer-operated 24-hour phone line, is ideal for large trials and especially multicentre trials. Although potentially more efficient,

internet-based randomisation systems continue to generate concerns about ensuring security and confidentiality of patient details. Practical problems with randomisation may arise in surgical and laboratory-based trials where randomisation may need the assistance of nursing or technical staff.

While simple randomisation techniques will, on average, allocate equal numbers to each arm, occasionally, even in large trials, groups of different sizes can result. Block randomisation can be used to keep the numbers in each group very close at all times. In a trial of two alternative surgical treatments for menorrhagia we might want to ensure that each surgeon treats similar numbers of women by either method. Stratified randomisation produces a separate randomisation list for each surgeon (stratum) so that we get very similar numbers of patients receiving each treatment within each stratum. If envelopes are used, this may involve separate lists of random numbers and separate piles of sealed envelopes for each surgeon. We may additionally use blocks to ensure that there is a balance of treatments within each stratum. While stratified randomisation can be extended to two or more stratifying variables, we have to be careful to include only a few strata, to prevent generating extremely small subgroups. Stratification by centre is standard practice in multi-centre trials.

In small studies with several important prognostic variables such as infertility trials, random allocation may not provide adequate balance within the groups. The lack of numbers may make it difficult to stratify for all the important variables. Here, it is still possible to achieve balance using minimisation, which is based on the concept that the next patient to enter the trial is allocated to whichever treatment would minimise the overall imbalance between groups at any stage of the trial. Even in small trials this provides groups that are comparable across several prognostic factors. It is important to specify exactly which prognostic variables are to be used and to say how they are to be grouped. For example age, previous pregnancy and duration of infertility are important prognostic factors for fertility. Minimisation in this context will require a statement about the actual age groups, for example <30 years and ≥30 years. Minimisation is crucial in infertility trials where a clinically significant difference in live birth rates associated with alternative treatments is small and easily overpowered by the effect of prognostic factors such as age, parity and previous pregnancy.

Occasionally we allocate a group of subjects together rather than individuals to treatments. For example, in a health promotion study carried out in general practices, we might need to apply the intervention to all patients in the practice. This may involve display of publicity material in the waiting room, for example. In this situation, we may need to keep groups of patients separate in order to avoid contamination. In a different setting, if we are providing a special physiotherapist to advise patients in a ward, it would be difficult for the nurse to visit some patients and not others. If we are providing training to the patients or their carers, we do not want the subjects receiving training to pass on what they have learned to controls. This might be desirable in general, but not in a trial. A group of subjects allocated to a treatment together is called a cluster. Clusters must be taken into account in the design as the use of clusters reduces the power of the trial and so requires an increase in sample size.

A practical problem relating to randomisation concerns the emotive nature of some of the conditions under evaluation such as infertility or termination of pregnancy. Some women may be unwilling to accept the extra stress of participating in a trial over and above what is already a complex and psychologically challenging experience. There may also be compelling social reasons why women undergoing termination are less likely to opt for randomisation, comply with trial protocols and follow-up arrangements. Infertile couples may be required to fund their treatment themselves. This could influence their decision to refuse to participate in a trial where the experimental arm (such as assisted hatching) is substantially more expensive than standard treatment, unless the trial organisers offer to absorb the extra

costs. Often there is an imperative to provide 'treatment' at the request of the couples. This makes it difficult to recruit couples into a clinical trial where one of the options is 'expectant management'.

CONCEALMENT OF ALLOCATION

The unpredictability of the randomisation process can only be successful if followed by allocation concealment, i.e. concealment of the sequence until patients have been assigned to their groups.[59] This ensures strict implementation of a random allocation sequence without foreknowledge of treatment assignments. Awareness of the next treatment allocation could lead to exclusion of certain women based on their prognosis because they would have been allocated to the perceived inappropriate group. For example, in a trial of unexplained infertility, women with a prolonged duration of infertility could be excluded if the next treatment allocation were known to be a 'no treatment' arm. Adequate concealment would ensure that the decision to accept or reject a participant should be made and informed consent obtained without prior knowledge of the nature of the assignment.

Trials that use inadequate or unclear allocation concealment have tended to yield 40% larger estimates of effect compared to those which used adequate concealment.[60-62] Trials with poorly concealed allocation also generated greater heterogeneity in results, i.e. the results fluctuated extensively above and below the estimates from better studies.[60]

BLINDING

Double blinding seeks to prevent ascertainment bias, protects the sequence after allocation and cannot always be implemented.[1] As in the case with allocation concealment, lack of blinding may lead to exaggerated estimate effects of treatment. A survey of trials in gynaecology found that investigators could have used double blinding more often.[1] When used, methods of double blinding were poorly reported and rarely evaluated. It is recommended that authors provide adequate information about the methods used to ensure double blinding. This should include details such as the type of intervention (capsules/tablets), and efforts made to duplicate the characteristics of the treatment (taste, appearance, route of administration). In addition it is important to be explicit about the methods used to control the allocation schedule, such as location of the schedule during the trial, details of when the code was broken for analysis and the circumstances under which the code could be broken for individual cases (adverse reactions). Finally there should be a statement about the perceived success or failure of the double blinding efforts.

EXCLUSIONS

Exclusions can occur due to eventual discovery about ineligibility, deviations from protocol, withdrawals or losses to follow-up. Exclusions before randomisation do not affect the internal validity of the trial but can compromise generalisability. For most pragmatic trials it is important to keep the eligibility criteria to a minimum. In practice it is unusual to find significant qualitative differences between women in trials and those in the general population. Exclusions after trial entry represent a further source of bias within an RCT as any erosion over the course of the trial from those initially randomised groups is not likely to be random in nature. The accepted method of primary analysis in all cases is by 'intention to treat', i.e. analysis of patients in the originally assigned groups regardless of any breaches of protocol.[63] This can prove unnerving for clinicians especially in the context of surgical trials. For example in a trial comparing hysterectomy versus endometrial ablation many clinicians would find it difficult to accept results of analysis of amenorrhoea rates by intention to treat arguing that it is inappropriate to include hysterectomised women in the ablation group as this would lead to an overestimation of amenorrhoea rates. Investigators can also do secondary analyses, preferably pre-planned based on only those participants who fully complied with the trial protocol (per protocol) or who received a particular

treatment irrespective of randomised assignment (analysis by treatment received). Secondary analyses are acceptable, as long as researchers label them as such, and as non-randomised comparisons. The advantage of randomisation is entirely lost when investigators exclude participants and in effect present a non-randomised comparison as the primary result, i.e. similar to a cohort study. Exclusions of participants can lead to misleading results.[64] Researchers sometimes exclude patients on the basis of outcomes that happen before treatment has begun such as pregnancy in a couple with infertility. Although this may seem sensible in as much as the event of interest occurred independent of the treatment, the same argument could be used for excluding pregnancies in a no intervention arm of the trial.

It is important to attempt to minimise exclusions and be explicit about those cases where exclusions occurred. This can be enforced by minimising the delay between randomisation and initiation of treatment. This can be particularly relevant to infertility trials where couples could fall pregnant before treatment can start or where the intervention is conditional on a set of clinical criteria. For example, in couples randomised to IVF or ICSI it may be more efficient to delay randomisation until after oocyte recovery so that women who have failed to respond to gonadotrophin stimulation are not included.

FOLLOW-UP

It is important to pre-determine the length and type of follow-up for each trial. The precise circumstances and the time interval will depend on the nature of the trial. In fertility trials the traditional method was to express outcomes as pregnancy rates per cycle. This meant the duration of follow-up was brief. For more robust outcomes like pregnancy rate per woman, it may be necessary to extend the follow-up for three to six cycles depending on the nature of the treatment. A further 9 months need to be added on to allow live birth per couple to be used as an outcome. For menorrhagia trials, 80% of re-treatments occur within 2 years, making this an acceptable duration for follow-up in the first instance. A prolonged period of follow-up of up to 5 years would be ideal as many women could expect the effects of their treatment to wane over time and long-term complications of therapy to surface. This would appear to be equally true for urogynaecology trials. For termination of pregnancy, follow-up has to be kept short as the loss to follow-up is high and many women may not wish to be contacted at a later date. For HRT trials, which genuinely wish to address crucial outcomes such as rates of fracture, cardiovascular disease or Alzheimer's disease, follow-up may need to be extended to tens of years. This obviously raises significant ethical, logistic and financial issues which may well need to be taken into account whilst planning such trials.

DATA COLLECTION

Data in a trial are usually collected from sources such as case notes, local clinic databases and patient questionnaires. Occasionally interviews may be used to explore areas which are not capable of being probed adequately with questionnaires. General practitioners, local and national databases may also be accessed to obtain clinical information such as retreatment rates or serious complications about patients who are lost to follow-up.

CONDUCT

Recruitment

To avoid recruitment bias, it is important to target all eligible women and record all refusals. It may be helpful to obtain some baseline clinical details about them in order to explore any major differences between participants and non-participants, which could affect the external validity of the trial.

Trial Co-Ordination

Following informed consent, it is important to obtain baseline information by filling in datasheets or questionnaires prior to randomisation. Subsequent data collection should occur at the pre-specified times and an efficient system of timely

reminders put into place. In pragmatic trials it is often important to distinguish those women who no longer wish to continue with the allocated treatment from those who wish to terminate their involvement with the trial and do not wish to be contacted for follow-up or have questionnaires sent to them. Hopefully the numbers in this latter group should be small but their wishes should be respected.

Data Entry and Analysis

This is an important aspect of the trial and errors here can lead to significant bias. As mentioned above, analysis should be by intention to treat. Each woman should be analysed as though she had received the intervention to which she had been randomised. This minimises any bias due to non-random removal of participants from the trial. The exception is explanatory trials, usually phase I and II drug trials, where strict rules of exclusion for protocol violation apply. Occasionally it may be important from a clinical point of view to perform as separate analysis by treatment received. This should be clearly described as such and should be used to assess the primary outcome. Intention to treat can cause much consternation among clinicians particularly in surgical trials where some outcomes may seem absurd—for example continuing menstrual loss in women allocated to hysterectomy who did not undergo the operation but were analysed by intention to treat.

Presenting Results

Analysis should follow the original plan set out in the protocol and the CONSORT recommendations should be observed. Particularly helpful is a trial chart which sets out in an explicit manner any exclusions or loss to follow-up. Results of subgroup analyses should be treated with caution and used mainly as hypothesis-generating exercises in most modest-sized trials. There should be a conscious attempt to limit discussion to the results generated by the trial and avoid speculation.

ETHICS OF TRIALS

The scientific rationale for conducting trials is collective equipoise. Clinicians need to be genuinely uncertain about the best treatment. In such a clinical situation, there should be no conflict between the interests of those participating in a trial and those who stand to gain in the future. The important issue is that participants are also in personal equipoise and give informed consent.

Despite awareness of its importance, there is evidence that some doctors do not seem to take informed consent as seriously as they should.[65] This may well be because participants seem to be less willing to be randomised, when they are given more preliminary data, and made aware of any accumulating evidence of effectiveness. In many trials, a significant number of participants emerge from consultations expecting to benefit personally by their participation.

Some infertility-related procedures are described as 'licensed treatment' under the aegis of the Human Fertilisation and Embryology Authority (HFEA) in the United Kingdom. Clinical data pertaining to licensed treatments (including donor insemination, IVF and ICSI) are confidential and may not be revealed to researchers (including clinicians) who are not covered by the institutional HFEA treatment licence, without the explicit permission of the couple. This can create problems in accessing data, particularly follow-up data from notes or databases. Furthermore, trials involving manipulation of gametes and embryos need separate approval from the HFEA in addition to approval from the local ethics committee.

For all clinical trials, it is sensible from an ethical and financial point of view to have clear stoppage rules as part of the original study design. An independent data monitoring committee should be available to review the results of an interim analysis. Early stopping should only occur under pre-planned, well-specified circumstances such a marked superiority or toxicity of one arm of the study which is greater than that originally hypothesised. Examples include stopping a trial evaluating the use of prophylactic antibiotics during hysteroscopic surgery where the control arm demonstrates a significantly higher rate of infection.[66] Alternatively, in a trial comparing a policy of single versus double embryo transfer (in order to prevent twin pregnancies) it may be appropriate to stop if the pregnancy rate in the single embryo group becomes unacceptably low.

CONCLUSION

Clinical trials in gynaecology have lagged behind those in other disciplines in terms of overall numbers as well as quality. There are few large multi-centre trials, particularly surgical trials. The clinical population is heterogeneous and interventions under scrutiny diverse. Some treatments, such as those for infertility and unwanted fertility target women (and their partners) who have specific reproductive health needs but are otherwise in good health. Trials also need to be able to compare interventions that cross different treatment boundaries. Trialists in this field need to design more pragmatic trials with clinically meaningful outcome measures. In gynaecology these should be quality of life and satisfaction; in infertility, live birth rates per couple/woman. Finally, the importance of collecting cost data cannot be overstated in terms of planning gynaecological services which are effective, acceptable and affordable.

REFERENCES

1. Schulz KF, Grimes DA, Altman DG, Hayes RJ. Blinding and exclusions after allocation in randomised controlled trials: survey of published parallel group trials in obstetrics and gynaecology. *BMJ* (1996) **312**(7033): 742–4.
2. Out HJ, Schnabel PG, Rombout F, Geurts TB, Bosschaert MA, Coelingh Bennink HJ. A bioequivalence study of two urinary follicle stimulating hormone preparations: Follegon and Metrodin. *Human Reprod* (1996) **11**(1): 61–3.
3. El-Refaey H, Rajasekar D, Abdalla M, Calder L, Templeton A. Induction of abortion with Mifepristone (RU 486) and oral or vaginal Misoprostol. *N Engl J Med* (1995) **332**: 983–7.
4. The Aberdeen Endometrial Ablation Group. A randomised trial of hysterectomy versus endometrial ablation for the treatment of dysfunctional

bleeding: clinical psychological and economic outcome at four years. *Br J Obstet Gynaecol* (1999) **106**: 360–6.

5. Cooper KG, Jack SA, Parkin DE, Grant AM. Five-year follow up of women randomised to medical management or transcervical resection of the endometrium for heavy menstrual loss: clinical and quality of life outcomes. *BJOG: Int J Obstet Gynaecol* (2001) **108**(12): 1222–8.

6. Roland M, Torgerson DJ. Understanding controlled trials: what are pragmatic trials? *BMJ* (1998) **316**: 285.

7. Goverde AJ, McDonnell J, Vermeiden JPW, Schats R, Rutten FFH, Schoemaker J. Intrauterine insemination or in-vitro fertilisation in idiopathic subfertility and male subfertility: a randomised trial and cost-effectiveness analysis. *Lancet* (2000) **355**: 13–18.

8. Khan KS, Daya S, Collins JA, Walter SD. Empirical evidence of bias in infertility research: overestimation of treatment effect in crossover trials using pregnancy as the outcome measure. *Fertil Steril* (1996) **65**(5): 939–45.

9. Fender GRK, Prentice A, Gorst T, Nixon RM, Duffy SW, Day NE, et al. Randomised controlled trial of educational package on management of menorrhagia in primary care: the Anglia menorrhagia education study. *BMJ* (1999) **318**: 1246–50.

10. Morrison J, Carroll L, Twaddle S, Cameron I, Grimshaw J, Leyland A, et al. Pragmatic randomised controlled trial to evaluate guidelines for the management of infertility across the primary care–secondary care interface. *BMJ* (2001) **322**: 1–7.

11. Kerry SM, Bland JM. Sample size in cluster randomisation. *BMJ* (1998) **316**: 549.

12. Kerry SM, Bland JM. The intracluster correlation coefficient in cluster randomisation. *BMJ* (1998) **316**: 1455.

13. Donner A, Klar N. *Design and analysis of cluster randomization trials in health research*, 1st edn. London: Arnold (2000).

14. Aboulgar MA, Mansour RT, Serour JI, Amin YM, Kamal A. Prospective controlled randomised study of in-vitro fertilisation versus intracytoplasmic sperm injection in the treatment of tubal factor infertility with normal semen parameters. *Fertil Steril* (1996) **66**: 753–6.

15. Ruiz A, Remohi J, Minguez Y, Guanes P, Simon C, Pellicer A. The role of in vitro fertilisation and intracytoplasmic sperm injection in couples with unexplained infertility after failed intrauterine insemination. *Fertil Steril* (1997) **68**: 171–3.

16. Bhattacharya S, Hamilton MPR, Shabban M, Khalaf Y, Seddler M, Ghobara T, et al. A randomised controlled trial of in-vitro fertilisation (IVF) and

intra-cytoplasmic sperm injection (ICSI) in non-male factor infertility. *Lancet* (2001) **357**: 2075–9.

17. Torgerson D, Sibbald B. Understanding clinical trials: what is a patient preference trial? *BMJ* (1998) **316**: 360.

18. Brocklehurst P. *Br J Obstet Gynaecol* (1997) **104**: 1332–5.

19. Brewin CR, Bradley C. Patient preferences and randomised clinical trials. *BMJ* (1989) **299**: 313–15.

20. Henshaw RC, Naki SA, Russell IT, et al. Comparison of medical abortion with vacuum aspiration; women's preferences and acceptability of treatment. *Br Med J* (1993) **307**: 714–17.

21. Ashok PW, Kidd A, Flett GM, Fitzmaurice A, Graham W, Templeton A. A randomised comparison of medical abortion and surgical vacuum aspiration at 10–13 weeks gestation. *Human Reprod* (2002) **17**(1): 92–8.

22. Cooper KG, Parkin DE, Garret AM, Grant AM. A randomised comparison of medical and hysteroscopic management in women consulting a gynaecologist for treatment of heavy menstrual loss. *Br J Obstet Gynaecol* (1997) **104**: 1360–6.

23. Torgerson DJ, Klaber-Moffett J, Russell I. Patient preferences in randomised trials: threat or opportunity? *J Health Serv Policy* (1996) **1**(4): 194–7.

24. Piaggio G, Pinol APY. Use of the equivalence approach in reproductive health clinical trials. *Stat Med* (2001) **20**: 3571–87.

25. Jones B, Jarvis P, Lewis JA, Ebbutt AF. Trials to assess equivalence: the importance of rigorous methods. *BMJ* (1996) **313**: 36–9.

26. Röhmel J. Therapeutic equivalence investigations: statistical considerations. *Stat Med* (1998) **17**: 1703–14.

27. Ebbutt AF, Frith L. Practical issues in equivalence trials. *Stat Med* (1998) **17**(15 & 16): 1691–1701.

28. Pandian Z, Bhattacharya S, Nikolaou N, Vale L, Templeton A. In-vitro fertilisation for unexplained subfertility (Cochrane Review). In: *The Cochrane Library*, Issue 4. Oxford: Update Software (2002).

29. Roland M, Torgerson DJ. Understanding controlled trials: what outcomes should be measured? *BMJ* (1998) **317**: 1075–80.

30. Cranney A, Welch V, Adachi JD, Guyatt G, Krolicki N, Griffith L, Shea B, Tugwell P, Wells G. Etidronate for treating and preventing postmenopausal osteoporosis (Cochrane Review). In: *The Cochrane Library*, Issue 2. Oxford: Update Software (2002).

31. Patrick DL, Bergner M. Measurement of health status in the 1990s. *Ann Rev Public Health* (1990) **11**: 1165–83.

32. Gill TM, Feinstein AR. A critical appraisal of the quality of life measurements. *JAMA* (1994) **272**(8): 619–26.

33. Fayers PM, Sprangers MAG. Understanding self-rated health. *Lancet* (2002) **359**: 187–8.

34. Ware JE, Sherbourne CD. The MOS 36-item short form health survey (SF-36). Conceptual framework and item selection. *Med Care* (1992) **30**: 473–83.

35. McGee H, Hannah M, O'Boyle CA, Hickey A, O'Malley K, Joyce CRB. Assessing the quality of life of the individuals: the SEIQOL with a health and gastroenterology unit population. *Pschol Med* (1991) **21**: 749–59.

36. Guyatt GH, Bombardier C, Tugwell PX. Measuring disease specific quality of life in clinical trials. *Can Med Assoc J* (1986) **134**: 889–95.

37. Kelleher CJ, Cardozo LD, Khullar V, Salvatore S. A new questionnaire to assess the quality of life of urinary incontinent women. *Br J Obstet Gynaecol* (1997) **104**(12): 1374–9.

38. Moos RH. Typology of menstrual cycle symptoms. *Am J Obstet Gynecol* (1969) **103**: 390–402.

39. Jones G, Kennedy S, Barnard A, Wong J, Jenkinson C. Development of an endometriosis quality-of-life instrument: The Endometriosis Health Profile-30. *Obstet Gynecol* (2001) **98**(2): 258–64.

40. Schneider HP, Heinemann LA, Rosemeier HP, Potthoff P, Behre HM. The Menopause Rating Scale (MRS): comparison with Kupperman index and quality-of-life scale SF-36. *Climacteric* (2000) **3**(1): 50–8.

41. Sanders C, Egger M, Donovan J, Tallon D, Frankel S. Reporting on quality of life in randomised controlled trials: bibliographic study. *BMJ* (1998) **317**: 1191–4.

42. Graham WJ. Outcomes and effectiveness in reproductive health. *Social Sci Med* (1998) **47**(12): 1925–36.

43. Williams B. Patient satisfaction: a valid concept? *Social Sci Med* (1994) **38**: 509–16.

44. Sitzia J, Wood N. Patient satisfaction: a review of issues and concepts. *Social Sci Med* (1997) **45**(12): 1829–43.

45. Bury M. Doctors, patients and interactions in health care. In: *Health and Illness in a Changing Society*. London: Routledge (1997).

46. Department of Health. *The New NHS: Modern and Dependable*. London: HMSO (1998).

47. Williams B, Coyle J, Healy D. The meaning of patient satisfaction: an explanation of high reported levels. *Social Sci Med* (1998) **47**(9): 1351–9.

48. Hopton JL, Howie JGR, Porter MD. The need to look at the patient in General Practice satisfaction surveys. *J Fam Prac* (1993) **10**: 82–7.

49. Williams SJ, Calnan M. Key determinants of consumer satisfaction in general practice. *J Fam Prac* (1991) **8**: 237–42.

50. McIver S, Meredith P. There for the asking: can the government's planned annual survey really measure patient satisfaction? *Health Serv J* (1998) **19**: 26–7.

51. Leimkuhler A, Muller U. Patient satisfaction–artifact or social fact. *Nervenarzt* (1996) **67**: 765–73.

52. Owens DJ, Batchelor C. Patient satisfaction and the elderly. *Social Sci Med* (1996) **42**: 1483–91.

53. Drummond MF, Davies L. Economic analysis alongside clinical trials. Revisiting the methodological issues. *Int J Technol Assess Health Care* (1991) **7**: 561–73.

54. Barber JA, Thompson SG. Analysis and interpretation of cost data in randomised controlled trials: review of published studies. *BMJ* (1998) **317**: 1195–200.

55. Fayers PM, Hand DJ. Generalisation from phase III clinical trials: survival, quality of life and health economics. *Lancet* (1997) **350**: 1025–7.

56. Briggs A. Economic evaluation and clinical trials: size matters. *BMJ* (2000) **321**: 1362–3.

57. Bowling A. *Measuring Disease: A Review of Disease Specific Quality of Life Measurement Scales*. Mitton Keynes: Open University Press (1994).

58. Peto R, Collins R, Gray R. Large scale randomised evidence: large sample trials and overviews of trials. *J Clin Epidemiol* (1995) **48**: 23–40.

59. Schulz KF and Grimes DA. Generation of allocation sequences in randomised trials: chance not choice. *Lancet* (2002) **359**: 515–19.

60. Schulz KF, Chalmers I, Hayes RJ, Altman DG. Empirical evidence of bias: dimensions of methodological quality associated with estimates of treatment effects in controlled trials. *JAMA* (1995) **273**: 408–12.

61. Moher D, Pham B, Jones A, *et al*. Does quality of reports of randomised trials affect estimates of intervention efficacy reported in meta-analysis. *Lancet* (1998) **352**: 609–13.

62. Juni P, Altman D, Egger M. Assessing quality of controlled trials. *BMJ* (2001) **323**: 42–6.

63. Pocock SJ. *Clinical Trials: A Practical Approach*. Chichester: John Wiley & Sons (1983).

64. Schulz KF, Grimes DA. Sample size slippages in randomised trials: exclusions and the lost and wayward. *Lancet* (2002) **359**: 781–5.

65. Edwards SJ, Lilford RJ, Hewison J. The ethics of randomised controlled trials from the perspectives of patients, the public and health care professionals. *BMJ* (1998) **317**: 1209–12.

66. Bhattacharya S, Parkin DE, Reid TMS, Abramovich DR, Mollison J, Kitchener HC. A prospective randomised study of the effects of prophylactic antibiotics on the incidence of bacteraemia following hysteroscopic surgery. *Eur J Obstet Gynaecol Reprod Biol* (1995) **63**: 37–40.

RESPIRATORY

22

Respiratory

ANDERS KÄLLÉN
AstraZeneca, Lund, Sweden

AIRWAYS DISEASES

Airway obstruction is a common and important feature of some respiratory diseases. It can be acute, 'semi-chronic' (e.g. due to cancer) or chronic. The chronic obstructive airway diseases can be divided into whether the obstruction is reversible or not. In the former case the patient usually has asthma, in the latter case chronic obstructive pulmonary disease, abbreviated COPD. These disease concepts lack precise definitions, and the division is only meant as a first approximation. Both diseases are inflammatory diseases mainly of the lower respiratory tract: in asthma there is an inflammatory process mainly in the central airways, whereas the inflammation of COPD is predominantly peripheral with progressive destruction of lung tissue. Inflammation in the upper respiratory tract, i.e. rhinitis, is characterised by both acute and chronic conditions, the most distinctive being seasonal hayfever.

This chapter will discuss clinical trials in the three diseases asthma, COPD and rhinitis, with the focus on the first of these.

MEDICAL BACKGROUND

Asthma

From a clinical point of view, asthma presents itself by recurrent breathlessness, cough or wheeze caused by variable or intermittent narrowing of the intra-pulmonary airways. The severity of these symptoms has a wide range, from very mild intermittent with symptoms only upon provocation, to severe persistent with large impact on daily life. There is no precise definition of asthma, and therefore the prevalence is hard to establish. We know, however, that it is commoner in children than in adults, and more common in boys than in girls.[1] A figure for children around 10% and half that for adults is probably close to reality in most of the western world. There is however a definite regional inhomogeneity with regions with much higher prevalence and regions where the disease is rare. Most epidemiological studies seem, however, to agree that the prevalence is rising.[2]

The high prevalence of asthma gives a poor prediction of the impact of the disease on the community, because the overwhelming majority

Textbook of Clinical Trials. Edited by D. Machin, S. Day and S. Green
© 2004 John Wiley & Sons, Ltd ISBN: 0-471-98787-5

of asthmatics are mild sufferers with symptoms confined to wheezing after exercise or breathlessness in association with an upper respiratory tract infection. At the other end of the spectrum, asthma is a crippling, life-threatening disease with acute severe attacks requiring emergency room treatment. In the western world, about 1% of adults and 2% of children need medical attention for asthmatic symptoms.[3,4]

Many factors are known to cause narrowing of intra-pulmonary airways. The sensitivity to such stimuli varies between individuals but under normal circumstances the concentration of such substances is too low to produce symptoms in healthy subjects. Asthmatic patients are more or less characterised by a high sensitivity to such stimuli, a phenomenon called *non-specific bronchial hyperresponsiveness*. The most common cause of non-specific bronchial irritation is exercise and, for many, this may be the only manifestation of their asthma.

It is essential to make a clear distinction between this non-specific hyperresponsiveness and the allergic reactions. Allergy is an immunological reaction to a specific environmental agent. Hyperresponsive bronchi, in addition to responding in an exaggerated fashion to exogenous stimuli, will also respond in an enhanced fashion to inflammatory mediators released in the bronchial wall as a result of an allergic reaction. Thus a trivial allergic reaction in a hyperresponsive bronchus may provoke a large bronchoconstrictive response. There is little, if any, relationship between the degree of atopy and non-specific hyperresponsiveness. Instead the degree of non-specific hyperresponsiveness is associated with the degree of inflammation in the respiratory tract.[5]

Asthma may start at any age. When starting during childhood and adolescence it is likely to be associated with atopy, as compared to when symptoms start later in life. Most asthmatic patients have perennial symptoms, but a minority shows a seasonal variation, sometimes confined to periods with air-borne pollen, sometimes to the winter months. Thus different asthmatics may have symptoms during different periods of the year, with long periods of absolute or relative relief between attacks of varying severity.

In general, asthma carries a favourable prognosis because the bronchial inflammation does not usually cause permanent tissue damage. However, in a subgroup of subjects, irreversible bronchial obstruction develops later in life.[6]

COPD

Chronic obstructive pulmonary disease is characterised by long-term, in general progressive, irreversible obstruction of the flow of air out of the lungs. To a large extent it is comprised of two related disease:

1. Chronic bronchitis, whose clinical definition is productive cough (from bronchial secretion) on most days for 3 months/year for two consecutive years. The mucus hypersecretion comes from hypertrophied bronchial glands and increases the risk of bacterial lung infections.
2. Emphysema, which has a pathological definition with enlargement of the alveoli due to the destruction of the walls between them. These walls contain elastic fibres, so their destruction reduces the elasticity of the lung, leading to collapse, and thus obstruction, of airways.

The disease entities asthma, chronic bronchitis and emphysema are in no way mutually exclusive: a given patient can have symptoms from more than one. The definitions of the last two does not imply that the patient has airway obstruction, so not everyone with these diseases has COPD.

COPD is believed to affect more than half a billion people worldwide, causing perhaps 3 million deaths annually. When diagnosed, this is often in a relatively late stage of the disease, with less than 50% of lung function remaining, so the majority of cases are at any specified point in time undiagnosed. The prevalence of diagnosed COPD is about 5%, and is increasing.

Pathologically COPD is a disease with periferal inflammation (thus rather a bronchiolitis than bronchitis) with progressive lung tissue destruction. In the western world, by far the most important factor responsible for COPD is smoking; it has been said to be responsible for up to 90% of COPD patients.[7] However, only about 15–20% of all cigarette smokers develop COPD. The mechanism seems to be that cigarette smoke attracts cells (neutrophils, macrophages and cytotoxic T-cells as opposed to eosinophils and T-helper cells in asthma) to the lungs that promote inflammation, and these are stimulated to release elastase, an enzyme that breaks down the elastic fibres in lung tissue. Normally the lungs are protected against this enzyme by the elastase inhibitors, among them α_1-antitrypsin, which is produced in the liver (congenital deficiency of this enzyme is another, but rare, causation for emphysema). Air pollution has been suspected to have similar effects as smoking, but it is unclear to what extent that is an important aetiological factor for COPD. Also, there is a high COPD incidence in women in Asia attributed to cooking fumes.[8]

The typical COPD patient has been smoking 20 or more cigarettes a day for more than 20 years and presents with a chronic cough, shortness of breath (dyspnea) and frequent respiratory infections. If the underlying disease is mainly emphysema, shortness of breath may be the only symptom. Initially the dyspnea only comes during physical exercise, but as the disease progresses it occurs already on minimal exertion. For the patient with chronic bronchitis dominating, the major symptoms are chronic cough and sputum production. The sputum may be clear but is usually coloured and thick as bacterial colonisation is common.

Rhinitis and Nasal Polyposis

The upper respiratory tract is to some extent like terminal bronchioli without smooth muscles. Instead the nose has venous sinusoids and the major reason for obstruction of the upper airway tract is vasodilation of capacitance vessels and oedema while secretion can contribute. Another difference to the lower tract is that stimulation of nervous irritant receptors in the nose results in sneezing, which is the cleaning reflex of the upper airways corresponding in a way to coughing, which is the cleaning reflex of the lower airways.

Inflammation in the upper respiratory tract, rhinitis, presents as one or more of the symptoms nasal congestion, rhinorrhea (i.e. runny nose), sneezing and itching. Chronic inflammatory conditions can in predisposed individuals result in benign protrusions of nasal polyps into the nasal cavity, polyposis.

Rhinitis can be allergic or non-allergic, where the latter is characterised by presence of symptoms of varying severity. Allergic rhinitis can be seasonal as hay fever (SAR = Seasonal Allergic Rhinitis), or perennial. In the latter case the symptoms can be due to continuous exposure to allergens like the house dust mite, or may present themselves intermittently as episodes triggered by allergens like, e.g., grass pollen. Despite the common inflammatory denominator for allergic rhinitis and polyposis, there is no evidence that the two conditions are closely linked, or that allergy plays a major role in the aetiology of nasal polyposis.

Rhinitis is a very common disease, but surprisingly little is known about its epidemiology. The nose has a filter function, and is therefore exposed to a much larger amount of inhaled allergens per square centimetre than bronchi, especially when the allergens are large. SAR is due to air-borne plant pollen. From a clinical point of view the most widely distributed ones are those of grasses, but some tree pollen, including birch and olive tree, are also important, as is ragweed. It is important to note that the pollen season for an individual plant species varies from one country or region to another. Also, whereas the season for air-borne pollen is limited to perhaps half a year in temperate zones, in warmer climates it is so long that what seems to be perennial symptoms may be provoked by multiple and sequential seasonal allergies.

Patients with nasal polyposis suffer from a series of symptoms, just as in rhinitis but in particular nasal blockage and an absence of smell. The prevalence is not known, there are few epidemiological studies, but it is probably in the range of 1–4%. The diagnosis of polyps requires appropriate inspection of the nasal cavities by a trained physician.

CURRENT TREATMENTS

The respiratory tract has a limited repertoire of responses to irritation or other stimulation. In the nose vasodilation leads to decreased airway calibre and nasal blockage. The bronchi may change their calibre or alter the amount of glandular secretion produced, leading to obstruction. There is oedema, hyperaemia and cellular infiltration of the wall of the tract. Afferent nerves may signal information to the brain stem to produce sneezing (upper tract) or cough or the sensation of breathlessness (lower tract). The relative importance of these factors varies between individuals, and different drugs interfere with different factors.

Drugs for chronic obstructive respiratory diseases are given either systemically, as tablets, or by local administration using an inhalation device. When it comes to inhaled products, it is important to note that a treatment consists of two objects, a drug to be delivered to the body and an inhalation device used for this deliverance. We will not discuss devices here, only drug classes. It is however important to understand that the amount of drug delivered to the airways may vary considerably from one inhalator to another.[9] The same might be true of the distribution pattern within the lungs, with potential consequences for the effectiveness of the treatment.

Bronchodilator Drugs

There are three basic groups of bronchodilator drugs—β_2-agonists (today by far the largest), xanthines and anticholinergics.[10] Their modes of action differ somewhat. We discuss each class of drugs separately.

β_2-**Agonists** bind to the β-adrenergic receptor and stimulate the intracellular accumulation of the signal substance cAMP (cyclic adenosine monophosphate). There are now three known types of β-adrenergic receptors in the human body: stimulation of the β_1-receptor causes

cardiac stimulation and intestinal inhibition, whereas stimulation of the β_2-receptor results in bronchodilatation, vasodilatation, stimulation of skeletal muscles and uterine contractile inhibition. A third type, β_3-receptors, cause lipolysis.[11]

The development within this drug class has been towards more and more potent and selective β_2-agonists. The first generation of drugs were short-acting with a duration of action of, at most, 4–6 hours. Lately a few long-acting drugs, with duration of action superseding 12 hours, have been introduced.[12]

β_2-agonists are of benefit to the majority of asthmatic patients because of the bronchodilator property; rapid-acting ones are often given as rescue medication for relief of symptoms. The drug class does however have actions other than smooth muscle relaxation that may contribute to their long-term therapeutic effect in asthma and motivate their use in COPD: they stimulate mucociliary function in the airways, restore normal clearance of bronchial secretion and inhibit microvascular permeability in the airways leading to decreased mucosal oedema.

Side-effects are a consequence of the binding to receptors in tissues and organs outside the lung: tremour by binding to receptors in skeletal muscle, tachycardia by binding to receptors in the heart (this problem has been reduced as the drugs became highly selective, but there are some β_2-receptors in the heart as well) and hypokalemia, due to a redistribution from extra- to intracellular spaces. In general tolerance develops rapidly to the extra-pulmonary effects, so these are usually mild or absent in patients, though individual variation in the sensitivity can make the use of these drugs impossible in the occasional patient.

Xanthines, the most well-known member of which is caffeine but the most widely used one as treatment for airway obstruction is theophylline, are potent smooth muscle relaxants by acting directly in the intracellular messenger cAMP. Thus they have about the same pharmacological actions as β_2-agonists. But since they act intracellularly and not by binding to a receptor on the cell surface, the effect is more generalised and the side-effects are somewhat different and potentially more serious than those of β_2-agonists. The most important ones relate to the gastrointestinal, cardiovascular and central nervous systems. At the start of treatment with oral theophylline, most patients will experience some caffeine-like symptoms including irritability and nausea, symptoms which usually fade away after a few days. For that reason, however, treatment is usually initiated in subtherapeutic doses and progressively increased over a period of 1–2 weeks.[13]

The serious side-effects, in contrast to the caffeine-like ones, are well correlated to plasma concentrations. In clinical practice theophylline concentration in plasma has to be monitored and dose adjusted so that the plasma concentration lies within a therapeutic window. Because of this the use of xanthines has diminished over the last 10 years as alternative treatment has become available.

Anticholinergic drugs have been used since ancient times for the treatment of asthma. The use of various plant derivatives has evolved through synthetic atropine to more selective bronchodilating anticholinergic agents with fewer side-effects than atropine.[14]

The bronchodilating effect of this drug class is due to their antagonism of the binding of acetylcholine (from the vagal nerve) to the muscarinic receptors of bronchial smooth muscle. These drugs are particularly used in treating reversible airway obstruction in COPD.

The side-effects of anticholinergic agents are due to blockade of muscarinic M_2-receptors in other organs and include dryness of the mouth, blurred vision, urine retention and difficulty in micturition, tachycardia, flushing and lightheadedness.

Corticosteroids

That glucocorticosteroids (GCSs) have a therapeutic effect on asthma, rhinitis and other anti-inflammatory diseases has been known for a long time and is due to their being manmade analogues of an endogenous anti-inflammatory steroid–cortisol. Cortisol is in a way nature's own remedy for inflammation: if we remove the adrenal glands inflammatory reactions are greatly exacerbated. Regulation of endogenous cortisol is complex, involving the hypothalamic–pituitary–adrenal (HPA) axis. During a severe inflammatory response, elevated levels of cytokines stimulate centres in the brain, leading to an increase of cortisol in the circulation thereby attenuating the inflammatory response. It is now believed that even at normal levels, endogenous hormones will regulate inflammation. The GCS mode of action is by binding to a glucocorticoid receptor within the cell's cytosol. When used for treating, e.g., asthma GCSs lead to a reduction of airway inflammation, mucous hypersecretion and airway reactivity while restoring the integrity of the airways.[15]

Originally GCSs were given systemically as asthma treatment. There are however well known side-effects of high does of oral GCSs over a long time that limits that usage. These include, but are not limited to, osteoporosis, hypertension, adrenal insufficiency and Cushingoid features as well as growth retardation in children. Concern about these side-effects diminished the use of oral GCS as an asthma treatment. Inhaled GCSs have improved the benefit/risk ratio. Since administration is aimed directly at the site of inflammation, lower doses can be used, giving lower GCS concentrations in plasma with largely negligible systemic side-effects as a result. Inhaled GCSs are now widely accepted as first-line anti-inflammatory therapy for asthma.[16]

To evaluate the long-term side-effects of inhaled GCSs is difficult. They are rare at doses given in asthma treatment, so large numbers of patients and long-term clinical studies are needed. Some information can be gained by studying the endogenous cortisol levels. As already mentioned, the endogenous cortisol level is controlled by the highly complex HPA axis. Introduction of exogenous GCS in the plasma will affect this axis and lead to a suppression of the endogenous cortisol levels, the degree of which is determined by the plasma concentrations and the potency of the drug. Thus, the degree of suppression is a measure of the amount of active (on the HPA axis) exogenous GCS in the body.

Other Drugs

Vasoconstrictors are used extensively in rhinitis. Topical α-agonistic sympatomimetics effectively and promptly alleviate the nasal blockage. They have no effect on rhinorrhea, nasal itch or sneezing.[17]

Antihistamines are used for rhinitis, mainly as rescue medication. Their main effect is to block peripheral H_1-receptors which limits vasodilatation in the nasal mucosa. They have an effect on nasal itching, sneezing and discharge, but little or no effect on nasal congestion and blockage.[18]

Disodium cromoglycate (DSCG) and nedocromil sodium DSCG has been used as a prophylactic anti-asthma drug, mainly by children and young adults.[19] To be effective it should be administered four times per day. Originally its mechanism of action was proposed to be stabilisation of mast cells, though that is probably not the case. Taken immediately before exposure, DSCG affects the asthmatic reactions induced by various stimuli. However, after discontinuation of long-term treatment, DSCG seems not to have modulated the bronchial hyperresponsiveness or the underlying inflammatory reaction.

Nedocromil sodium is another non-steroidal substance with anti-inflammatory properties *in vitro*. It acts as an inhibitor at several levels of neurogenic inflammation in asthma. Clinical studies have demonstrated improvements in airway functions, including a reduction of bronchial hyperreactivity, but it does not protect against maximal airway narrowing, which is an important feature of inhaled corticosteroids.

Both DSCG and nedocromil are remarkably free from side-effects. They are also used for rhinitis, with effects similar to antihistamines.

Leukotriene modifiers The cysteinyl leukotrienes are products of the arachidonic acid metabolism with effects that mimic many features of asthma, e.g. by increasing eosinophil migration, mucus production, airway wall oedema and causing bronchospasm. Oral leukotriene receptor antagonists, to be administered once or twice daily, are available along with an oral leukotriene synthesis inhibitor, which has to be administered four times daily.

Leukotriene modifiers improve airway function and decrease the need for additional maintenance and rescue asthma therapies. Leukotriene modifiers also attenuate bronchospasm induced by allergens, exercise, cold air, salicylates and exercise. In patients with chronic, persistent asthma, results from clinical studies indicate that inhaled corticosteroids have a more consistent and greater average effect than antileucotriene drugs.[20]

The long-term safety of leukotriene modifiers is still not clear. Some patients reducing their oral corticosteroids when treatment with antileukotriene drugs has been initiated have developed a special type of vasculitis called Churg–Strauss syndrome. However, it might be the unmasking of a pre-existing condition and not induced by the leukotriene modifier *per se*.

MEASUREMENT SCALES

When measuring the status of the chronic obstructive airways disease in a subject we can rely either on data obtained at a visit to the clinic, or we can monitor the patient over a longer period by daily recordings at home.

At a visit to the clinic the primary focus is usually to obtain an objective, indirect, measure of airways narrowing – a lung function test. Such a test measures some functional index of the airway calibre in some kind of experimental setting. We will discuss various such indices and experimental settings and what they measure.

In the latter case, long-term daily recordings, we provide the patient with a diary card and usually ask him/her to record twice daily information relating to symptoms of the disease under study. In addition patients are often given a device to obtain an objective measurement of lung function at home, traditionally a peak flow meter.

These two approaches are in no way mutually exclusive – in a long-term study we can make experimental manoeuvres of the first kind. As an example there is virtually no long-term asthma trial that does not measure FEV_1 on visits to the clinic. However, for the present discussion we consider experimental approaches and diary card approaches separately, except that single FEV_1 measurements at the clinic will be discussed along with diary cards.

Lung Function Measurements

Airway narrowing leads to an increased resistance to the airflow. The airway resistance can be measured directly with body plethysmography (in a 'body-box'), an expensive and rather complicated procedure. Another way of measuring lung function is by flow measurements, which uses much more inexpensive apparatus, a spirometer. However spirometric measurements, to be discussed below, depend not only on airways resistance, but also on lung volumes.

When doing a spirometric manoeuvre the patient takes a maximum deep breath and then exhales as rapidly as possible as much as possible. The spirometer records the exhaled volume as a function of time, $V(t)$. From this curve (Figure 22.1) a number of spirometric indices can be obtained. The most widely used measure is the forced expiratory volume in one second ($V(1)$, denoted FEV_1), followed by the forced vital capacity ($V(\infty)$, denoted FVC). If the expiratory effort has been markedly inadequate it is usually obvious from the trace.

By calculating numerically the derivative of $V(t)$ we obtain the expiratory airflow. Its maximum value, which usually occurs within 100 ms, is the peak expiratory flow (PEF). Often the spirometric result is shown by plotting the flow against the volume exhaled. From this curve we can identify both PEF and FVC (but not FEV_1), but can also define new measurements, like $FEF_{25\%}$, which is the flow when 25% of the FVC has been exhaled. Another measure of current interest is $FEF_{25-75\%}$, which is the amount of volume expired per second when the exhaled volume increased from 25% to 75% of FVC. It is considered to measure effects in the small airways.

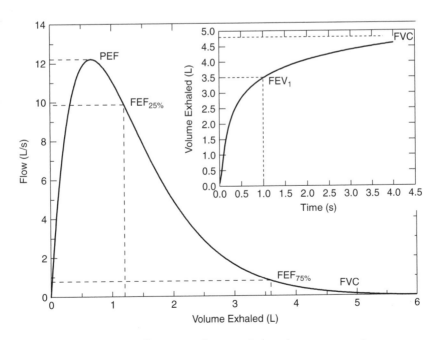

Figure 22.1. Illustration of some spirometric measurements

A full spirometric manoeuvre consists of measurement of the inspiratory part also. The inspiratory vital capacity (IVC) is a measure of the functional residual capacity (FRC) and is an important measure in COPD patients.

If performed correctly, the spirometric test is highly reproducible but somewhat effort-dependent. Different parameters are effort-dependent to different degrees: e.g. FEV_1 is less dependent than FVC, since it only needs maximum effort for 1 s. The direct measurement of airway resistance (R_{aw}), which is done in the body box, is effort-independent, but has a poor reproducibility. Since the spirometry has a good reproducibility, and uses fairly simple and portable equipment, it is most useful for clinical purposes. In special situations, however, the assessment of resistance might be preferable.

PEF is much more effort-dependent than FEV_1, but it can also be measured by a much cheaper apparatus than a spirometer. Such a peak flow meter is often provided to the patients for self-monitoring at home. Instructions are then given to fill in a diary card and to contact the healthcare service when PEF has dropped for a few consecutive days below prespecified levels. In the same way, PEF can be monitored with this simple device in a long-term study by recording, often twice daily, in a diary card.

There is a diurnal variation in FEV_1 and other lung function measurements. It is therefore important when comparing different such measurements obtained at different visits to the clinic for the same patient, that these measurements are taken at approximately the same time of the day.

Lung function measurements can be followed in order to assess effects, but also to characterise disease severity. However lung function is a function of both gender, age and 'size of patient'. Therefore a lung function parameter cannot be judged on an absolute scale – an FEV_1 of 2.4 L means different things for a young, tall boy and an old, tiny woman. A measure of disease severity would be the ratio of the actual FEV_1 and the would-be, and unmeasurable, FEV_1 the patient should have without the obstructive airway disease. As a remedy for the latter

various predicted formulas have been obtained for different lung function parameters. Thus, e.g., a key disease severity parameter is the FEV_1 in percent of predicted normal, both for asthma and COPD. There are a number of such formulae available, generally depending on demographic variables like race, gender, age and height.[22] It should be emphasised, however, that these measures cannot be anything but rather approximative ones, since the predicted normal values are not exact counterparts to the unknown lung function without disease! If the lung function is between 80% and 120% of the predicted normal value, it is in general considered to be 'normal'.

Another disease characteristic obtained from lung function measurements is the reversibility. This is an index obtained from a very simple single-dose monitoring experiment: we measure FEV_1, give a rapid-acting β_2-agonist and wait 30 min (typically) to measure FEV_1 again. The classical reversibility is then obtained as

$$\text{reversibility} = 100 \times \frac{FEV_1(\text{after}) - FEV_1(\text{before})}{FEV_1(\text{before})}$$

A value in excess of 15% was previously considered indicative of reversible airways obstruction, though later guidelines[21] use 12%. The basis for these numbers is somewhat unclear – it is probably chosen in order to be 'certain' that there is an effect: the variability in FEV_1 is such that a numerical increase *per se* is not a definite proof of an improved lung function.

Upper Airway Function Tests

There are also upper airway function tests similar to the lung function indices discussed above. They are however much less used, since symptom scores are considered of overriding importance in rhinitis studies. Resistance can be estimated by two different techniques: posterior rhinomanometry in which values are obtained by probes placed in the mouth, and anterior rhinomanometry in which a device in the nose is used. Less complicated, and expensive methods for assessing nasal patency rely on the measurement of peak nasal flow either on inspiration (PNIF) or expiration (PNEF). We do not discuss these methods in any further detail.

DESIGNS FOR EXPERIMENTAL ASTHMA TRIALS

For asthma studies, there are a number of experimental designs to measure various aspects of the therapeutic effect based on objective lung function measures. For this section, let E denote an index of lung function. In most real-life cases this is FEV_1, but the discussion is not restricted to this case.

We can group the designs in two groups: either the response after administration(s) of a study drug is followed, which can be done by time or by increasing doses, or the protective effect of the study drug to some provocation is assessed.

Single Dose Monitoring

This type of experiment is simple. Consider one individual on one occasion when this experiment is performed. We first take a baseline measurement, E_0, give the study drug and then follow lung function at predetermined timepoints after study drug administration. This provides us with an approximation of a response curve $E(t)$, where we use $E(0) = E_0$ (though technically it was obtained at a timepoint $t < 0$). From this curve a number of measures can be obtained for further analysis. The two most important measures derived from the curve $E(t)$ are

1. The average level, defined as area under the curve (of the polygonal approximation we have observed to the response curve) divided by observational time. This we denote by E_{av}.
2. The maximal level, E_{max}.

We can also compute t_{max}, the time at which E_{max} occurred. This is sometimes useful. Other potential measures are related to the concept responders 'onset of action' and 'duration of effect'. Tradition has it that for FEV_1, effect

is declared at a timepoint t if there is a 15% increase compared to baseline at that time. Based on such a concept, we can define: the time of onset as the timepoint (if any) at which the polygonal curve cuts the line $E = 1.15 \times E_0$ for the first time (for rapid-acting bronchodilators one usually added the restriction that this should occur within 30 min). The ending of effect occurs at the timepoint on the polygonal approximation which is followed by at least two observations below the line $E = 1.15 \times E_0$, provided that two measurements were taken. If only one was taken, that will suffice and if no measurement was found below the line, censor the end of effect to the last measured time. The duration is then the time from onset of action to end of effect.

The main problem with these definitions of onset and duration of action is not the arbitrary number 15%, but the fact that effect is measured by relating to baseline. This is not appropriate, since lung function has a clear diurnal variation. It might be a reasonable approximation for a few hours, the perceived time of clinical efficacy of a short-acting β_2-agonist, but will produce an incorrect result if used for a longer period. In fact, there are studies in which a patient receiving placebo as treatment has had a definite increase in lung function already on the first measurement after treatment administration (changes in the means – not individual spurious events), so the use of baseline as a reference when declaring effects should very much be questioned.

A related problem is to define responders. As the name suggests, a responder is a subject who responds to the treatment. Traditionally this has been decided based on the maximal increase from baseline. The discussion above implies that this is not necessarily a good way to go. To actually measure effect, we need to relate the measurements to the measurements obtained without drug administration. However, since asthma is not a stable disease, these must be taken simultaneously. And this is impossible! In clinical trials we do not really need this concept at all, except for descriptive purposes. We will return to the question of duration in the discussion of an example.

One lesson, however, from the discussion is that effect for many of these variables is often clinically measured as percent change. This means that

$$\Delta \text{effect} = \Delta E / E \approx \Delta \ln(E)$$

which by integration motivates why many lung function indices should be analysed on a logarithmic scale. We analyse these types of trials with multiplicative models, which is justified by this observation.

Challenge Tests

A challenge test is similar to the single dose monitoring test, except that most of the monitoring takes place after a provocation of some kind. Two important cases of challenge are exercise, either a treadmill test or using a cycle ergometer, and an allergen to which the patient is allergic. A baseline measurement E_0 is taken, often after administration of study drug. Then the provocation is done and lung function followed. In most cases there are two phases in the reaction found. First there is an immediate reaction with bronchoconstriction within minutes which lasts 1–2 hours. Several hours later there is a delayed reaction with a much slower and sustained time course.

Typically an exercise test is followed only during the immediate reaction, the actual existence of a delayed reaction is controversial. The protective effect of the study drug can be measured by maximal decrease in lung function from baseline:

$$Index_{EIB} = 100 \times (E_0 - E_{\min})/E_0$$

and we only need to follow the patient until we know he has attained the low turning point, whereafter he is given a high dose of a bronchodilator in order to restore lung function. Because of the intrinsic variability in lung function measurements spurious local minima can occur in the measurement series – it is important that the investigator has certified that the global minima has occurred before stopping. The most common lung function measurement here is again FEV_1. It should be noted that a better definition of the index would be $Index_{EIB} = 100 \times E_{\min}/E_0$, since then the analysis could be done on the multiplicative scale as discussed above!

For allergen challenge test we are more interested in the whole response for 10–12 hours, in order to study both the immediate reaction and the late reaction. The immediate reaction (EAR = early asthmatic reaction) is an episode of acute bronchoconstriction which peaks between 10 and 20 min after inhalation and resolves within 1.5–2 hours. The late reaction (LAR = late asthmatic reaction) is probably an inflammation mediated bronchoconstriction which starts about 3 hours after allergen inhalation and does not resolve for many hours. Allergen challenge tests are potentially dangerous, and are therefore not much favoured as a mode of studying asthma.

If they are, we need to measure FEV_1 repeatedly during the first hour, and then more sparsely during the next 7–8 hours (perhaps once an hour). The EAR is most often defined as the maximum percent reduction in FEV_1 (from baseline) occurring in the first hour after challenge, whereas the LAR is defined as the maximum percent reduction in FEV_1 (again from baseline) occurring between 3 and 7 hours after challenge. Alternatively we compute the area under the curve for the first hour and for the period between 3 and 7 hours after challenge and use that as an efficacy measure in much the same way as for the single dose monitoring experiment.

Hyperresponsiveness Studies

The level of airway responsiveness to a non-specific stimulus is measured by exposing subjects to the stimulus and measuring the response. There are a number of dialects of this test, by varying the selected stimulus, the mode of administration of it and the method of assessing the response.

The most commonly used stimuli are methacholine and histamine, though small doses of allergens can also be used. Methacholine and histamine produce similar responses, but the latter has more side-effects and can only be administered safely in concentrations up to 32 mg/ml, whereas methacholine can be used safely in concentrations up to 256 mg/ml (these numbers should be compared to the clinical definition of hyperresponsiveness which is that the provocation dose (PD_{20}, see below) is $\leq$ 8 mg/ml). The stimuli is administered from an aerosol which can be done in different ways. Suffice it to note that one can either do it with or without a dosimeter which controls the dose. Response is generally measured either as FEV_1 or as airway resistance (or its inverse, conductance).

Technically the subject first inhales saline and then inhales progressively increasing, often doubled, doses of the stimuli from the aerosol at 3-min intervals. There is a measurement after each dose administration, so we can consider the response to be a function of the last concentration or dose given. In both cases the saline inhalation produces the baseline value. From this dose–response curve (I call it that, though sometimes it is a concentration–response curve) different characteristics can be computed. A general dose–response curve is sigmoidal in shape which is well approximated with a loglinear portion over most of its response range. We can, however, not clinically obtain information on much more than the lower part of this dose–response curve, which means that traditional measures for dose–response curves (ED_{50} and slope) are not usually estimatable. We can think of the effect of the drugs as a parallel shift of the response curve so that if a given response is obtained with dose D without the drug, it takes dose ρD (with, hopefully, $\rho > 1$) to get that response with the drug. To estimate ρ in this type of study we fix a level, expressed as percent decrease in the response, and estimate the dose of stimuli needed to obtain that level. The dose which gives a decrease of $x\%$ in the response variable is denoted PD_x (or PC_x if we do not control doses). For FEV_1 we usually compute PD_{20}, whereas for R_{aw} a higher percentage can be used.

The actual algorithm for estimation of PD_x can vary. The following suggestion is justified by this description of the dose–response curve.

1. If there is a dose with less than $x\%$ decrease followed by a dose with more than $x\%$, loglinear interpolation (of log D vs. response) is done.
2. If the first dose provoked a fall in excess of $x\%$, we cannot do loglinear interpolation. In that case we do a linear interpolation back to baseline and obtain a dose corresponding to a fall of $x\%$ from this. However, we never go back more than to half the first dose given.
3. If the last dose produced a fall of less than $x\%$, we extrapolate loglinearly, but only up to twice the highest dose given.

What to use as dose can also be discussed. If we do not control the dose, we must use the concentration given. If we control the dose, we can choose to use cumulative doses or last dose without much difference in the final results, when provocation doses are compared (because for a geometric series, the sum is essentially proportional to the next dose, and we compare ratios). In general the use of the cumulative dose seems to be favoured.

The measure PD_{20} is not limited to the possible interpretation discussed above (as the relative dose potency ρ of the stimuli). If the effect is due to changes in both position and shape, the measure can still be used. For epidemiological purposes another index has been introduced, the two-point slope, which is the percent decline from baseline to last dose, divided by last dose. Though this index has a clear interpretation (as percent decrease per unit dose), this interpretation is wrong since the decrease is not linear with dose – instead it is virtually zero until it becomes linear with log-dose.

Note: It has been suggested that you cannot estimate PD_x if there has not been a fall of $x\%$. Technically this means that we should note it as missing. This might be sensible for the caring of the patient, where this is perceived as no hyper-responsiveness. However, for a clinical study, where treatments are compared, it is imperative to do an estimation. Setting it to missing means that the analysis loses the information that a high dose is needed to achieve the specified decrease!

EXERCISE TESTS IN COPD

Since a progressive decline in physical fitness is the main characteristic of COPD, exercise tests are useful for a proper evaluation of treatment effects in these patients. In these tests exercise can be either walking, running (treadmill tests) or bicycling. The basic design of the test can be, in its purest form

1. to determine the maximal workload sustainable, or
2. to fix the workload at some level, and determine the endurance time.

An example of the first kind is to measure the distance walked in a prespecified time, like 6 or 12 min. The second kind counterpart would be to fix (individually) the pace which at walking should be done and then measure time walked. It is believed that the second kind of experiment is more relevant in the study of COPD – that it correlates better with breathlessness and disability. The first kind of test is probably much influenced by attitude and expectation. We should also note that the second kind of test should provide a lower metabolic and respiratory stress than the first one and that the limiting factor in an exercise test does not have to be the physical fitness – COPD patients may well fail due to muscular fatigue before general fatigue.

In practice many tests used constitute a compromise between these two approaches: a specific time schedule is designed so that the work load is held fixed for some fixed time, then increased for 'a step' for another period of time, etc. Typical cycle-ergometry and treadmill tests have this design, as has the so-called shuttle walking test in which the patient walks at a given pace for one minute, then increases the pace for another minute, etc., all according to a well-defined protocol. The natural outcome of

these experiments is an endurance time, though for some cycle-ergometry tests you could alternatively use the total workload (but these should be heavily correlated).

For a comparison of some exercise tests in COPD, see Ref.[23].

In conjunction with these tests measurements of breathlessness are usually done. There are different tests available. A much used dyspnoea score is the Modified Borg scale,[24] in which dyspnoea is scored on a 0–10 scale before and after the exercise test. Alternatively one can use a visual analogue scale with the same effect. An alternative scale is the Transitional Dyspnoea Index,[25] for which we first rate three factors (functional impairment, magnitude of task and magnitude of effort) on baseline, each on scales 0–4 (well, 4–0 actually – the scale is reversed), and then rate the changes over the exercise directly on a scale from −3 to +3.

EXPOSURE STUDIES ON RHINITIS

For allergic rhinitis there are two study designs of the experimental type available. Both are exposure studies, one in the natural season, one in an artificial season:

1. The Park study. In this study the subjects are exposed to pollen over a 1–2 day period by walking around in a park. There are two main problems with this type of study – it is highly dependent on season and the patients often find it very boring.
2. The experimental Nasal Allergen Challenge Artificial Season model. In this type of study the subjects are artificially exposed to pollen for some period. This can be either as spray application for a few consecutive days, or in an Environmental Exposure Unit (EEU) in which subjects are exposed to pollen in a special room for, typically, 3 hours on a number of consecutive days. In this room there is a flow of air to which the pollen is added and evenly distributed in the air by fans.

In both cases we measure nasal symptoms as outcome variable. Both these studies are parallel groups in design, but effects can often be demonstrated with rather small patient numbers.

LONG-TERM CLINICAL STUDIES WITH DIARY CARDS

In a diary card study, the patient is provided with a diary card to fill in various information about the status of his disease under investigation, often twice daily. For most asthma/COPD studies, the patients also measure PEF. It is important that the patient uses the same peak flow meter throughout the study, since different brands have different scales, and there is a considerable within-brand variability as well. In addition to this, some symptom scoring is requested. This can be either an overall assessment of symptoms, or assessments of specific symptoms, like wheezing, shortness of breath and cough for asthma. Finally, for asthma/COPD studies, the use of rescue medication, usually a short-acting β_2-agonist, should be entered into the diary card. With the increased use of IT, paper-based diary cards are more and more replaced with electronic counterparts, which has the potential benefit of monitoring when the recordings are done. Some such devices can also contain a spirometer, which makes it possible to replace the somewhat variable PEF measurement with the more accepted FEV_1 measurement. The fact that the electronic device can be programmed so that it only accepts data obtained at the timepoint when it should be obtained, increases the validity of this type of data. The FEV_1 measurements recorded with a portable spirometer should be more valid than PEF data obtained by a peak flow meter and manually recorded on a paper-based diary card. Our discussion will primarily relate to the old paper-based diary cards with a concomitant peak flow meter. We leave it to the reader to assess potential changes that occur for electronically fetched data.

In terms of basic design we have two types of long-term clinical studies in asthma:

1. Studies in which treatments are fixed throughout the period under investigation. An arm in

such an study might be, e.g., budesonide Turbuhaler 200 μg b.i.d.

2. Studies in which the treatment is not fixed throughout the period under investigation. In such studies we can either vary the dose of the investigational product, or vary the dose of some concomitant treatment. One typical such study has an arm in which treatment is initiated with a high dose of a given GCS, which is then reduced according to some scheme until the patient is no longer controlled on the present dose. A variant are the steroid sparing studies, in which a fixed dose of some investigational treatment is given throughout the study period and concomitant with this treatment some GCS is given, the dose of which is then reduced in steps. For inhaled GCS, oral steroid sparing studies have been performed in this way, for other anti-inflammatory drugs like leukotriene modifiers inhaled steroid sparing studies are relevant.

The usage of the diary card data varies between these two types of data. In studies with fixed treatments they define the primary efficacy variables, whereas in studies with varying treatment doses, dose changes are conditioned on the diary card variables and these therefore act only as control variables.

Diary card data in a long-term clinical study often represents a considerable amount of data, as measured in megabytes on disk. The number of megabytes, however, does not truly reflect its information value. Data is not obtained in a very controlled fashion. Morning values are generally considered slightly sharper than evening values, since sleep is comparatively similar among patients and data should be obtained and recorded immediately after waking up.

For that reason, peak flow obtained in the morning is often considered the primary variable of interest in a long-term diary card study on asthmatics. The day-to-day variability, for a symptomatic asthmatic, can be considerable. However, using the mean of all values over a prespecified period, as long as possible, generally provides us with a measure that has proven to be useful in many clinical studies. An alternative efficacy measure is to use FEV_1 measurements obtained at visits to the clinic. Though each individual FEV_1 measurement so obtained is much more reliable than a single PEF measurement, the overall mean over a treatment period of daily recorded PEF measurements obtained in the morning is, in our experience, a more efficient variable for demonstrating differences between treatments in lung function. Since most treatments are mainly symptomatic, integrated measures over time are the relevant 'endpoint' measures.

When using FEV_1 obtained at visits to the clinic as primary variable in a long-term clinical trial, we must take the diurnal variation of lung function into account. Thus it is important that FEV_1 is measured at approximately the same time of day on each visit. To obtain maximal efficiency we also need to schedule the patients for visits to the clinic early in the morning (around 8 a.m.), with approximately the same argument as given for peak flow morning measurements above. The possibility of enforcing this will very much determine the effectiveness of the FEV_1 variable in discriminating between treatments.

In COPD studies lung function is also of interest, but for this disease the symptomatic benefit is stressed more. For COPD, rating of night sleep, breathlessness, coughing and chest tightness seem to be accepted symptoms to include in diary cards.

For rhinitis, the symptoms recorded are nasal blockage, rhinorrhea, sneezing and/or itchy nose which sometimes are combined into the nasal index score, which is the sum of them. In addition to this, eye symptoms are recorded as a secondary variable. The most readily available objective measure in the clinical trial setting is either the Peak Nasal Inspiratory Flow (PNIF) or Peak Nasal Expiratory Index. Of these the PNIF parameter seems to be the most discriminative.

The data in diary cards can be used in different ways to compute variables for use in statistical comparisons. As already indicated, in fixed dose studies period mean values are often computed, not only of PEF measurements, but also of symptom scores and of the use of rescue medication. Because of the intrinsic variability in the underlying disease it is important to compute means over long periods, preferably the full treatment period. This means that, for some drugs at least, the mean will contain data from a period of onset of action, though the effect of that will be minor in long-term studies.

Mean values of symptom scores do not seem very meaningful to most clinicians in assessing the actual response. An alternative is to compute the percentage of symptom-free days, which is somewhat simpler to interpret clinically. Similarly it might be useful to compute the percentage of days with no rescue medication.

When many symptoms are recorded individually, one approach to the analysis of the data is to compute the sum of the symptoms (as the nasal index score), but an alternative is to analyse them simultaneously in a multivariate analysis.

Even more useful, sometimes, is to collect data within a day, or adjacent days, to form new measures. One simple such measure for asthma is to define a patient to have control of the asthma, if there are no symptoms and the patient did not use rescue medication. The percentage of such days with asthma control can be a useful summary measure for some patient populations, typically rather mild ones. A variant of this is to define mild exacerbations, or episodes, of asthma from diary cards by looking for worsening of lung function and/or increase in rescue consumption and/or symptoms. The exact criteria for such episodes probably need to be adjusted to the patient population under study, and to the study design. In order to avoid spurious events, it might be a good idea to define an event to have occurred for two consecutive days in order to be labelled an episode. From an analysis point of view we can analyse time to first such exacerbation or the percentage of episode-free days. Analysis of exacerbation is even more relevant in COPD studies than in asthma studies.

One final note on response data in studies on asthmatic patients, especially PEF, and the disease asthma in general. When we interpret diary card data, obtained over a longer period, we must interpret it on a group mean level. A discussion on individual responders is virtually meaningless. A responder refers to a patient that responds to the investigational treatment. This cannot be assessed on the basis of diary card data, since the underlying disease is, by definition, varying – what seems to be a clear response could well be a period of good asthma control totally unrelated to drug effect (in some cases a study effect) and the converse. This is obvious once one has inspected placebo data in a long-term study. However this does not exclude that one can define responders according to some criteria and compare percent responders between treatments, since that is a comparison on group level.

So far we have considered studies with fixed treatments during the investigational period. In a study which tries to identify the minimal dose on which the patient is controlled, the obvious endpoint for analysis is this minimal dose. This is true irrespective of whether the dose in question refers to the investigational drug or to some concomitant drug (as e.g. in the oral sparing studies alluded to above).

More explicit examples of this will be demonstrated later.

QUALITY OF LIFE

Asthma and COPD are chronic disorders that can place considerable restrictions on the physical, emotional and social aspects of the lives of patients. Assessments of the patient's own perception of the impact of asthma on their life, of general well-being, is known as measurement of quality of life. Quality of life may be useful for assessing the degree of morbidity, e.g. in order to evaluate the health economic impact of the diseases in the community. It is assessed by questionnaires that include a large set of physical and psychological characteristics assessing the general functioning and well-being in the context of lifestyle. Quality of life scales are either general and not specifically designed for patients with asthma or COPD, or they are more specific disease-related but, as of today, in general not applicable to the general population due to cultural differences.

General health status scales such as the Sickness Impact Profile with 136 items[26] have been proposed. A compromise between lengthy questionnaires and single-item measures of health has also been proposed. The Nottingham Health Profile with 45 items and SF-36 (a Measures of Sickness short-form general health survey) are now widely used and validated. The SF-36 Health Status Questionnaire is based on 36 items selected to represent eight health concepts (physical, social and role functioning; mental health; health perception; energy/fatigue; patin; and general health).[27] Its quality of life scales have been shown to correlate with the severity of asthma, but it has yet to demonstrate any superiority over the simpler, diary card-based symptom scores for demonstrating effect in clinical trials.

For COPD the St. George's Respiratory Questionnaire has gained importance in later years. It is perhaps the most comprehensive questionnaire for evaluation of quality of life in airways diseases and allows for direct numerical comparisons to be made among patients, study populations and therapies, and has sensitivity when applied to mild as well as severe disease.[28] It was developed by Paul Jones at St. George's Hospital in London in 1990 and is designed to measure impact on overall health, daily life and perceived well-being. The measure consists of 50 (76 responses) items that produce three domain scores and one overall score. The domains are: symptoms (severity and frequency), activity (that cause or are limited by breathlessness) and impact (on social life and psychological disturbances caused by the airways disease).

CLINICAL TRIAL METHODS

HOW TO AVOID BIAS

Blinding

Most effect measurements of the respiratory diseases discussed here are influenced to a non-negligible degree by the patients' expectations. One typical example of this is that in some double-blind, placebo-controlled single dose trials measuring bronchodilation, there is an immediate response in lung function also in the placebo group, which probably is due to (false) expectations. The classical methods to avoid expectation bias, blinding and randomisation, are therefore important. A clinical study in this area should follow a double-blind approach in which study drugs are prepacked in accordance with a suitable randomisation schedule, and supplied to the trial centre(s) labelled only with the subject number and the treatment period so that no one involved in the conduct of the trial is aware of the specific treatment allocated to any particular subject, not even as a code letter.[29] The code should not be broken until all decisions concerning data validity have been taken and documented.

Many studies in the respiratory area concern inhalation products, where there are not only, say, two different drugs involved, but also two different inhalers (or perhaps one drug in two different inhalers). To maintain blinding in those situations one often needs to resort to the 'double-dummy' technique. This means that for each inhaler there has to be two clones: one with active drug and one with placebo. On each inhalation occasion, the subject has to inhale not only from the inhaler with active substance, but also from the other inhalers, but containing placebo. This might lead to a large number of inhalations per occasion, which in turn might lead to incomplete compliance. Note that the use of different inhalers implies a consideration on the order in which these should be taken. Carry-over effects from one type of inhaler might dictate which should be taken first/last, whereas in other situations a balanced scheme might be called for.

Rhinitis studies pose a special problem in terms of blinding because the double dummy technique is not considered appropriate – there is a fear that additional placebo material may clear the airways of drug so that the response is different with and without simultaneous placebo administration. This is a problem mainly when two different drugs inhaled through different devices are to be compared. The partial remedy that is most often used is to include a placebo group, and let half the group have one device and the other half the other device. That way, at least, the patient does not know whether he gets active drug or not.

Open labelled studies might be acceptable for some systemic effects studies where the outcome variable is the plasma concentrations of some marker, or in long-term safety studies.

Randomisation

Studies in respiratory diseases must also be properly randomised, so that prognostic factors are distributed between groups by chance alone, which minimises selection bias. For many outcome variables some prognostic factors are known, and it is important for the credibility of the result that the choice of group for individual patients has not been made by the investigator. The observed outcome can still be due to an imbalance of prognostic factors between groups, but randomisation at least means that this was produced by chance alone, not by the parties involved in the study (provided the study is also blinded).

By the way, this last point is why it is meaningless to do group comparability testing at baseline. The p-value computed from a statistical test is a measure of how certain one is that the 'null hypothesis' is wrong, how improbable the result is assuming that the null hypothesis is true. For a test comparing baseline data (i.e. data obtained before randomisation), say the mean, for two treatments, the p-value is a measure of how unlikely the observed group mean difference is. If this is small, say $p < 5\%$, this means that an unlikely event has occurred, or that the groups are not equal on average. However, if we trust our randomisation procedures, there is no factor that can explain why the two groups should not be equal except for chance alone, so we must conclude that an unlikely event has occurred. The unlikely event, i.e. the difference observed at baseline, might have consequences on the results. But the extent of that effect does not depend on the p-value of a test at baseline, it depends on the correlation of the effect variable with the baseline variable in question. This means that a large baseline difference might have no consequences at all, or a small difference at baseline might have large consequences. In the respiratory area it is very rare that the latter is the case. If observed differences at baseline causes concern, the robustness of the results should be checked with respect to this issue, not a separate test at baseline.

Other Sources of Bias

Another way to risk selection bias, also in a randomised, double-blind study, is to exclude data obtained on treatment. To exclude patients on data obtained prior to first dose cannot in itself produce bias. However the prognostic factors for respiratory trials, like FEV_1 in percent of predicted normal and reversibility, are only estimates of time-varying entities and are not precise enough that we can actually claim that a patient violating some inclusion criteria is not necessarily an appropriate patient for the trial. They are essential in order to focus the investigator on the appropriate patient population, but once a violation to the protocol criteria has emerged it might be appropriate to use the patient in the statistical analysis. With Senn,[30] I consider the protocol a guide to the physician, not the statistician.

Protocol violations after the first dose should not in general invalidate the patient for the statistical analysis. If such a protocol violation is confounded with treatment effects, their omission might bias the result. However, the fact that they are protocol violations might in itself imply that the measurements are improper measurements, which is another type of bias. This problem is illustrated in respiratory trials by the use of rescue medication.

During an asthma or COPD trial patients are usually provided with short-acting β_2-agonists to use as rescue medication. This means that some measurements of lung function and symptoms will be influenced by this add-on therapy, and the validity of those measurements (as direct treatment measures) will therefore be questioned. If treatments have the same effect they pose no

problem, since they should occur with similar frequency in different groups. However, a more effective treatment is expected to have less consumption of rescue medication. As a consequence there is a bias towards no effect by including those measurements when computing period means for instance. If we ignore them (i.e. consider them to be missing) we introduce a bias in the same direction, since we only count the days when the patient was, relatively speaking, symptom-free. There seems to be no easy way out of this dilemma, and the approach we have taken is to ignore the additional information on recently taken rescue medication for the analysis, but instead plot, descriptively only, for each day the proportion of patients that takes rescue close enough to peak flow measurement. Hopefully, and this is usually the case, the main result and this graph gives the same message on effect. At least this approach should be conservative.

TRIAL DESIGN CONSIDERATIONS

From a bird's-eye perspective, there are two types of responses for respiratory diseases:

1. Immediate responses that disappear within a short period of time. This includes the fast bronchodilating effect of β_2-agonists, responses to various provocations and specific systemic effects that are measured by markers in the blood (like plasma cortisol for glucocorticosteroids and serum potassium for β_2-agonists). Many of these studies are single dose studies.
2. Long term studies addressing effects on symptoms or average lung function of the underlying condition.

Crossover Trials

For the first type of studies, the crossover design is well suited. In such a study each subject is randomised to a sequence of treatments, and acts as his own control for treatment comparisons. In many cases this is attractive, because the within-subject variability is smaller than the between-subject variability which means that a smaller study is required for the same power, as compared to a parallel group study. Numerous variations exist, e.g. trials in which each subject receives only a subset of the treatments studied (incomplete design), and trials where the same treatment is repeated within a subject.

However, there are caveats with crossover studies. The primary caveat is the possible presence of carry-over effects (in fact, non-equal carry-over effects), which might bias treatment comparisons. When deciding if a crossover design is appropriate for a particular study, we therefore must convince ourself, beforehand, that we can get rid of possible carry-over effects by separating the various treatment periods with washout periods during which no treatment is given. For a single-dose short-acting β_2-agonist trial a washout period need in general only be a few days. A trial which studies cortisol depression after short periods of GCS administration should have washout periods of 1–2 weeks, though shorter ones are acceptable in single dose studies.

When periods in crossover trials contain repeated dosing over a few weeks, and the actual experiment is performed at the end of such a period, it is often unnecessary to have drug-free washout periods between periods. But to take that step, one must make plausible that taking a new treatment directly after another does not by itself have any effects on the variables to analyse.

Parallel Group Trials

Since the treatment for respiratory diseases in general is to achieve a prolonged improvement of the underlying condition, the most important trials need to extend over longer periods. The most natural design for them is the parallel group design, where the subjects are randomised to one of a number of arms, each arm being allocated a different treatment. These treatments will include the investigational product at one or more doses, possibly including a placebo (dose = 0) arm, and possibly some active control treatments at one or more doses.

Sequential Trials

Sequential trials are not much used in the respiratory area. A long-term study can obviously not be done this way, since the total study period would be enormous. For experimental studies, on the other hand, the setup is often of such complexity that the clinic need to have clear specifications on patient numbers before the start of the study for their planning.

Interim Analysis

Interim analyses should not be needed in trials in the respiratory area, except possibly for first dose in man studies on new drugs – but then it is a drug issue and not a therapeutic area issue. Interim surveys of safety data might well be justified in the beginning of clinical programmes, but for efficacy issues they are seldom needed.

HANDLING OF MISSING VALUES

The experimental type of studies are often very difficult to perform clinically. To get good quality data, it is extremely important that the investigator with staff has a good knowledge and experience in this type of study. It is in general better to do such studies in one or two experienced centres with many patients, as compared to using many centres with fewer patients – despite the fact that the study might take longer to perform. With those premises missing values are, in our experience, a negligible problem since in general experimental sequences are complete. When missing values occur, they are due to discontinuations between experimental sessions and these are few and there is no problem in analysing the resulting unbalanced study.

It is a completely different issue with the long-term clinical studies. Here patients not only discontinue treatment, but there are also missing observations during the period. For the fixed treatment trial the purpose is in general to achieve a steady state, on group level, on the treatment and then compare the level of the measured variable in steady state between groups. For patients reaching steady state we therefore in general have a number of data points measuring steady state level, in the case of diary cards quite a few. The efficacy variable is then usually a summary statistic of these data points, like a period mean of a diary card variable. Missing values during this period does therefore not constitute a major problem – we take the mean of available data.

Sometimes a long-term clinical study contains experimental procedures, like a methacholine provocation test. Or just spirometry at the clinical visit, at least FEV_1. This is then done at least once pre-randomisation and then again only a few times on treatment, in particular on the last protocol visit. The effect variable should not be defined as the change from baseline to last protocol visit, but as the change from baseline to the last visit on treatment the patient attended. Specifically, instead of analysing the change in $\log PD_{20}$ from visit 2 to visit 8, we define the efficacy variable as the change from visit 2 to the last visit on treatment, which might be visit 4, 6 or 8 in a particular study. Technically this is equivalent to what is called the last value carried forward, or the last value extended, principle, but there is no need to use that label if we define the efficacy variable appropriately.

This still leaves us with one key problem – what if we do not have any efficacy measurements on treatment to use. To avoid that problem in diary card studies, it is often better to define the full treatment period as the period over which to compute summary statistics. At least that provides an effect measurement for each individual who has started to fill in the diary cards. The drawback is that the period mean for one patient can be the mean of 90 data points, whereas for another it is the mean of only a few data points. The next step is in general to analyse these period means with an ANOVA, and then the information of the precision of the computed mean is lost. On balance, it seems better to have an effect measurement on each patient.

For data obtained on clinical visits, the risk of having no measurement at all on treatment is not negligible. The omission of such patients from the analysis means that there might be a potential bias in the end result. To understand this, assume that there are no withdrawals in group A, but half the patients withdraw from group B because of insufficient efficacy. The remaining patients in group B are then the ones who needed less treatment. That patient group has a corresponding subgroup in group A of approximately the same size (as a consequence of proper blinding and randomisation procedures), but group A also contains another subgroup of patients, corresponding to the ones that dropped out from group B. The remaining groups are therefore not really comparable, and inference drawn from available data might be misleading!

However, there is no simple, trustworthy, remedy for this. Our approach is to use available data for the analysis, hoping that the potential bias is conservative (which it probably is in most cases for respiratory trials). However, if there is a large difference in withdrawal rates between the groups, it is logical to do the primary analysis on withdrawal data to assert group differences.

When describing diary card data, daily mean value curves by treatment are useful. When computing these mean values, missing values pose great problems in that raw mean values can produce very misleading impressions on group behaviour. To see why, consider a placebo arm in a diary card study in asthma in which the patients with worsening of symptoms drop out progressively (the worse the symptoms, the earlier they drop out). As the patients with low response values drop out, the group mean will increase, so the temporal behaviour of the mean values will indicate that the placebo group increases in effect with time. However, this effect is solely due to withdrawals!

To avoid this culprit when plotting the temporal behaviour of variables some kind of imputation of data is needed, in order to keep the denominator the same when computing mean values within a treatment group. The simplest such imputation is to use the last value extended (LVE) approach, in which the last value for a withdrawal is extended to later timepoints. Using this principle, the mean values plotted can be interpreted as follows: the mean at time t is the mean of the last recorded measurements up to and including time t. When using this principle for diary card variables like PEF it is often better not to take only the last measurement, but rather a mean of a few measurements. More sophisticated approaches based on some kind of multiple imputation technique for missing data can also be considered, but the add-on value of doing that is probably very small for the average study in respiratory diseases.

MULTIPLE COMPARISONS

A respiratory trial usually contains a number of effect variables, and often also a number of different treatments. Thus there are multiple comparisons to be done. This poses a major problem, because of the risk of over-emphasising fluke significances because of many comparisons.

To handle the many effect variables we therefore have to predefine which one is to be considered the primary one. It is from the result on this variable that the overall statistical conclusion from the study can be drawn. In general one study can have a few different objectives that are not closely related (like efficacy and safety), and then a primary variable for each objective should be appropriate. However, it is probably a too statistical approach to focus only on the primary variable when trying to understand the results of a clinical trial. No variable fetches all aspects of a respiratory disease, and the approach should be to select the most sensitive variable as primary variable, to decide on the overall conclusion, but then a number of secondary variables should be so described that one gets an overall picture of what is 'going on'.

When it comes to the problem of multiple treatment comparisons, the study logic should be structured in terms of well spelled out objectives. To prove efficacy might mean one comparison, to estimate a relative dose potency another analysis. With precisely formulated questions the multiplicity problem here should at least diminish substantially. This approach will be illustrated in what follows.

SAMPLE SIZE DETERMINATIONS

In order to certify that a proposed study is of an appropriate size, a sample size justification is needed in the protocol. It cannot be justified ethically to succumb a number of patients to a study protocol if there is no hope whatsoever to demonstrate what you want to demonstrate. Similarly, if the study is heavily overdimensionalised we have put an unnecessary number of patients at whatever risk the study can carry with it, and that is not ethical too. However, sample size determination is there to ethically justify the study in advance – it has no consequences when the results are obtained.

In the respiratory area many test hypotheses are stated in terms of mean values, and for such variables the sample size is (essentially) proportional to the ratio $(\sigma/\Delta)^2$, where σ is the residual standard deviation and Δ is the mean difference we do not want to miss. When using a multiplicative model for a variable, these entities refer to the logarithm of the variable in question. Note that σ means different things in a crossover trial and in a parallel group trial – in the former case it refers to a within-patient variability (more exactly $\sqrt{2}\times$ the residual standard deviation of the ANOVA) and in the latter to a between-patient variability. Also what is relevant is the residual standard deviation from the proposed analysis of variance, which might contain a baseline adjustment.

The following table shows some typical values of the sample size parameters that can be used for asthma trials. Each example will be discussed in more detail below.

Increase in	Design	σ	Δ	$(\sigma/\Delta)^2$
PEF morning (L/min)	PG	40–45	10–20	4–20
Symptom score (0–3 scale)	PG	0.4–0.5	0.05–0.15	6–100
FEV_1 (L)	PG	0.4–0.5	0.05–0.1	15–100
$\ln(AUC\ FEV_1)$ (L)	XO	0.07–0.10	0.05–0.10	0.5–4
$^2\log(PD_{20})$	XO	0.9–1.1	1–2	0.8–4

Here the range is not a range – the lower number for σ represents an optimistic number, the larger number a conservative one. Similarly, for Δ the range is more of a typical range for which to dimensionalise, not a range on what can be obtained. To obtain numbers (per group in the parallel group case) from this we should multiply by approximately 25.

For the crossover measurements of the table, we just note that the AUC refers to AUC-based average over the full period and that for that variable the pre-dose FEV_1 value is used as covariate in the analysis. For the PD_{20} case no baseline covariate is used.

For the parallel group measurements we use baseline covariate. For PEF morning a baseline is obtained as the mean value over a number of measurements, typically 1–2 weeks, and then the effect variable as the mean of 1–3 months of data. The shorter the periods, the larger the residual standard deviation. Similarly, for FEV_1 the table refers to a measurement both at baseline and end of treatment, but the treatment value could well be a mean of a number of measurements. Moreover, the FEV_1 data refers to the situation when visits to the clinic are spread out over the morning, the European style, as discussed earlier. With visits scheduled at 8 a.m. precisely larger effects can be expected.

Concerning symptoms scores, these too are obtained from period means of diary card data, and relate to a typical asthma study. Changes in symptom scores are often small in studies in asthmatics with mild–moderate severity, since they do not have many symptoms on entry. In rhinitis studies a combination of symptom scores is often done. If we use the TNS discussed earlier we typically have a standard deviation of about 1.3 and effect sizes of 0.5–1, giving a $(\sigma/\Delta)^2$ of 2–8. Typically, therefore, rhinitis studies can be smaller than asthma studies.

For COPD, exacerbation rates are more important as outcome variable. A rate of one exacerbation per year can be used in sample size calculations.

SUBGROUP ANALYSIS

When doing statistics on trials in respiratory medicine, the question of subgroup analysis inevitably presents itself, as in so many areas of medical statistics. It is however no more sensible to do such analysis on data on lung function than in the general case.[30] Ultimately it has to do with the generalisability of the results of a trial.

In airways diseases, asthma in particular, the disease severity varies among patients. Thus the magnitude of the response attainable will vary between patients. How much will partly depend on what we measure. If we measure lung function, patients with small lungs, like little women, will be expected to have smaller numerical effects than patients with large lung volumes, like tall men. This does not mean that the actual benefit to the patient is less, only that the outcome variable suffers from this deficiency. We could remedy this partially by measuring lung function in percent of predicted normal, which tries to capture size differences, instead. But that is only a partial remedy to a larger problem – that there is a large heterogeneity in response sizes for some outcome variables, which does not necessarily reflect different clinical responses. Compliance to study procedures might also influence the measured responses.

This heterogeneity in the disease population is not a problem for the proper conclusions of a clinical trial. Consider a randomised parallel group study in which treatments A and B are compared. If properly conducted observed treatment differences should be explained by different treatment effects alone, and any claim from the study should relate to the relative effect of the two treatments. If it turns out that the effects differ, say, between men and women, that should not jeopardise the outcome of the trial, since a proper randomisation implies that the sex distribution is similar in the two groups. We get problems only when we try to compare effect sizes between studies. Differences in effect sizes could well be explained not only by different patient populations, including gender distribution, but also by different compliance to study procedures in the trials.

This discussion implies that estimated treatment effects, at least for lung function variables, should be interpreted with caution. It is often much better to try to transform the information on the effect scale to a dose scale, as will be extensively discussed in sections to come.

Another implication of the discussion is that if we start to compare different subgroups in an asthma trial we can expect to find different responses. One such example is the multi-centre trial, in which we have many centres, often from different countries, with different patient populations and medical traditions. Different effect sizes should not come as a surprise, and do not necessarily indicate interpretational problems in terms of overall effects. We would also expect that if we compare the effects in a subgroup of mild asthmatics to a subgroup of more severe asthmatics within the trial, they will not be identical.

Subgroup analysis will by definition be less powered than the analysis of the full analysis data set. As a consequence, subgroup analysis is not a sensible thing to do in a single trial, unless well specified in advance, and then the study size should be large enough for this subgroup analysis. If not specified in advance, the risk of a fluke significance because of the ever-present multiplicity problem is too large, leading to false conclusions.

However, subgroup analysis is in general totally unnecessary. If we want to see if the response differs between men and women, as an example, the proper approach is not to analyse the subgroup of men and the subgroup of women separately. It is to analyse the full data set with an interaction factor for treatment and sex. If this interaction test is statistically significant, we know that there is a difference in the response for men and women. We can even quantify it, if we so choose. Similar adjustments can be done for disease indices like lung function in percent of predicted normal or reversibility. But the add-on value of doing this remains to be proven, except that it might reduce the residual variance in the analysis of variance model.

PHASE I/II STUDIES

EFFICACY STUDIES

In terms of efficacy, not much can be done in a phase I trial. These trials, mainly concerned with tolerability and pharmacokinetics, give no real clue to whether a new drug actually works or not. Note that in general a respiratory drug must be very well tolerated to be useful, since there are so many efficacious and safe drugs on the market.

When trying to establish that a new drug is effective in asthma or not and to estimate clinically relevant doses, the approach differs between the drugs that have more or less immediate effect on lung function, typically bronchodilators, and the ones that work more indirectly on lung function, via the inflammatory process, as glucocorticosteroids. For bronchodilators we can use small-scale experimental studies, whereas for anti-inflammatory drugs we typically need long-term studies from the very start.

To establish efficiency is conceptually simple: all we need to do is to show that a given dose of the drug is superior to placebo. There is however no true placebo treatment in long-term asthma or COPD trials – at a minimum the patients need to be provided a short-acting β_2-agonist to be used as rescue medication. All new drugs are therefore studied on top of some baseline treatment, which in most cases is not very constant. For example, a GCS treatment is taken in addition to rescue medication. It potentially becomes a problem when you want to introduce a new rescue treatment, which is to be taken when needed, and you need to document long-term effects.

The next question, possibly posed in the same study, is which is the relevant dose-span for further investigation? For a dose–response study (including the simple one with only placebo and one dose) the choice of patients is important. The majority of asthmatics, the mild ones, do not need much therapy and because of the relative imprecision in the measurement tools, many patients will have no measurable response in many of the tests discussed. For a bronchodilator study of the crossover type, where the design contains a number of experimental days when response is followed after a dose, some bronchoconstriction is needed in order to see an effect. By definition the bronchoconstriction varies with time for an asthmatic, so the measured response will not only depend on the dose of the bronchodilator, but also on the degree of airway narrowing on the particular day the experiment is done. Thus it is difficult to assess efficacy for the individual patient, which we handle in clinical studies by considering means. But more importantly, in order to achieve dose–response we need sufficiently many patients with sufficiently many days on which they can respond. The selection of such patients is not easy!

For long-term diary card studies we have a similar problem. The effect measures are rather noisy, and we generally need somewhat large studies to measure a signal through all the noise. In parts of the world with a widespread health care system most asthmatics are rather well treated. In particular the use of GCS already in fairly mild asthma in Europe, Australia and Canada seems to have made the majority of asthmatics more or less symptom-free for most of the time. That in turn means that the traditional diary card might have difficulty in catching any responses.

From the foregoing discussion it should be clear that the magnitude of response in a particular variable is very difficult to assess: if it is small, is it because the patients studied did not have much room for improvement or was it because the drug was of minor efficacy? The only way, it seems, to actually assess the degree of response is to compare it to something we know, by experience, to work – to include an active control in the clinical trial. In my personal view, a clinical dose – response trial in asthmatics without an active control has very little information value. Also note that we should not need placebo in order to prove efficacy – it should suffice if we could prove that there is a dose–response relationship (this is in fact the point with the expression 'show dose–response': to prove that the drug has a pharmacological

effect). This does not rule out (if the slope is positive) that small doses have a negative effect and larger doses a positive effect, something that should be borne in mind when interpreting the result.

What can be done in a placebo-controlled dose–response study without an active control is to estimate the minimal effective dose (MED). This addresses the question: 'Which is the lowest dose, of those studied, that is proven effective' and tests, in a recursive manner to control significance level, the doses from highest to lowest with placebo. There are a number of algorithms available that can be used, but the key point about MED is that it is the lowest dose that we *from this study* can claim is effective. Thus the result depends heavily on the size of the study and choice of patient population, a property the average physician probably would not like MED to have. Thus there is a great danger in using MED as defined here for decision making. In my view MED is more likely to lead to false decisions than correct ones.

The information we actually want from a dose–response study is the shape of the dose–response curve, to allow us to pick the 'best' dose. Not a detailed shape, a simple approximation which can be used to derive insights from. As long as there is a monotonous dose–response curve a more complicated description than the one provided by the formula

$$E = E_0 + E_{\max}/(1 + (ED_{50}/D)^{\gamma}) \qquad (1)$$

is rarely needed. This formula contains four parameters: E_0 is the baseline level of the response variable, corresponding to placebo. $E_{\max}$ is the maximal effect attainable, ED_{50} is the dose required to obtain 50% of this and finally, γ is a sensitivity parameter which measures how much the response changes with changes in dose. The shape of this function is a sigmoidal curve with the extremely important property that over much of the range (say from $E_0 + 0.2E_{\max}$ to $E_0 + 0.8E_{\max}$) it can be well approximated by a straight line $E = a + b \ln D$. A description of such a dose–response curve should be the purpose of the dose–response trial, not to discuss the individual doses that were actually chosen to be used in the study.

Identifying the dose–response curve, however, does not give you a hint on how well the treatment compares to competing treatments. For that purpose it is wise to include an active control in the trial. We can then use the dose–response curve to estimate the dose of the new drug that produces the same effect as the active control does, hopefully with confidence limits.

Example: Bronchodilation

The bronchodilating effects of two long-acting β_2-agonists, we call them A and B, each with its own inhalation device, were compared by giving single dose administrations, followed by repeated measurements of FEV_1 over a 12-hour period. The following five treatments were

studied in a randomised, double-blind, double-dummy crossover study: 6, 12 and 24 μg of drug A, 50 μg of drug B and placebo.

In Figure 22.2 we see the geometric mean values, expressed as percent increase from the measurement taken prior to treatment administration. The reason for plotting geometric, and not arithmetic, means is that results are often to be expressed as percent increases, and then data should be analysed on a logarithmic scale and geometric means are therefore more natural than arithmetic ones. As a consequence, differences are unnatural entities to discuss and should be replaced by ratios.

To actually analyse the data we want some overall summary statistic that includes both the maximal effect and the duration of response and we use the area-based average $FEV_{1,av}$ over 12 hours. If we want to keep the idea of analysing on a multiplicative scale, we need to compute the

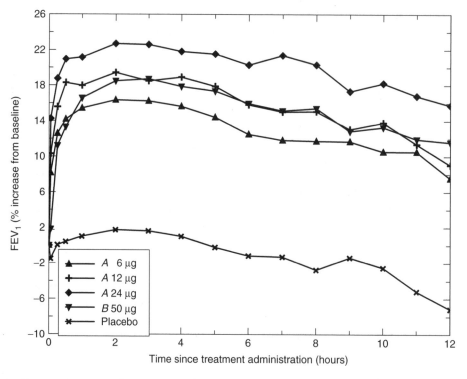

Figure 22.2. Geometric mean values, expressed as percent increase from the baseline measurement, of FEV_1 measurements over 12 hours for individual treatments

area all the way down to zero. Alternatively, we could integrate over the baseline measurement, but then the area could be negative and we would be forced to do the final analysis on the original scale. We have chosen the former approach.

The ANOVA uses the model

$$\ln(FEV_{1,av}) = \text{patient} + \text{treatment}$$
$$+ \text{period} + \ln(FEV_{1,base})$$

To have baseline as a covariate in a single dose study is rather essential. If we observe lung function over a short time period, baseline is very important and we could probably just as well use $FEV_{1,av}/FEV_{1,base}$ as effect variable. However, when we observe over a longer time period, the influence of baseline should diminish and after many hours could probably just as well be ignored. By using it as a covariate, we get a reasonable compromise between these two extremes.

Based on the results from this analysis we can address various questions:

1. Which doses of drug A can we claim to be effective? To find this out we compare them, from highest to lowest dose, with placebo. Here is the result in tabular form:

Treatment	Mean ratio	95% Confidence limits
24 μg of A	1.214	1.177, 1.252
12 μg of A	1.176	1.140, 1.212
6 μg of A	1.154	1.119, 1.190

Mean ratio relates to placebo. We see that the mean effect is 15–21% larger than it is for placebo, and the confidence intervals clearly show that all these comparisons were statistically significant. So we can claim that 6 μg is an effective dose of drug A, without compromising the significance level (see the discussion on MED).

2. Which dose of drug A has the same mean effect as the reference treatment, 50 μg of

drug B? To do this, we fit (weighted linear regression to keep track of the uncertainties of the means[31]) a straight line to drug A means vs. log-dose and estimate the dose that has the same mean effect as the reference treatment. This is illustrated in Figure 22.3. The actual dose estimate was 9.3 μg with 95% confidence limits 3.4–19 μg. As a consequence we find that 24 μg of drug A as a single dose has greater bronchodilating effect over 12 hours than 50 μg of drug B.

3. What about duration of effect? Looking at Figure 22.2 we see from the placebo curve indications of the diurnal variation that is known for lung function. To define duration by identifying when individual curves cross a line, say 15% above baseline, does not seem appropriate – if the placebo curve drops, you might still have a good response even when you are back to baseline. A more statistically sound approach would be to rephrase the question as 'is there still an effect after 12 hours' and then compare the treatments to placebo at that point in time. This is done in the following table:

Treatment	Mean ratio	95% Confidence limits
24 μg of drug A	1.246	1.187, 1.309
12 μg of drug A	1.176	1.120, 1.234
6 μg of drug A	1.168	1.112, 1.226
50 μg of drug B	1.200	1.144, 1.260

Again mean ratio relates to placebo and we have responses that are between 17% and 25% larger than that after 12 hours. Thus all active treatments clearly have a duration in excess of 12 hours.

SYSTEMIC EFFECTS

Effects of anti-asthma drugs are in general not confined to the lungs. Both β_2-agonists and GCSs have receptors on/in cells throughout the body. Since the drugs are cleared through the bloodstream they will therefore have systemic

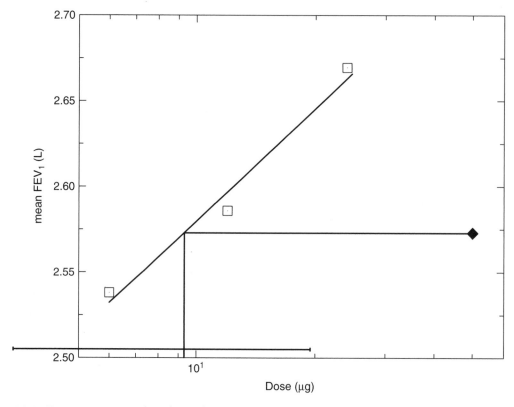

Figure 22.3. Treatment mean values for 12-hour average FEV$_1$ with fitted log–linear dose–response curve for drug A and estimation of D_{eq} relative to 50 µg of drug B

effects (albeit perhaps not measurable). In contrast to the anti-asthmatic effects, these effects can be measured both in healthy volunteers and in patients.

GCSs are synthetic cousins to an endogenous, anti-inflammatory, substance, cortisol. Given this, we can compare the pharmacodynamic systemic effects of different GCSs by comparing their effects on endogenous cortisol levels. This has the added advantage over drug plasma concentrations that it accounts for differences in potency in decreasing plasma levels of cortisol (which is done by negative feedback on the HPA axis). It is important to state at this point that we do not study endogenous cortisol levels because they themselves represent a dangerous side-effect. They are studied because they are sensitive markers for the 'amount' of exogenous GCS in the body!

With this model in mind we can use cortisol in plasma as an index of the systemic burden of therapeutically given GCS. By measuring the effect on cortisol we get a rather direct measure of the overall potency and concentration in plasma of the GCS. We can however not measure it timepoint by timepoint and compare to measurements without drug, since the level of cortisol is determined as a balance between production and elimination (with a half-life of about 1.5 hours) and the GCS acts on the production side. We therefore need to study a longer period. The cortisol levels in plasma have a diurnal rhythm which is very pronounced, so the most appropriate study to do is to give repeated doses of the GCS until a new steady state has been reached and then measure p-cortisol for 24 hours. A typical schedule is every other hour. The most useful variable to study is the area under the curve for those 24 hours. In steady state, when there is a 24-hour periodicity, this is proportional to the amount produced during 24 hours.

The actual clinical consequences of the levels attained are very hard to assess. They are surrogate measures of the long-term effects, but as such they should provide useful relative information on different GCSs, though we can never expect effects on p-cortisol to be a perfect predictor of say relative risk of osteoporosis. The distribution pattern in the body of the GCS might be of some consequence for this.

Example: Comparison of Plasma Cortisol Dose–Response Curves

We want to compare two inhaled steroids (with inhalation devices), call them A and B in terms of their degree of suppression on the plasma cortisol level. The comparison is done in healthy volunteers in a randomised, open seven-way crossover study. Each treatment period consists of 4 days, and there was a washout period of at least 2 days between each such treatment period. Each steroid was given in three doses: 200, 400 and 1000 μg b.i.d. for A and 200, 375 and 1000 μg b.i.d. for B. The seventh treatment was a placebo treatment. Blood samples were measured every second hour during the last 24 hours in each treatment period (10 p.m. to 10 p.m.). In all 21 healthy volunteers participated in the study and all completed all treatment periods.

The effect of the fact that the study is open is hard to assess. If the administration of one of the drugs is associated with more stress than the administration of the other, this might bias the result. However, this seems unlikely, and doing the study open has the benefit that fewer inhalations are required on each occasion.

To analyse the study, we first do an ANOVA. It is done on the logarithm of the concentrations with standard factors for a crossover study: subject, treatment and period. As a first presentation of the results we can compare all active treatments to placebo:

Treatment	Mean ratio (%)	95% Confidence limits	p
200 μg of A	97.4	73.3, 129.3	0.85
400 μg of A	94.1	70.9, 125.0	0.67
1000 μg of A	70.0	52.7, 92.9	0.014
200 μg of B	76.4	57.6, 101.5	0.063
375 μg of B	53.5	40.3, 71.1	0.00003
1000 μg of B	9.1	6.9, 12.1	<0.00001

Here the mean ratio is presented as a percentage. For instance, 76.4% for 200 μg of drug B means that there is a suppression of $100 - 76.4\% = 23.6\%$.

This result does not tell much about how the drugs compare. To do that we can fit parallel non-linear dose–response curves to the mean effect data, adjusting for precision by using a weighted non-linear regression.[31] We assume for this analysis that given enough steroids, the cortisol levels go down to zero. The result is graphically shown in Figure 22.4.

With the appropriate parametrisation here, we obtain that the relative dose potency is estimated to be 3.7, with 95% confidence limits 2.7 and 6.4. Thus, in terms of depressing cortisol levels, B is estimated to be about four times more potent than A (remember that a letter stands for a GCS plus a device – change device and this relation might change). Or put in other words: to achieve the same average depression in cortisol, we can use a four times larger dose of A than of B.

Having obtained this result, the immediate question is: 'How relevant is this result to the target group of the drug – the asthmatic patient?'. We cannot extrapolate these results to patients 'as is'. There is a basic difference between a healthy volunteer and an asthmatic – the latter has an ongoing inflammatory process. This means that the dynamic system regulating cortisol is disturbed (compared to healthy) and we can expect smaller absolute effects of a given dose of the GCS. So a typical patient might have a larger ED_{50} than a typical healthy volunteer. By the same token we can expect different patients to vary considerably in this respect.

However, there is no reason to expect that different GCS should act differently in patients

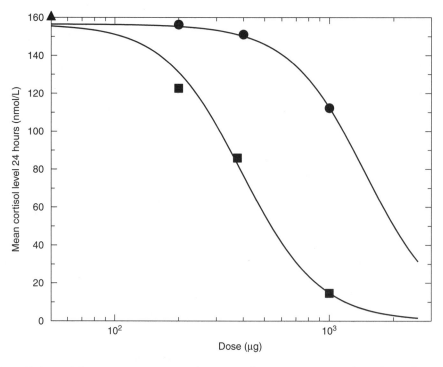

Figure 22.4. Estimated dose–response mean value curves for treatments *A* (to the right) and *B* (to the left)

and in healthy volunteers, i.e. there is no reason to claim that the relative effect of two GCS, as measured by the potency ratio, ρ, should differ between patients and healthy volunteers, or between different categories of patients for that matter. If such differences turn out to be the case, the reason must be that the systemic dose differs between healthy volunteers and patients, and then, most likely, between patients of different degrees of severity in their disease.

PHASE III STUDIES

DOCUMENTING EFFICACY AND SAFETY

Most drugs for obstructive airway diseases are given for maintenance treatment, and the main point to document is the level of disease control of the proposed treatment. At the same time it is important to document the adverse event profile, since most of the drugs in this therapeutic area are considered very safe, and safety must

not be an issue of a new drug. Thus the pivotal confirmatory trials for the airway diseases asthma, COPD and rhinitis are parallel group, diary card studies typically spanning from a month up to a year.

Asthma Trials

For asthma the typical study length for an efficacy study seems to be 3 months, though occasionally longer studies are needed. As already discussed, there is a continuous scale of severity of each of the respiratory diseases. The severity of asthma can be classified into a few groups, each of which has its recommended medical treatment. Both the classification and the recommended treatment are, like the disease under study, somewhat varying with time. The following classification is meant only to be indicative on what type of criteria are used for such classification.

Intermittent: These patients have normal lung function between occasional exacerbations with symptoms at most once a week. FEV_1 in percent of predicted normal should be $\geq 80\%$.

Mild persistent: Now symptoms appear weekly, but not many times a day and exacerbations may affect both activity and sleep. FEV_1 in percent of predicted normal should be $\geq 80\%$.

Moderate persistent: Symptoms appear daily, and affect both activity and sleep. There are night-time symptoms weekly and FEV_1 is within 60–80% of predicted normal.

Severe persistent: These patients have continuous symptoms, frequent exacerbations and night-time symptoms, which limits physical activity. FEV_1 in percent of predicted normal is $\leq 60\%$.

This classification borrows from the GINA classification.[32] However, that classification also uses a concept of variability which we do not discuss.

To describe the patient's disease severity in a clinical trial we use data obtained at a visit to the clinic before randomisation. In addition, a diary card is provided for a run-in period to assess symptoms and use of rescue medication. Inclusion into a study is often based on these measurements. A more practically, oriented classification of the severity of asthma is based on the use of GCS in the patient's regular treatment: no GCS (intermittent–mild), inhaled GCS up to 400 µg/day (mild persistent), inhaled GCS in the range 400–1000 µg/day (moderate) and inhaled GCS ≥ 1000 µg/day (severe). So the daily dose of background GCS treatment can be used as an indicator of asthma severity. Another classification is based on PC_{20}.[33]

The best way to use the information in diary cards might vary between patient groups. As already explained, the traditional use of diary card data is to assess changes in period means. This is expected to work best in patients with moderate asthma. In the intermittent group one should not expect effects of any considerable magnitude because the lung function is close to normal, and the patient is, for most of the time, symptom-free. In the group of the most severe patients, patients often have obtained an irreversible component to the disease and therefore show little improvement in lung function. Instead the focus for studies in severe patients might be on how a new treatment can substitute for an old treatment without compromising the patient: e.g. how much oral steroids can be spared by taking inhaled GCS, or how much inhaled steroids can be spared when taking a concomitant leucotriene modifier.

The main objective of the confirmatory trials is to show efficacy, and thus require a placebo control. This was discussed earlier. Concerning doses, for the majority of drugs for airway diseases, there is not one dose that is appropriate for all patients. Instead a range of doses has to be justified and documented in the clinical programme. The general discussion on MED and dose–response is relevant here too.

Example: A Diary Card Study with Fixed Treatment Arms

The main outcome variable in a diary card trial with fixed treatment arms is some kind of summary measure (typically a mean value) over a longer period, presumed to represent, on a group level, for most part a steady state situation. We also need a corresponding measure during the baseline/run-in period for the statistical analysis.

Figure 22.5 shows the estimated daily means of a 3-month clinical trial in asthma. The study was a multi-centre, double-blind, double-dummy study of 3 months' treatment with investigational drugs. There were 52 centres in seven different countries worldwide and the randomised treatments were placebo, two dose levels, 100 and 600 µg daily dose, of the GCS A and one dose level, a daily dose of 200 µg of the GCS B. In all 547 patients were enrolled, of which 472 were randomised and 383 completed the study. There were twice as many withdrawals in the placebo group as in the other groups. The mean age was 44 years, the mean FEV_1 in percent of predicted normal was 70% and the mean reversibility was 24%. All patients were on inhaled steroids when entering the study – the mean daily dose was 850 µg ranging from 500 to 1500. Thus the population must be characterised as being moderate–severe.

To plot the temporal behaviour of the effect of the four treatments, simple mean values are expected to produce a bias towards no effect. At least when comparison is done to placebo: in this group there were more withdrawals and many of these can be expected to be due to reasons that are correlated to (lack of) treatment effects. Some weeks into the treatment period, raw mean values for this group will therefore mainly include patients that are not in desperate need of GCS treatment. This will introduce a selection bias which will partly hide the effect of the treatments. To avoid this problem, that different days will contain different patients, we have pre-processed data when plotting Figure 22.5 to make sure all days contain data from all patients. The way this is done is as follows:

1. Linear interpolation is done in order to impute all missing values between the first and the last recorded day for each patient.

2. If the patient withdrew from the study before the 90th treatment day, the mean of the last three recorded days is extended from the last recorded day plus one to day 90 post-randomisation.

Then daily means are computed by treatment. In Figure 22.5 an additional operation has been made: for each treatment we compute a baseline by taking the average of the run-in means and subtract that from all daily means. This is done in order to highlight changes since that is what the analysis focuses on.

The statistical analysis of this data uses the period means from the individual patients: the mean is computed for the run-in period, which is used as a baseline, and then for the treatment period (from the day of randomisation and onwards). The change from baseline is used as effect variable, and the analysis is an ANOVA with treatments and centre as factors and baseline

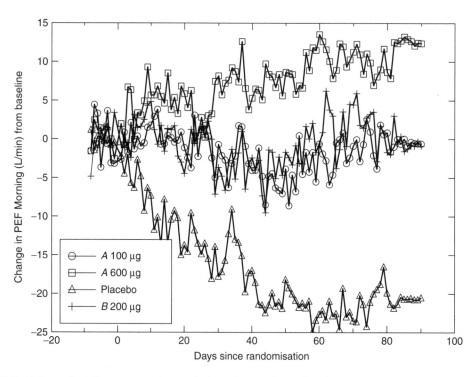

Figure 22.5. Estimated daily mean values of the change from baseline in PEF morning. See text for computational details

as covariate. The following table shows the adjusted mean values for the effect variable for the four treatment groups, adjusted to a common baseline value (the mean over the full study population):

Treatment	Mean	SEM	95% Confidence limits
placebo	−10.5	3.3	−17.0, −4.0
A 100 µg	−0.3	3.3	−6.8, 6.2
A 600 µg	7.4	3.3	1.0, 13.9
B 200 µg	2.0	3.4	−4.7, 8.8

From this analysis we also find that there is a statistically significant, negative, dependence of the change in PEF on the baseline PEF and that the estimated residual standard devotion was 35.9 L/min. As is common for this kind of data, the explanatory power of the analysis is small: only 8% of the variability is explained by the model.

Other diary card variables are often analysed the same way as was shown for PEF morning, by first computing individual period means. Symptom scores and rescue medication are however variables for which the average value is not necessarily easy to interpret. Symptom scores are really ordered categorical data, and even though the average gives a hint of the amount of symptoms, it is not clear that e.g. $(2 + 2)/2$ means the same as $(1 + 3)/2$. For rescue medication, the problem is mainly that we use the mean as a measure of location for a distribution which, for some patients, might be skew. Also the distribution of period means over patients may well be skew.

For symptom scores and rescue medication it is therefore often useful to compute the percentage of symptom-free days, or the percentage of days with no rescue, instead of period means. At least the former is often for mild patients a more efficient measure than the corresponding period mean. And it is clinically easier to interpret. This idea can be carried one step further: we can introduce the concept of an 'asthma controlled day', as one in which there are

no asthma symptoms and no rescue medication was needed. The percentage of such days is often a useful variable, at least in studies on mild–moderate asthmatics. Modification to a 'well-controlled' day for more severe patient populations is possible.

Another approach to diary card data is to measure time to first exacerbation. In a population like this, this is not expected to produce better results than the ones presented but, as already discussed, this approach might be useful in milder populations. For illustration, we have used the following definition of an exacerbation for the present study (which was in moderate–severe patients): for there to be a mild exacerbation one of the following three criteria should be fulfilled on two consecutive days:

1. Morning or evening PEF should be more than 20% below the period mean during run-in.
2. Rescue medication should be up at least four inhalations above the period mean during run-in.
3. The patient woke up during night-time and took rescue medication.

By scanning the diary cards we can, for each patient, compute the time to first exacerbation, if there is one, otherwise the patient is censored.

With this definition, we can present results as Kaplan–Meier plots for the time to event, as in Figure 22.6. We see a picture similar to that conveyed by the period means. Statistically we can compare groups either by log-rank tests or semiparametric Cox regression. In the table below treatments are compared to placebo based on a Cox regression model:

	Hazard ratio	95% Confidence limits	p-Value
A 200 µg vs placebo	0.7813	0.5642, 1.082	0.137
A 600 µg vs placebo	0.6731	0.4812, 0.9414	0.0207
B 200 µg vs placebo	0.717	0.5127, 1.003	0.0519

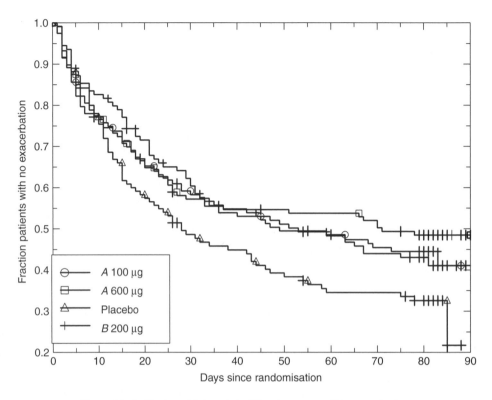

Figure 22.6. Kaplan–Meier plot of the time to a mild exacerbation

We see that the hazard for a mild exacerbation for the high dose of A, e.g., is estimated to be about 67% of that of placebo. As expected in this patient group, the results are, from a statistical point of view, somewhat weaker than the ones obtained from the analysis of period means.

A Dose Reduction Study

To compare the efficacy of two GCSs, a randomised, double-blind parallel group study with two treatment arms (one for each GCS) was designed. The objective is to estimate the relative dose potency by starting each arm on a high dose of the GCS, treating for some weeks, stepping down the dose and treating for some weeks, making a further step down, etc. This is done until the asthma is no longer controlled. This way we obtain for each patient the lowest dose on which the patient had asthma control (the one previous

to the last one). This we call the MED (Minimal Effective Dose) for the patient.

Such a study needs a detailed definition of what is meant by asthma control. There is no such universal definition, but lack of asthma control is essentially the same thing as a mild exacerbation, as discussed above. So the working definition above could be used, and the algorithm is to step down until a mild exacerbation occurs.

In such a study the diary card variables *per se* are not of independent use, they should not be compared between groups, except possibly the data on the highest dose. Instead it is expected that the mean values are similar in the two arms over the treatment period, what varies is the underlying dose producing those effects. The effect variable of interest is the MED, which is to be compared between the groups.

The nature of MED is such that the best way of analysing it is not immediate. On the one hand it will be rather discrete in nature, with only a few possible levels. On the other hand the most informative way of expressing the result is to say how much more was needed on average for one as compared to the other (like that the MED for A was on average 125% that for B). We advocate for that reason that MED is analysed under a multiplicative ANOVA model, i.e. after log transformation of the dose, provided that MED > 0 in all cases. The most appropriate way to do this is to regard the data as interval censored data for the analysis.

One final comment on the design of long-term asthma trials. In many instances, especially for dose–response studies, it is informative for the interpretation of the results to relate the observed effects to the 'highest effects attainable'. This can be done within a study, so that the patients are put on a heavy treatment, consisting of a high dose of a GCS and a long-acting β_2-agonist (or whatever is considered necessary to get the patient in as good a condition as possible), either during run-in, in a period after a run-in period or by adding on a period at the end of the study with a similar treatment. The purpose of this is to be able to quantify the response in terms of what can actually be achieved in the patients under study. If we put this reference period at the end of the study, we must make certain that all patients, including withdrawals, pass it in order to avoid having problems with a selection bias. If we put this reference period before randomisation, we might have carry-over effects into the randomised treatments with their potential problems. But having such a period as reference often helps in the interpretation of the results.

COPD Studies

For COPD the classification of disease severity can be made as follows:[34]

Mild: This is what is called the smoker's cough. The patient has FEV_1 > 60% of predicted normal, no breathlessness and is in general unknown to the health care system.

Moderate: The patient has breathlessness on exertion and FEV_1 in the range 40–60% of predicted normal.

Severe: The patient has breathlessness on everyday activities and FEV_1 < 40% of predicted normal.

What is to be proved in a clinical programme for a COPD drug depends on what the claim of the drug is. We can crudely divide effects on COPD into two groups: symptomatic effects and disease modifying effects. The natural history of COPD is one of an accelerated progressive decline in lung function leading up to a distressful, premature, death. This decline in lung function leads to progressive symptoms and diminished exercise endurance. Symptomatic effects relate to the alleviation of symptoms and improvement of quality of life, whereas disease modifying effects are effects that lessen the decline rate in lung function.

A drug with symptomatic effects on COPD should work on a rather short time-scale. It should lead to improved symptoms, fewer exacerbations and better performance on exercise tests. Many drugs that were originally anti-asthma drugs have been tried, and licensed, for the COPD indication. Part of their effect may well be due to the reversible component that many COPD patients have in their disease – in other words an anti-asthma effect within the COPD. In order to claim effects above this, studies have been performed in which one tries to exclude patients with reversible components by using exclusion criteria on patients with a reversibility test above 15% of baseline. To claim that short-term effects seen in the population are due to non-anti-asthma effects because of such exclusion criteria is obviously not correct – a patient with reversible airways obstruction can well have a reversibility of less than 15% on a particular occasion. Since COPD is a disease affecting small airways, it seems more logical to base short-term effects on measurements related to these airways, as opposed to FEV_1. However, regulatory requirements make FEV_1 the primary efficacy variable in COPD studies – at least as of this writing – though emphasis is made on the symptoms and/or exercise tests also. In fact the CPMP guidelines require two primary efficacy variables in COPD studies – one should be FEV_1 and the other a symptom score.[35]

A COPD study for a drug with primarily symptomatic effects is in general a long-term study, probably with diary cards, not very different from the asthma trial discussed above. Prevention of exacerbations is perhaps the most important aspect of COPD treatment, so a 6-month study is the minimum.

A COPD drug which claims disease modifying properties has a heavier burden of proof on it. The effect of disease modifying is that the rate of decline in lung function is reduced. To prove this, we need to do long-term studies over 3–5 years, or perhaps more, in which lung function is measured repeatedly. The statistical analysis should focus on the rate of decline, which could be done using a linear mixed effects model.

Rhinitis Trials

Classification of rhinitis patients into groups according to severity is lacking. The accepted division is between occasional and continuous expression of symptoms, i.e. between seasonal allergic rhinitis and perennial rhinitis. The rhinitis symptoms are the same, so the measurements, notably symptom scores, are the same. As already indicated symptoms are often recorded in diary cards for blockage, runny nose, sneezing/itchy and eye symptoms, and the sum of the first three make up the Combined Nasal Symptom score or Nasal Index Score, which is a useful primary variable for clinical trials.

The difference between seasonal and perennial rhinitis lies more in the study design/conduct. For perennial rhinitis the situation is similar to that for asthma or COPD in that the patient can start the trial almost any time. For hay fever, however, the study must be conducted over a rather short period of pollen exposure. What makes these trials more difficult is that ideally the patients should be included during the onset of the pollen season to get baseline data, then followed over one to several pollen peaks with treatment. The

intensity of the rhinitis is dependent on pollen counts in the air, and lack of treatment effects can well be due to insufficient pollen exposure. Therefore concomitant collection of pollen data is not only useful but almost necessary when trying to understand lack of effect in such studies.

THERAPEUTIC EQUIVALENCE

One of the challenges for drug development is to prove that a new treatment is therapeutically equivalent to a reference treatment. In the area of respiratory diseases this problem appears in two different settings – when we want to register a new formulation, most often a new inhaler, and in market claims of equality of two treatments. The background and motivation of these differ somewhat, so we discuss them separately.

Bioequivalency of Two Devices

Bioequivalency refers to a specific problem. Assume that a drug is delivered as a tablet or in some other form, such that it must pass through the bloodstream before reaching its site of action. Then the plasma concentration profiles of the drug define the clinical effect. This reasoning is the rationale for the bioequivalence concept: to prove that two formulations are bioequivalent, show that the plasma concentration profiles are sufficiently similar. From that we could then logically infer that the therapeutic effects are sufficiently similar to have the same therapeutic effect. This is in general a rather straightforward problem, requiring only small pharmacokinetic studies.

For many years there has been a well-defined method to establish bioequivalency in this situation. We reduce the general question of similar plasma concentration curves to key measures of rate and extent of absorption, including AUC. The ratio of two AUCs measures the relative bioavailability of the two formulations and the requirement is that the ratio of the means (analysed under a multiplicative model) should have confidence limits within 80–125%.

For inhaled respiratory products, however, the site of action, the lungs, lie prior to the bloodstream (i.e. when the drug appears in the blood it has in general had its desired pharmacological effect). Thus plasma concentrations cannot predict effect by pure logic! Equal delivered dose does not by logic imply the same effect for different inhalers, because different inhalers could deposit the drug in different parts of the lungs. For that reason, to bridge from one inhalation device to another is not necessarily a simple case of measuring plasma concentrations. As of this writing there is substantial confusion on how to proceed with bioequivalence studies for inhalers. We will discuss some aspects of the problem here.

The first aspect is that what you inhale are particles, and these will be deposited differently depending on size. To give an equivalent effect, we therefore need equivalent *in vitro* performance of the two inhalers. For the rest of the discussion we assume that *in vitro* data is similar for the two inhalers.

The basic assumption is that since what appears in the bloodstream does not have to have passed the site of action, systemic exposure, as measured by drug concentrations in the circulation, is not necessarily enough to conclude efficacy. However, similar systemic exposure should be sufficient to deduce similar systemic effects, and therefore reduce much of the question of bioequivalent side-effects to the classical bioequivalence method.

Logically, if we measure blood concentrations and conclude that the systemic exposure is the same, the outstanding question is if the drug has been delivered to the site of action. For a nasal spray it is hard to see how it can fail to do so. For a nasal spray, therefore, to require anything beyond *in vitro* data and pharmacokinetic data might be an overkill. For an orally inhaled drug the situation is more complicated.

If we consider a bronchodilator as an example, we need the drug to hit the receptors of the contracted muscles. To check that the drug has hit these, we can therefore do a pharmacodynamic study, e.g. a single dose study in which FEV_1 is followed for a number of hours, or a bronchoprovocation study if that is preferred. A suggested design is to study two or three doses of each inhaler, in order to see not only that the response is similar, but also that there is a similar sensitivity to changes in dose. These are, relatively speaking, simple studies to perform.

The next question is, which should the decision rule be for bioequivalency for such a study – when are two inhalers considered to be similar? There seems to be two approaches used over the last few years. One is to use the word comparability. This is, for good reasons, not well defined and essentially means that there is a dose–response relationship on each device and that, numerically, the mean on each dose level is similar in the eye of the regulator. Thus there is no true statistical decision plan associated with the study and it is not used as proof *per se*, only as supportive information to what *in vitro* and PK data provides. The other approach is strictly statistical. In this case we should compute the relative dose potency with confidence limits. At present, in the case of bioequivalency for pMDIs for albuterol (salbutamol in the US), FDA requires that the 90% confidence limits for this parameter should be contained in the interval 2/3–1.5. The justification for these limits is not clear, but they imply that the mean effect is so similar for the two pMDIs that they could be switched on the market.

When it comes to decide bioequivalency for orally inhaled anti-inflammatory drugs the problem is even more difficult, since there are, as of today, no designs available that can provide the kind of answers discussed for bronchodilators, to a reasonable price. The problem is that in most studies the dose–response appears rather flat, so very large studies are needed for the type of decision plan that was indicated above.

Marketing Therapeutic Equivalence

The other aspect of therapeutic equivalence is to show that a new treatment is as effective as an old one, whereas it has some other benefits compared to it.

Proving that two treatments are equivalent has, however, a long history in the context of medicine. The traditional way was to misuse the *p*-value technology – if we could not demonstrate a difference ($p > 5\%$) the treatments are equal. This is obviously wrong (it is similar to 'not proven guilty' in court, which means only that, not that one is proven innocent), which is by now acknowledged by most, but not all, workers in the field. A theoretically valid approach became legitimised by the ICH guidelines,[29] which defines an algorithm borrowed from the original bioequivalency concept for plasma concentrations. First you prespecify some limits (corresponding to the 80–125% above) and if your 95% (sic!) confidence interval for the mean difference is contained within this prespecified interval, you can declare therapeutic equivalence. This approach is however complicated, when your effect scale has no obvious interpretation, like a lung function scale or a symptom scale. To be a sensible approach, the prespecified limits must imply that clinicians do consider such a small difference to be of no clinical consequence – the predetermined limits must be agreed on. It is hard to forsee that this can actually be done in the field of respiratory medicine, since many effect changes mean different things depending on what population is studied.

There is however a sensible, though expensive, approach available – the one used for demonstrating bioequivalency of bronchodilators. The key there is to translate from the effect scale to the dose scale, by studying dose–response. Almost all drugs in the respiratory area (though there are exceptions) are available in multiple doses, and when two treatments (drug plus inhaler) are to be compared, at least one of them can in general be varied on some kind of dose scale.

The simplest such design is as follows. To prove that dose a of a treatment A is therapeutically equivalent to a treatment B (dose need not be specified), we can study doses $a/2$ and $2a$ of A (not dose a!) and treatment B. By assuming a linear dose–response relationship (versus log-dose) for A, we can estimate the dose of A that has the same effect as treatment B. Illustrations of this, with more than two doses of A were illustrated earlier. Now, if the 90% confidence limit for the dose of A that has the same effect as treatment B lies between $a/2$ and $2a$ it is reasonable that dose a of A is equivalent from a clinical point of view to treatment B from an efficacy point of view. This is because half the dose has less effect and twice the dose more effect. Implicitly this assumes that the clinical response to a suboptimal dose is to double this, which is what is done with most drugs in the respiratory area. In general, to draw the conclusion of therapeutic equivalence, large studies might be needed.[36]

Often one tries to establish the therapeutic equivalence in one clinical study, and compare benefits in the other. Basically I do not think this is the way to go about this kind of problem – in most cases it is probably a problem that should be discussed in terms of therapeutic ratio, as discussed in the next section.

The Real Issue – The Therapeutic Ratio

Dose–response studies provide us, at best, with doses for further investigation. However, whether a drug ends up being superior or inferior to what is on the market is not determined by what dose it is given in. What is the point in halving the nominal dose, if you get twice as much adverse effects?

The appropriate measure here is the therapeutic ratio. The therapeutic ratio for a drug relates the positive effect to the negative effect. To understand it, assume that effects, both positive and negative, are measured on a scale from 0 to 100. Also assume, for the time being, that the dose–response curves for positive and negative effects are parallel. Then a therapeutic ratio for this drug of 2 means that twice as large a dose is needed to get the same negative effect as positive effect. Thus we can define the therapeutic ratio for drug A as $TR(A) = ED_{50}(\text{side-effect})/ED_{50}(\text{effect})$. If we have two drugs, we can define the relative therapeutic index of A to B as $TR = TR(A)/TR(B)$, which is equivalent to the ratio $\rho(\text{effect})/\rho(\text{side-effect})$, where ρ is the relative dose potency for the two drugs with respect to the indicated effect. This means that we can estimate not only the relative therapeutic index, but also confidence intervals to the estimate, by assessing the relative dose potencies. Moreover, we can define the therapeutic index as a ratio of relative dose potencies without assuming that the effect and the side-effect curves are parallel. To be meaningful it only requires that the dose–response curves for efficacy are parallel and the dose–response curves for the side-effect are parallel. We can estimate the therapeutic index by combining effects from two studies – one on efficacy and one on side-effect, but better still is to obtain all the information in one study.

The first problem to solve is the precise definition of outcome variables, both positive and negative. Different results can be obtained by using different outcome variables. It is therefore important that the precise objective is spelt out and the outcome variables related to this. The following example is an illustration.

Example: Estimating the Relative Therapeutic Index

In order to assess the relative usefulness of a long-acting β_2-agonist, call it A, and a short-acting one, which we call B, we want to compare one topical effect, bronchodilation, and one systemic effect, suppression of serum potassium. The study was of crossover design with single-dose administrations and serial measurement of both variables taken.[37] In order to be able to get meaningful estimates of the relative therapeutic index we need many patients, relatively speaking, and in order to obtain a simpler study we choose to measure the maximal effect on each parameter and compare that.

Thus a randomised, double-blind, six-period crossover study was designed with the following single dose treatments: placebo, 6 µg, 24 µg and 72 µg of drug A and 200 µg and 1800 µg of drug B. Each treatment period consisted of a single dose administration which was followed for 4 hours and from each experimental sequence the maximal FEV_1 value and the minimal S-potassium value was extracted for statistical analysis.

Figure 22.7 demonstrates the main result. We see (period and baseline adjusted) treatment means together with straight line approximations to the dose–response curves for each variable. In order to make the results more interpretable mean values (and lines) are expressed as a percentage of the mean value for placebo. From these straight lines we can estimate the relative dose potency, as discussed earlier, for each variable separately:

Variable	ρ	95% Confidence limits
FEV_1	147	65, 534
S-potassium	60	41, 91

Thus we see that in terms of efficacy, the long-acting drug A is almost 150 times more efficient than the short-acting B. On the side-effect side, A is 60 times more potent, so from this data we see that the relative therapeutic index is estimated to be $146.6/59.75 = 2.4$. To obtain confidence limits is somewhat involved since we need to take into account the covariation of the two variables. How to do this is outlined in Ref.[38] The result is that the relative therapeutic index is estimated to be 2.5 with (approximative) 95% confidence limits 1.02 and 9.0 ($p = 0.046$).

The conclusion from this is, that in terms of the variables of this analysis treatment A is estimated to be 2.5 times 'better', but it is certified that it is 'better' than treatment B. Of course, this result is not better than data. From Figure 22.7 we see that the lowest dose of each drug has a very small average effect on serum potassium. It could (and should) be questioned if these really are on the log-linear part of the dose–response curve. We can repeat the analysis by only incorporating the doses 24 and 72 µg of A and 1800 µg of B for serum potassium.

OTHER ISSUES

PHASE IV

Much phase IV work focuses on comparisons with competitor products in order to demonstrate the advantages of the new product. This has been

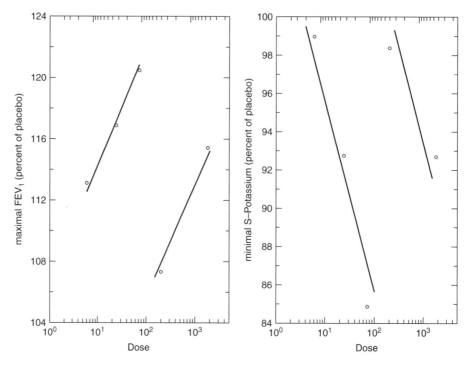

Figure 22.7. Adjusted mean values for each treatment and outcome variable

discussed in previous chapters and will not be repeated here. In addition to that, special safety issues might have to be addressed, which might call for large-scale studies in order to study some rare event.

PHARMACO-ECONOMICS

Asthma is a costly illness – its costs can account for as much as 1–1.5% of all resources in the health care sector. The costs are, however, unevenly distributed among the asthmatics; it is not uncommon that 10% of the most severe cases (usually patients with uncontrolled asthma) account for over 50% of the total cost. There should thus be room for a significant cost reduction by improving disease control.

The costs can, basically, be divided into three categories (usually only the first, although sometimes also the second category is measured):

1. *Direct costs*, defined as health care resources consumed, include costs associated with drugs, devices, consultations with physicians, emergency room visits and hospitalisations.
2. *Indirect costs*, defined as lost productivity, include time off work or school, either patient or relative, premature retirement and death. Indirect costs may account for up to 50% of the cost of asthma.
3. *Intangible costs*, contain factors related to quality of life (grief, fear, unhappiness, pain, etc.).

Within the direct costs, drugs and general practitioner visits can, crudely, be considered costs of managing controlled asthma, whereas emergency room and hospital costs can be assumed to relate to treatment failure. Assuming this to be about 75% of the total cost, the major part of the costs of asthma appear to be a result of inadequately controlled disease. Thus, the goal is to get control of the asthma, which (for example) can be done by patient education[39] and prophylactic therapy. As an example of the latter, it has been demonstrated that the introduction of high-dose inhaled steroids in patients with severe asthma reduced the number of days of hospitalisation by 80%.[40] It should also be noted that a part of the drug costs consists of rescue medication, like short-acting β_2-agonists, and is in itself a sign of the disease not being adequately under control, and that an increase in prophylactic therapy, like inhaled steroids, might decrease these costs.

So, the economics of asthma inform us that a large population of mild-to-moderate asthmatics has a low daily cost. For some of these patients, the disease becomes uncontrolled and costly, with hospitalisations and time off work or school, possibly progressing into early retirement or death. Some of these cases are probably due to bad compliance with treatment regimens. International guidelines therefore stress that prophylactic treatment should be introduced at an early stage in asthma treatment, resulting in an increase in drug and general practitioner costs, but hopefully leading to reduced hospitalisation costs and indirect costs. As an observation on this topic, it can be mentioned that the cost of the avoidance of one admission to hospital will pay for about 3 years of treatment with inhaled steroids.[41]

Apart from collecting data on costs, it is also important to measure the individual's quality of life and the effectiveness of various interventions (where effectiveness, as compared to efficacy, ideally should measure the effects of an intervention in clinical practice and also in units the patients care about). This is perhaps especially important if a new medical treatment increases the total costs, as it then becomes important to relate these extra costs to the additional effectiveness gained. Currently recommended effectiveness variables include the number of symptom- and episode-free days. In cost-effectiveness analyses, if both costs and effectiveness are higher for one of the treatments, the difference in costs is divided by the difference in effectiveness to obtain a cost–effectiveness ratio. This ratio is, for example, expressed as: compared to treatment A, treatment B costs $\$x$ per symptom-free day gained. That ratio thus gives

support in answering the question on whether the additional effectiveness (or quality of life or asthma control) can justify the extra costs.

Furthermore, it is important to keep in mind that costs often are country-specific, e.g. in the case of an international clinical trial, and some adaptation is needed before translating results from one country to another. This is so because the outcome of a new treatment will depend on the local medical tradition, drug pricing and the unit costs of other health care resources, and a number of social conditions like the labour market. In general, though, as the interest for 'value for money' and cost-containment in the health care sector grows, the importance of these kind of evaluations is likely to increase. From clinical trials it is thus important to measure these kind of variables (both costs and effectiveness), which then can be used as the basis for a cost–effectiveness analysis.

META-ANALYSIS

Meta-analysis is in general useful when the focus is on an issue for which data is available in a number of studies, but each individual study is underpowered for that particular issue. Such issues might be questions related to special subgroups or issues of rare events. Obvious examples of the latter are special, and rare, adverse events. In this respect the respiratory area does not differ much from other areas. The results obtained so far within the respiratory area from meta-analysis are not impressive.[42]

REFERENCES

1. Beasley R. Worldwide variation in the prevalence of symptoms of asthma, allergic rhinoconjunctivitis and atopic eczema. *Lancet* (1998) **351**: 1225–32.
2. Chadwick DJ, Cardew G. *The Rising Trends in Asthma, Ciba Foundation*. Chichester: John Wiley & Sons (1997).
3. Peat J, Li J. Reversing the trend: reducing the prevalence of asthma. *J Allergy Clin Immunol* (1999) **103**: 1–10.
4. Sears MR. Epidemiology of childhood asthma. *Lancet* (1997) **350**: 1015–20.

5. Barnes PJ. The changing face of asthma. *Q J Med* (1987) **63**: 359–65.

6. Lange P, Parner J, Vestbo J, Schnohr P, Jensen G. A 15-year follow-up study of ventilatory function in adults with asthma. *N Engl J Med* (1998) **339**: 1194–200.

7. Sherman CB. The health consequences of cigarette smoking. Pulmonary diseases. *Med Clin N Am* (1992) **2**: 355–75.

8. Buist SA. Smoking and other risk factors. In: Murray JF, Nadel JA, eds. *Textbook of Respiratory Medicine*, 2nd edn. Philadelphia: WB Saunders (1994) 1259–87.

9. Selroos O, Pietinalho A, Riska H. Delivery devices for inhaled asthma medication Clinical implications of differences in effectiveness. *Clin Immunother* (1996) **6**: 273–99.

10. Selroos O. Bronchial asthma, chronic bronchitis and pulmonary parenchymal diseases. In: Morén F, Dolovich MB, Newhouse MT, Newman SP, eds. *Aerosols in Medicine. Principles, Diagnosis and Therapy*, 2nd edn. Amsterdam: Elsevier Science (1993) 261–89.

11. Bartnes PJ. Beta-adrenergic receptors and their regulation. *Am J Respir Crit Care Med* (1995) **152**: 838–60.

12. Löfdahl CG, Chung KF. Long-acting β_2-adrenoceptor agonists: a new perspective in the treatment of asthma. *Eur Respir J* (1991) **4**: 218–24.

13. Rall TW. Drugs used in the treatment of asthma: the methylxanthines, cromolyn sodium, and other agents. In: Gilman AG, Rall TW, Nies AS, Taylor P, eds. *Goodman and Gilman's The Pharmacological Basis of Therapeutics*, 8th edn. New York: Pergamon Press (1990) 618–37.

14. Gandevia B. Historical review of the use of parasympatholytic agents in the treatment of respiratory disorders. *Postgrad Med J* (1975) **51**(Suppl 7): 13–20.

15. Brattsand R, Selroos O. Glucocorticosteroids. In: Page CP, Metzger WJ, eds. *Drugs and the Lung*. New York: Raven Press (1994) 101–220.

16. The British Guidelines on asthma management. *Thorax* (1997) **52**(Suppl 1): S1–21.

17. Howarth PH. The medical treatment of chronic rhinitis. In: Busse WW, Holgate ST, eds. *Asthma and Rhinitis*. Boston: Blackwell Scientific (1995) 1415–28.

18. Simons FER. Antihistamines. In: Mygind N, Naclerio R, eds. *Allergic and Non-allergic Rhinitis. Clinical Aspects*. Copenhagen: Munksgaard (1993) 123–36.

19. Bernstein JA, Bernstein IL. Cromones. In: Barnes PJ, Grunstein MM, Leff AR, Woolcock AJ, eds. *Asthma*. Philadelphia: Lippincott-Raven (1997) 1647–66.

20. Barnes NC. Effects of antileukotrienes in the treatment of asthma. *Am J Respir Crit Care Med* (2000) **161**: S73–6.

21. ATS guidelines.

22. Quanjer PH, Tammeling GJ, Cotes JE, Pedersen OF, Peslin R, Yernault JC. TI: lung volumes and forced ventilatory flows. Report Working Party: Standardization of Lung Function Tests. European Community for Steel and Coal. *Eur Respir J* (1993) **6**(Suppl 16): 5–40.

23. Oga T, Nishimura K, Tsukino M, Hajiro T, Ikeda A, Izumi T. The effects of oxitropium bromide on exercise performance in patients with stable chronic obstructive pulmonary disease. A comparison of three different exercise tests. *Am J Respir Crit Care Med* (2000) **161**: 1897–901.

24. Borg GAV. Psychophysical bases of perceived exertion. *Med Sci Sports Exercise* (1982) **14**: 377–81.

25. Mahler DA, Wells CK, Feinstein AR. The measurement of dyspnea. Contents, interobserver agreement, and physiologic correlates of two new clinical indexes. *Chest* (1984) **85**: 751–8.

26. Berger M, *et al.* The Sickness Impact Profile: development and final revision of a health status measure. *Med Care* (1981) **19**: 787–805.

27. Stewart AL, Hays RD, Ware JE Jr. The MOS short-form general health survey. Reliability and validity in a patient population. *Med Care* (1988) **26**: 724–35.

28. Jones PW, Quirk FH, Baveystock CM. The St George's Resp questionnaire. *Resp Med* (1991) **85**: 25–31.

29. ICH Harmonised Tripartite Guideline. Statistical principles in clinical trials. *Stat Med* (1999) **18**: 1905–42.

30. Senn S. *Statistical Issues in Drug Development*. Statistics in Practice. Chichester: John Wiley & Sons (1997).

31. Källén A, Larsson P. Dose response studies: how do we make them conclusive? *Stat Med* (1999) **18**: 629–41.

32. Global Initiative for Asthma. National Institutes of Health. National Heart, Lung, and Blood Institute Publication 95-3659 (1995).

33. Woolcock AJ. Therapies to control the airway inflammation of asthma. *Eur J Respir Dis* (1986) **69**(Suppl 147): 166–74.

34. BTS Guidelines for the management of chronic obstructive pulmonary disease. *Thorax* (1997) **52**(Suppl 5): S1–28.

35. Committee for proprietary medicinal products (CPMP). Points to consider on clinical investigation of medicinal products in the treatment of patients with chronic obstructive pulmonary disease (COPD). London: EMEA (1998).

36. Källén A, Larsson P. On the definition of therapeutic equivalence. *Drug Inform J* (2000) **34**: 349–54.

37. Rott Z, Böcskei C, Poszi M, Juhasz G, Larsson P, Rosenborg J. On the relative therapeutic index between formoterol Turbuhaler and salbutamol pressurized metered dose (pMDI) inhaler in asthmatic patients. *Eur Respir J* (1998) **12**(Suppl 28): 324s.

38. Källén A. A note on therapeutic equivalence and therapeutic ratio with application to studies in respiratory diseases. *Drug Inform J* (2001) **35**: 1495–505.

39. Liljas B, Lahdensuo A. Is asthma self-management cost-effective? *Patient Educ Counsel* (1997) **33**: 97–104.

40. Adelroth E, Thompson S. Advantages of high-dose inhaled budesonide. *Lancet* (1988) **i**: 476.

41. Blainey D, Lomas D, Beale A, Partridge M. The cost of acute asthma: how much is preventable? *Health Trends* (1991) **22**: 151–3.

42. Jadad RJ, Moher M, Brownman GP, Booker L, Sigouin C, Fuentes M, Stevens R. Systemic reviews and meta-analyses on treatment of asthma: critical evaluations. *BMJ* (2000) **320**: 537–40.

Index

Note: page numbers in *italics* refer to figures and tables and boxes

Textbook of Clinical Trials. Edited by D. Machin, S. Day and S. Green
© 2004 John Wiley & Sons, Ltd   ISBN: 0-471-98787-5